Autism: From Theory to Practice

Autism: From Theory to Practice

Edited by Martha Welch

AMERICAN
MEDICAL PUBLISHERS
www.americanmedicalpublishers.com

American Medical Publishers,
41 Flatbush Avenue,
1st Floor, New York,
NY 11217, USA

Visit us on the World Wide Web at:
www.americanmedicalpublishers.com

ISBN: 978-1-63927-283-9

Cataloging-in-Publication Data

Autism : from theory to practice / edited by Martha Welch.
p. cm.
Includes bibliographical references and index.
ISBN 978-1-63927-283-9
1. Autism. 2. Autism spectrum disorders. 3. Hyperlexia. I. Welch, Martha.
RC553.A88 A98 2022
616.858 82--dc23

Table of Contents

Preface

This book aims to highlight the current researches and provides a platform to further the scope of innovations in this area. This book is a product of the combined efforts of many researchers and scientists, after going through thorough studies and analysis from different parts of the world. The objective of this book is to provide the readers with the latest information of the field.

Autism spectrum disorder is a complicated condition that includes problems with communication and behavior. Disorders in the part of the brain that interprets sensory input and processes language is one of its suspected causes. There are several disorders which fall under the umbrella of autism spectrum disorders such as Asperger's syndrome, autistic disorder, childhood disintegrative disorder, and pervasive developmental disorder. Autism can be diagnosed by a developmental screening test, and autism diagnostic observation schedule test. There is no cure for autism; however, some therapies and medications can be used to manage its symptoms. These therapies include behavioral and communication therapy, applied behavior analysis, occupational therapy, sensory integration therapy, and speech therapy. This book discusses the fundamentals as well as modern approaches to autism. It presents researches and studies performed by experts across the globe. This book will provide comprehensive knowledge to the readers.

I would like to express my sincere thanks to the authors for their dedicated efforts in the completion of this book. I acknowledge the efforts of the publisher for providing constant support. Lastly, I would like to thank my family for their support in all academic endeavors.

Editor

1

Autism: the micro-movement perspective

Elizabeth B. Torres[1,2*], Maria Brincker[3], Robert W. Isenhower[4], Polina Yanovich[5], Kimberly A. Stigler[6], John I. Nurnberger[7], Dimitris N. Metaxas[8] and Jorge V. José[9]

[1] Psychology Department, Rutgers Center for Cognitive Science, Center for Computational Biomedicine Imaging and Modeling (Computer Science), Movement Disorders, Neurology, Rutgers University School of Medicine, Rutgers University, New Brunswick, NJ, USA
[2] Movement Disorders, Neurology Department, Indiana University School of Medicine, Indianapolis, IN, USA
[3] Philosophy Department, University of Massachusetts, Boston, MA, USA
[4] Psychology Department, Rutgers University, Piscataway, NJ, USA
[5] Computer Science Department, Rutgers University, Piscataway, NJ, USA
[6] Department of Psychiatry, Indiana University School of Medicine, Indiana University, Indianapolis, IN, USA
[7] Department of Psychiatry, Christian Sarkine Autism Treatment Center, Riley Hospital for Children, Indiana University School of Medicine, Indiana University, Indianapolis, IN, USA
[8] Computer Science Department, Center for Computational Biomedicine Imaging and Modeling, Rutgers Center for Cognitive Science, Rutgers University, Piscataway, NJ, USA
[9] Physics Department Bloomington, Department of Cellular and Integrative Physiology, Indiana University School of Medicine, Indiana University, Bloomington, IN, USA

Edited by:
Anne M. Donnellan, University of San Diego, USA

Reviewed by:
Jayanth Banavar, University of Maryland, USA
Erin Manning, Concordia University, Canada

****Correspondence:***
Elizabeth B. Torres, Psychology Department, Rutgers University, Busch Campus, 152 Frelinghuysen Rd., Piscataway, NJ 08854, USA
e-mail: ebtorres@rci.rutgers.edu

The current assessment of behaviors in the inventories to diagnose autism spectrum disorders (ASD) focus on observation and discrete categorizations. Behaviors require movements, yet measurements of physical movements are seldom included. Their inclusion however, could provide an objective characterization of behavior to help unveil interactions between the peripheral and the central nervous systems (CNSs). Such interactions are critical for the development and maintenance of spontaneous autonomy, self-regulation, and voluntary control. At present, current approaches cannot deal with the heterogeneous, dynamic and stochastic nature of development. Accordingly, they leave no avenues for real time or longitudinal assessments of *change* in a coping system continuously adapting and developing compensatory mechanisms. We offer a new unifying statistical framework to reveal re-afferent kinesthetic features of the *individual* with ASD. The new methodology is based on the non-stationary stochastic patterns of minute fluctuations (micro-movements) inherent to our natural actions. Such patterns of behavioral variability provide re-entrant sensory feedback contributing to the autonomous regulation and coordination of the motor output. From an early age, this feedback supports centrally driven volitional control and fluid, flexible transitions between intentional and spontaneous behaviors. We show that in ASD there is a disruption in the maturation of this form of proprioception. Despite this disturbance, each individual has unique adaptive compensatory capabilities that we can unveil and exploit to evoke faster and more accurate decisions. Measuring the kinesthetic re-afference in tandem with stimuli variations we can detect changes in their micro-movements indicative of a more predictive and reliable kinesthetic percept. Our methods address the heterogeneity of ASD with a personalized approach grounded in the inherent sensory-motor abilities that the individual has already developed.

Keywords: autism spectrum disorders, stochastic kinesthetic re-afference, Gamma probability distribution, spontaneous behavioral variability, non-stationary statistics

INTRODUCTION

A core challenge facing research of spectral disorders has been the highly heterogeneous clinical presentation, with manifestation of symptoms varying greatly from individual to individual. In the case of autism spectrum disorders (ASD), individuals show an inherent lack of flexibility, a reliance on sameness, and problems with social interactions. However, even two individuals with the same diagnosis score are rarely alike. The developmental trajectories of ASD can be highly non-linear, ranging from early regression associated with large delays to relatively rapid development associated with advanced skill sets. The adaptive compensatory mechanisms of the autistic individual continuously coping with developmental disturbances are not well-understood.

Current diagnostic practice involves the use of subjective observational inventories (SOIs) based on clinical observations with shifting criteria (e.g., see recent DSM-5 *vs.* DSM-IV-TR debate). Such SOIs provide no objective handle on the heterogeneity of the presentation, and might even obscure individual compensatory capabilities already developed by a coping-adaptive system. In autism the SOI's are primarily rooted in studies involving high functioning boys, with little inclusion of girls, possibly contributing to a steady nearly 5:1 boys-to-girls diagnostic ratio over the years (Volkmar et al., 1993; Lord and Bishop, 2010; Mandy et al., 2012; Dworzynski et al., 2012). Under the current practices many children are missing the optimal window for intervention. There is no way to *objectively* subtype idiosyncratic differences in ASD and/or to dynamically track individual changes in performance *in real time* during behavioral therapies or longitudinally. New methods are also needed to dynamically track the effectiveness of drug therapies on an individual basis.

The SOI's provide criteria for a triad of ASD symptoms that up to now have remained disconnected: (1) problems with social interactions; (2) communication impairment; and (3) repetitive-restrictive behaviors (reliance on sameness). These criteria are based on observation of behaviors. Although behaviors necessarily involve movements, movement disturbances have not been included in the criteria for ASD.

Movements can be performed under voluntary control or occur spontaneously beneath full intentional awareness (Torres, 2011, 2013b). Spontaneous movements and reflexes exist embedded in natural movement sequences and carry rhythms that in typical neonates can be entrained socially e.g., with adult speech (Condon and Sander, 1974) even before perception has fully matured. Retrospective studies of reflexes and spontaneous movements have shown that their disruption precedes the diagnosis of ASD (Teitelbaum et al., 1998; Karmel et al., 2010). On the voluntary side, intentional motions have been documented in neonates as early as 10 days old (van der Meer et al., 1995) continuing along a maturation process that leads to stable goal-directed reaches (Von Hofsten, 1982, 2004; Thelen et al., 1993, 1996; Bhat and Galloway, 2006; Lee et al., 2008; van Wermeskerken et al., 2011). In autism however, typical volitional control is highly compromised often with a striking disconnect between the intentions and the actions of the affected individual (Robledo et al., 2012).

Throughout typical development innate reflexes may initially play a role in the identification of systematic patterns during spontaneous exploratory behaviors by providing reliable referencing anchors. Under typical evolution of reflexes goal-less movements transition into well-coordinated goal-directed acts under volitional control (Thelen and Smith, 1994; Rovee-Collier et al., 2001). In this regard, a hallmark of typical development and maturation is the acquired ability from a young age to flexibly adapt to new contextual situations and interchangeably use and fluidly navigate through spontaneous and intentional patterns of behavioral variability (Torres, 2011, 2013b). This ability might be absent in ASD according to studies of natural motions. We found that the clear distinction quantified in typical controls between goal-directed and spontaneous, goal-less segments of movements was blurred in an individual with ASD (Torres, 2012).

Motor research in ASD has reported life-long persistence of early reflexes, reflexes that typically disappear within weeks of birth (Minderaa et al., 1985; Reed, 2007) as well as other motor disturbances (Damasio and Maurer, 1978; Maurer and Damasio, 1979, 1982; Hill and Leary, 1993; Donnellan and Leary, 1995; Leary and Hoyle, 2009; Donnellan et al., 2013). Yet movement impairments have failed to provide a homogenizing "endophenotype" for ASD. Movement disturbances have not been considered a core symptom of ASD and as such are not part of the diagnostic criteria. Perhaps those who diagnose the disorder consider movement disturbances as secondary because of the non-rigorous and subjective ways in which movement has typically been studied in ASD.

Unlike other fields specializing in modeling motion control (Marsden et al., 1989; Doyle et al., 2009) with applications to human behaviors (Todorov, 2005; Bays and Wolpert, 2007; Wolpert, 2007), the ASD sub-field that studies some aspects of motion in human movements has not conceived the stochastic feedback-control nature of motion in biological systems. Along these lines there have been recent attempts to link prior computational models of motor control to autism research (Gowen and Hamilton, 2013). Yet these attempts continue to focus exclusively on intended, goal-directed behavior, consequently disregarding spontaneous behavioral variability and the potential role that it could play in autism. In their present form, computational approaches to motor control cannot address the heterogeneity of the disorder as these models have not been grounded on the empirical estimation of the stochastic signatures of sensory-motor noise/signal of the *individual*. The latter however, are necessary to design personalized therapies tailored to the individual's best abilities.

Here we propose that considering the stochastic nature of both *voluntary* and *spontaneous* motions as separable forms of sensory feedback will shed light on the general question of how we attain spontaneous autonomous control over our actions and make them volitional.

To achieve control and regulation of the motor output in its simplest form, any biological system will require a minimum of afferent sensory feedback in real time. This continuous efferent-afferent flow exchange would enable proper guidance and anticipatory planning of sensory-motor consequences (Kawato and Wolpert, 1998). But besides the goal-driven directionality of the output flow, the temporal transduction and transmission delays inherent to any biological system in the face of sensory-motor noise should also be considered. In the past some of these issues in human motor control have been studied under the general umbrella of internal models (Kawato and Wolpert, 1998; Wolpert et al., 1998) with a focus on goal-directed actions. We posit, however that internal transduction and transmission delays may occur at different time scales for intended and spontaneous motions and that this differentiation, which must be acquired through maturation, may help a system discriminate between levels of intentionality or spontaneity for the same action (Torres, 2013b). Without such separable kinesthetic re-afferent feedback it is hard to understand how a system could turn movement into a tangible percept, fluidly integrate it with other sensory modalities and become cognizant of its own motions, let alone of the motions of others. These ingredients are all crucial for understanding and executing social dynamics in real time. Yet, they have not been considered in movement research in general and in ASD research in particular.

In autism research, movement has been essentially conceived as a form of efferent motor output with a unidirectional flow from the central nervous system (CNS) to the periphery (Jones and Prior, 1985; Rogers et al., 1996; Rinehart et al., 2001; Williams et al., 2001; Noterdaeme et al., 2002; Teitelbaum et al., 2002, 2004; Minshew et al., 2004; Jansiewicz et al., 2006; Mostofsky et al., 2006; Gowen et al., 2008; Fournier et al., 2010a,b) neglecting in more than one way the dynamics of spontaneous behavioral variability patterns inherently present in our motions (Gidley Larson et al., 2008; Haswell et al., 2009; Izawa et al., 2012) and their non-stationary statistics, as pointed out early on by Bernstein (1967).

To truly understand and appreciate the potential roles that our movements and their inherent variability could play in re-shaping the intentional control of our actions and decisions, we have proposed to treat movements and their variability also as a form of kinesthetic re-afferent input, flowing from the peripheral to the CNSs (Torres, 2013b) (**Figure 1A**). We have recently introduced the notion that this re-afferent feedback signal gives rise to precise stochastic signatures of movement fluctuations over time (that we have coined "micro-movements"). These micro-movements are proposed to contribute to the regulation, coordination, and control of multiple layers of functionality, in correspondence with a gradient of statistical variability that ranges from autonomic to voluntary levels of control (Torres, 2011) (**Figure 1B**). At the two extremes of this gradient, behavioral variability from motions voluntarily performed would have different stochastic signatures than behavioral variability from involuntary motions. This is a feature that has enabled blind classification of motion segments of typical subjects (Torres, 2011, 2013b) but failed in a subject with ASD (Torres, 2012).

Parts of the peripheral information involving position, movement, touch, and pressure along with their patterns of variability are routed through general somatic afferent (GSA) fibers: some flow through the so-called "conscious" proprioceptive channels that reach the neocortex via the thalamus, whereas others flow through "unconscious" proprioceptive channels with targets at the cerebellum, striatum, and limbic systems (O'Rahilly and Müller, 1983) (**Figure 2**). Typically there is balance and flexible exchange between these re-afferent forms of feedback that facilitate central regulation, anticipatory planning, and predictive control of the motor output and its consequences. In autism it is very unlikely that this balance and flexibility remains. Several of the cortical and sub-cortical structures that are targeted by GSA fibers

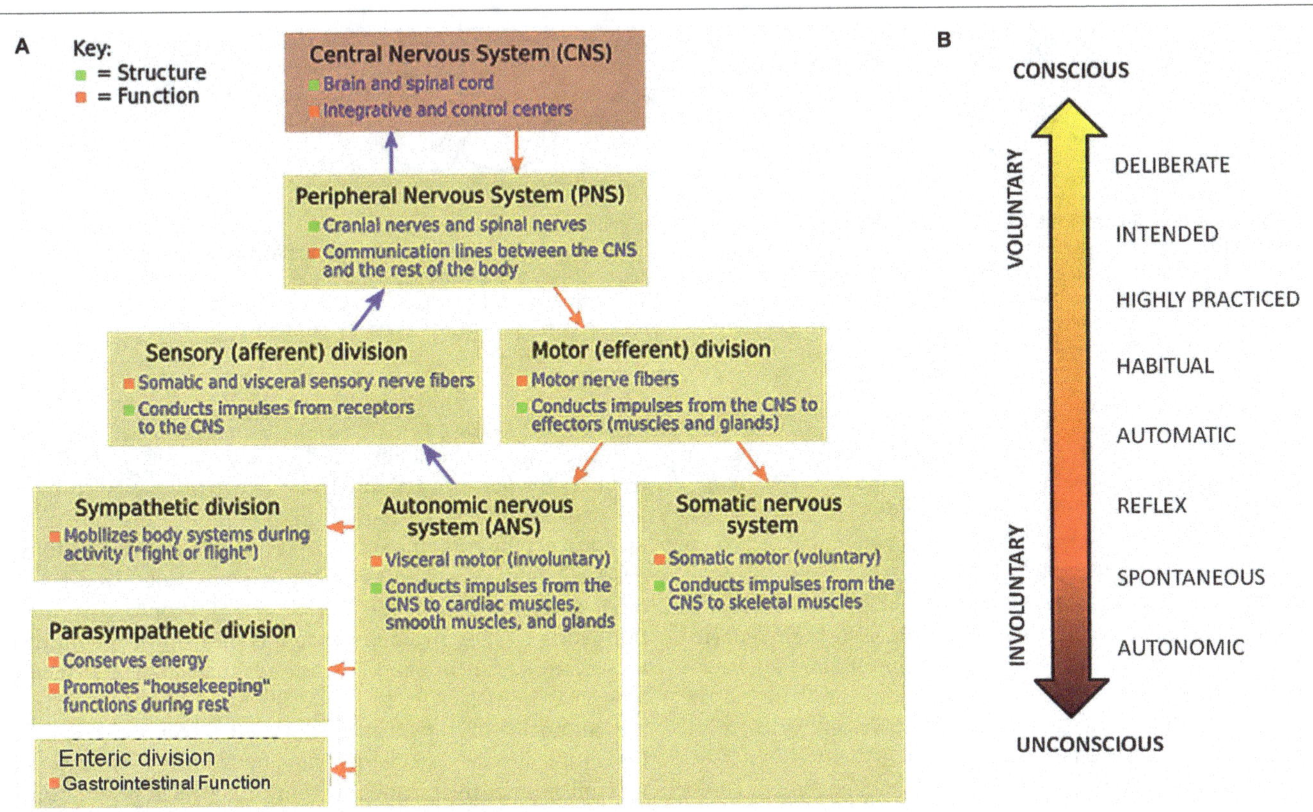

FIGURE 1 | Levels of the nervous system impacted by sensory-motor noise and gradient of movement variability mapped onto spectrum of movement functionality. (A) The labels of the simplified schematics represent only some of the many known functionalities of the system. Current autism research primarily focuses on centrally driven goal-oriented tasks typically performed under voluntary control and ignores the dynamics of the peripheral nervous systems (with their autonomic and somatic subdivisions). **(B)** Schematic to show a spectrum of movement functionalities that map onto a gradient of statistical variability. We highlight the need to study movement at all these levels and how autonomic and somatic functions scaffold and contribute to the maintenance of adaptive volitional control and intentional behavior. Both typical development and potential aberrancies are objectively quantifiable in the stochastic rhythms of *all* our motions at accessible levels (e.g., speech gestures, eyes, facial micro-expressions, head, body, limbs, etc.).

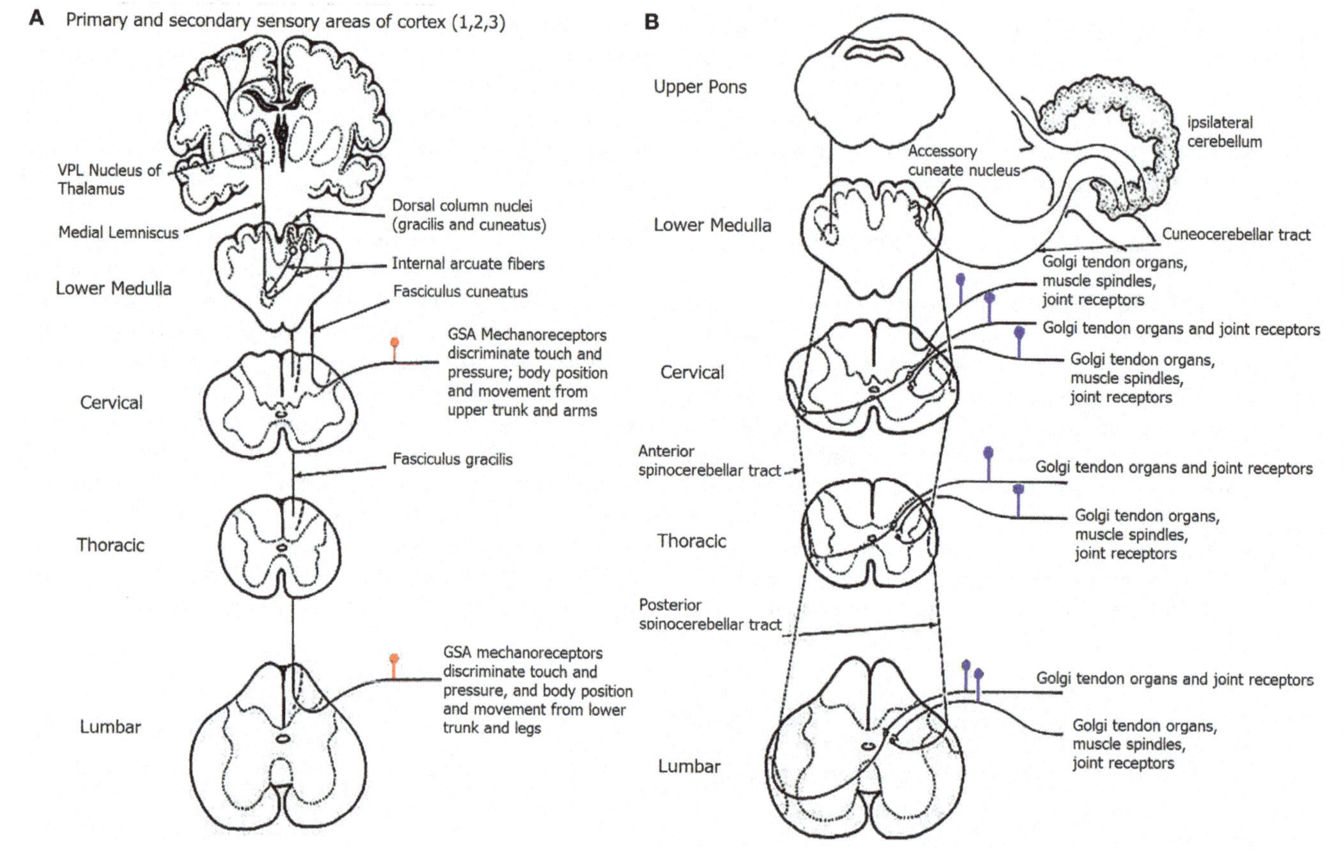

FIGURE 2 | General Somatic Afferent (GSA) pathways for proprioception. (A) The so-called conscious proprioception conveying information about touch and pressure and body position and movement through the GSA mechanoreceptors sensitive to discriminating among various levels of the input patterns. Synapses at several points conduct information via the thalamic relay station onto the primary and secondary somatosensory cortices (Broadman areas 1, 2, and 3). **(B)** The so-called unconscious proprioception conveying information about position and movement including dynamics (mass-, forces-, gravity-, and fine internal timing-related information) through Golgi tendon organs, joint receptors, and muscle spindles. Synapses along the way carry information with targets at cerebellar structures.

are reported to be impaired along with anomalies involving central and peripheral synapses (Damasio and Maurer, 1978; Maurer and Damasio, 1979, 1982; Jacobson et al., 1988; Rinehart et al., 2002; Amaral and Corbett, 2003; Schumann et al., 2004; Takarae et al., 2007; Amaral et al., 2008; Mostofsky et al., 2009; Qiu et al., 2010; Breece et al., 2012; Nordahl et al., 2012). Problems with the autonomic nervous system (ANS) have also been reported in ASD. These involve the enteric (gastro-intestinal) subsystems (Ashwood et al., 2003; Molloy and Manning-Courtney, 2003; Buie et al., 2010; de Magistris et al., 2010; Kushak et al., 2011; MacFabe et al., 2011; Mazurek et al., 2013) as well as issues with the circadian rhythms (Bourgeron, 2007; Glickman, 2010). Unusual and unpredictable pain and temperature deregulation are well-documented, particularly in autism of known etiology (Nader et al., 2004; Tordjman et al., 2009; Dubois et al., 2010; Klintwall et al., 2011; Zeidan-Chulia et al., 2011; Bandstra et al., 2012).

These disturbances involve motion control at many functional levels of **Figure 1B**. In ASD such aberrancies are likely to impede *spontaneous autonomy* of the body, body self-awareness, arousal, affective-emotive behaviors, and overall impair volitional control over the person's actions. The above mentioned disturbances are often bundled as "co-morbid" symptoms and downplayed or discarded by contemporary psychological approaches to ASD, despite being widely reported by parents, self-advocates, and other researchers (Donnellan et al., 2013). Proper instrumentation exists to objectively measure many of these disruptions at these various functional levels but adequate statistical methodology has been lacking to tackle these issues in real time and longitudinally in a personalized manner. We show here that the non-stationary stochastic signatures of micro-movements variability and their rates of change in each person can be precisely measured and dynamically tracked over time. They constitute a signature unique to each individual that will help us address the heterogeneity of ASD. They will also help us unveil the best somatosensory-motor capabilities that each person inherently developed along a unique coping and compensatory, adaptive developmental trajectory. We propose ways to use micro-movements' variability as a gateway into the best abilities of each individual with autism.

METHODS

PARTICIPANTS

We examined a cohort of 78 participants (34 ASD and 44 typically developing TD) ranging from 3.5 to 61 years of age with varying reported IQ. These individuals all were diagnosed as autistic by professionals/agencies qualified to do so and who had no affiliation with our laboratory or this research. Demographic information across participants is listed in **Tables A1–A3**.

They performed two versions of a basic pointing task, one which we call "baseline pointing" to a dot. The other one we will refer to as "decision-making pointing" as it is a match to sample task where the target stimuli requiring a decision changes (**Figure 3**). Reported IQ of individuals with ASD ranged from 40 to 110. For TD individuals IQ is reported 90 and above, with education spanning from pre-school to college levels (22 TD were of college level). The TD children attend the same school as the children with ASD and both are exposed to similar curricular activities. Parents signed parental consent for the children and young adults provided their consent. The protocol was approved by both the Institutional Review Board at Rutgers University and at Indiana University in compliance with the Declaration of Helsinki.

TASK AND APPARATUS

Collecting goal-directed vs. goal-less pointing segments

A motion caption system (Polhemus Liberty, 240 Hz) recorded the movements and software [MouseTracker (Freeman and Ambady, 2010)] concurrently time stamped the touches and stimuli presentation, all synchronized to the same CPU. The hand positional trajectories were harnessed. To assess velocity-dependent parameters first-order (velocity) changes in position over time were obtained using the smoothing and derivative functions from the Spline toolbox in MATLAB (MATLAB version 2012a, Natick, MA, The MathWorks Inc.) with software developed in-house. For each velocity trajectory the instantaneous length of the three dimensional velocity vectors along the curve

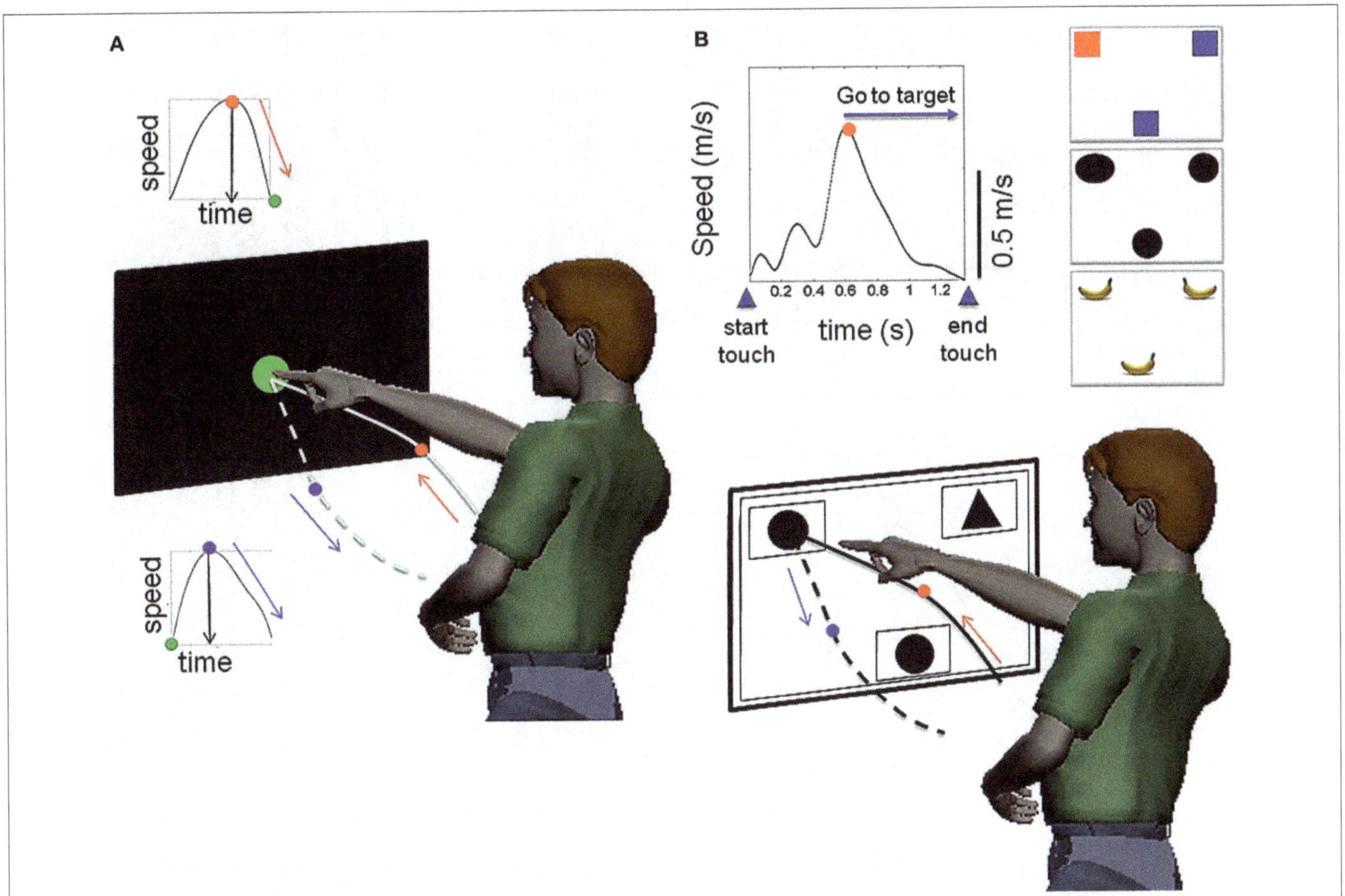

FIGURE 3 | Two variants of the pointing task to examine goal-directed and incidental goal-less movements in closed loop with decision-making processes. (A) Variant 1: basic pointing task, measuring the goal-directed motion to touch a target on the touch screen and spontaneous retraction away from it. The arrows mark the flow of motion. The speed profiles are also plotted as insets, with the dot marking the peak velocity and the arrow marking the time at which the peak is attained. **(B)** Variant 2: decision-making pointing during a match to sample task (upper-left and upper-right corners) matches the sample (bottom-center). A representative speed profile is also plotted as insets with the landmarks used to navigate the behavior. The touch at the bottom-center of the touch-screen simultaneously presents the sample and two possible targets. After the decision has been made, the hand goes to the targeted choice and touches the screen again. Examples of other stimuli—of varied cognitive load—used in the match-to-sample task are shown as well.

was obtained using the Euclidean norm. A speed profile as a function of time was obtained. In a subset of the participants of college level the MotionMonitor suite from SportsInn, was used to collect data using the Polhemus Liberty (240 Hz) as well. The positional data was filtered using Butterworth filter, 20 Hz cutoff.

The baseline pointing paradigm is depicted in schematic form in **Figures 3A,B** shows the decision-making pointing schematics for the match-to-sample task with representative stimuli types depicted in the top-right corner of panel **3B** (e.g., circles, oval, and rotated bananas). Movements were unconstrained in three-dimensional physical space and performed naturally—self-paced and without pre-defined temporal constraints—in a setup similar to that of the children's classroom settings involving a desk and computer screens that the children typically interact with. **Figure 4A** shows representative hand trajectories from natural motions in one block of trials lasting 16.7 s (40,000 frames recorded at 240 frames per second) including the continuous flow of motion throughout this block. The pointing motion segments had to be extracted from this natural flow and separated from the rest (the incidental transitional segments).

During the experiments the children freely moved and interacted with the touch screen. They triggered the trials by touching the screen which displayed the sample to match. The targets (2 choices) appeared and they chose the target by pointing. The landmarks in **Figure 4A** are the speed minima (blue circles) and the speed maxima (black stars). The black trajectories are

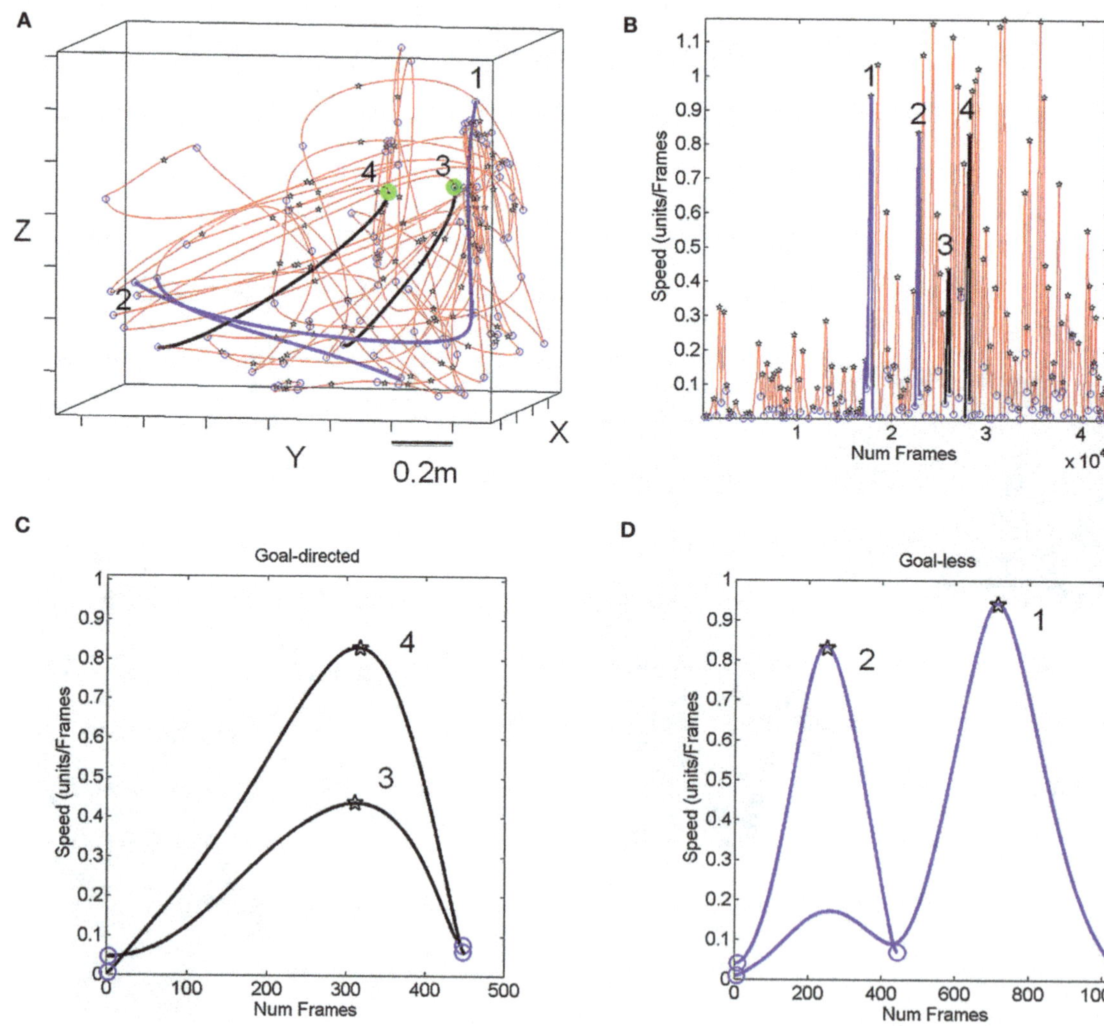

FIGURE 4 | Navigating through the continuous flow of natural motions and separating goal-directed from goal-less segments of behavior. (A) Hand movement trajectories from a typical child collected during 16.7 s of the match-to-sample task (at 240 frames/s) which required deciding between two stimulus choices. The blue circles mark the speed minima (pauses) while the black stars mark the speed maxima. The black curves denote the pointing trajectories to the green target at two different positions on the monitor facing the child. The blue curves are incidental to the task, goal-less movements in transition to other goal-directed motions. **(B)** Corresponding speed profiles along the trajectories in **(A)**. Numbers and colors correspond to the curves in **(A)**. The speed temporal profile permits to navigate through the acceleration and deceleration phases of the continuous flow of motion. **(C)** Zooming into the goal-directed speeds and **(D)** the goal-less speed profiles which were automatically harnessed by a computer interface (see methods in the main text).

representing pointing movements toward the green target locations (the target on the touch screen). Such movements will be termed "goal-directed" throughout the paper. The blue trajectories are representative of incidental movements that connected the goal-directed ones. These will be termed throughout the paper "goal-less" movement segments. These movements occur spontaneously, largely beneath awareness. Both movement classes were automatically extracted from the continuous flow of the behavioral trajectories by a software interface developed in house.

The **Figure 4B** shows the speed profiles corresponding to the trajectories in **Figure 4A** lasting 16.7 s. The blue and black segments correspond to the goal-less and goal-directed segments highlighted in **Figure 4A**. The panels **4C,D** zoom in these sample speed profiles and show the speed minima (blue circles) and maxima (black stars) as those plotted along the trajectories. The numbers identify the segments.

A computer interface logged and time stamped the screen touches to automatically navigate the behavior and separate the goal-directed segments from the goal-less ones. The screen touches were the behavioral landmark delimiting these segments. Backtracking along the valleys and peaks of the hand speed profile from the screen touch to the previous stop of the hand yielded the goal-directed segments. The movements away from the target starting right after the screen touch until the next full stop yielded the goal-less segments. The speed profiles from each movement type were harnessed and examined under a new statistical platform for behavioral analyses (SPBA) (Torres and Jose, 2012).

Sample trajectories from the baseline pointing are shown in **Figure 5A** for the goal-directed (left) and goal-less (right) segments. In this case (an adult) the movements were more structured than those of the children (e.g., shown in **Figure 4**). Along the trajectories we also plot the speed maxima corresponding to the single peak in **Figure 5B**. We are interested in the statistical properties of the spread of the speed maxima and on the spread of the time to reach the maximum speed for both movement types.

The SPBA treats the speed-dependent variations from trial to trial as a stochastic process over time. Specifically we are interested in the *micro-movements* that these parameters describe from one trial to the next. Taken in isolation, these small fluctuations in the value of the movement parameter say nothing about the person's behavior. Yet, over time, they accumulate evidence of the continuous flow of physical behavior, which we can study as a stochastic process. Based on their frequency distributions we can experimentally estimate their probability distributions and examine the evolution of the stochastic signatures in real time as well as longitudinally across different sessions.

This framework does not assume a priori that the data distributes normally (so as to take an average of a given parameter over n trials). This assumption is common in ASD motor

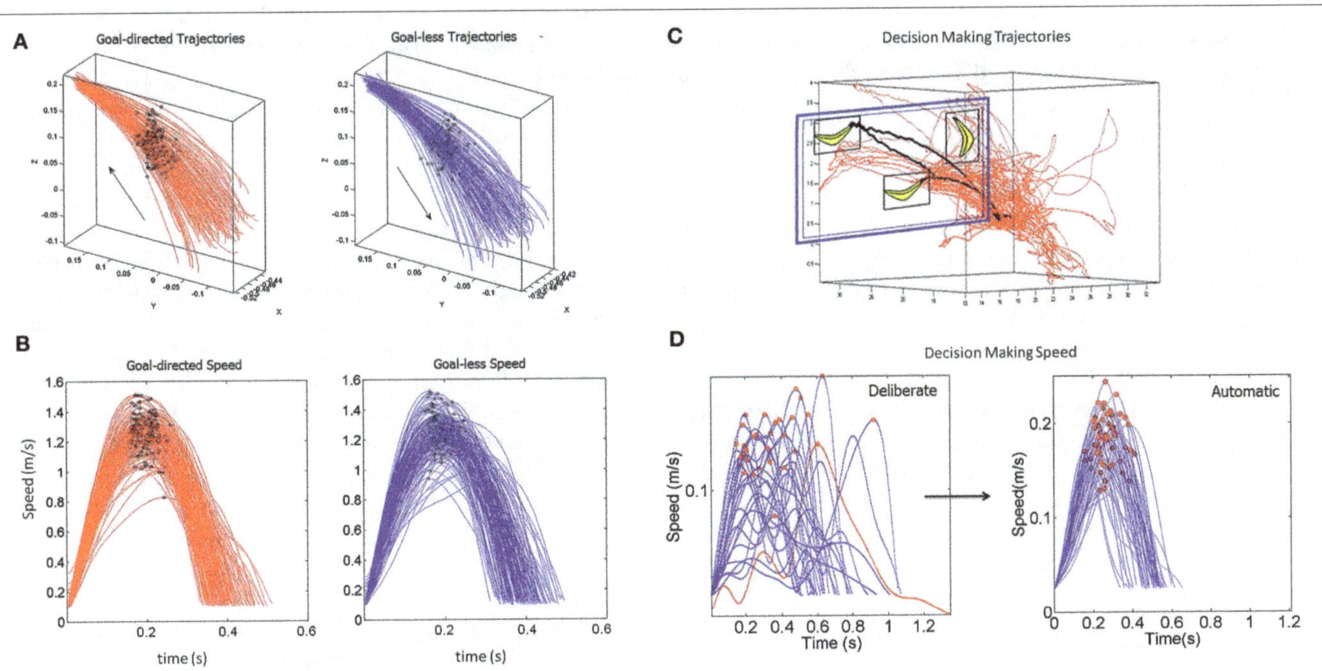

FIGURE 5 | Sample hand trajectories and speed profiles from the two variants of the pointing task. (A) Forward movements to the goal and incidental goal-less segments of the basic pointing task performed by an adult participant. The arrow marks the direction of the movement. The stars mark the spatial location of the peak velocity along the trajectories. **(B)** The corresponding instantaneous speed profiles along the trajectories in **(A)**. Notice that these are deceptively similar as the differences lie in their stochastic signatures across trials. **(C)** Decision-making hand trajectories from a child participant. Black trajectories highlight the extraction of goal-directed paths in contrast to goal-less segments. **(D)** Sample speed profiles during the goal-directed decision-making paths. Red dots mark the peak velocity. Red speed is featured in **Figure 3B**. Notice the evolution from slow and multimodal to fast and unimodal profiles within seconds. The former appear with higher cognitive loads and evolve toward the unimodal "bell-shaped" profiles that are the hallmark of automatic point-to-point behavior in primates.

research, where the theoretical Gaussian distribution is often used to describe the behavioral outcome by the mean and the variance of the parameters of interest and/or perform ANOVA (analyses of variance) and regression analyses on the movement data. Instead, we here experimentally estimate, for each person, the probability distribution most likely describing the movement trajectory parameter. This must be done, as we have previously shown that these velocity-dependent micro-movements do not distribute normally in young healthy adults (Torres, 2011). Normality is a requirement for justifiable use of the mean, variance, and parametric models (Limpert et al., 2001; Limpert and Stahel, 2011), but it has not been properly tested in ASD motor research.

The micro-movements permit proper estimation of the underlying distributions of motor control parameters in a personalized manner and serve to reliably predict different levels of intentionality in the individual's actions (Torres, 2013b). Using the SPBA it is possible to statistically index the predictability and the reliability of the probability distribution estimated from the experimental data as the actions continuously unfold.

To navigate the continuous flow of natural behaviors we had to consider additional issues in pointing during decision-making. The natural trajectories of the hand shown in **Figures 4A, 5C** contained both multimodal and unimodal profiles (**Figure 5D**). The latter had smooth slow-down-speed-up sub-segments with no full stops and were associated with exploratory motions as the decision was being made. In such cases the change in the slope of the speed curve was not abrupt—as when the hand comes to a full stop—and above the 5% cutoff from the speed maximum of the segment. Over repetitions of the pointing act, the unimodal speed profiles were re-acquired, indicating that the motions became ballistic and had the signature of automatic reaches. We quantified such adaptive transitions in the speed profiles and in the decision-making parameters. These features enabled automatic segment extraction during decision-making. MATLAB software was developed in-house to detect such subtle differences in densely sampled data.

Parameters of interest

Micro-movement parameters. Micro-movement parameters included the maximum value of the speed (*m/s*) and time (*s*) at which these occurred (computed in each trial). The average speed of each trial was also obtained. To remove allometric effects of body-size across ages in each trial we gathered the normalized peak velocity (the peak velocity divided by the sum of the peak velocity and the averaged trial speed) (Mosimann, 1970; Lleonart et al., 2000).

Decision-making parameters. Decision-making parameters included the accuracy of the decision in the match-to-sample task (measured as the % correct) and the movement decision latency (*s*). Movement decision latency was measured as the time (*s*) from the onset of the stimulus (evoked by the participant touching the bottom-center of the screen **Figure 3B**) to the screen touch at the targeted choice. This includes the reaction time, the time spent deciding, and the actual movement time. Subtracting the movement time (which the speed profile yields between the two relevant minima) provides the decision latency (*s*). Changes in decision accuracy and latency over time were measured in response to different stimuli (**Figure 3B**) by comparing the first 150 trials to the last 150 trials for each subject. This comparison also enabled us to assess possible fatigue and/or attentional distraction effects. Non-parametric statistics were used to assess significance, as the distributions of these parameters turned out to be highly skewed.

DISTRIBUTIONAL ANALYSES

These analyses are explained elsewhere (Torres, 2011, 2013a,b). Briefly, we used the continuous two-parameter Gamma family of probability distributions to empirically estimate the probability distribution underlying each person's velocity-dependent micro-movements. **Figures 6 A–D** provide examples of frequency distributions from the micro-movement parameters of interest from the experimental data of 2 participants, one with ASD and one TD. The two parameters (shape and scale) of the Gamma probability distribution were obtained using maximum likelihood estimation (MLE) with 95% confidence intervals. The shape (a) and scale (b) parameters can then be plotted in the Gamma plane. They uniquely characterize, with high confidence, the stochastic signatures of the micro-movements as they accumulate evidence across trials on the behavior of each individual under each given condition (**Figures 6E,F**).

DYNAMICALLY TRACKING THE UNIQUE RATE OF CHANGE OF THE MICRO-MOVEMENTS' STOCHASTIC SIGNATURES FOR EACH INDIVIDUAL

Across different task contexts, we can also track the changes in these stochastic signatures and build a stochastic trajectory in parameter space over time as a function of different stimuli. Each point in the stochastic trajectory is a 2D vector that over time changes direction and magnitude. These rates of change of position in the Gamma plane can also be dynamically tracked in real time and longitudinally. They are unique to each individual. In **Figure 6E** we show samples of two extreme limits of the Gamma family of probability distribution for two children, one with ASD and one TD. The blue curve (ASD) is an Exponential probability distribution and the red curve (TD) is a skewed distribution tending toward the Gaussian distribution limit. The former describes a totally random process where previous events do not contribute to the prediction of later events, whereas in the latter previous events do contribute to the prediction of future events. The baseline stochastic signatures for these children are shown with confidence intervals in **Figure 6F** and the stochastic trajectories of each child corresponding to three different stimuli in the match to sample task are shown in **Figure 6G**.

Lastly there are two important additional methodological steps: we performed (1) a Blind Classification of the cohort, and (2) a Verification step.

Within a cohort, the individuals with similar micro-movement variability will automatically cluster together, as their (a,b) stochastic signatures will be close in the Gamma plane. In contrast, those with dissimilarities in the variability of their micro-motions will fall far apart on the Gamma plane. This is an

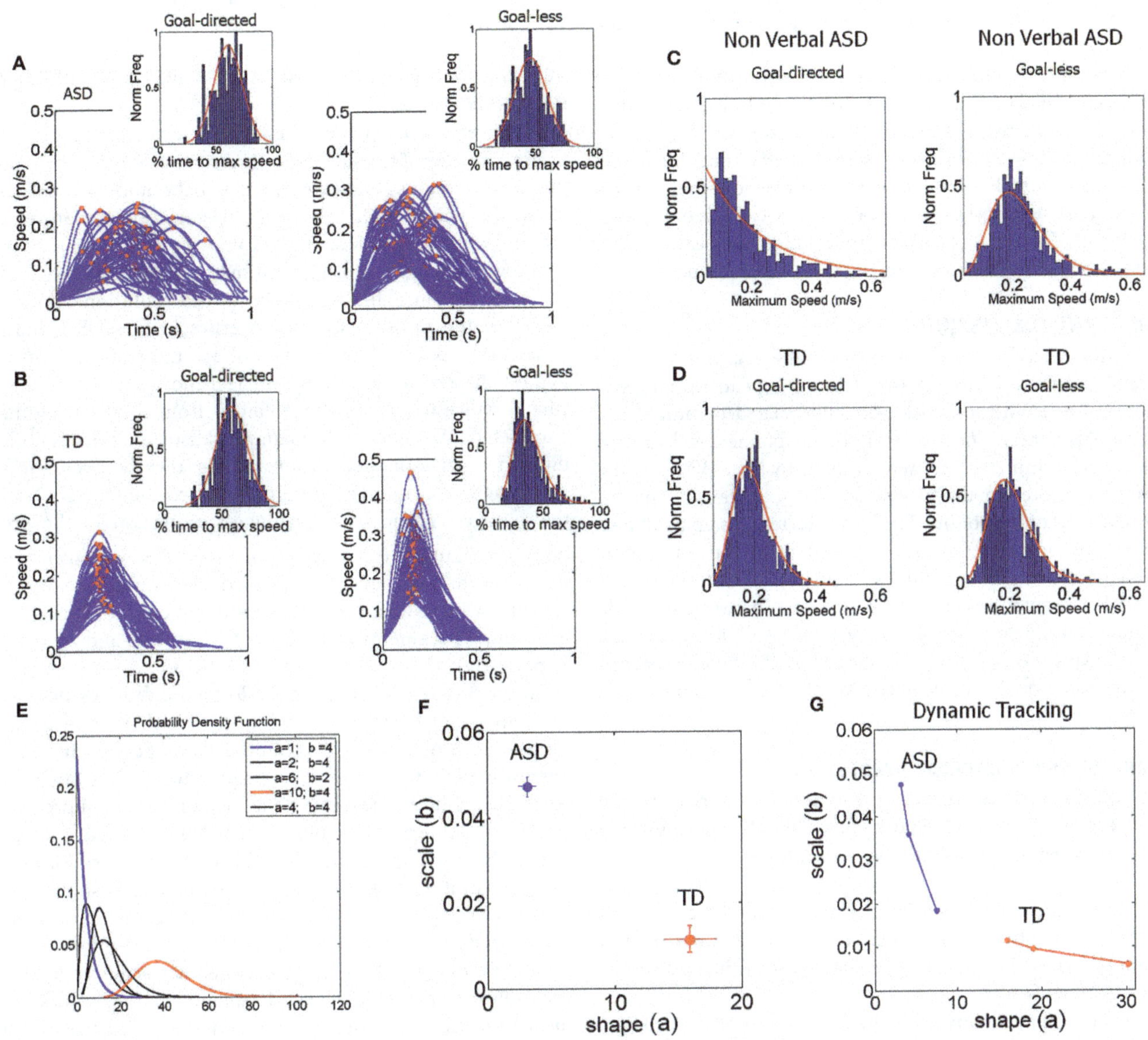

FIGURE 6 | Simple objective metric to screen idiosyncratic differences and to dynamically track progress in ASD. (A) Instantaneous speed profiles from a low-functioning non-verbal child with ASD across a subset of trials in one session. Red dots mark the maximum speed value of each trial, goal-directed-forward (left) *vs.* incidental goal-less segments (right). Insets are the normalized frequency distributions of the percent of movement time (s) to reach the maximum speed compiled across sessions. Over thousands of repetitions, this parameter distributes normally in the child with ASD for goal-less reaches. **(B)** Speed profiles of a TD child from a subset of trials in a session (age matched control). The distribution of the percent of time to reach the maximum speed for goal-less segments is skewed. This was the general trend across groups. **(C)** Refers to **(A)**, normalized frequency distribution of the value of the speed maximum compiled across sessions for thousands of trials (goal-directed reaches ASD) well-fit by an Exponential distribution. Retraction segments span an asymmetric distribution. **(D)** Refers to **(B)**, normalized frequency distributions of speed maxima for the goal-directed and goal-less motions of the TD child. **(E)** Schematics of the continuous probability Gamma family with shape (*a*) and scale (*b*) parameters to illustrate that the continuous two parameter Gamma family of probability distributions captures the broad range of cases, spanning from low-functioning, non-verbal ASD to high-functioning, verbal ASD to TD children and young adults (blue curve is the ASD and red the TD cases). **(F)** The MLE of (*a*,*b*) uniquely localize each child on the Gamma-plane with the 95%-confidence intervals. **(G)** Examples of personalized stochastic trajectories constructed by measuring the stochastic signatures of velocity-dependent hand micro-movements in response to each stimulus type in the match to sample task. Notice that the rate of change of the stochastic trajectory is unique to each child.

important advantage of this method, as subjects are not grouped a priori (using e.g., K-means algorithm or related clustering methods with preset cluster numbers). Rather it is the inherent statistics of the parameters that determine the groupings (Blind Classification step). Various subjective clinical assessment scores can then be used to find which one best fits within each and across the self-emerging clusters of micro-movement phenotypes. Thus, in assessing ASD the subjectively determined scores and the objective micro-movement metrics can complement each other. Together they would provide an important improvement over the current methods.

Atypical micro-movements might be perceptible to some experienced clinicians (through their own fine-tuned visual perception of movement), but cannot be captured under the current diagnostics categories, which focus on intended and high-level cognitive behaviors. However, under this framework these movements that occur largely beneath awareness can be objectively documented. This is of particular importance in assessing individuals who may not be able to report their self-inferences.

RESULTS AND DISCUSSION

This section describes the results from the analyses of hand kinematics with a focus on the velocity-dependent parameters, as well as from the decision-making related parameters of latency and accuracy. The scatter of points obtained as described above in the Gamma plane were colored by age. We used the reported IQ scores in the validation step to obtain a qualitative assessment of the cohort. The blind clustering step produced self-emerging aggregates, which we used to obtain an ensemble plot on the Gamma plane for both the goal-directed and the goal-less segments. An empirical relation between the scale and shape parameters revealed a power-law fit for each case using the expression $f(x) = mx^n$. We report the exponents (linear regression slope) and goodness of fit of the parameters in **Table A3**.

SUPPORT FOR METHODOLOGICAL HYPOTHESES

These experimental results that we will describe shortly provide support for our proposed methodological hypotheses (**Figure 1**) and carry several important specific implications:

(1) The trajectories of the stochastic signatures and their rates of change with stimulus type were unique to each person and best described by a range of probability distributions within the Gamma family.
(2) Based on inherent similarities in their movement parameters sub-groupings self-aggregated. These were confirmed using the SOI criteria.
(3) Given that micro-movements are affected by sensory stimuli, we can drive the system with different forms of sensory guidance. We can then record the motor and cognitive-decision output parameters and readily determine which form of guidance is the most efficient. Efficient here refers to the steering of re-afferent kinesthetic input toward higher predictive and more reliable statistics of the velocity-dependent micro-movements. The latter accompany faster and more accurate decision-making.
(4) Since the rate of change of the stochastic signature is unique to each individual and since the variability in goal-directed and in goal-less segments can be studied in tandem with decision-making, we can determine which of these types of processes a person uses most efficiently.
(5) This implies that we can very precisely and objectively tailor interventions to each person (even non-verbal participants) and dynamically adapt these new personalized therapies as a function of the inherent capabilities of the person, as their progress unfolds.

ACQUISITION OF PREDICTIVE AND EXPLORATIVE MICRO-MOVEMENTS IN TD INDIVIDUALS

We uncovered a scaling power law characterizing the typical maturation process of the stochastic signatures of velocity-dependent micro-movements (**Figure 7A**). We note the automatic clustering along the line of unity of the (a,b) stochastic signatures estimated from the normalized peak velocity. In the bottom panel we show the actual empirically estimated probability distribution for each person. This figure shows the evolution and maturation of the noise-to-signal properties of these distributions. In all participants under 4 years of age the curves showed the highest dispersion according to the Fano Factor (Fano, 1947) [the variance to mean ratio obtained from the (a,b) estimated parameters]. Specifically the Gamma statistics revealed significant differences in estimated mean and variance between the self-emerging clusters shown in **Figure 7A** according to age. Notably the youngest group had the highest dispersion in the probability distribution (*noise to signal ratio*) $F = \frac{\sigma_w^2}{\mu_w}$ taken within the time window between the movement onset and the peak velocity, which was very different between the forward and withdrawing segments (on average 190 ± 50 ms and 70 ± 40 ms, respectively).

In the 3–4 year olds, not only do the movements have a significantly higher variance (leading to a higher noise to signal ratio) than adults ($p < 10^{-5}$) but they also operate within a very narrow bandwidth window (low exploration). This implies that regardless of limb size, these young children have unpredictable velocity-dependent variations in their hand movements and do not yet have the systematic diversification necessary for an efficient exploratory trial-and-error learning. This is shown by the broad overlapping green curves in the **Figure 7C**. Each curve corresponds to a child. Notice that the micro-movements for each child of more than 4 years of age has acquired a broader exploratory range (blue curves) (spanning more values of the mean) for this parameter and the variance (width) significantly decreases. With age the reliability with which the peak velocity can be estimated from trial to trial based on the probability distribution significantly increases (i.e., the Fano Factor decreases). Pair-wise comparisons performing Wilcoxon ranksum test ($p < 0.0001$ comparing children <4 and children >4; $p < 7.3 \times 10^{-5}$ comparing children <4 and young adults; $p < 1.9 \times 10^{-4}$ comparing children >4 and young adults).

Across the developmental lifespan these properties and the goodness of fit remained for both goal-directed and goal-less segments. Using the general fitting function $f(x) = mx^n$ we obtained $m = 0.77$ and $n = -1.02$ with 95% confidence intervals [0.6523, 0.9016] and [−1.058, −0.9918], respectively. The goodness of fit parameters were, Summed-Squared-Error SSE $= 5.9 \times 10^{-8}$, $R^2 = 0.999$, adjusted $R^2 = 0.999$ and Root Mean Squared Error, RMSE $= 6.6 \times 10^{-5}$. Notably the mean value for the Gamma distribution is $\mu = a * b$ and the variance is $\sigma^2 = a * b^2$. Thus, the Fano Factor, $FF = b$, which provides the dispersion of the distribution, is also the scale parameter. The higher the value of the scale parameter, the higher the dispersion (i.e., the lower the

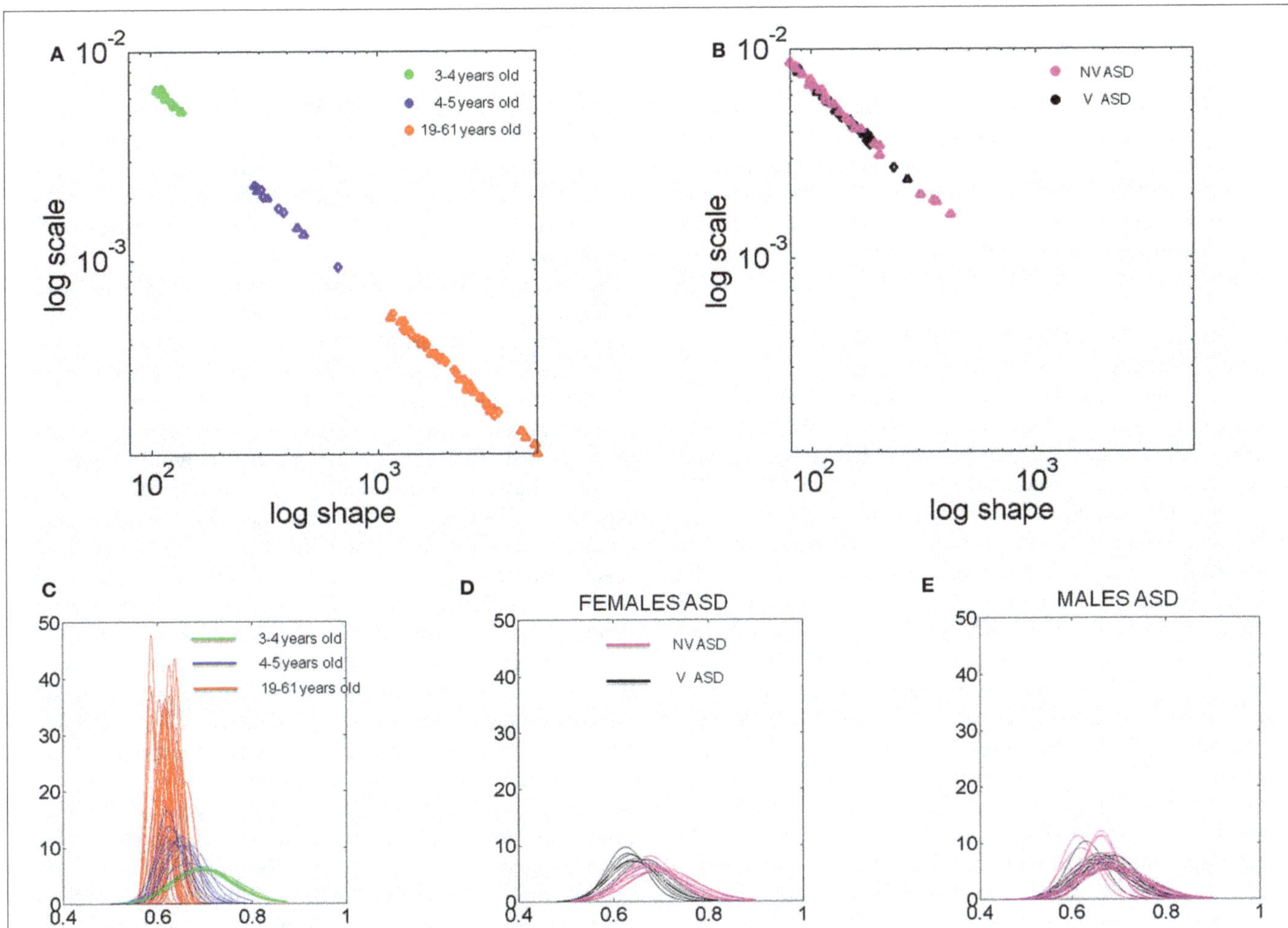

FIGURE 7 | Typical and atypical development of micro-movement patterns. The stochastic signatures of velocity-dependent variability captured in the normalized maximum speed ($V_{max}/(V_{max} + V_{avrg})$) of hand pointing motions across different ages. The shape and scale estimated parameters of the continuous two-parameter Gamma probability distribution family uniquely labels each individual in the group (78 participants total). **(A)** Fourty-four typical controls self-cluster by age along the line of unity on the log-log Gamma plane according to a scaling power law. **(B)** Thirty-four participants with ASD also align on the line of unity. Notice that the 34 ASD participants include verbal and non-verbal subjects, spanning from 4 to 25 years of age, yet they all fall along the statistical region of the TD 3–4 years old. **(C)** Estimated probability distributions of the velocity-dependent parameter for all TD subjects using their empirically obtained hand speed profiles. Notice that the noise-to-signal ratio changes dramatically from 3–4 to 4–5 years of age along with the bandwidth of parameter values that the distribution spans across subjects ($p < 10^{-5}$). All the 3–4 year old subjects collapsed on the same curve with the noise overpowering the signal but the 4–5 year old subjects have acquired a kinesthetic percept with significantly lower noise-to-signal ratio and broader bandwidth. Such diversification of the kinesthetic input is maximal in the adults who have highly reliable and predictive kinesthetic input. **(D,E)** The kinesthetic input of the ASD participants—unlike that of the 3–4 TD—was unreliable and noisy with narrow bandwidth of parameter values. However, some of the verbal females with ASD separate from the non-verbal females with ASD and from all other subjects (black curves with lower dispersion and centered at 0.62) but do not quite reach the level of kinesthetic input reliability of the TD. The micro-movements in the ASD males are indistinguishable between verbal and non-verbal participants.

reliability of the prediction of future events) which is what we see in the youngest children of the group (green dots in **Figure 7B** and green curves in **Figure 7C**).

These results suggest that a pivotal maturation in kinesthetic re-afference occurs in TD children around the age of 3–4 years. We consistently found three fundamental developments in the kinematics micro-movements from trial to trial: (1) the value of the shape parameter increases (higher predictability); (2) the noise decreases (higher reliability); (3) the bandwidth of reliable values broadens, thus allowing for efficient exploration. In brief, the development of higher predictive power for future velocities based on past velocities (what is referred to as priors in Bayesian statistics), allows reliable explorative variations: a stable kinesthetic percept is acquired.

We propose that these three factors together make the kinesthetic variations truly perceptual as the predictability along with the reliability of exploratory "sampling" makes it possible through active movements to seek and notice "broken expectations." They carry information about internal and external environmental constraints. In parallel, decision-making about cognitive stimuli becomes significantly faster (**Figure 9F**) and more accurate (**Figure 10**). It is thus no coincidence that TD children universally acquire the "bell-shaped" speed curve around this age (Thelen et al., 1993; Konczak and Dichgans, 1997; Von Hofsten, 2009) which, as we will see shortly, from this age also flexibly re-adapts when faced with new cognitive loads to then return once again to the stable unimodal or "bell-shaped" state. It is important here to note that all children in both groups, TD and ASD, performed this goal-directed task. However, the levels of predictability, reliability, and the bandwidth of their stochastic signatures increased with age, suggesting the above mentioned maturation process.

MICRO-MOVEMENTS GO AWRY IN ASD: RANDOM, NOISY, RESTRICTIVE KINESTHETIC INPUT

In drastic contrast to TD development we found that the normalized peak velocity of all 34 participants with ASD across ages and verbal or non-verbal status remained on the region of the Gamma plane corresponding to younger TD (**Figure 7B**). These included adolescents (14–16 years old) and young adults (18–25 years old). While the noise-to-signal ratio had significantly decreased in the TD 4–5 year olds as compared to that of TD 3–4 years olds (**Figure 7A**), here there were no significant differences between any of the ASD age-groups (pair-wise comparisons ranksum 4–10 years old *vs.* 16–25 years old test $p > 0.14$), neither between the verbal *vs.* non-verbal types (pair-wise comparisons ranksum test $p > 0.19$). Furthermore, there were significant differences in the noise-to-signal ratios of the participants with ASD and those of the TD participants (rank sum test $p < 7.2 \times 10^{-8}$).

Besides the noise overpowering the signal in ASD, we also found a lack of diversity in the kinesthetic input. This is appreciated in the **Figure 7D** where the curves of the Gamma probability distribution of most ASD participants as with the TD 3–4 years old span a very narrow bandwidth of values. Note the contrast to TD 4–5 years old and TD adults who span a large range of values of the mean parameter of the distributions. Thus, whereas the TD cases show a clear transition toward more predictive power, to the right of the Gamma plane, the participants with ASD never transition to lower noise-to-signal ratios and remain with a very narrow range of speed values. The results consistently show that the motions of the participants with ASD do not spontaneously gain the predictability that emerges from and further allows for active autonomous exploration.

This is a crucial finding as all ASD (and no TD) participants showed such unusual normalized peak velocities. It therefore appears to be a unifying characteristic—or endo-phenotype—for the entire autism spectrum irrespective of the heterogeneity of overall clinical presentation. Further, such non-predictability of micro-movements can be hypothesized as directly linked to the pervasive difficulties in ASD with flexibly switching from a set of stable behaviors to another set. We consider this to be one of the most significant and important findings of our studies.

VELOCITY-DEPENDENT BLIND CLUSTERING AND VALIDATION OF TD vs. ASD PARTICIPANTS

Motivated by the results from the normalized peak velocity we assessed the stochastic signatures of the average trial speed. The **Figure 8B** shows the self-aggregate scatters that automatically emerged according to the micro-movements' fluctuations metric. To gain insights into the clinical nature of each aggregate we colored the dots by age and IQ. This validated the results according to the reported IQ scores in ASD since the orientation of the self-emerging clusters revealed a trend in reported intellectual capabilities (as currently judged by standardized tests) according to verbal skills. This is shown in the zoomed-in panels below **Figure 8B**.

The coloring gave rise to the empirical frequency histograms in **Figure 8A** well-fit by estimating the two Gamma parameters in each cluster of **Figure 8B**. The resulting distribution estimated curves are superimposed in red on the empirical frequency distributions of **Figure 8A**. Notice that the TD children younger than 4 years old show an Exponential distribution similar to the one observed in the speed maxima for individuals with ASD (**Figure 6C** goal-directed pointing). This is important, since the Exponential distribution is a memoryless, random distribution, indicating that the fluctuations in the average speed of goal-directed movements are not predictive of the impending speed. Yet in the TD participants older than 4 years of age this statistical feature changes toward a skew distribution so that the kinesthetic percept to which these re-afferent fluctuations give rise becomes more stable (verifiable). By college age the average speed in a past trial does contribute in a predictive manner to indicate future performance according to the more symmetric nature of the frequency distribution of this cluster.

In marked contrast to the young TD 4–5 year old, in the ASD groups older than 8 years old the clusters are closer to Exponential than to Gaussian. See panel **8B** on the Gamma plane. The findings thus mirror those regarding the bandwidth of velocity maximum values in TD *vs.* ASD development. However, notice that the non-verbal 4–6 year old ASD group is closer to the 4–5 years old TD group than to the older—both verbal and non-verbal—ASD groups. This is also appreciated in the ensemble data of **Figure 8C** which is well-fit by a power relation $f(x) = mx^n$ with $m = 0.028$ and $n = -0.420$, with 95% confidence intervals $[0.025, 0.030]$ and $[-0.492, -0.347]$, respectively. (The goodness of fit parameters were $SSE = 4.63 \times 10^{-6}$, $R^2 = 0.992$, adjusted $R^2 = 0.991$ and $RMSE = 0.0010076$). These averaged trial speed results were thus consistent with those from the normalized maximum speed, yet they added more information: (1) the 4–6 year old participants with ASD, were the only ones to approach the area of the TD 4–5 year old, and (2) older individuals with ASD settled into non-predictive and non-exploratory variation patterns further from the TD developmental trajectory than the younger group.

The clusters found in the line-fit (**Figure 8C**) span several orders of magnitude. They may serve to blindly characterize the pre-school-to-college transition with respect to this metric within a typical developmental trajectory. See further details for each cluster in **Table A3**. The zoomed-in lower panels of **Figure 8B** show the suggested orientation axes from the validation procedure. The reported-IQ direction of the blindly determined clusters coincided with the reported clinical scores in both ASD and TD. Validating the axes for the ASD population by age again showed a reversed orientation compared to TD. Notably, even the

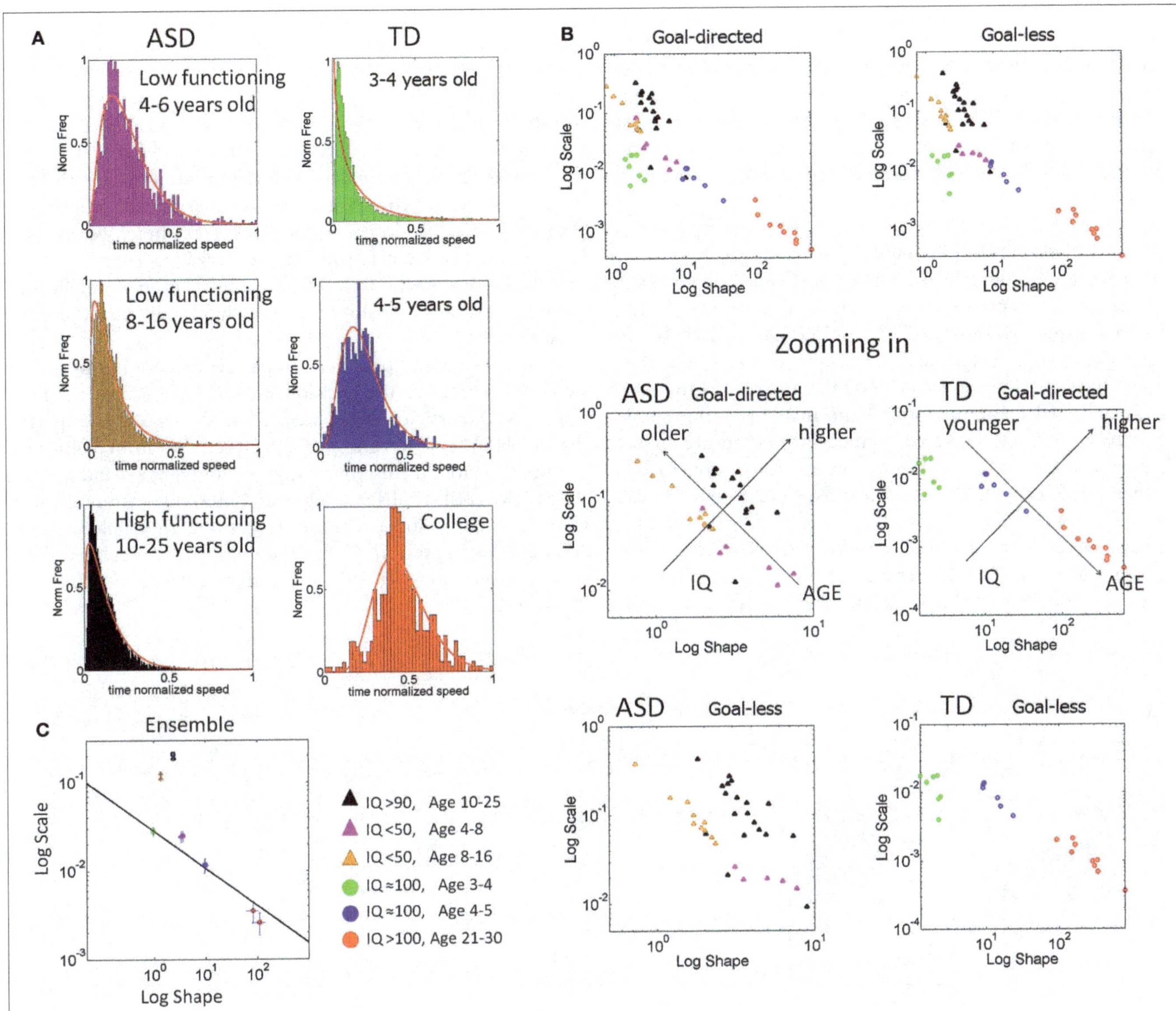

FIGURE 8 | Self-emerging statistical subtypes for TD and ASD cohorts as a function of age and intellectual abilities. (A) Normalized frequency distributions from each self-emerging micro-movements' based cluster in **(B)** is shown for the averaged speed in goal-directed segments and incidental goal-less motions. Each distribution is comprised of several thousand trials. Note that the changes in the shape and scale of each frequency histogram are captured well by the continuous Gamma family described in **Figure 6E** ~15 min into the session upon change in stimulus. **(B)** Scatter of points, where each point represents a participant uniquely labeled by the (*a*-shape, *b*-scale) parameters on the Gamma plane [**Table A4** list MLE (*a*,*b*) values with 95% confidence regions]. Log-log scales are used to depict several orders of magnitude in both axes covering the typical human continuum from pre-school to college. The self-emerging clusters were blindly revealed by the patterns of micro-movements according to the average motion speed. The validation step coloring the scatter according to age and IQ, depicted in the legend, revealed a correspondence with the self-grouping. Bottom panels zoom in the scatters from forward and retraction hand movements. Notice that in ASD the age axis orients the older children away from the typical course of development. **(C)** The stochastic signatures of each cluster are well-characterized by a power relation fit through six points (goal-directed and goal-less for each TD group). The power relation spans several orders of magnitude on both axes (details of the goodness of fit in the main text). Notice again that the young ASD participants fall closer to the TD trajectory in stark contrast to the older verbal and non-verbal ASD participants who stray off the TD path.

verbal ASD group veers-off the typical trajectory. We return to this reversed developmental trend in ASD micro-movements in the conclusions, as it highlights the importance of early detection and intervention. It also raises the issue of whether certain symptomatic behaviors in ASD are actually due to active coping as part of an adaptive mechanism in these individuals.

Notice also that the procedure of validating (and coloring) clusters by reported-IQ and age revealed 3 outliers from the verbal ASD cluster. See the zoomed-in lower panel of goal-less segments in **Figure 8B**. Note that the 2 outliers to the left were the ones scoring highest on the repetitive-stereotypical behavior subscale of the ADOS. Their IQ scores were in the 80–90 range and they have some verbal abilities, yet their somatosensory-motor stochastic signatures placed them in the cluster with the non-verbal individuals with IQs below 50. The third outlier whose signatures fell close to the young TD cluster was recently mainstreamed to a regular kindergarten. Thus, the discovery of those outliers by our approach before knowing their previous test results highlights the individual precision of the micro-movement perspective.

DECISION MAKING-DEPENDENT CLUSTERING

The inherent variability in the velocity-dependent parameters from the hand kinematics thus revealed self-emerging clusters which unambiguously separated ASD and TD individuals of comparable chronological ages and IQ. These clusters were then used to assess the decision latency and the accuracy of the decision as the participants performed the match-to-sample task. The decision latency increased significantly according to the Friedman's test when going from color discrimination to discrimination of shapes and rotated objects. Column effects were observed across stimulus type ($p < 4.9 \times 10^{-102}$, χ^2 482.41) and rows effects were observed across cluster type ($p < 8.5 \times 10^{-97}$, χ^2 458.16). The **Figure 9A** reveals the empirical frequency distributions of this decision-making parameter while **Figure 9B** shows the localization of the different clusters on the Gamma plane. Here we note that ASD participants above 4 years of age cluster closer to TD participants younger than 4 years than to their same age TD peers. Thus, the cognitive decision latency parameter reveals an atypical developmental trajectory precisely compatible with what we found via the micro-movement parameters. It is important to clarify that the use of term "cognitive" here is reserved for non-motor parameters tied to decision-making. For example, we examine the accuracy and the latency of the decision. This is in contrast to the use of the term cognitive in relation to intellectual capabilities—as we do not know exactly how to measure those in ASD.

Another cognitive parameter impacted by the stimulus change was the accuracy of the decision, which decreased in the non-verbal ASD participants as well as in the young TD participants. The % of errors generally increased from color discrimination to the discrimination of ambiguous and rotated shapes (Kruskal–Wallis $p < 0.05$, χ^2 14.99) but with more variability in the color condition errors for the children with ASD and no significant changes for the verbal adults and the college level group (Friedman's test $p < 0.86$, χ^2 0.03). See **Tables 1–2**.

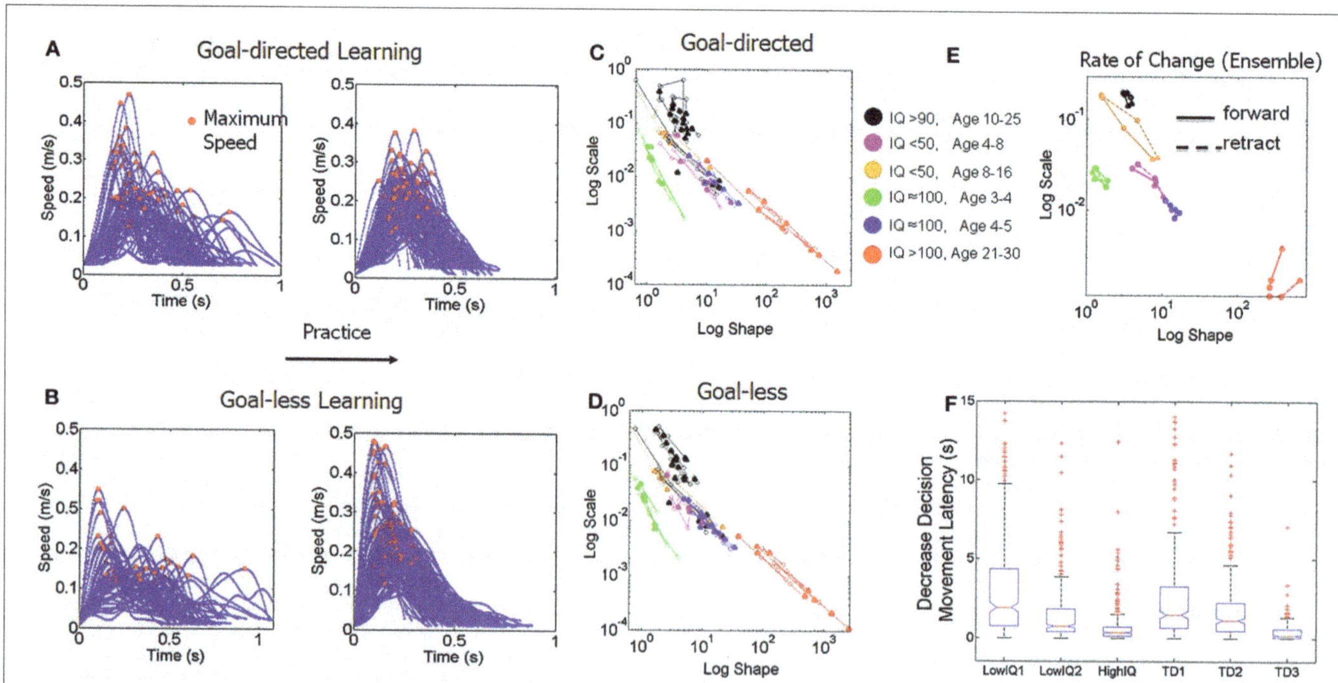

FIGURE 9 | Dynamically tracking the micro-movements as a function of decision-making. (A) Speed profiles from a pre-school TD participant showing how changes in cognitive load of the decision-making task initially evoked multiple peaks in the hand velocities to the target, yet unimodality returned within minutes of practice. The stabilization also manifested in the goal-less segments **(B)**. **(C)** log-log plot of trajectories of the rate of change in the stochastic signatures of the average movement speed in the goal-directed hand motions in each self-emergent statistical subtype of **Figure 8A** (depicted in the legend). Each individual manifested different responses to the change in cognitive load on the micro-movements, and these effects were objectively tracked in each session (open circles represent color and shape, followed by triangle representing rotation). **(D)** The shifts in the stochastic signatures were also tracked in the goal-less non-instructed hand retractions. **(E)** The ensemble data shows greater shifts for the older non-verbal ASD groups. **(F)** With movement practice, the decision-making latencies (shown in seconds) significantly decreased across clusters when comparing the 150 later to the 150 earlier trials of each session (details in main text). Participants with lower IQ and younger TD participants showed the strongest effects. Similar trends on the increase in accuracy are reported in the main text.

Table 1 | Systematic changes in cognitive decision-making performance occurring in parallel with motor (speed) learning.

	Color	Shape	Orientation
	Mean (*SD*)	**Mean (*SD*)**	**Mean (*SD*)**
Percent correct	0.97 (0.18)	0.95 (0.21)	0.91 (0.29)
Decision time (ms)	2285.4 (2370.1)	2570.8 (2926.9)	2739.8 (3527.8)
ASD-DT reduction (ms)	2887 (2168)	1538 (1382)	1344 (843.8)
P-value ASD-DT reduction	6.7×10^{-7}, $\chi^2 = 28.41$	0.003, $\chi^2 = 11.3$	0.05, $\chi^2 = 5.87$
TD-DT reduction (ms)	1556 (1048)	1757 (1480)	2798 (3325)
P-value TD-DT reduction	4.5×10^{-5}, $\chi^2 = 20$	1.2×10^{-9}, $\chi^2 = 41.02$	2.1×10^{-13}, $\chi^2 = 58.37$

Percent correct is the total percentage of correct responses for all individuals for each stimulus type. Decision Time (DT) is the length of time from stimulus onset to when the participant touched one of the two targets. DT reduction is the average number of milliseconds by which participants got faster when comparing their performance for the first 50 trials to the last 50 trials for each stimulus type. This gives a measure of performance gains over time. P-values are reported for Kruskal-Wallis comparisons. Number of trials used across stimulus types and subjects: 2546 color; 3588 shape; 2996 rotation. Reductions in latency are reported on the table for the ASD and the TD groups overall. For the individual self-emerging clusters they were significant across conditions for cluster 1 (non-verbal ASD 4–6 years old, $p < 0.0002$, $\chi^2 = 17.97$); cluster 2 (non-verbal ASD 8–16 years old, $p < 5.8 \times 10^{-5}$); but not significant for cluster 3 (verbal ASD 10–25 years old, $p < 0.80$, $\chi^2 = 0.45$). The TD cluster 4 also had a significant reduction in the latency of the decision-making motion (TD 3–4 years old, $p < 0.0003$ χ^2 16.53) but not significant in cluster 5 (TD 4–6 years old, $p < 0.49$, $\chi^2 = 1.42$) and in cluster 6 (TD 21–30 years old, $p < 0.52$, $\chi^2 = 1.28$).

Table 2 | Systematic changes in cognitive decision-making performance occurring in parallel with motor (speed) learning: condition's pair wise comparison.

	Color vs. Shape	Shape vs. Orient	Color vs. Orient
	Tukey HSD	**Tukey HSD**	**Tukey HSD**
Percent correct	0.0001	0.05	0.0001
Decision time (ms)	0.001	0.0001	0.0001

Tukey's HSD post-hoc tests revealed that each group was different from each other group for both Percentage Correct and Decision Time. The direction of significance reveals that Orientation was the most difficult task (fewer correct, longer decision time), whereas color was the easiest task.

DYNAMIC, REAL TIME TRACKING OF INDIVIDUAL ADAPTIVE PROGRESS

The changes in decision-making stimuli affected hand speed profiles, which gave rise to a re-learning process that we dynamically tracked. As new variants of the task were introduced the hand speed profiles systematically changed from unimodal to multimodal, decreased the accuracy in the children (Kruskal–Wallis $p < 0.05$, χ^2 14.99), and increased the latency of their decision-making responses (Friedman test, stimulus effect $p < 4.9 \times 10^{-102}$, χ^2 482.41, cluster effect $p < 8.5 \times 10^{-97}$, χ^2 458.16). Yet within minutes the speed profiles returned to their stable unimodal feature. Thus the introduction of new tasks with different cognitive loads gave rise to a tractable real time learning-adaptation process. This process also revealed that the stochastic signatures of the average hand speed shifted at a different rate, a rate that was unique to each individual in the cohort.

Examples of multimodal speed profiles are shown in the left panels of **Figures 9A** (goal-directed) and **9B** (goal-less). These changes manifested in both TD and ASD groups. After minutes of practice, the speed profiles recovered their unimodality and the movements themselves became faster. This is shown on the right panels of **Figures 9A,B**. In particular, notice that the time (ms) to reach the maximum speed value was within different time scales in the goal-directed and goal-less motions. The latter had latencies of time to peak velocity on the order of 60–90 ms, which is too fast to reach visual awareness as the hand-eyes are still processing touch-visual information about the chosen target. Statistically significant differences were found across participants in this kinematic latency parameter when comparing goal-directed and goal-less segments (Wilcoxon ranksum test $p < 10^{-6}$) whereby in the goal-directed reach the median time to the maximum speed was between 172.95 and 210.53 ms in ASD and between 109.50 and 179.81 ms in TD. In contrast the goal-less segments were between 93.28 and 108.30 ms in ASD and between 60.34 and 152.11 ms in TD. From this result we conjecture that the fast, automated goal-less motions may be routed differently through the sub-cortical "unconscious" proprioceptive GSA fibers (e.g., such as those in **Figure 2B.**). The forward reaches, where the movement is deliberately launched as a person decides on a matching target show longer latencies to reach the maximum speed. These may be routed through the cortical "conscious" proprioceptive GSA fibers in (**Figure 2A**).

We also tracked the stochastic signature of each individual by math-to-sample discrimination task: color, geometric shapes, and rotated objects (**Figures 9C,D**). Here we show the longitudinal trajectories across weeks for the youngest groups (3–16 years old). On the same Gamma plane we show the real time shifts within one session for the older participants (16–30 years of age) from both ASD and TD groups performing the task within one and/or two sessions. Interestingly, some systematically shifted toward the Gaussian range (positive predictive gain), while others moved back (negative random-memoryless gain) or had near-zero gain on the Gamma plane with variable rates that depended on the stimuli. The overall behavior of the ensemble could also be objectively quantified. See **Figure 9E** for each of the self-emerging clusters. Notice that on this logarithmic scale the older non-verbal ASD cluster showed the largest overall shift toward the typical ranges. Importantly, as the perceptual stimulus changed this was the cluster whose shifts in the stochastic signatures of the goal-less motions maximally differed from the shifts for the goal-directed motions. This distinction became maximal for the decisions on geometric shapes. A possible interpretation of this finding is that this non-verbal ASD group prefers spatial/geometric stimuli in the very precise sense that these allow a better distinction of their goal-directed and goal-less micro-movements than other stimuli. Applied to behavioral training regimens this suggests that these individuals would benefit from usage of geometric type stimuli, which made their motions more predictable and more functionally differentiable in the least amount of time.

Figure 9F shows the decrease in latency (s) for the initiation of the goal-directed movement when comparing the 150 earlier trials to the 150 later trials. The improvements in speed and accuracy of the decision as well as those in the speed of the hand pointing motions render fatigue or attentional effects unlikely in these experiments.

The non-verbal children with ASD and lower reported-IQ experienced the largest improvements in combination with the largest shifts in micro-movements and a different course of performance gains for the goal-less segments incidental to the task (**Figure 9E**). **Table A3** reports further details of this learning progression in the decision-making parameters. **Figure 10** shows the distributions of the decision latency using the clusters obtained from the velocity-dependent micro-movements in **Figures 7, 8**. Thus, through rehearsing, this simple decision-making task, independent of the level of task understanding, reveals statistical shifts toward more predictable micro-movements of their incidental goal-less motions.

Table 1 lists the means and standard deviations for the learning-based reduction in the decision latency across trials and longitudinally for each task. Median values for the reduction in latency per cluster are: TD kindergarten (1601 ms); TD preschool (1203 ms); TD college level (172 ms); non-verbal ASD 4–6 years old (1937 ms); non-verbal ASD 8–16 years old (710.5 ms); verbal ASD 10–25 years old (437 ms). Practice registered significant reductions in the overall movement time for each self-emerging cluster (ranksum test, $p < 0.05$). Along with the reductions in latency, there were corresponding increases in choice-accuracy as measured by the percent correct, $F_{(2,\ 9130)} = 52.37$, $p < 0.0001$. As indicated by *post-hoc* tests, each group was significantly different from each other group for both parameters. See **Table 2** for *P*-values of Tukey's range *post-hoc* tests (Honest Significant Difference tests).

Individuals improved their overall performance longitudinally with practice as evidenced by a significant reduction in the decision time once the speed profile became unimodal and the movement duration was steady (**Table 1**). As the speed profiles evolved to the unimodal signature of automatic reaches so did their proficiency at the cognitive decision-making task. Both TD and ASD participants showed cognitive effects of having to adjust to new tasks. However, both the older verbal ASD and the college-level TD group adjusted to the change in stimulus faster than the children and their accuracy rate was nearly 100% for each stimulus type (Wilcoxson ranksum test across thousands of trials $p < 0.46$).

These similarities between the adults with ASD and the TD adults are interesting given the findings that the stochastic signatures of their micro-movements were fundamentally different during the decision-making pointing. This suggests that rather different mechanisms were used to attain accuracy in each case. Proprioceptive input was random, (unpredictable), noisy

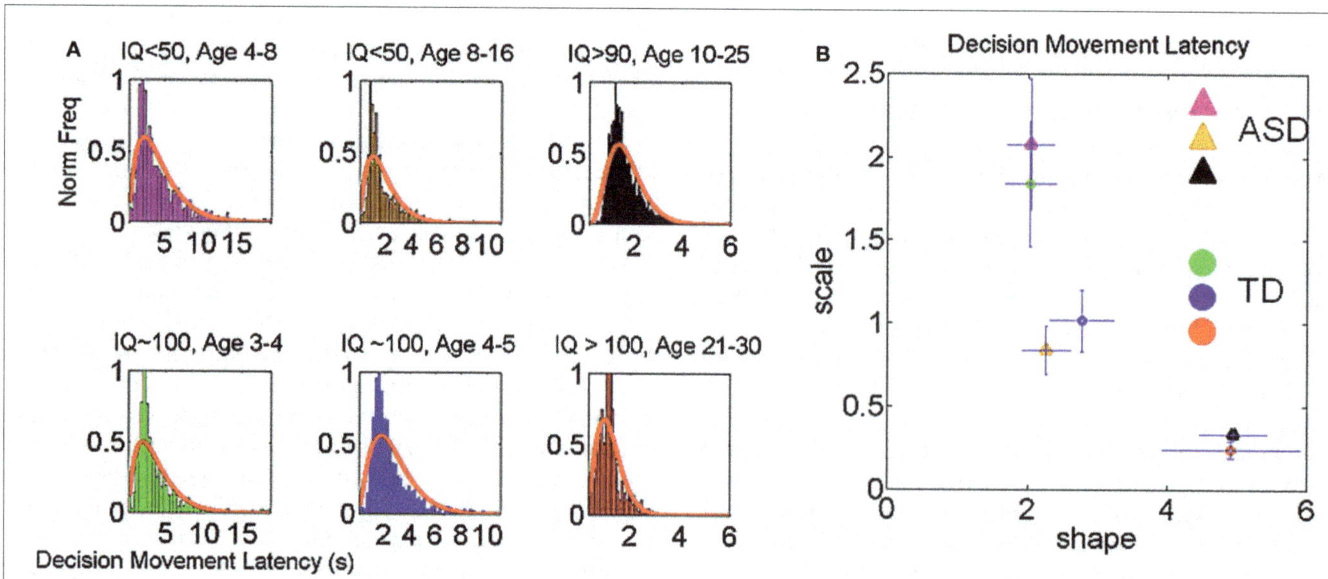

FIGURE 10 | Decision movement latency across self-emerging clusters. **(A)** Frequency histograms of the decision movement time from the self-evoked onset of the sample stimulus to the end of the forward motion at the touch of the screen on the targeted choice. Clusters are from the self-emerging aggregates of the velocity-dependent kinematics parameters. **(B)** Stochastic signatures of this parameter on the *(a,b)* Gamma plane. Notice here that 4–8 year old ASD participants are closer to the 3–4 year old TD participants than to the TD group closer to their own age.

(unreliable), and non-diversified in ASD. They were able to maximally distinguish goal-directed from goal-less motions only in the spatial geometric stimulus set. Given these results, it is possible that they were relying on the actual spatial physical stimulus present throughout the decision. This is in contrast to reliance on an automated, embodied version of it, as we believe was the case for the TD participants. Further testing of this supposition is warranted given also that other researchers have reported that people with ASD rely on visuospatial strengths to perform cognitive tasks that do not, with neurotypicals, require such skills (Samson et al., 2012). In that report Mottron and his team (which, interestingly, includes individuals with autism) have suggested that the over-reliance on complex visualization may be a successful adaptation and, indeed, provide further support for the neurodiversity model of autism.

CONCLUSIONS AND FUTURE STEPS

Our work introduces a new unifying statistical framework and a set of objective metrics to tackle the heterogeneity of spectral disorders. This is a personalized approach to the analyses of real time behavior and to assess longitudinal changes in general. Using this approach it is possible to dynamically track not only the natural developmental trajectories of the individual but also the rates of accelerated change as a function of sensory stimuli in general. The new conceptualization of micro-movements not only as efferent signal but also as kinesthetic re-afferent signal is bound to have a broad impact for the study of behavior across various disciplines. From movement neuroscience to sports science to computer science and robotics, this new biologically plausible notion of behavioral variability along with the new statistical platform for dynamic stochastic tracking could transform the ways in which we study and assess learning, adaptation, normal development, and normal aging. The new framework will also enable us to detect atypical patterns and track those patterns as they evolve both in real time and longitudinally.

The micro-movements are here hypothesized to reflect layers of multi-directional internal and external influences on the central and peripheral nervous systems (**Figures 1A,B**). The re-afferent nature of the velocity-dependent micro-movements paired with their precise measurements at the motor output open the possibility of unveiling potential regulatory control and adaptive mechanisms of the typical system as well as their different manifestations in the specific case of ASD.

This approach can thus inform the search for "endo-phenotypes" across the autism spectrum. Studying physical hand movements allowed us to rapidly detect autistic traits and track the idiosyncratic rates of change in micro-movements *for each individual*. Our methods permitted tackling such issues in real time during decision-pointing actions, as well as longitudinally across different experimental sessions. We found that micro-movements serve as a putative biomarker of typical proprioceptive-motor development in the limbs as well as to flag deviations from the typical developmental path. Applied to 34 individuals with a diagnosis of ASD we blindly detected clusters of individuals with similar micro-movement features and validated that these anomalies in micro-movements corresponded to degrees of verbal capabilities as well as to clinically reported IQ scores.

The classification approach developed here demonstrated that the new framework can address the heterogeneity of the disorder and blindly sub-type autism severity according to the subject's verbal capabilities without a priori choosing the clusters or trying to homogenize the various groups. Our approach also addresses the non-stationary statistical nature of natural behaviors.

An important aspect of the new metrics is that they enable the identification in real time of the type of sensory input which can accelerate learning by steering the person's proprioception toward more predictive behavioral regimes with faster and more accurate decisions. This is because we have precise ways to detect changes in such stochastic patterns toward predictive or toward random regimes. We can assess the statistical reliability (noise-to-signal ratios) in the context of all natural movements—goal-directed segments or goal-less segments occurring beneath awareness. We can selectively find and use the form of sensory-motor guidance that makes the individual more efficient at choosing and controlling adequate motor programs in the face of sensory-motor noise. Micro-movements therefore offer a new way to automatically track improvements, and reinforce the re-afferent sensory-motor input that leads to predictive proprioception. Micro-movements also allow automatic discounting of the input that makes the proprioception noisier and more random.

In short, through movement variability, understood not only as efferent motor output but also as kinesthetic re-afference in the context of stochastic processes, we offer a new unifying framework to (1) idiosyncratically quantify different levels of ASD in real time; (2) dynamically track real time and longitudinal performance in the context of decision-making; and (3) develop new personalized therapies that may exploit the sensory-motor capabilities of the autistic individual.

The micro-movement methodology does not depend on explicit instructions. It can track spontaneous behavioral variability and variability from deliberate behaviors. This means that individuals with ASD who are non-verbal or who may have difficulties acting on command will be able to benefit from personalized therapies that use their micro-movement statistics. This is important because many non-verbal individuals have already developed their own compensatory strategies undetectable by conventional methods. Our methods can detect and harness patterns from spontaneous behaviors that fall beneath the person's awareness and reflect some of those strategies.

We are at present using these methods to track longitudinal changes in spontaneous behavior before, during and after treatment of an FDA-approved clinical trial drug using insulin-like growth factor 1 in children with a diagnosis of autism of known etiology [specifically, in children with Phellan-McDermid syndrome (Phelan and Rogers, 1993)].

We have discovered that the continuous two-parameter Gamma family of probability distributions captures with high confidence level the velocity-dependent variability inherent to all human movements throughout typical and atypical development and adulthood. This developmental path is well-characterized with a scaling power-law relation that objectively captures a connection between patterns of micro-movements and performance in decision-making related to cognitive control. Points corresponding to neighboring individuals on the Gamma plane had similar micro-movement signatures and similar verbal capabilities. Each person's signatures shifted at a different rate as a function of stimulus and task context, potentially signaling different levels of behavioral flexibility unique to each individual. This result offers a new form of flexibility-based classification for neurodevelopmental—and neurodegenerative (Torres, 2013a)—disorders in general. This further enables flagging early on atypical signatures of kinesthetic re-afference. It also shows the tangible possibility of developing objective target therapies tailored to each person's predispositions, capabilities, and flexibility so badly needed in autism research and treatments.

TOO MUCH NOISE: THE CORRUPTED KINESTHETIC RE-AFFERECE IN ASD

As noted, the unveiled body micro-movements are also the immediate object of internal kinesthetic sensations as they shift signatures over time. Notice here that the problem may be at the motor output due, for example, to low muscle tone; it may be at the afferent synapses; it may be at the central level where commands are issued, etc. The point is that we can capture a read-out of the somatosensation of the person at the motor output—even without knowing the exact origins of the disturbances. We know that these stochastic fluctuations are being kinesthetically sensed by the system over time and impinged by external and internal influences. Thus, we can track those effects and efficiently, *in real time*, steer the system using adequate input. Our methodology objectively quantifies the dynamic sensation of re-afferent movements and thereby quantifies a form of proprioception. Our findings show a developmental trajectory wherein TD micro-movement proprioception undergoes maturation that results in specific probabilistic expectations. In the language of Bayesian statistics, such acquired "priors" allow the agent to make meaningful categorizations and sense unexpected internal and external disruptions through their own movements. We have also found that mature TD micro-movements can be separated into functional classes with different levels of intentionality. They operate at different time scales in their latencies to reach critical points (e.g., maxima) along the kinematic trajectory.

The measured experimental data shows that the path of micro-movement development is fundamentally different for the individuals diagnosed with ASD. Their hand movements appear to remain at the kinesthetic stage of TD 3–4 year old children and to some extent even regress as they veer off the typical developmental path. The data shows that regardless of age, the individuals with ASD do not acquire their own reliable statistical expectations from their behavioral variability (i.e., do not acquire reliable kinesthetic priors). Their sensory-motor signal is overpowered by noise and never diversifies.

LINKING KINESTHETIC RE-AFFERENT MICRO-MOVEMENTS, LACK OF SOCIAL COMMUNICATION, AND OTHER BEHAVIORAL SYMPTOMS IN ASD

Lack of flexibility

Reliable kinesthetic priors are needed as anchors to measure new movement fluctuations; i.e., to establish an implicit embodiment of the statistics in the external signal. The empirical finding that ASD individuals do not acquire such expectations implies that they cannot discriminate different levels of functionality in their physical movements. A testable hypothesis is that it is unlikely that they would be able to discriminate different levels of functionalities in the movements of others, e.g., distinguish when a gesture is intentional from when the same gesture is spontaneous. Further, the lack of kinesthetic priors means that the individual with ASD lacks an implicit reference frame for new variations in different contexts. Thus, they cannot discriminate the variability of their own movements from contextual internal and external influences. Where the TD individual can purposefully sample and adapt to sensed changes, any attempt to diversify the input would amplify the noise and maximize uncertainty for the autistic individual. The reliance on sameness can be, at least in part, traced back to the lack of movement expectations or "kinesthetic priors." These may also have downstream effects on perceptual and mental navigation. It forces the autistic system to rely on the concrete "here and now" of perceived body position and environment. All in all, we conjecture that these experimental findings may begin to unify and explain several of the key symptoms of ASD.

Sensory integration

The lack of reliable priors, the excess noise, and the lack of re-afferent diversity are likely to impede the integration of sensory inputs from different sensory modalities as there is no internalized sensory-motor frame of reference to organize the sensory integration. If so, this would restrict the autistic individual to rely on the modality that best works for his/her system, actively ignoring other modalities that would only amplify the sensory-motor noise and increase uncertainty. The sensory issues in ASD are multipronged. They often have an impact on their ability to sort information from single modalities at low-level processing. Likewise, for a hyper sensitive system, if everything is signal in certain sensory domains, how does that system filter out interfering signal (noise) from the relevant signal within a given sensory modality? Our new methods will allow further investigations of other potential underlying causes for the disruptions quantified here, including possible malfunctioning of the ANS and their relation to circadian rhythms regulating food-intake, sleep cycles, and gastro-intestinal functions. It may be possible to assess contributions of the peripheral noise-to-signal re-afferent feedback to the central regulation, coordination, and control of anticipatory sensory-motor integration.

Cortical and peripheral anchors

We propose the hypothesis that the typical development of "kinesthetic priors" is essential not only for anchoring kinesthetic sensing but also for the typical development of cortical sensorimotor circuits; circuits critical for flexible hierarchical action planning, shifts of attention, and establishing counterfactuals in symbolic problem solving. Experiencing kinesthetic re-afference as a stable percept serves as an abstract generalization that allows us to navigate and track action opportunities "off-line" without constant concurrent perceptual guidance. This hypothesis finds some support in the current hand micro-movement variations. The TD children younger than 4 years did not reliably show internalized priors—a result congruent with the maturation stages necessary to perform traditional theory of mind tasks (Baron-Cohen et al., 1985). The new methodology will enable further explorations into the nature of the shifts in stochastic signatures characterizing the morphing of noise into signal during flexible exchanges between intentional and spontaneous mode of behavior.

Accumulative social and communicative issues

It is very unlikely that individuals with ASD can make anticipatory decisions and estimate the consequences of their own impending actions in a timely fashion. This is suggested by the quantified random, noisy, and restrictive proprioception, prevailing across ages in the data set. Much less probable would be that they could apply fine-tuned discriminations to the actions and emotional facial micro-expressions of others during real time social interactions. Given the stochastic signatures of kinesthetic re-afference found here, it may be possible to investigate more precisely why it seems impossible for individuals with ASD to visually perceive intentional motions and weight their potential consequences, e.g., to "see" in real time the intentional movements in cartoons with geometric figures as shown in the classic Heider and Simmel experiment (Heider and Simmel, 1944).

It is our conjecture that the noisy, random, and restrictive proprioception of their own physical micro-movements impedes as well their visual perception of micro-movements in others during real time interactions. A congruent map between physical and visual perception of motion may be necessary for the correct interpretation of external movement patterns inherently present in social dynamics (Johnson et al., 2012a,b). Without basic kinesthetic re-afference in place it is very unlikely that flexible and timely discrimination between intentional and spontaneous gestures develops.

The proposed framework will permit us to deconstruct impairments in social interactions via the stochastic approach to assess in real time the non-stationary signals generated by our bodies and by the bodies of others in a social scene. These include speech, gestures, body poses as well as the velocity-dependent kinematics of the micro-expressions of the faces conveying emotional content. Micro-movements thus conceived as kinesthetic re-afference are present across all functional levels of the nervous system (in **Figure 1B**). If this input is noisy and unstable, the required map between visual and kinesthetic percepts of our own motions and those of others would be disrupted. This would make it impossible to co-adapt social interactions in real time and, in general to mentally navigate through social dynamics with successfully confirmed outcomes.

Coping and compensatory adaptive mechanisms

Lastly, we conjecture that the observed behavioral symptoms are dynamic byproducts of an individual coping with low-level corrupted signals. Similar to any other biological system, the autistic system may have found compensatory strategies to deal with corrupted re-afferent input and close the feedback loops to sustain a rudimentary form of (non-anticipatory) motor control. An intriguing result from this work is the effect of aging on the micro-movements of individuals with ASD. In the initial stages around 4–6 years of age the children with ASD studied were closer to the TD children of similar chronological age than to the children with ASD older than 8 years of age. Then their micro-movements' stochastic signatures not only veered-off the typical developmental path, it also reversed direction away from it. The empirical data suggests that as individuals with autism age, their micro-movements become even more random, noisier, and more restricted. Why this reversal? We hypothesize that this reversal is part of a dynamic *coping strategy* that ends up reinforcing a narrow bandwidth of sensory input embedded in unreliable re-afferent information from their physical actions. If sensory-motor integration fails and the system cannot spontaneously form proper maps of the body in space and time and filter relevant perceptions, then exploration can only bring more uncertainty.

TD individuals can anchor their explorations in implicit predictable priors that allow variations to become informative signals. They can then adaptively reshape these priors on demand. For individuals with nearly "memoryless" statistics and little implicit sense of their own bodies—every variation becomes noise. Thus, the intense desire for sameness—and to some extent the avoidance of social interactions—can be seen as active attempts to limit uncertainty (noise) in an already noisy and non-diversified input. Some repetitive motions can be understood as part of a search for current verification of body position in space, which would help not only the impaired implicit body map but also could be used to "keep out" confusing and perplexing noise from the broader environment. Restricted interests can be seen as higher-level attempts to create predictable environmental pockets where expectations hold. This yields a memory/world-based predictability and a sense of safety whereby nearly no adjustment is needed for successful actions.

In accordance with the idea of successful coping, we saw that individuals with ASD often had a high accuracy in the match-to-sample decision, in spite of their corrupted proprioception. This suggested that they rely on an alternative strategy. Where the embodiment of the statistics of the external physical input is likely to underlie the fast and accurate decisions in TD individuals, the improvements in decision-making accuracy in the ASD individuals must depend on alternative means such as the concrete physical input (e.g., the visual feedback present throughout the decision period).

Future research and therapies will need to be more alert to disentangle the atypical behavioral phenotypes of people with ASD into original impairments and/or active successful coping behaviors. Whereas, our actions rely on anticipatory and mentally controlled and regulated physical motor outputs rooted in highly expected variability, the ASD individual must rely on the concrete here and now with minimum likelihood for anticipation and mental control and regulation of the efferent motor output.

One could argue that the way forward will involve an analysis of idiosyncratic micro-movement challenges and an individualized treatment approach that exploits not only whatever movements a particular individual on the spectrum can manage but also whatever adaptations his/her different neurology and experience have afforded him/her. Here individuals with autism could play an active role in helping us figure out why they have been able to come so far with the movement challenges they obviously have (Savarese, 2013).

FUTURE STEPS

While we provide here a new framework and a set of objective metrics to dynamically study both typical and autistic traits, we are still far from explaining the causes of these atypical micro-movements to get closer to the true underlying causes of autism. Our results suggest that there is a lack of spontaneous autonomy in the autistic system that impedes adaptive and co-adaptive volitional control. These may be largely contributed by corrupted afferent peripheral information, including input from the autonomic and somatic nervous systems of which we specifically tackled hand movement proprioception here. Our work highlights that autism is a systemic neurodevelopmental disorder with concrete, measurable physical bases. Autism should not be exclusively portrayed as a psychological, abstract cognitive/social problem of a *"disembodied"* brain. That would be merely a static snapshot of a person whose sensory-motor systems are clearly evolving and changing in adaptive and compensatory ways.

The metrics and framework offered here provide a complementary and new way to unify brain and body interactions rather dynamically. We can now study the dynamic contributions from peripheral afferents in tandem with centrally sent signals and aim at evoking and maintaining in the autistic individual better regulation and anticipatory control of the efferent output signals. We need to exploit the capabilities inherent in individuals coping with and adapting to sensory-motor problems of genetic and/or epigenetic origins. By connecting and being able to measure central and peripheral contributions objectively we can redefine autism in relation to phylogenetic constraints involving synapses and networks at all levels of the nervous systems (not just at the cortical level). More importantly, we can find new avenues for personalized target treatments—*even before we get at the causes of autism.*

It is clear, nonetheless, that we need to look beyond the limb movements explored in this current study. In the future we need to explore the possibility that the noisy and narrowed-bandwidth proprioception of the limbs and hand motions may extend to all functional levels of micro-movements including those embedded in speech and facial micro-expressions. Sensory-motor orofacial nerves are phylogenetically and anatomically different from those of the limbs. We hypothesize different developmental timelines and cognitive effects for orofacial proprioception than those which we have found for hand and arm-based movements. This is a testable hypothesis under the present framework. Further, conceiving motion across multiple functional levels as a *change of position over time*, we can apply the current statistical metrics to objectively measure all sensory levels of biological beings in real time (**Figure 2**). Thus, we propose to further use the present methods to understand autism above and beyond perceptible differences with TD controls.

Despite the systemic problems identified with movement-based proprioceptive information, a positive result emerged from the decision-making experiment. Most participants with ASD experienced a shift of their micro-movements as a function of changes in match-to-sample stimuli. In several cases and for specific stimulus types this shift was toward the predictive limits of the Gamma plane. This implies that, at least transiently, changes in sensory input can (1) be detected by the autistic systems and (2) help anchor movements in such a way as to make pointing motions more predictable. Even though internal feedback is corrupted, reliance on the concrete physical reality allows external anchoring to close the feedback loops and support adaptive exploration: i.e., a form of sensory substitution that we can link to patterns of spontaneous micro-movements. In another paper of this Research Topic (by Torres et al.) we show how in a matter of seconds computerized behavioral interventions requiring no instructions can lead non-verbal children with ASD toward the spontaneous self-discovery of a goal and the autonomous and more anticipatory control of motions: They attain a reward and sustain it under a form of *acquired* adaptive volitional control. The participants in that study retained their shifts weeks later. Even without practice their micro-movements shifted toward anticipatory, intentional features. We were able to automatically and objectively track these changes longitudinally using the current framework and metrics. In this sense we already know that in several of these children there were long-term gains in predictability and reliability of their actions, not just transient changes within a given session.

In the present work we also registered negative gains toward the Exponential range of the Gamma plane as the individual adapted to the new task context. We can test *selectively* in real time which sensory modality may better guide each person toward predictive or preferred performance. In other words, we can automatically detect which form of sensory input most likely accelerates the learning progression with minimum resistance by the child's sensory-motor systems. This would be the sensory input with the largest rate of change toward higher predictability (highest value of the shape parameter toward the Gaussian limit of the Gamma plane) and highest reliability (the lowest dispersion which corresponds to the lowest Fano Factor given by the variance to mean ratio). We can reinforce that source of sensory guidance and discount the sensory modality that makes the kinesthetic percept noisier and more random.

To the best of our knowledge this is a new way to objectively and dynamically track in real time the shifts in stochastic signatures of the non-stationary statistics of the continuous flow of natural behavior. We have developed a methodology that permits very precise and automatic assessment of the form of guidance that most rapidly improves re-afferent kinesthetic input and accelerates learning. This in turn leads to an enhanced volitional control of the child over his/her motions and the development of better autonomy over the connection between his/her intentions and actions. This is the first inclusive methodology that harnesses the sensory-motor capabilities and the adaptive learning predispositions that are already present in the individual with ASD.

Our work differs fundamentally from current behavioral training techniques which rely on commands and a priori selected stimuli. Our next immediate goal is to design new metrics that can tell us exactly the path of least resistance [in a very precise physical sense (Lanczos, 1966; Feynman et al., 2006)]: the path which accelerates learning and moves the child's kinesthetic re-afference away from the rim of maximum uncertainty. Overall, we found that each individual in the spectrum is *unique* and learns at a unique rate, a result that we would have missed had we assumed homogeneity a priori, formed groups accordingly, and assumed a priori an underlying probability distribution common to the entire ASD cohort.

Although we have used here human participants to illustrate the use of the new framework, micro-movements are inherent to any biological organism with sensory transducers, which autonomously moves to survive and reproduce. Our framework can also be applied to objectively analyze behavioral phenotyping assays in animal models of autism (and other spectral disorders) to evaluate important contemporary emerging theories that will guide our quest for the causes of ASD and for clinical treatments (Markram and Markram, 2010; Silverman et al., 2010).

In summary, we have shown that studying the statistics of micro-movements' variability provides a powerful tool to build a new generation of objective diagnostic assessments of ASD. These include new metrics to assess the long-term flexibility and plasticity of sensory-motor systems in the face of compensatory adaptive mechanisms self-discovered by the person with ASD on a short-term basis. The new methodology will enable the development of new personalized interventions tailored to the individual's inherent capabilities. The individual with ASD does not develop by default the predictability of micro-movements that allows for anticipatory, adaptive, and explorative behavior. However, applying our new methods has allowed us to uncover new ways to evoke real time transient changes toward predictive behaviors with long-lasting effects retained weeks later (Torres, 2013a,b in this issue).

We have quantified ways to evoke shifts toward predictive statistical movement regimes as well as changes toward faster and more accurate decisions. This, despite the quantification of movement sensing that appears to be overpowered by noise and lacking diversification. With this new methodology we can now explore the heterogeneity of ASD and enhance cognitive learning predispositions inherently present in each child. We studied not only goal-directed movements but also spontaneous behavioral variability present in incidental motion segments (largely beneath the person's awareness). Such motion segments pursued no concrete goals. They provide new means to objectively quantify changes in a type of cognitive learning that occurs without explicit instructions and largely without concrete purpose. Future work will extend this quantification to other automatic and autonomic levels across other populations of neurodevelopmental spectral disorders of known and of unknown etiology.

ACKNOWLEDGMENTS

We thank Harriet Coles for very valuable comments on the manuscript. We thank Dr. Sandy Harris, Dr. Lara Delmolino, Dr. Kate Fiske, Jennifer Biddick, and Meredith Bamond from the Douglass Developmental Disability Center (DDDC) at Rutgers University, and all the staff members at the DDDC for assistance with participants, data collection, and clinical records. We thank Carrie Fisher and Dawn L. Graham for assistance with participants and their medical records at the Institute for Psychiatric Research and also the Riley Hospital for Children, both part of Indiana University School of Medicine. We thank Di Wu for suggestions as to how to properly renormalize all the velocity data. This work was funded by NSF Cyber-Enabled Discovery and Innovation Type I (Idea) grant # 094158 to Elizabeth B. Torres and Dimitris N. Metaxas "A novel quantitative framework to study lack of social interactions in ASD Spectrum Disorders" and by the New Jersey Governor's Council for Medical Research and Treatment of Autism grant # 10-403-SCH-E-0 "Perceptual Motor Anticipation in ASD."

REFERENCES

Amaral, D. G., and Corbett, B. A. (2003). The amygdala, autism and anxiety. *Novartis Found. Symp.* 251, 177–187; discussion: 187–197, 281–197.

Amaral, D. G., Schumann, C. M., and Nordahl, C. W. (2008). Neuroanatomy of autism. *Trends Neurosci.* 31, 137–145.

Ashwood, P., Anthony, A., Pellicer, A. A., Torrente, F., Walker-Smith, J. A., and Wakefield, A. J. (2003). Intestinal lymphocyte populations in children with regressive autism: evidence for extensive mucosal immunopathology. *J. Clin. Immunol.* 23, 504–517.

Bandstra, N. F., Johnson, S. A., Filliter, J. H., and Chambers, C. T. (2012). Self-reported and parent-reported pain for common painful events in high-functioning children and adolescents with autism spectrum disorder. *Clin. J. Pain* 28, 715–721.

Baron-Cohen, S., Leslie, A. M., and Frith, U. (1985). Does the autistic child have a "theory of mind"? *Cognition* 21, 37–46.

Bays, P. M., and Wolpert, D. M. (2007). Computational principles of sensorimotor control that minimize uncertainty and variability. *J. Physiol.* 578, 387–396.

Bernstein, N. (1967). *The Co-ordination and Regulation of Movements.* Oxford: Oxford Press.

Bhat, A. N., and Galloway, J. C. (2006). Toy-oriented changes during early arm movements: hand kinematics. *Infant Behav. Dev.* 29, 358–372.

Bourgeron, T. (2007). The possible interplay of synaptic and clock genes in autism spectrum disorders. *Cold Spring Harb. Symp. Quant. Biol.* 72, 645–654.

Breece, E., Paciotti, B., Nordahl, C. W., Ozonoff, S., Van de Water, J. A., Rogers, S. J., et al. (2012). Myeloid dendritic cells frequencies are increased in children with autism spectrum disorder and associated with amygdala volume and repetitive behaviors. *Brain Behav. Immun.* doi: 10.1016/j.bbi.2012.10.006. [Epub ahead of print].

Buie, T., Fuchs, G. J. 3rd., Furuta, G. T., Kooros, K., Levy, J., Lewis, J. D., et al. (2010). Recommendations for evaluation and treatment of common gastrointestinal problems in children with ASDs. *Pediatrics* 125(Suppl. 1), S19–S29.

Condon, W. S., and Sander, L. W. (1974). Neonate movement is synchronized with adult speech: interactional participation and language acquisition. *Science* 183, 99–101.

Damasio, A. R., and Maurer, R. G. (1978). A neurological model for childhood autism. *Arch. Neurol.* 35, 777–786.

de Magistris, L., Familiari, V., Pascotto, A., Sapone, A., Frolli, A., Iardino, P., et al. (2010). Alterations of the intestinal barrier in patients with autism spectrum disorders and in their first-degree relatives. *J. Pediatr. Gastroenterol. Nutr.* 51, 418–424.

Donnellan, A. M., Hill, D., and Leary, M. R. (2013). Rethinking autism: implications of sensory and movement differences for understanding and support. *Front. Integr. Neurosci.* 6:124. doi: 10.3389/fnint.2012.00124

Donnellan, A. M., and Leary, M. R. (1995). *Movement Differences and Diversity in Autism/Mental Retardation: Appreciating and Accommodating People with Communication and Behavior Challenges.* Madison, WI: DRI Press.

Doyle, J. C., Francis, B. A., and Tannenbaum, A., (2009). *Feedback Control Theory.* Mineola, NY: Dover.

Dubois, A., Rattaz, C., Pry, R., and Baghdadli, A. (2010). Autism and pain - a literature review. *Pain Res. Manag.* 15, 245–253.

Dworzynski, K., Ronald, A., Bolton, P., and Happe, F. (2012). How different are girls and boys above and below the diagnostic threshold for autism spectrum disorders? *J. Am. Acad. Child Adolesc. Psychiatry* 51, 788–797.

Fano, U. (1947). Ionization yield of radiations. II. The fluctuations of the number of ions. *Phys. Rev.* 72, 26.

Feynman, R. P., Leighton, R. B., and Sands, M. L. (2006). *The Feynman lectures on physics.* San Francisco, CA: Pearson/Addison-Wesley.

Fournier, K. A., Hass, C. J., Naik, S. K., Lodha, N., and Cauraugh, J. H. (2010a). Motor coordination in autism spectrum disorders: a synthesis and meta-analysis. *J. Autism Dev. Disord.* 40, 1227–1240.

Fournier, K. A., Kimberg, C. I., Radonovich, K. J., Tillman, M. D., Chow, J. W., Lewis, M. H., et al. (2010b). Decreased static and dynamic postural control in children with autism spectrum disorders. *Gait Posture* 32, 6–9.

Freeman, J. B., and Ambady, N. (2010). MouseTracker: software for studying real-time mental processing using a computer mouse-tracking method. *Behav. Res. Methods* 42, 226–241.

Gidley Larson, J. C., Bastian, A. J., Donchin, O., Shadmehr, R., and Mostofsky, S. H. (2008). Acquisition of internal models of motor tasks in children with autism. *Brain* 131, 2894–2903.

Gilliam, J. (2006). *GARS-2: Gilliam Autism Rating Scale-Second Edition.* Austin, TX: PRO-ED.

Glickman, G. (2010). Circadian rhythms and sleep in children with autism. *Neurosci. Biobehav. Rev.* 34, 755–768.

Gotham, K., Pickles, A., and Lord, C. (2009). Standardizing ADOS scores for a measure of severity in autism spectrum disorders. *J. Autism Dev. Disord.* 39, 693–705.

Gowen, E., and Hamilton, A. (2013). Motor abilities in autism: a review using a computational context. *J. Autism Dev. Disord.* 43, 323–344.

Gowen, E., Stanley, J., and Miall, R. C. (2008). Movement interference in autism-spectrum disorder. *Neuropsychologia* 46, 1060–1068.

Haswell, C. C., Izawa, J., Dowell, L. R., Mostofsky, S. H., and Shadmehr, R. (2009). Representation of internal models of action in the autistic brain. *Nat. Neurosci.* 12, 970–972.

Heider, F., and Simmel, M. (1944). An experimental study of apparent behavior. *Am. J. Psychol.* 57, 243–259.

Hill, D. A., and Leary, M. R. (1993). *Movement Disturbance: a Clue to Hidden Competencies in Persons Diagnosed with Autism and Other Developmental Disabilities.* Madison, WI: DRI Press.

Izawa, J., Pekny, S. E., Marko, M. K., Haswell, C. C., Shadmehr, R., and Mostofsky, S. H. (2012). Motor learning relies on integrated sensory inputs in ADHD, but over-selectively on proprioception in autism spectrum conditions. *Autism Res.* 5, 124–136.

Jacobson, R., Le Couteur, A., Howlin, P., and Rutter, M. (1988). Selective subcortical abnormalities in autism. *Psychol. Med.* 18, 39–48.

Jansiewicz, E. M., Goldberg, M. C., Newschaffer, C. J., Denckla, M. B., Landa, R., and Mostofsky, S. H. (2006). Motor signs distinguish children with high functioning autism and Asperger's syndrome from controls. *J. Autism Dev. Disord.* 36, 613–621.

Johnson, G., Yanovich, P., Difeo, G., Yang, L., Santos, E., Ross, N., et al. (2012a). "Congruent map between the kinesthetic and the visual perceptions of our physical movements, even with noise," in *Annual Meeting of the Society for Neuroscience* (Washington, DC).

Johnson, G., Yanovich, P., Difeo, G., Yang, L., Santos, E., Ross, N., et al. (2012b). "What do we see in each other: How movement drives social interaction," in *IGERT-NSF Video and Poster Competition: Award Winning* (Washington, DC). Available online at: http://posterhall.org/igert2012/posters/220

Jones, V., and Prior, M. (1985). Motor imitation abilities and neurological signs in autistic children. *J. Autism Dev. Disord.* 15, 37–46.

Karmel, B. Z., Gardner, J. M., Meade, L. S., Cohen, I. L., London, E., Flory, M. J., et al. (2010). Early medical and behavioral characteristics of NICU infants later classified with ASD. *Pediatrics* 126, 457–467.

Kawato, M., and Wolpert, D. (1998). Internal models for motor control. *Novartis Found. Symp.* 218, 291–304; discussion: 304–297.

Klintwall, L., Holm, A., Eriksson, M., Carlsson, L. H., Olsson, M. B., Hedvall, A., et al. (2011). Sensory abnormalities in autism. A brief report. *Res. Dev. Disabil.* 32, 795–800.

Konczak, J., and Dichgans, J. (1997). The development toward stereotypic arm kinematics during reaching in the first 3 years of life. *Exp. Brain Res.* 117, 346–354.

Kushak, R. I., Lauwers, G. Y., Winter, H. S., and Buie, T. M. (2011). Intestinal disaccharidase activity in patients with autism: effect of age, gender, and intestinal inflammation. *Autism* 15, 285–294.

Lanczos, C. (1966). *The Variational Principles of Mechanics.* Toronto, ON: University of Toronto Press.

Leary, M. R., and Hoyle, R. H. (2009). *Handbook of Individual Differences in Social Behavior.* New York, NY: Guilford Press.

Lee, H. M., Bhat, A., Scholz, J. P., and Galloway, J. C. (2008). Toy-oriented changes during early arm movements IV: shoulder-elbow coordination. *Infant Behav. Dev.* 31, 447–469.

Limpert, E., and Stahel, W. A. (2011). Problems with using the normal distribution–and ways to improve quality and efficiency of data analysis. *PLoS ONE* 6:e21403. doi: 10.1371/journal.pone.0021403

Limpert, E., Stahel, W. A., and Abbt, M. (2001). Log-normal distributions across the sciences: keys and clues. *Bioscience* 51, 341–352.

Lleonart, J., Salat, J., and Torres, G. J. (2000). Removing allometric effects of body size in morphological analysis. *J. Theor. Biol.* 205, 85–93.

Lord, C., and Bishop, S. L. (2010). Autism spectrum disorders: diagnosis, prevalence and services for children and families. *Soc. Res. Child Dev.* 24, 1–26.

Lord, C., Risi, S., Lambrecht, L., Cook, E. H. Jr., Leventhal, B. L., Dilavore, P. C., et al. (2000). The autism diagnostic observation schedule-generic: a standard measure of social and communication deficits associated with the spectrum of autism. *J. Autism Dev. Disord.* 30, 205–223.

MacFabe, D. F., Cain, N. E., Boon, F., Ossenkopp, K. P., and Cain, D. P. (2011). Effects of the enteric bacterial metabolic product propionic acid on object-directed behavior, social behavior, cognition, and neuroinflammation in adolescent rats: relevance to autism spectrum disorder. *Behav. Brain Res.* 217, 47–54.

Mandy, W., Chilvers, R., Chowdhury, U., Salter, G., Seigal, A., and Skuse, D. (2012). Sex differences in autism spectrum disorder: evidence from a large sample of children and adolescents. *J. Autism Dev. Disord.* 42, 1304–1313.

Markram, K., and Markram, H. (2010). The intense world theory - a unifying theory of the neurobiology of autism. *Front. Hum. Neurosci.* 4:224. doi: 10.3389/fnhum.2010.00224

Marsden, J. E., Krishnaprasad, P. S., and Simo, J. C. (1989). "Dynamics and control of multibody systems," in *Proceedings of the AMS-IMS-SIAM Joint Summer Research Conference held July 30-August 5, 1988, with support from the National Science Foundation* (Providence, RI: American Mathematical Society).

Maurer, R. G., and Damasio, A. R. (1979). Vestibular dysfunction in autistic children. *Dev. Med. Child Neurol.* 21, 656–659.

Maurer, R. G., and Damasio, A. R. (1982). Childhood autism from the point of view of behavioral neurology. *J. Autism Dev. Disord.* 12, 195–205.

Mazurek, M. O., Vasa, R. A., Kalb, L. G., Kanne, S. M., Rosenberg, D., Keefer, A., et al. (2013). Anxiety, sensory over-responsivity, and gastrointestinal problems in children with autism spectrum disorders. *J. Abnorm. Child Psychol.* 41, 165–176.

Minderaa, R. B., Volkmar, F. R., Hansen, C. R., Harcherik, D. F., Akkerhuis, G. W., and Cohen, D. J. (1985). Snout and visual rooting reflexes in infantile autism. *J. Autism Dev. Disord.* 15, 409–416.

Minshew, N. J., Sung, K., Jones, B. L., and Furman, J. M. (2004). Underdevelopment of the postural control system in autism. *Neurology* 63, 2056–2061.

Molloy, C. A., and Manning-Courtney, P. (2003). Prevalence of chronic gastrointestinal symptoms in children with autism and autistic spectrum disorders. *Autism* 7, 165–171.

Mosimann, J. E. (1970). Size allometry: size and shape variables with characterizations of the lognormal and generalized gamma distributions. *J. Am. Stat. Assoc.* 65, 930–945.

Mostofsky, S. H., Dubey, P., Jerath, V. K., Jansiewicz, E. M., Goldberg, M. C., and Denckla, M. B. (2006). Developmental dyspraxia is not limited to imitation in children with autism spectrum disorders. *J. Int. Neuropsychol. Soc.* 12, 314–326.

Mostofsky, S. H., Powell, S. K., Simmonds, D. J., Goldberg, M. C., Caffo, B., and Pekar, J. J. (2009). Decreased connectivity and cerebellar activity in autism during motor task performance. *Brain* 132, 2413–2425.

Nader, R., Oberlander, T. F., Chambers, C. T., and Craig, K. D. (2004). Expression of pain in children with autism. *Clin. J. Pain* 20, 88–97.

Nordahl, C. W., Scholz, R., Yang, X., Buonocore, M. H., Simon, T.,

Rogers, S., et al. (2012). Increased rate of amygdala growth in children aged 2 to 4 years with autism spectrum disorders: a longitudinal study. *Arch. Gen. Psychiatry* 69, 53–61.

Noterdaeme, M., Mildenberger, K., Minow, F., and Amorosa, H. (2002). Evaluation of neuromotor deficits in children with autism and children with a specific speech and language disorder. *Eur. Child Adolesc. Psychiatry* 11, 219–225.

O'Rahilly, R., and Müller, F. (1983). *Basic Human Anatomy: a Regional Study of Human Structure.* Philadelphia, PA: Saunders.

Phelan, K., and Rogers, C. (1993). "Phelan-McDermid Syndrome," in SourceGeneReviews™ [Internet]. eds R. A. Pagon, T. D. Bird, C. R. Dolan, K. Stephens, and M. P. Adam (Seattle, WA: University of Washington).

Qiu, A., Adler, M., Crocetti, D., Miller, M. I., and Mostofsky, S. H. (2010). Basal ganglia shapes predict social, communication, and motor dysfunctions in boys with autism spectrum disorder. *J. Am. Acad. Child Adolesc. Psychiatry* 49, 539–551, 551.e1–551.e4.

Reed, P. (2007). "The return of the reflex: considerations of the contribution of the early behaviorism to understanding, diagnosing, and preventing autism," in *New Autism Research Developments*, ed B. S. Mesmere (Hauppauge, NY: Nova Science Publishers), 19–24.

Rinehart, N. J., Bradshaw, J. L., Brereton, A. V., and Tonge, B. J. (2001). Movement preparation in high-functioning autism and Asperger disorder: a serial choice reaction time task involving motor reprogramming. *J. Autism Dev. Disord.* 31, 79–88.

Rinehart, N. J., Bradshaw, J. L., Tonge, B. J., Brereton, A. V., and Bellgrove, M. A. (2002). A neurobehavioral examination of individuals with high-functioning autism and Asperger's disorder using a fronto-striatal model of dysfunction. *Behav. Cogn. Neurosci. Rev.* 1, 164–177.

Robledo, J., Donnellan, A. M., and Strandt-Conroy, K. (2012). An exploration of sensory and movement differences from the perspective of individuals with autism. *Front. Integr. Neurosci.* 6:107. doi: 10.3389/fnint.2012.00107

Rogers, S. J., Bennetto, L., Mcvoy, R., and Pennington, B. F. (1996). Imitation and pantomime in high-functioning adolescents with autism spectrum disorders. *Child Dev.* 67, 2060–2073.

Roid, G. H. (2003). *Stanford-Binet Intelligence Scales.* Itasca, IL: Riverside Pub.

Rovee-Collier, C. K., Hayne, H., and Colombo, M. (2001). *The Development of Implicit and Explicit Memory.* Amsterdam; Philadelphia: John Benjamins Pub. Co.

Samson, F., Mottron, L., Soulieres, I., and Zeffiro, T. A. (2012). Enhanced visual functioning in autism: an ALE meta-analysis. *Hum. Brain Mapp.* 33, 1553–1581.

Savarese, R. J. (2013). Moving the field: the sensorimotor perspective on autism (Commentary on "Rethinking autism: implications of sensory and motor differences," an article by Anne Donnellan, David Hill, and Martha Leary). *Front. Integr. Neurosci.* 7:6. doi: 10.3389/fnint.2013.00006

Schumann, C. M., Hamstra, J., Goodlin-Jones, B. L., Lotspeich, L. J., Kwon, H., Buonocore, M. H., et al. (2004). The amygdala is enlarged in children but not adolescents with autism; the hippocampus is enlarged at all ages. *J. Neurosci.* 24, 6392–6401.

Silverman, J. L., Yang, M., Lord, C., and Crawley, J. N. (2010). Behavioural phenotyping assays for mouse models of autism. *Nat. Rev. Neurosci.* 11, 490–502.

Takarae, Y., Minshew, N. J., Luna, B., and Sweeney, J. A. (2007). Atypical involvement of frontostriatal systems during sensorimotor control in autism. *Psychiatry Res.* 156, 117–127.

Teitelbaum, O., Benton, T., Shah, P. K., Prince, A., Kelly, J. L., and Teitelbaum, P. (2004). Eshkol-Wachman movement notation in diagnosis: the early detection of Asperger's syndrome. *Proc. Natl. Acad. Sci. U.S.A.* 101, 11909–11914.

Teitelbaum, P., Teitelbaum, O., Nye, J., Fryman, J., and Maurer, R. G. (1998). Movement analysis in infancy may be useful for early diagnosis of autism. *Proc. Natl. Acad. Sci. U.S.A.* 95, 13982–13987.

Teitelbaum, P., Teitelbaum, O. B., Fryman, J., and Maurer, R. (2002). Infantile reflexes gone astray in autism. *J. Dev. Learn. Disord.* 6, 15.

Thelen, E., Corbetta, D., Kamm, K., Spencer, J. P., Schneider, K., and Zernicke, R. F. (1993). The transition to reaching: mapping intention and intrinsic dynamics. *Child Dev.* 64, 1058–1098.

Thelen, E., Corbetta, D., and Spencer, J. P. (1996). Development of reaching during the first year: role of movement speed. *J. Exp. Psychol. Hum. Percept. Perform.* 22, 1059–1076.

Thelen, E., and Smith, L. B. (1994). *A Dynamic Systems Approach to the Development of Cognition and Action.* Cambridge, MA: MIT Press.

Todorov, E. (2005). Stochastic optimal control and estimation methods adapted to the noise characteristics of the sensorimotor system. *Neural Comput.* 17, 1084–1108.

Tordjman, S., Anderson, G. M., Botbol, M., Brailly-Tabard, S., Perez-Diaz, F., Graignic, R., et al. (2009). Pain reactivity and plasma beta-endorphin in children and adolescents with autistic disorder. *PLoS ONE* 4:e5289. doi: 10.1371/journal.pone.0005289

Torres, E. B. (2011). Two classes of movements in motor control. *Exp. Brain Res.* 215, 269–283.

Torres, E. B. (2012). Atypical signatures of motor variability found in an individual with ASD. *Neurocase* 1, 1–16.

Torres, E. B. (2013a). The rates of change of the stochastic trajectories of acceleration variability are a good predictor of normal aging and of the stage of Parkinson's disease. *Front. Integr. Neurosci.* 9:10 doi: 10.1186/1744-9081-9-10

Torres, E. B. (2013b). Signatures of movement variability anticipate hand speed according to levels of intent. *Behav. Brain Funct.* 9, 10.

Torres, E. B., and Jose, J. V., (2012). *Novel Diagnostic Tool to Quantify Signatures of Movement in Subjects with Neurobiological Disorders, Autism and Autism Spectrum Disorders.* New Brunswick, NJ: US patent application.

van der Meer, A. L., van der Weel, F. R., and Lee, D. N. (1995). The functional significance of arm movements in neonates. *Science* 267, 693–695.

van Wermeskerken, M., van der Kamp, J., Te Velde, A. F., Valero-Garcia, A. V., Hoozemans, M. J., and Savelsbergh, G. J. (2011). Anticipatory reaching of seven- to eleven-month-old infants in occlusion situations. *Infant Behav. Dev.* 34, 45–54.

Volkmar, F. R., Szatmari, P., and Sparrow, S. S. (1993). Sex differences in pervasive developmental disorders. *J. Autism Dev. Disord.* 23, 579–591.

Von Hofsten, C. (1982). Eye-hand coordination in the newborn. *Dev. Psychol.* 18, 450–461.

Von Hofsten, C. (2004). An action perspective on motor development. *Trends Cogn. Sci.* 8, 266–272.

Von Hofsten, C. (2009). Action, the foundation for cognitive development. *Scand. J. Psychol.* 50, 617–623.

Williams, J. H., Whiten, A., Suddendorf, T., and Perrett, D. I. (2001). Imitation, mirror neurons and autism. *Neurosci. Biobehav. Rev.* 25, 287–295.

Wolpert, D. M. (2007). Probabilistic models in human sensorimotor control. *Hum. Mov. Sci.* 26, 511–524.

Wolpert, D. M., Miall, R. C., and Kawato, M. (1998). Internal models in the cerebellum. *Trends Cogn. Sci.* 2, 338–347.

Zeidan-Chulia, F., Gursoy, U. K., Kononen, E., and Gottfried, C. (2011). A dental look at the autistic patient through orofacial pain. *Acta Odontol. Scand.* 69, 193–200.

Conflict of Interest Statement: The authors declare that the research was conducted in the absence of any commercial or financial relationships that could be construed as a potential conflict of interest.

2

Motor development and motor resonance difficulties in autism: relevance to early intervention for language and communication skills

Joseph P. McCleery*, Natasha A. Elliott, Dimitrios S. Sampanis and Chrysi A. Stefanidou

School of Psychology, University of Birmingham, West Midlands, Birmingham, UK

Edited by:
Elizabeth B. Torres, Rutgers University, USA

Reviewed by:
Djoher N. Abrous, Institut des Neurosciences de Bordeaux, France
James B. Ackman, Yale University, USA
Jafri M. Abdullah, Universiti Sains Malaysia, Malaysia
Rochelle Ackerley, University of Gothenburg, Sweden
Elger Abrahamse, University of Ghent, Belgium
Judy Flax, Rutgers University, USA

****Correspondence:***
Joseph P. McCleery, School of Psychology, University of Birmingham, Frankland Building, Edgbaston, Birmingham, West Midlands B15 2TT, UK.
e-mail: joe.mccleery@gmail.com

Research suggests that a sub-set of children with autism experience notable difficulties and delays in motor skills development, and that a large percentage of children with autism experience deficits in motor resonance. These motor-related deficiencies, which evidence suggests are present from a very early age, are likely to negatively affect social-communicative and language development in this population. Here, we review evidence for delayed, impaired, and atypical motor development in infants and children with autism. We then carefully review and examine the current language and communication-based intervention research that is relevant to motor and motor resonance (i.e., neural "mirroring" mechanisms activated when we observe the actions of others) deficits in children with autism. Finally, we describe research needs and future directions and developments for early interventions aimed at addressing the speech/language and social-communication development difficulties in autism from a motor-related perspective.

Keywords: autism, motor, early intervention, communication, language

INTRODUCTION

Autism is a pervasive developmental disorder that is diagnosed based upon behavioral criteria for impairments in social skills, communication and language skills, and restricted interests and repetitive behaviors. Autism is currently considered to be a "spectrum" disorder, with three Pervasive Developmental Disorders now being termed Autism Spectrum Disorders (ASDs): Autistic Disorder, Aspergers Disorder, and Pervasive Developmental Disorder-Not Otherwise Specified (PDD-NOS). Individuals with these three different ASDs differ somewhat in regards to the nature and/or severity of their early language and intellectual difficulties. However, individuals with these three ASDs are similar in that they share impairments in social and communication skills, and that the onset of their difficulties begins by three years of age (American Psychiatric Association, 2000).

The only motor abnormalities currently included in the diagnostic criteria for ASDs are stereotypical repetitive behaviors (American Psychiatric Association, 2000; see also Lord and Jones, 2012). These repetitive behaviors include motor stereotypies, such as hand and finger mannerisms, body rocking, and arm flapping (Lord et al., 1994; Loftin et al., 2008). However, impairments in motor development commonly observed in children and adults with ASDs are not limited to motor stereotypies (Kopp et al., 2010; Linkenauger et al., 2012). Early motor delays, gait abnormalities, and difficulties with gross and fine motor coordination, postural control, and imitation have been found to constitute significant neurological co-morbid conditions in this population (Provost et al., 2007; Bhat et al., 2011; Maski et al., 2011). For example, Nobile et al. (2011) examined motor dysfunction in ASDs and found that children diagnosed with Autistic Disorder presented with stiffer gait, difficulties maintaining a straight line while walking, and postural abnormalities. Similarly, other studies have reported an "ataxic" gait in adults with autism (Hallett et al., 1993), and reduced postural stability, especially when somatosensory input was disrupted (Minshew et al., 2004). Deficits in postural stability and motor coordination in individuals with ASDs were confirmed through a recent meta-analysis conducted by Fournier and colleagues (Fournier et al., 2010). Children and adults with autism have also been found to exhibit praxis and imitation difficulties, including manual, postural, and orofacial imitation (Rogers et al., 1996, 2003; Stone et al., 1997; Stone and Yoder, 2001; Williams et al., 2004; Mostofsky et al., 2006; Dziuk et al., 2007; Vanvuchelen et al., 2007, 2010; Stieglitz Ham et al., 2008; Dowell et al., 2009). Critically, evidence suggests that deficits in motor skills, coordination, and balance are not limited to individuals with ASD experiencing cognitive delays (Jansiewicz et al., 2006). A variety of mechanisms have been proposed to account for the motor functioning differences observed in individuals with ASDs, including abnormalities in the cerebellum (Fatemi et al., 2012), impairments in frontal-striatal connections (Fournier et al., 2010), difficulties in self-other mapping (Williams et al., 2001), impaired sensory input (Gowen and Hamilton, 2013), and impaired multisensory integration (Gowen and Hamilton, 2013).

The aim of the current review is to outline the evidence for ASD-related motor development and motor resonance difficulties, and to examine current research on interventions that attempt to apply motor-related approaches to improve speech/language and social communication skills in children with autism. Similar to recent reviews by others (e.g., Iverson, 2010; Bhat et al., 2011), we first describe the existing evidence for early delayed, impaired, and atypical motor development in autism. In this review, we place particular emphasis on research related to several motor development mechanisms and milestones believed to be associated with concurrent and later speech/language and social communicative functioning. Next, we address current evidence for impairments in motor resonance (i.e., "mirror neuron") functioning in individuals with autism, which has implications for social engagement during communication interactions. After this, we carefully examine and evaluate the existing motor-related autism intervention research that targets speech/language and social-communication skills. This includes augmentative and alternative communication (AAC) interventions, more directly motor-based behavioral interventions, electromagnetic brain stimulation interventions, and interventions that utilize synchronous motor activities to increase speech/language and social communication skills. The current review differs distinctly from previous reviews, which have focused primarily on interventions for sensorimotor skills themselves (e.g., Baranek et al., 2008; Bhat et al., 2011), as opposed to motor-related attempts to specifically target speech/language and communication skills. We conclude our review by describing research needs and future directions for research on early interventions for speech/language and social-communication skills from a motor-related perspective.

EARLY MOTOR DEVELOPMENT IN AUTISM

Evidence suggests that autism is caused by a complex combination of multiple genetic and environmental factors. Twin studies examining the concordance of autism in monozygotic versus dizygotic twins provide evidence that genetics play a key role (Folstein and Rutter, 1977; Ritvo et al., 1989; see also Hallmayer et al., 2011). In addition to strong genetic influence on the development of autism itself, milder versions of the social, communication, and other difficulties experienced by individuals with ASD have also been documented in unaffected first-degree relatives (i.e., siblings, parents) of those with ASDs (Landa et al., 1991; Bolton et al., 1994; Hughes et al., 1997; Piven and Palmer, 1997; Piven et al., 1997; Folstein et al., 1999; Murphy et al., 2000; Pickles et al., 2000; Bishop et al., 2004; Adolphs et al., 2008; Smith et al., 2009). These results provide evidence that the complex genetic mechanisms that contribute to the development of autism also impact upon other members of families affected by autism. This, then, creates an opportunity to explore the effects of familial/genetic risk factors on various brain and behavioral mechanisms early in life in ASD, through the study of infant siblings of children already diagnosed with ASDs (Rogers, 2009; Yirmiya and Charman, 2010).

Extensive research has been conducted on motor behaviors and motor-related skills in infants who are at high risk for developing autism, with solid implications for our understanding of motor development associated with autism (Iverson and Wozniak, 2007; Rogers, 2009). In a comprehensive review of the autism high-risk infant literature, Rogers (2009) concludes that delays in motor development have been a consistent finding in this population. Of particular note is her conclusion that some important, albeit subtle, repetitive movements, and unusual sensory behaviors appear to emerge earlier in development than impairments in social and communication skills in this population (Rogers, 2009). In this section of the review, we focus on the key findings of the autism early motor development literature, with an emphasis on those motor and motor-related behaviors that are believed to be most relevant to successful communication and language development.

One of the earliest developing motor-related behaviors having associations with language development is the vocal-motor and facial-motor coordination that emerges during face-to-face interactions in the first half of the first year of life (Iverson and Fagan, 2004). During this time, infants begin to engage in coordinated vocal and facial motor activity routines (such as reciprocal vocalizations, imitation of mouth opening, positive/negative facial expressions, and gaze) on a second-by-second timing scale, with both familiar and unfamiliar communicative partners. This motor synchrony reflects interpersonal coordination of listening to and producing vocal-motor activity, which can be considered developmental precursors to the timing pragmatics of interpersonal interaction during conversation (Colonnesi et al., 2012). Existing evidence suggests that the nature and degree of this early infant coordination and tuning of motor activity with others predicts later infant social-emotional and cognitive development in typically developing infants (Feldman et al., 1996).

Yirmiya et al. (2006) measured communicative synchrony in 4-month-old infant siblings of children diagnosed with autism and low-risk infants without a family history of autism during mother-infant interactions. They uncovered evidence for weaker synchrony for infant-led interactions in the high-risk group (see also Brisson et al., 2011). Furthermore, the authors reported that these infants at risk for autism displayed fewer non-verbal requesting behaviors (such as pointing), and performed worse than low-risk infants on the language scales of the Bayley Scales of Infant Development, in follow-up at 14 months of age (Yirmiya et al., 2006). These findings support the hypothesis that risk for autism is associated with impaired vocal-motor coordination synchrony at 4-months of age, and that this has relevance to the later development of linguistic and pre-linguistic behaviors.

Another major stage of links between motor activity and language development occurs during the second half of the first year of life (Bates et al., 1999; Bates and Dick, 2002). Studies have shown that sharp increases in coordinated and repetitive arm movement and hand banging co-occur with the onset of reduplicative babble (i.e., canonical babble; e.g., "baba") between 6- and 11-months of age in typically developing infants, likely reflecting entrainment of the vocal and manual motor systems (Locke et al., 1995; Iverson et al., 2007; see also Petitto and Marentette, 1991; Petitto et al., 2004). This relationship is robust across typical infants of widely varying age of reduplicative babble/hand banging onset (Eilers et al., 1993; Iverson et al., 2007), as well as children with delayed language, including those with

Down Syndrome and those with Williams Syndrome (Cobo-Lewis et al., 1996; Masataka, 2001). Finally, delayed onset of reduplicative babble has been found to be a marker for delays in speech and language in the general population of infants (Oller et al., 1998).

In 2007, Iverson and Wozniak examined the rate of rhythmic arm movements during pre-babble and babble onset sessions in high-risk and low-risk infants. Rates of rhythmic arm movements increased from the pre-babble sessions to the babble-onset sessions in both high-risk and low-risk infants; however, this increase was lower in the high-risk group (Iverson and Wozniak, 2007). In addition, the high-risk infants exhibited delays in reduplicative babble onset and first word use between 5 and 14 months of age, as well as delays in language development at 18 months of age (Iverson and Wozniak, 2007). A related study by Gernsbacher et al. (2008) found that scores on oral-motor (e.g., blowing bubbles) and manual-motor skills (e.g., pointing to request) during home videos distinguished infants who later developed autism from those who were typically developing, as well as infants who were later minimally and highly fluent. Together, these findings suggest that oral-motor and manual-motor skills may contribute to both social-communication and speech/language skills deficits in this population.

Another major stage of links between motor, speech, and language development occurs from approximately 10- to 20-months of age. There is evidence to suggest that typically developing infants learn to understand word-object relationships through repeated episodes of shared joint visual attention to an object (e.g., following a point to look at the ball together) paired with adults verbally labeling the objects (e.g., "ball") during this period (Baldwin, 1995). This represents a complexity of emerging skills in following and comprehending the motor actions of others in relation to increasingly specific distal targets, and in increasingly dynamic activities and contexts (e.g., Tomasello and Farrar, 1986; Baldwin et al., 1996; Flom et al., 2004).

There is extensive evidence that both young children diagnosed with autism and young toddlers at risk for autism exhibit pervasive impairments in joint attention behaviors. In 2005, Goldberg and colleagues identified deficits in social-communicative behaviors, including responding to joint attention bids, in both 17-month-old high-risk infants and 2-year-old children already diagnosed with autism, compared with typically developing infants and children (Goldberg et al., 2005). In another study, involving 20-month olds diagnosed with autism, Charman (2003) found that declarative, triadic gaze switching was correlated with both language ability and autism symptom severity outcomes at 42 months of age (see also Yoder et al., 2009). Together, these results provide evidence to support the hypothesis that early deficits in the understanding of the gestures and actions of others are present from early in life in this population, and that these deficits are predictive of later social-communication and language deficits in children with autism (see also Rogers, 2009). Given the evidence from typical development, it will also be important to examine potential relationships between early exploratory and locomotor activity and later joint attention and language skills in infants at high risk for autism (see e.g., Campos et al., 2002).

Alongside the development of these social coordination and social-communication aspects of action perception and understanding, there is extensive evidence for more direct, *in vivo* links between gesture and language development in infants and children. Specifically, once infants have mastered the basic understanding of the gestures and actions of other people, they begin to regularly produce and employ increasingly complex communicative and symbolic gestures of their own, furthering their own communications and their language development (Bates and Dick, 2002). For example, the onset of recognitory gesture production, such as putting a cup to one's mouth and pretending to drink, correlates with the onset of vocal naming, both within and across infants between 11- and 16-months of age (Volterra et al., 1979; Shore et al., 1990). Between 18- and 20-months of age, gestures with one meaning are used in combination with words with other meanings, in order for the child to begin to be able to produce longer communications (e.g., point to chair and say "mom" to request that mom sits down; see Bates and Dick, 2002, for discussion). Impairments in the production of recognitory gestures as well as the coordination of speech and gesture during communication are core diagnostic measures of early childhood autism, which are included in the Autism Diagnostic Observation Schedule and the Autism Diagnostic Interview (Lord et al., 1994, 2000).

In this section, we have reviewed evidence that suggests that infants and young children with autism exhibit deficits and/or delays in a number of motor-related milestones that are believed to reflect critical stages in speech/language and communication development. Indeed, several of these deficits and delays have been found to be concurrently and/or predictively associated with important speech/language and social communication abilities in these infants and children. These motor and motor coordination milestones are likely to be supported by the core motor system and its mediators, including the primary motor cortex, cerebellum, motor-related frontal-striatal connections, visual regions involved in action perception, and a distributed system for sensorimotor integration (see **Figure 1** and **Table 1** for more information). These findings have clear implications for how motor-related interventions might be used to facilitate and support speech/language and communication development in this population, which is the focus of this review. Before we address this, however, we discuss the evidence for deficits in the motor resonance (i.e., "mirror neuron") system in individuals with autism. This system, which is involved in "mirroring" the actions of others within our own motor planning (i.e., premotor cortex) system, has been proposed to impact upon language development directly (Oberman et al., 2005), or to index social engagement with relevance for speech/language and social communication development in ASD.

MOTOR RESONANCE DEFICITS IN INDIVIDUALS WITH AUTISM

Extensive research, particularly over the past 15 years, has provided convincing evidence that our motor system "resonates" the actions of others that we view, hear, or view and hear (di Pellegrino et al., 1992; Rizzolatti et al., 1996; Iacoboni et al., 1999; Kohler et al., 2002; Gazzola et al., 2006). That

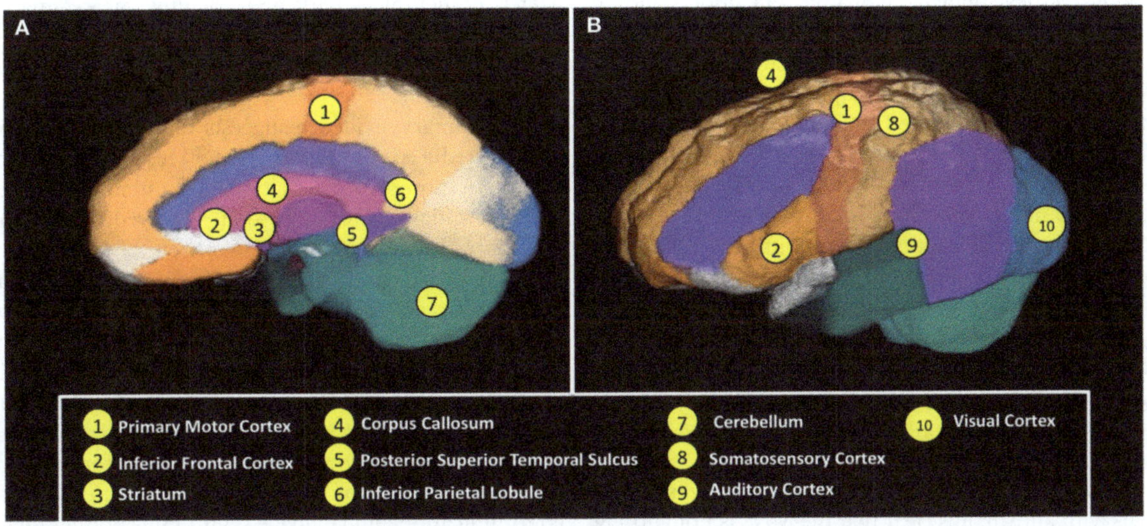

FIGURE 1 | Neural regions and mechanisms involved in (A) motor functioning and action perception, and (B) neural coordination and connectivity for sensorimotor and speech/language functioning. See **Table 1** for brief descriptions of these regions and associated mechanisms. Images of an average of 6-year-old child brain generated via the Magnetic Resonance Image database of Sanchez et al. (2012).

Table 1 | Brain regions and mechanisms associated with motor aspects of language development.

Number (see Figure 1)	Brain region or mechanism	Description
1	Primary motor cortex	Primary cortical generator of motor activity, both simple and complex.
2	Inferior frontal cortex	Motor planning region, and key region of the frontal mirror neuron system; also includes Broca's area. Includes representations of hand and mouth actions, and has been implicated in links between hand and mouth actions that facilitate speech/language production and development.
3	Striatum	Portion of the subcortical basal ganglia system, involved in the modulation of movement; affected by inputs from motivational systems.
4	Corpus callosum	Bundle of neural fibers that connect the left and right hemispheres of the brain, facilitating inter-hemispheric communication and coordination.
5	Posterior superior temporal sulcus	Cortical region involved in biological motion perception. Key region of the posterior mirror neuron system, which has been specifically implicated in perceptual aspects of action encoding and understanding.
6	Inferior parietal lobule	Cortical region involved in the association and integration of sensory information. Key portion of the posterior mirror neuron system, which has been specifically implicated in goal-related aspects of action understanding.
7	Cerebellum	Neural region involved in the coordination, precision, and timing of movement, motor learning, and motor integration.
4, 8, 9, 10	Neural integration and connectivity	Both motor and language functioning require coordination and integration across multiple sensory modalities and hemispheres. For example, motor planning and motor coordination require integration of information from visual and motor cortices. Similarly, speech perception requires visual-motor/auditory integration (e.g., mouth movement, speech sounds), and meaningful/iconic language involves the integration of multiple real-world experiences with objects that are encoded within and across the visual, somatosensory, motor, and auditory cortices.

is, our motor planning and related action production systems in pre-motor and other regions of the cortex appear to "mirror" the actions of observed others onto our own action/motor planning system (e.g., Inferior Frontal Gyrus, Inferior Parietal Lobule, Superior Temporal Sulcus; see **Figure 1** and **Table 1**), presumably allowing us to better represent and understand the nature and details of the actions and activities of others (Rizzolatti and Craighero, 2004). This "mirror neuron" system (MNS) has been proposed to underlie a number of critical social-interactive and social-communicative skills, including imitation, language development, empathy, and understanding the social perspectives and intentions of others (Iacoboni and Dapretto, 2006). Following an initial suggestion that impairments in mirror neuron functioning may play an important role in the behavioral deficits observed in individuals with autism in 2001 (Williams et al., 2001), behavioral and neuroimaging research has sought to test this hypothesis. Although the findings are somewhat mixed, and there is particular debate about behavioral data on MNS functioning and its proposed relationship to imitation functioning in the literature (Southgate and Hamilton, 2008; see also Hamilton, 2009), the hypothesis of impaired motor resonance in individuals with ASD has generally been supported in the experimental behavioral and brain imaging literatures (Oberman and Ramachandran, 2007; Becchio and Castiello, 2012; Enticott et al., 2012; Oberman et al., 2012).

Despite extensive evidence for reduced visuomotor resonance in individuals with autism, it is clear that the MNS is not entirely "broken" in this population. For example, individuals with ASD have been found to exhibit normal motor interference during simultaneous execution-observation of meaningless arm movements (e.g., Gowen et al., 2008; see Becchio and Castiello, 2012, for review). Most relevant to the current review, Oberman et al. (2008) used electroencephalography (EEG) mu suppression to uncover evidence for normal MNS activation during the observation of the actions of familiar people, but reduced MNS activation during the observation of the actions of unfamiliar people, in children with autism. These data provide direct evidence that the MNS of children with autism is, in fact, capable of responding normally to the actions of others. Along these same lines, a study by Pierce and Redcay (2008) used functional Magnetic Resonance Imaging (fMRI) to uncover evidence that the Fusiform Face Area (FFA) is also activated normally in response to familiar faces, but not in response to unfamiliar faces, in children with autism.

Like the MNS, evidence had generally supported the hypothesis of impaired FFA functioning in individuals with autism prior to this. Together, these findings on familiarity effects in social processing (i.e., MNS, FFA) are consistent with the hypothesis that lack of social and/or emotional familiarity with, or interest in, unfamiliar others may be driving reduced activation of social brain networks, including the MNS, in children with autism. One distinct possibility is that children with autism exhibit reduced social interest and/or social-cognitive attention for strangers, relative to other children. This hypothesis receives support from event-related potentials (ERPs) EEG evidence that very young children with autism exhibit reduced late frontal cortex activity in response to unfamiliar faces (Dawson et al., 2002). More specifically, Dawson et al. (2002) found that both typically developing children and children with developmental delays without autism showed larger amplitude ERPs in response to unfamiliar relative to familiar faces, suggesting increased neural activity for the processing of unfamiliar people. However, children with autism did not exhibit this "interest in strangers" effect. In the same study, all three groups of children did exhibit differential brain responses to familiar versus unfamiliar toys, suggesting that this difference in children with autism reflected a lack of neural activity and cognitive processing specifically for unfamiliar people (see also Oberman et al., 2008; Pierce and Redcay, 2008; Becchio and Castiello, 2012; Dawson et al., 2012).

In summary, evidence suggests that individuals with autism exhibit reduced or absent motor resonance activity during the observation of the actions of unfamiliar others. While it was initially suggested that this reduced/absent activity reflects a "broken" MNS (Williams et al., 2001; Oberman and Ramachandran, 2007), more recent results and analysis suggests that reduced/absent mirror neuron activity may reflect reduced social engagement in this population (Oberman et al., 2008; Becchio and Castiello, 2012). Taking the latter view, in the current review, we consider early behavioral interventions that teach speech/language and social communication skills in the specific context of socially engaging synchronous motor activities as a potential motor-related pathway to increasing social-communication and language skills in this population.

INTERVENTIONS

Delays and impairments in motor and motor-related development in infants and children with autism have implications for early intervention in this population. Whereas previous reviews have focused on interventions aimed at improving sensory and motor functioning (Baranek et al., 2008) and other ASD-related behaviors (Sowa and Meulenbroek, 2012), here we review and discuss existing and emerging motor interventions that are more directly relevant for increasing social-communication and language skills in toddlers and children with autism. We focus particular attention on their theoretical and practical relationships to motor theories of social-communication and language development, as well as to their existing evidence base. In examining the evidence base, we consider several types, or levels, of evidence (see **Table 2**). These include case study reports, which can involve descriptions of multiple children but without experimental controls. Next, we consider experimental single subject designs, which exert experimental control through the use of baseline recordings of varying lengths across multiple children, thus more reliably attributing intervention effects to intervention onset. Along with these, we include small-scale pseudo-experimental research designs, whereby children are assessed pre- and post-intervention, but without a comparison control group to account for potential naturally occurring developmental improvements in the target behaviors. Finally, we consider large-scale experimental group studies, Randomized Controlled Trials (RCTs; efficacy trials), and RCTs conducted in community settings (effectiveness trials). As ASDs are a unique class of developmental disorders, we focus our review specifically on the evidence-base for the efficacy and effectiveness of each intervention for children with ASDs. Finally, we focus exclusively on interventions for non-verbal and minimally verbal children, because there are existing evidence-based interventions that are effective for more verbally able children with autism (Koegel, 2000). We start with sign language intervention, which has previously been proposed to be a mechanism for linking motor-based gesture and speech and language development in these children.

Table 2 | Levels of evidence for each intervention.

Intervention	Brief description	Case reports	Experimental single-subject designs (multiple baseline designs, reversal designs) and small-scale pseudo-experimental group designs	Large experimental study	Randomized controlled trial	Community-based randomized controlled trial	Summary of evidence
AUGMENTATIVE AND ALTERNATIVE COMMUNICATION (AAC) INTERVENTIONS							
Sign language (SLT)	Teaches child to use hand, arm, facial, and other actions to create symbolic communications	5+ 1. Fulwiler and Fouts (1976) 2. Brady and Smouse (1978)	15+ 1. Carr et al. (1987) 2. Barrera and Sulzer-Azaroff (1983) 3. Sundberg et al. (2000)	1 1. Layton (1988) 2. Yoder and Layton (1988)	0	0	Extensive research base. Weak but mixed evidence for learning of sign language. Weak evidence for learning of speech. Weak evidence for learning of speech via sign plus speech training. See Schwartz and Nye (2006).
Picture exchange communication system (PECS)	Teaches child to exchange pictures with others, in order to make requests and comment	5+ Speech: 1. Webb (2000) 2. Bondy and Frost (1994) Communication: 3. Anderson et al. (2007) 4. Malandraki and Okalidou (2007)	5+ Speech: 1. Charlop-Christy et al. (2002) 2. Carr and Felce (2007a) Communication: 3. Travis and Geiger (2010) 4. Greenberg et al. (2012)	1 Communication: 1. Lerna et al. (2009)	3+ Speech: 1. Yoder and Stone (2006a) Communication: 2. Yoder and Lieberman (2010)	1 Speech: 1. Gordon et al. (2011) Communication: 2. Howlin et al. (2007)	Extensive research base. Moderate evidence for both picture-based and verbal communication gains. See Sulzer-Azaroff et al. (2009).
MOTOR-BASED BEHAVIORAL INTERVENTIONS							
Prompts for restructuring oral muscular phonetic targets (PROMPT)	Uses physical prompts to the vocal apparatus, as well as social, kinesthetic, and proprioceptive awareness, to increase speech and language.	0	1 1. Rogers et al. (2006)	0	0	0	Limited evidence in ASD.
Auditory motor mapping treatment	Teaches the pairing of sounds with motor actions during picture-based word teaching in order to facilitate vocalization	0	1 1. Wan et al. (2011)	0	0	0	Limited evidence in ASD.

(Continued)

Table 2 | Continued

Intervention	Brief description	Case reports	Experimental single-subject designs (multiple baseline designs, reversal designs) and small-scale pseudo-experimental group designs	Large experimental study	Randomized controlled trial	Community-based randomized controlled trial	Summary of evidence
ELECTROMAGNETIC BRAIN STIMULATION INTERVENTIONS							
Transcranial direct current stimulation (TdCS)/Transcranial magnetic stimulation (TMS)	Electromagnetic brain stimulation procedures.	0	1 1. Schneider and Hopp (2011)	0	0	0	Limited evidence in ASD.
INTERVENTIONS TARGETING SYNCHRONOUS MOTOR ACTIVITIES							
Early start denver model (ESDM)	Integrative model of play-based behaviorist/operant teaching methods within a comprehensive developmental framework.	5 1. Voos et al. (2012) 2. Vismara and Rogers (2008)	20+ (includes PRT evidence) 1. Vismara et al. (2009) 2. Vismara and Lyons (2007) 3. Pierce and Schreibman (1995) 4. Stahmer (1995)	1 1. Baker-Ericzén et al. (2007)	1+ 1. Dawson et al. (2010)	1 1. Rogers et al. (2012)	Extensive research base (includes PRT evidence). Moderate evidence for verbal and non-verbal communication gains. See Warren et al. (2011).
Reciprocal imitation training (RIT)	Uses reciprocal imitation and behaviorist principles to teach the child to imitate the motor actions and gestures of others in a play context.	0	3+ 1. Ingersoll and Schreibman (2006) 2. Cardon and Wilcox (2011)	1 1. Ingersoll (2010)	0	0	Moderate evidence for non-verbal communication and imitation gains.

AUGMENTATIVE AND ALTERNATIVE COMMUNICATION (AAC) INTERVENTIONS

Sign language training

For non-verbal autistic children, training in augmentative and alternative communication (AAC) offers a route via which these individuals can begin to communicate. The two most widely accepted AAC strategies are Sign Language Training (SLT; Carr et al., 1978) and the Picture Exchange Communication System (PECS; Bondy and Frost, 1994; Frost and Bondy, 2002; see **Figure 2**). Research suggests that educators believe that both of these strategies are viable options for teaching communication skills to children with autism displaying severe deficits in communication skills (Stahmer et al., 2005).

Given the strong links between gesture and verbal communication in typically developing infants, including those described in the sections above, the use of SLT to facilitate speech in developmentally delayed populations has a logical theoretical basis. Indeed, early studies investigating the impact of SLT on children with autism yielded promising results, in both the communicative and social domains (Miller and Miller, 1973; Bonvillian and Nelson, 1976; Fulwiler and Fouts, 1976; Brady and Smouse, 1978; Konstantareas, 1984). Contrary to expectations, however, these marked improvements in communication did not include speech development. Furthermore, the effectiveness of sign language alone as a means to facilitate speech in non-vocal autistic children was quickly called into doubt; as was the degree of experimental control employed by early research in this area (Carr et al., 1978; Carr, 1979; see **Table 2**).

Following the recognition that SLT did not lead to meaningful increases in speech in children with autism, studies utilizing training sessions that focused on coupling sign language with other forms of training (e.g., speech intervention plus SLT) were conducted. This combined intervention approach proved to be more effective than sign language alone for eliciting spoken vocabulary in nominally verbal autistic children (Brady and Smouse, 1978; Layton and Baker, 1981; Konstantareas, 1984; Yoder and Layton, 1988). However, when considering this research, it is important to note that the participants in these studies had existing verbal skills. Therefore, it has yet to be examined whether SLT in any form can elicit verbal communication gains in non-vocal autistic children. Moreover, outcomes following SLT are extremely and unusually variable. For example, although a small number of individuals with autism adopt sign language as their primary mode of communication and appear to readily learn signs (Barrera et al., 1980; Stull et al., 1980), others are unable to attain even the most basic signing skills (Webster et al., 1973; Brady and Smouse, 1978; Carr et al., 1978).

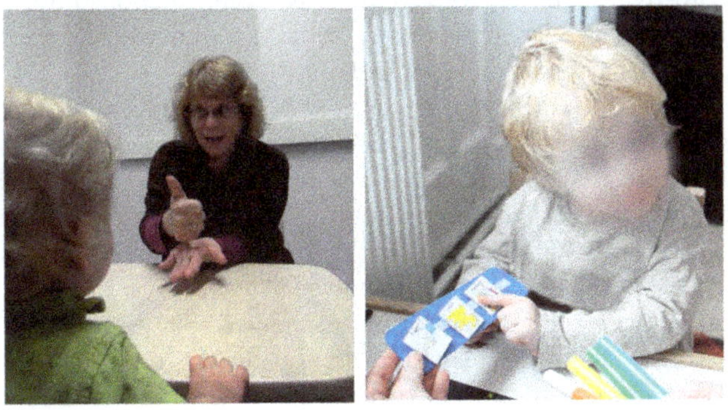

FIGURE 2 | Augmentative and Alternative Communication (AAC) interventions. Child and therapist engaged in Sign Language Training (left) vs. Picture Exchange Communication System (PECS) training (right). Sign Language Training (SLT) uses behaviorist imitation and prompting methods to teach children to use hand, arm, facial, and other body actions to produce symbolic communications. The Picture Exchange Communication System (PECS) uses behaviorist methods to teach children to hand one or more pictures to a variety of communicative partners, in order to request items/activities, respond to simple questions, and comment.

Despite decades of research into SLT as an effective tool for teaching those with ASD, the evidence that it leads to novel and/or increased functional uses of communication, speech, and language in this population is weak. Those who suggest that sign language, or total communication (sign plus speech), may serve to increase such skills in autistic individuals often base their arguments on single-subject research (Carr et al., 1978, 1987; Casey, 1978; Cohen, 1979; Schepis et al., 1982). Although rich in detail, the majority of these more promising SLT studies provide no measure of fidelity of implementation, few explored generalizability, and many fail to disclose sufficient detail for either clinical application or experimental replication (Millar et al., 2000; Schwartz and Nye, 2006). In their review of SLT in this population, Layton and Watson (1995) maintain that, despite extensive training, the majority of non-verbal children fail to develop any form of vocalization and, at most, learn a few basic signs, as a result of SLT. In a more recent review of sign language and communication gains in children with autism, Schwartz and Nye (2006) conclude that teaching communication through signing does not serve as an effective intervention to improve either sign or oral language communication in children on the autism spectrum (see also Millar et al., 2000).

While the poor results of SLT have often been overlooked in the literature, some attempt has been made to explain these findings. One proposed explanation for the relative failure of SLT is that the successful acquisition and use of sign language as a communicative tool is dependent on the ability to form a variety of manual-motor signs and there are many individuals with ASD who do not possess the fine motor skills required (Bonvillian and Blackburn, 1991; Seal and Bonvillian, 1997; National Research Council, 2001). Similarly, Mirenda and Erickson (2000) outline "the three I's" that contribute to successful sign language acquisition: *imitation*, *iconicity*, and *intelligibility*. They maintain that children with autism demonstrate a lack of imitation, symbolic representation, and motor coordination/planning skills, while the successful acquisition and use of sign language relies largely on the possession of these abilities (see **Table 1** and **Figure 1** for relevant neural mechanisms). In each of these proposed explanations, deficits and delays in motor and motor-related skills are key to explaining why children with autism generally fail to develop both sign language-based communication and speech and language skills as a result of SLT.

Picture exchange communication system (PECS)

Given the lack of meaningful progress as a result of SLT, it is unsurprising that the field has turned its attention to other AAC training practices. The PECS is a form of AAC that utilizes pictures as its primary medium of communication and, like SLT, has foundations in behaviorist principles. The primary goal of PECS is to establish and increase spontaneous communication within social contexts, which is initiated through picture-based communication (Bondy and Frost, 1998). PECS is a structured and manualized intervention program that is designed to teach children to communicate via a book containing detachable pictures (see **Figure 2**).

The PECS protocol is divided into six phases, each designed to expand upon the child's development during the previous phase. In Phase I, the child is taught to hand a single picture to another person, in exchange for a desired item or activity (e.g., a ball). In Phase II, the child is taught to exchange pictures with multiple people in multiple environments. Phase III teaches the child to discriminate and select among pictures for a number of desired items. Phase IV teaches the child to produce simple sentence structures (e.g., "I want ____.") using pictures, which are then handed to communicative partners using a sentence strip (see **Figure 2**). Finally, Phases V and VI teach responding to simple questions and commenting, using pictures. The child typically progresses from basic picture-based requesting, to more advanced picture-based responding and spontaneous commenting (Bondy and Frost, 1998). The surface appeal of PECS over sign language is understandable given that it does not rely on the communicator possessing complex fine motor skills, nor does it burden the communicator with learning a completely new language (Bondy and Frost, 1994). Furthermore, the gains facilitated by PECS do not appear dependent upon the child possessing preexisting skills (Bondy and Frost, 2002; Yoder and Stone, 2006a,b), and PECS appears to be readily learned by children with autism as well as other developmental disorders (Schwartz et al., 1998; Mirenda and Erickson, 2000; Charlop-Christy et al., 2002; Ganz and Simpson, 2004; Preston and Carter, 2009).

Although not initially developed to teach spoken language, a large and growing body of evidence demonstrates that PECS can assist with spoken language development in children with autism with existing, albeit limited, verbal skills (Bondy and Frost, 1994; Liddle, 2001; Charlop-Christy et al., 2002; Kravits et al., 2002; Magiati and Howlin, 2003; Anderson et al., 2007; Carr and Felce, 2007a; Carré et al., 2009; Jurgens et al., 2009; Preston and Carter, 2009; Sulzer-Azaroff et al., 2009; Greenberg et al., 2012). Early non-experimental, retrospective research by Bondy and Frost (1994) suggested that after one year of PECS usage, 76 percent of 66 young children developed speech either as their sole means of communication or alongside picture communication. Following a series of experimental single-subject design studies suggesting positive effects on both communication and speech as a result of PECS intervention, several large scale experimental studies have provided further strong and convincing evidence that PECS increases both social-communication and speech/language skills in children with autism. Indeed, increases in spoken and socio-communication skills through PECS training appear to be as prominent as in speech-based interventions (Yoder and Stone, 2006a,b; Lerna et al., 2012). For example, Yoder and Stone (2006a) compared the effects of PECS and Responsive Education and Prelinguistic Milieu Teaching (RPMT) in 36 toddlers and young children with autism. Both interventions were implemented for the same length of time, and at the same intensity. After six months of training, it was found that PECS training resulted in increased verbalizations, both in terms of frequency and range of words. Although children in both treatment groups were found to have made similar speech-related improvements by their six-month follow-up, the authors highlight that these results provide evidence that PECS leads to more swift speech development when compared to RPMT. Similarly, recent research by Lerna et al. (2012) compared the efficacy of PECS with Conventional Language Therapy (CLT) in a group of preschool children with ASD. Following six months of treatment, those receiving PECS demonstrated significant improvements in their joint attention, requesting, and imitation skills.

Although RCT's are severely lacking in the field of autism education research (Carter and Wheldall, 2008; Preston and Carter, 2009), the few large-scale examinations that have involved such advantageous designs have also replicated the promising data on PECS (**Table 2**). For example, a recent school-based RCT of PECS versus Treatment As Usual (TAU) by Howlin and colleagues highlighted gains in spontaneous requesting through picture use, speech, or both (Howlin et al., 2007). Gordon and colleagues (2011) examined these same data from 84 autistic children across 15 British schools, observing changes in spontaneous communication following immediate, delayed, or no PECS training. They found that children who had received immediate treatment demonstrated significant increases in both spontaneous speech/vocalizations, and in their usage of PECS. Furthermore, Carr and Felce (2007b) compared a PECS training group ($n = 24$) with a no treatment control group ($n = 17$), and uncovered evidence for significant increases in linguistic communicative initiations that included the use of spoken words within the PECS treatment group, and no improvements in such skills within the no-treatment control group. This, again, demonstrates the efficacy of PECS in eliciting both verbal and non-verbal communicative behaviors in children with autism.

It is worth noting that children with autism typically exhibit increases in speech during Phases IV and V of PECS training (Charlop-Christy et al., 2002; Ganz and Simpson, 2004). During these Phases, they are learning to use a larger number of pictures, and have also started to point rhythmically to sentences, often syllable by syllable (Frost and Bondy, 2002). Prior to Phase V, children are taught to (a) communicate with pictures (Phase I), (b) travel and seek their communication partner (Phase II), (c) discriminate individual pictures and what they each represent (Phase III), and (d) structure sentences through the use of a string of picture cards (Phases IV and V; Frost and Bondy, 2002). Phase IV is also the period during which a time delay procedure is used by the therapist, whereby she or he pauses after speaking the first portion of the picture-phrase (e.g., says "I want ...") and waits 3–5 s for the non-verbal or minimally verbal child to verbalize the label for the item they have requested (e.g., "ball") before providing the item to the child. In this instance, the child's rhythmic pointing to the pictures (e.g., I-want-BALL) continues as the therapist stops speaking, potentially facilitating the child's verbalization of the target item (e.g., "ball"). As mentioned, a plethora of research has demonstrated the link between the onset of speech, and the development of coordinated hand banging gestures. It is possible that the speech gains observed in many children during this phase of PECS are a reflection of this link, with implications for the potential importance and validation of hand-mouth motor plans, as described in relation to auditory motor mapping intervention below.

In sum, although there are strong links between motor-based symbolic gesture and speech development in typical infants and children, extensive research suggests that there is no robust link between SLT and increased speech in children diagnosed with autism. Although many children with autism do not readily learn the use of signs, a large body of evidence demonstrates the ease with which they acquire picture-based communication via PECS, suggesting that it is not an inability to learn that is attributable to their difficulties in sign language learning in this population. Furthermore, as outlined, research also suggests stronger links between speech development and PECS training vs. SLT, in children with autism. Some have proposed that difficulties in sign language learning are due to impairments in fine motor skills (Bonvillian and Blackburn, 1991; Seal and Bonvillian, 1997; National Research Council, 2001), whereas others have argued that it is a combination of *imitation skills*, *iconicity*, and *intelligibility* that present challenges to this population (Mirenda and Erickson, 2000). Next, we examine several more directly motor-based interventions that are currently under development to address social-communication and speech/language skills for this population.

MOTOR-BASED BEHAVIORAL INTERVENTIONS

While sign language is a gesture and motor-based intervention, there are other behavioral interventions that take an even more direct approach to addressing motor aspects of speech production. These include interventions that involve direct manipulations of the mouth and other sound-producing structures, and those that make more direct low-level links between hand and oral motor activity. Here, we describe research on the two interventions of this type that have been studied in relation to children with autism.

Prompts for restructuring oral muscular phonetic targets (PROMPT)

One intervention targeting the neuromotor underpinnings of speech production is the Prompts for Restructuring Oral Muscular Phonetic Targets (PROMPT; Chumpelik, 1984) model. PROMPT goes beyond auditory and visual input, integrating neuromotor principles with social, kinesthetic, and proprioceptive awareness to facilitate the production of clear sounds, speech, and language (Hayden, 2002). In addition to manipulating sound-producing structures, PROMPT places importance on body movement and stability. A typical PROMPT session involves play-based or naturally occurring activities that are likely to encourage interaction initiations from the child. Using these initiations or motivators as a therapeutic opportunity, the clinician then uses vocal modeling and physical manipulations of the child's speech mechanisms as they attempt verbalization. Such manipulations include touch, pressure, positioning, and movement to promote structural integration within the child's vocal apparatus (Hayden and Square, 1994; see **Figure 3**).

A PROMPT is available for every vowel or consonant in the English language, as well as for every single or combined speech-sound utterance. Specifically, therapists may use *parameter* prompts to provide support to the jaw and facial muscles; *surface* prompts to aid the formation of speech sounds and their associated timings and transitions; *syllable* prompts to teach the critical combination of jaw support and lip positioning required to produce legible syllables; and finally, *complex* prompts may be administered when teaching the formation of single sounds (Hayden, 2006) Due to these multiple types of prompts, the PROMPT model can be used to build upon the motor skills of children at all stages of speech production, from first-word attempts to the production of more intelligible speech. Throughout the course of intervention, manual prompts are gradually faded as the child demonstrates heightened oral awareness and control.

The PROMPT intervention method has been examined in a number of studies, although most report on individual case studies. For example, Square et al. (2000) examined six young children with language and phonological disabilities and, following PROMPT intervention, discovered increased accuracy of target word production, and generalization of abilities to untrained words. Gains were also noted in overall communication, social interaction, and intelligibility. Furthermore, Square et al. (1986) noted the efficacy of PROMPT training in three patients with acquired apraxia, whilst a recent study by Ward et al. (2009a,b) found gains in intelligibility, consonant accuracy, and generalized vocal improvements in children with cerebral

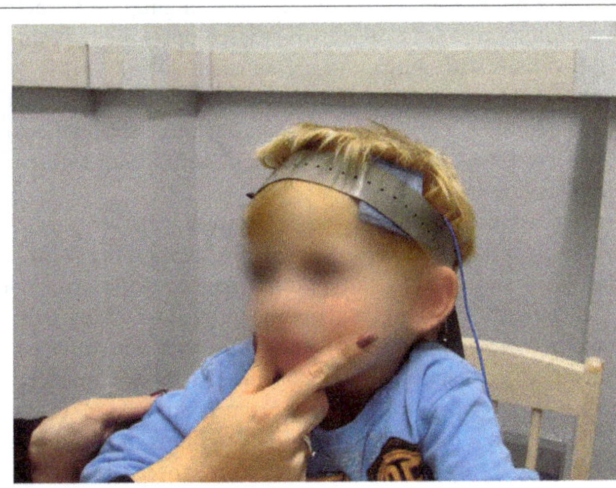

FIGURE 3 | Motor-based behavioral intervention and electromagnetic brain stimulation intervention. Child and therapist engaged in Prompts for Restructuring Oral Muscular Phonetic Targets (PROMPT) intervention. The child is also wearing a Transcranial Direct Current Stimulation (tDCS) electrode band. These two techniques are typically implemented separately. Here, the PROMPT therapist administers a physical prompt to the child's vocal-motor system, in order to facilitate production of a speech target, while the tDCS electrode applies a direct current to the left inferior frontal cortex.

palsy and speech impairments. In a case study of a severely apractic-aphasic male, PROMPT training for 41 weeks was associated with maintained articulation accuracy in a set of core functional words and phrases (Freed et al., 1997). Finally, although Dodd and Bradford (2000) found no effect of PROMPT intervention in three boys with phonological impairment without articulation disorders, Grigos et al. (2010) discovered increased articulation accuracy in a single subject with severe articulation impairment.

To date, only one published study has explored the effects of the PROMPT method in children with ASD. Rogers et al. (2006) randomly assigned 10 non-verbal children with autism to receive one of two interventions: the Denver Model (a play-based program based on reciprocal communication and social engagement; Rogers et al., 2000), or PROMPT. All participants received 12 weeks of treatment and were assessed for their use of novel words and phrases throughout the intervention, as well as for the maintenance of such functional communication at three weeks post-treatment. Assessments throughout and following intervention revealed that 80% of participants exhibited increases in spontaneous, functional words. In light of the small sample sizes, and in the absence of group comparisons, this study can only be considered a series of non-experimental case studies. Nevertheless, these preliminary findings do suggest potential promise for the use of the PROMPT model with autistic children, and future research should endeavor to examine a larger sample of autistic children in a RCT or other experimental assessment of the PROMPT intervention.

Auditory motor mapping training

Auditory-Motor Mapping Training (AMMT; Wan et al., 2009) is a recently developed multi-component intervention targeting the development of speech output through singing, motor activity, and imitation (Wan et al., 2010a). Based upon the hypothesis that individuals with autism have a deficient MNS, AMMT was designed to train sound-articulation associations by engaging multiple neural networks (Wan et al., 2010b). In essence, the goal of AMMT is to teach the pairing of sounds with motor actions in order to facilitate vocalizations.

During a typical AMMT session, a target word or phrase is introduced, and the therapist repeatedly intones the word or phrase while simultaneously tapping a pair of drums tuned to different pitches. The child is then encouraged or gently guided to imitate these actions, while being presented with images of the target object, action, or person. These three components are believed to work together to promote increased interactions between the auditory and motor systems, strengthening the likelihood of intelligible and functional speech production. For example, the use of intonation as opposed to simply speaking is designed to heighten bilateral fronto-temporal network activation—an area associated with components of the MNS (Brown et al., 2004; Ozdemir et al., 2006). Similarly, the engaging use of percussion has been implicated in the activation of a sensorimotor network responsible for articulatory and orofacial movements, as well as stimulating the mapping of sounds to actions through increased bilateral activation in the fronto-parietal motor-related network (Meister et al., 2003, 2009; Lahab et al., 2007). The third component, imitation, is designed to encourage learning, and is argued to alter the responses in the MNS (Catmur et al., 2007).

One small-scale study describing several cases has been reported on AMMT as an intervention for children with autism. Wan et al. (2011) examined 6 non-verbal children with autism who each received five AMMT sessions per week throughout an eight-week period. All children were assessed on their vocal production at baseline, during the therapy, and following completion of treatment. The authors report that word and phrase articulation improved notably in all of the children, with improvements including verbalizations of both trained and untrained words. Although promising, the results from this case study series must be interpreted with caution, particularly in regards to whether or not the intervention was driving the observed effects. To date, there has yet to be an experimental study examining the efficacy of AMMT for treating children with ASD. On the other hand, the results from these initial case studies serve as a promising starting point to initiate larger-scale and experimental studies of AMMT.

ELECTROMAGNETIC BRAIN STIMULATION INTERVENTIONS

Transcranial direct current stimulation and transcranial magnetic stimulation

Transcranial Direct Current Stimulation (tDCS) and Transcranial Magnetic Stimulation (TMS) are relatively new methods via which low intensity intracranial electrical current is applied to the cerebral cortex (see **Figure 3**). The current is the result of a fluctuating magnetic field that comes from external resources, and tDCS and TMS are considered non-invasive brain stimulation procedures (Pascual-Leone and Walsh, 2002; Gandiga et al., 2006). In tDCS, a relatively weaker direct current is applied constantly through electrodes attached to the scalp above a brain region of interest. This current alternates the neuronal excitability in either a positive or a negative manner, leading to changes in brain function (Nitsche et al., 2008). A combination of tDCS and other rehabilitative treatments has been studied in relation to motor training protocols (Hummel and Cohen, 2005). TMS has been successfully used to alleviate, or attempt to alleviate, neurological symptoms associated with stroke (Oliveri et al., 1999), epilepsy (Fregni et al., 2006), and a variety of psychiatric disorders (Lisanby et al., 2002). Most relevant to the current review, repetitive TMS (rTMS) has been shown to improve naming abilities in adults with chronic aphasia resulting from stroke (Martin et al., 2009; see also Mimura et al., 1998; Winhuisen et al., 2007).

In 2011, Schneider and Hopp applied tDCS to the left dorsolateral prefrontal cortex in a group of 10 minimally verbal children with autism, in order to examine the possibility of syntax acquisition as a result of tDCS (Schneider and Hopp, 2011). They found significant improvements in behavioral performance on a basic subject-verb-object sentence sub-test of the Bilingual Aphasia Test. Based on these promising group case study findings, the authors have proposed that additional research should be conducted in this area (see also Sokhadze et al., 2009). Furthermore, the results of a recent small-scale experimental study of adults with Asperger's Syndrome further suggest that the application of rTMS may, indeed, prove useful for improving language skills in those with ASD (Fecteau et al., 2011). It is important to note, however, that there are notable risks associated with both tDCS and TMS, some of which have particular practical, medical, and ethical implications for the application of these technologies to individuals with ASDs (see below for further information).

In sum, there are at least three relatively new strongly motor-related interventions for potentially treating speech and language skills in young non-verbal and minimally verbal children with ASD. Interestingly, each of these interventions has precisely one published paper on their usefulness in treating this population. Also of interest, is that the results of these studies all provide promising results. This being the case, however, none of these studies were experimental in nature and, instead, took the form of a small-scale pseudo-experimental design in each case. It is clear that experimental research is now warranted in order to examine the potential efficacy and effectiveness of these novel interventions. However, the application of one of these interventions, tDCS/TMS, presents some practical, medical, and ethical challenges in relation to children with autism (see Discussion and Future Directions, below, for further information).

INTERVENTIONS TARGETING SYNCHRONOUS MOTOR ACTIVITIES

Play-based intervention methods based upon the application of behavior analytic procedures are well-established and commonly used techniques for teaching children with autism difficulties to engage in new social, communication, play, language, and other behaviors. These interventions utilize operant teaching methods, including behaviorally-defined targets, contingent reinforcement (e.g., access to items and activities, descriptive praise), physical and verbal prompts, and shaping and fading procedures, to target skill development, while allowing the child a great deal of choice in play activities. Extensive and large-scale experimental research studies have shown that these interventions can increase generalized and spontaneous language and communication skills (Koegel and Koegel, 2006), improve social and play skills (Pierce and Schreibman, 1995; Stahmer, 1995), decrease inappropriate behavior (Koegel et al., 2005), and improve academic motivation and performance (Koegel et al., 2010).

More recently, researchers have worked to combine developmental and behavioral intervention approaches, whereby operant teaching methods are utilized to target skills within a strong developmental framework in a play-based context. Most relevant to the current review, two of these developmental-behavioral interventions specifically target social-reciprocity and social engagement in the context of synchronous motor activities, which may represent a potential motor-related pathway to increasing social-communication and language skills in this population.

Early start denver model (ESDM)

The Early Start Denver Model (ESDM) is an integration of a particular play-based behavior analytic approach, Pivotal Response Treatment (PRT), with developmental intervention methods designed to increase reciprocal social relationships and social engagement in young children with autism (Rogers and Dawson, 2009a). As with other play-based behavior analytic interventions, ESDM places a major focus on child motivation. Unique to the ESDM, however, is that the course of intervention for each child is based on a structured Curriculum Checklist, specifically targeting developmentally-based social-interactive skills, social communicative skills, cognitive skills, language, imitation, fine and gross motor skills, self-help skills, and adaptive behaviors (Rogers and Dawson, 2009b). The ESDM has an experimental evidence base, including an impressive and extensive set of previous experimental research studies on PRT and a large-scale RCT of the efficacy of the ESDM itself in toddlers on the autism spectrum (Dawson et al., 2010). In this study, 48 toddlers between 18 and 30 months of age were randomly assigning to either the ESDM intervention group, or to a group referred for community-provided intervention. Across the two-year training period, those in the ESDM intervention group demonstrated significant improvements in scores of adaptive behavior and IQ (including Verbal IQ/Language) when compared to both baseline scores and the community-referral group. These toddlers also exhibited more positive changes in the severity of their autism diagnosis. That is, in comparison with community intervention, ESDM intervention led to more children experiencing changes in their diagnosis from Autism to PDD-NOS.

Reciprocal imitation training (RIT)

Reciprocal Imitation Training (RIT) is a recently developed intervention that primarily targets object and gesture-based action imitation in children with autism (Ingersoll and Schreibman, 2006). Following the same basic principles as PRT and the ESDM, RIT is child-directed and incorporates motivational strategies to facilitate engagement and learning. However, RIT was developed on the grounds that naturalistic action imitation is a critical social learning tool that contributes to rapid advances in social and cognitive development in infants and children (Meltzoff and Moore, 1977; Bates et al., 1979; Fiese, 1990; Uzgiris, 1991; Carpenter et al., 1998; Charman et al., 2000, 2003; Stone and Yoder, 2001), and is significantly impaired in children with autism (Curcio, 1978; Dawson and Adams, 1984; Stone et al., 1997; Williams et al., 2004). In essence, the RIT intervention sessions are designed to create ongoing turn-taking situations whereby the therapist and child reciprocate imitation of each other's actions (see **Figure 4**). The RIT therapist imitates the child's actions with objects, gestures, movements, and vocalizations, and strategically incorporates the modeling of new developmentally-appropriate actions or gestures approximately once every one to two minutes. The child is provided with up to three actions to imitate in a naturalistic play context, before being physically prompted to imitate the fourth action if and when he or she does not engage in any imitation. As the child learns to reciprocate this imitation, and in turns becomes more attentive and socially engaged with the therapist, the need for prompting decreases until child-therapist imitation is a natural part of the play routine. The ultimate goal of RIT is to increase the generalized use of spontaneous imitation of both actions with objects and gestures, while facilitating gains in other social-communicative domains (Ingersoll and Schreibman, 2006).

The efficacy of RIT as an intervention for children with ASD is evidenced by multiple well-controlled research studies. Several experimental single-subject design experiments have demonstrate increases in object and gesture imitation, as well as highlighting gains in language and social skills as a result of

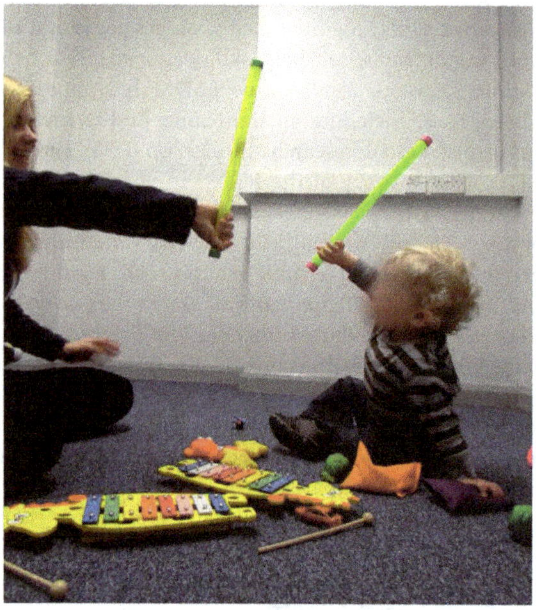

FIGURE 4 | Interventions targeting synchronous motor activity. Child and therapist engaged in Reciprocal Imitation Training (RIT). RIT involves the therapist imitating the child's actions and gestures, and also modeling developmentally-appropriate actions and gestures for the child to imitate, in a play context. The child is encouraged and prompted to imitate, until regular spontaneous reciprocal imitation is established.

RIT. For example, adopting a multiple-baseline design, Ingersoll and Schreibman (2006) found that after completion of the intervention phases, all five young children with ASD exhibited considerable improvements in object imitation, pretend play, joint attention and language. Importantly, such gains in imitation were found to generalize across materials, settings, and therapists (Ingersoll and Schreibman, 2006). Ingersoll and Gergans (2007) replicated these findings in a study investigating the effectiveness of parent-implemented RIT. Again, a multiple-baseline design across three families evidenced increased spontaneous object imitation in young children with autism, with effects exceeding the teaching period (Ingersoll and Gergans, 2007). Furthermore, in addition to object imitation, gains in gesture imitation have been demonstrated in a single-subject study by Ingersoll et al. (2007). In 2010, Ingersoll attempted to further validate these findings by conducting a pilot RCT into the effects of RIT on elicited and spontaneous imitation in autistic children (Ingersoll, 2010). Randomizing 21 young children into either RIT intervention or a control group, Ingersoll found larger imitation gains in the treatment group across all primary assessments, replicating previous single-subject findings. Thus, the large evidence-base for RIT as an effective intervention tool for autistic children is promising and, unlike other forms of ASD treatment, consists of multiple designs all demonstrating the same imitation, language, and social gains in this population.

Given the dynamic and effective nature of these play-based, reciprocal action and synchrony-oriented interventions, the ESDM and RIT appear to increase child-therapist social-motor synchrony (i.e., temporal coordination of movements) and social engagement (see also Landa et al., 2010). This increase in social-motor coordination and engagement may also increase social attention and motor resonance mechanisms in these children. Recall that there is evidence that activation of the MNS, FFA, and other social brain mechanisms may be limited in response to those individuals with whom children with autism are social-emotionally disconnected (e.g., unfamiliar people). Given that the ESDM and RIT increase social-communicative and language skills, one potential mechanistic pathway facilitating some of these behavioral changes is increased motor resonance through repeated social engagement with unfamiliar people. Evidence from a recent EEG/ERP study of face processing in toddlers with autism who received the ESDM vs. community-based services provides indirect support for this hypothesis. Specifically, the ESDM intervention increased late frontal activity in response to unfamiliar faces, relative to children who received TAU (Dawson et al., 2012). Because this was a study of static face processing, as opposed to human action processing, we cannot generalize these findings to the MNS without further research. However, direct experimental examinations of this hypothesis in the future, particularly experimental studies including measures of motor resonance, will be very informative in this regard.

DISCUSSION AND FUTURE DIRECTIONS

We have described several interventions aimed at increasing social-communication and language skills in young children with autism that have theoretical and/or practical roots in relationships of these skills to motor development. In doing so, we have given serious consideration to the intervention methods as well as the existing or emerging evidence-base for each such intervention. As outlined in this review, neither practical nor theoretical links between motor and communication/language development are sufficient to predict the efficacy of an intervention for children on the autism spectrum. For example, despite very strong practical and theoretical links between early symbolic gestures, such as the iconic manual and motor signs of sign language, and speech and language development in typically developing children, extensive research suggests that SLT is not a very effective way to teach either communication or speech/language skills to children on the autism spectrum. On the other hand, evidence suggests that these children can learn a picture-based social-communication system, PECS, rapidly and effectively. Furthermore, research suggests that PECS is a relatively more effective path to speech development in these children. There are multiple potential reasons for this seemingly contradictory finding, including the possibility that impairments in motor skills (e.g., fine motor skills), motor imitation, and/or iconicity make learning and producing the manual and motor signs of sign language particularly challenging for children with ASDs (see also **Figure 1** and **Table 1**).

We also reviewed and described several emerging intervention methods that take a more direct approach to motor aspects of speech production. These included PROMPT, which involves direct manipulations of the mouth and other sound-producing structures; AMMT, which aims to generate strong and direct temporal links between the child's auditory, motor, and speech production; and tDCS (and TMS), which involve directly stimulating motor and motor planning regions involved in speech production and other aspects of language. Although there is not yet existing experimental evidence for any of these interventions, reasonable pseudo-experimental/group case study reports on relatively well-characterized groups of children provide promising information to suggest that each of these interventions might prove effective for increase speech/language skills in this population. Therefore, experimental research is warranted on PROMPT, AMMT, and tDCS/TMS as potentially effective interventions for children with autism.

While the case study report on the group of minimally verbal children with autism receiving tDCS intervention is promising, there is also a need for caution in the pursuit of both research and practice involving the application of this technology to non-verbal or minimally verbal children with autism. While tDCS and TMS are generally believed to be safe procedures, there are also known risks (Wassermann, 1998; see also Loo et al., 2008; Rossi et al., 2009). For example, incorrect setting of electrical current or other parameters can trigger adverse events such as seizures, toxicity, headache, nausea, tissue damage, or burns. Furthermore, common adverse reactions include mild pain or sensitivity on the scalp, and headaches. It is, therefore, critically important to consider the ramifications involved with testing or treating non-verbal and minimally verbal children with autism with these technologies, given that they can neither provide informed consent nor effectively communicate injury or discomfort.

A risk of potentially even greater concern with the application of tDCS and TMS to children with autism is the potential for directly or indirectly causing seizure activity, or the onset of epilepsy. As characterized by Maski et al. (2011; see also Myers and Johnson, 2007), the prevalence of epilepsy is typically quoted in the literature as 30%. Identification of epilepsy in ASD is also challenging, due to the impact of ASD symptoms and behaviors on measurement/testing. As a result, assessing seizure risk would be very difficult to impossible for large numbers of non-verbal and minimally verbal children.

Despite the risks, tDCS and TMS have already been used to study children from a number of populations, including children who have experienced brain injury as a result of stroke (Frye et al., 2008; Kirton et al., 2010), children with language-learning disorders (Pugh et al., 2001), and children/adolescents with psychiatric disorders (Walter et al., 2001). Indeed, a clear strength of these technologies, and particularly tDCS, is that they are sufficiently streamlined and flexible in their application to be used with relatively young and relatively less able individuals. These techniques can even be used in conjunction with existing behavioral interventions (see **Figure 3**), potentially facilitating or enhancing their positive effects on speech and language development.

The possibility that the application of motor-related interventions might initiate the onset of even small to medium sized gains in speech development could have major long-term implications for quality of life. The results of several recent studies examining predictors of speech/language outcomes following early behavioral intervention suggest that a child producing even a few words prior to the start of intervention can play a key role in whether or not that child makes speech and language gains during the intervention (Gordon et al., 2011; Nahmias et al., 2012). Other research suggests that language abilities at 5- to 7-years of age are one of the key predictors of cognitive and adaptive skills outcomes in adulthood in this population (e.g., Gillespie-Lynch et al., 2012). At the same time, evidence suggests that relatively large percentages of autistic children who are completely non-verbal at 2-, 3-, and even 4-years of age develop speech and language skills fairly rapidly as a result of intensive early intervention (Koegel, 2000). Unfortunately, it is not currently possible to predict which non-verbal and minimally verbal young children will respond to any given early behavioral intervention (Stahmer et al., 2011).

As alluded to above, early intervention that targets speech and language skills by 2- to 4-years of age appear to be much more effective than those same interventions implemented after 5-years of age (Koegel, 2000), perhaps due to the existence of sensitive periods for speech/language and related skills (Fox et al., 2010; Windsor et al., 2011). Given the developmental complexity, and in some cases the seemingly strong biological nature, of motor development in relation to speech/language development, similar sensitive periods may exist in the relationships of motor and language/communication skills development. Therefore, the motor-related intervention pathways to language that have been discussed in this article, or others, may be most effective when intervention occurs in an ideal time window. Dependent upon the particular mechanism being targeted, this time window may be a sensitive biological/chronological age or developmental age period. For example, interventions that incorporate repetitive and coordinated hand banging may only be effective at facilitating speech when they occur during or shortly after the chronologically appropriate age of 7- to 12-months. Alternatively, intervening to increase these links may, as suggested by AMMT, still be effective at facilitating speech for any child below eight years of age who is in the pre-verbal or minimally verbal stage of development, for example. These are interesting clinical and empirical developmental questions, which can be directly examined in experimental studies.

CONCLUSION

In this article, we have reviewed the research on aspects of early motor development that are believed to be specifically relevant to speech/language and social communication in infants and children with autism. We have also reviewed motor-related interventions designed to increase speech/language and social-communication skills in young non-verbal and minimally verbal children with autism. This field is at an exciting time in this area of research and development. We now know from extensive research that SLT is not a very effective intervention for facilitating speech and language development in this population. Potential reasons for this include that children with autism exhibit specific difficulties in iconicity, imitation of the actions of others, and/or fine motor skills, which make it difficult for them to become effective signers. On the other hand, these children appear to learn a picture-based social-communication program relatively rapidly, and extensive evidence suggests that this type of communication training does facilitate the development of basic speech skills in many of these children. At the same time as this, small-scale pseudo-experimental studies on at least three types of recently developed motor-based speech/language interventions (PROMPT, AMMT, tDCS/TMS) have each produced very promising results. This provides an exciting opportunity for important new experimental research studies designed to directly examine the efficacy of these interventions with this population, for whom effective speech/language interventions have been challenging to identify and develop. Finally, researchers with expertise in traditional applied behavior analytic and developmental interventions have begun working together to develop interventions that combine these two approaches. The result is a combined intervention strategy that uses highly effective operant teaching methods with a socially and motorically interactive play-based approach to enhancing speech/language and social-communication skills. The effects of these interventions on the children appear to extend beyond simple skill learning, and to enhance social attention and social engagement in ways that may facilitate the activation of social brain networks, including the motor-resonance system. We are optimistic that the field is approaching a turning point, with potentially dramatic breakthroughs to come in both our treatment and our understanding of the speech/language and social-communication difficulties in this population, as well as their relationship to motor mechanisms and development.

ACKNOWLEDGMENT

The development and writing of this paper was facilitated by funding support from the UK-based charity, Autistica, to Joseph P. McCleery.

REFERENCES

Adolphs, R., Spezio, M. L., Parlier, M., and Piven, J. (2008). Distinct face-processing strategies in parents of autistic children. *Curr. Biol.* 18, 1090–1093.

American Psychiatric Association. (2000). *Diagnostic and Statistical Manual of Mental Disorders.* 4th Edn., text revision. Washington, DC: American Psychiatric Association.

Anderson, A., Moore, D. W., and Bourne, T. (2007). Functional communication and other concomitant behavior change following PECS training: a case study. *Behav. Change* 24, 173–181.

Baker-Ericzén, M. J., Stahmer, A. C., and Burns, A. (2007). Child demographics associated with outcomes in a community-based pivotal response training program. *J. Posit. Behav. Interv.* 9, 52–60.

Baldwin, D. A. (1995). "Understanding the link between joint attention and language," in *Joint Attention: Its Origins and Role in Development,* eds C. Moore and P. J. Dunham (Hillsdale: Lawrence Erlbaum Associates, Inc.), 131–158.

Baldwin, D. A., Markman, E. M., Bill, B., Desjardins, R. N., Irwin, J. M., and Tidball, G. (1996). Infants' reliance on a social criterion for establishing word-object relations. *Child Dev.* 67, 3135–3153.

Baranek, G. T., Wakeford, C. L., and David, F. J. (2008). "Understanding, assessing, and treating sensory-motor issues in young children with autism," in *Autism Spectrum Disorders in Infancy and Early Childhood: Diagnosis, Assessmetn, and Treatment,* eds K. Chawarska, A. Klin, and F. Volkmar (New York, NY: Guilford Press), 104–140.

Barrera, R., and Sulzer-Azaroff, B. (1983). An alternating treatment comparison of oral and total communication training programs with echolalic autistic children. *J. Appl. Behav. Anal.* 16, 379–394.

Barrera, R. D., Lobato-Barrera, D., and Sulzer-Azaroff, B. (1980). A simultaneous treatment comparison of three expressive language training programs with a mute autistic child. *J. Autism Dev. Dis.* 10, 21–37.

Bates, E., Benigni, L., Bretherton, I., Camaioni, L., and Volterra, V. (1979). *The Emergence of Symbols: Cognition and Communication in Infancy.* New York, NY: Academic Press.

Bates, E., and Dick, F. (2002). Language, gesture, and the developing brain. *Dev. Psychobiol.* 40, 293–310.

Bates, E., Thal, D., Finlay, B., and Clancy, B. (2002). "Early language development and its neural correlates," in *Handbook of Neuropsychology.* Vol. 6, Child neurology, 2nd Edn., eds I. Rapin and S. Segalowitz (Amsterdam: Elsevier).

Bates, E., Thal, D., Finlay, B. L., and Clancy, B. (1999). "Early language development and its neural correlates," in *Handbook of Neuropsychology.* Vol. 7, Child neurology 2nd Edn., Series eds F. Boller and J. Grafman; Vol. eds I. Rapin and S. Segalowitz (Amsterdam: Elsevier).

Becchio, C., and Castiello, U. (2012). Visuomotor resonance in autism spectrum disorders. *Front. Integr. Neurosci.* 6, 1–6. doi: 10.3389/fnint.2012.00110

Bhat, A. N., Landa, R. J., and Galloway, J. C. (2011). Current perspectives on motor functioning in infants, children, and adults with autism spectrum disorders. *Phys. Ther.* 91, 1116–1129.

Bishop, D. V. M., Maybery, M., Maley, A., Wong, D., Hill, W., and Hallmayer, J. (2004). Using self-report to identify the broad phenotype in parents of children with autistic spectrum disorders: a study using the Autism-Spectrum Quotient. *J. Child Psychol. Psychiatry* 45, 1431–1436.

Bolton, P., MacDonald, H., Pickles, A., Rios, P., Goode, S., Crowson, M., et al. (1994). A case-control family history study of autism. *J. Child Psychol. Psychiatry* 35, 877–900.

Bondy, A., and Frost, L. A. (1994). "The delaware autistic program," in *Preschool Education Programs for Children with Autism,* eds S. L. Harris and J. S. Handleman (Austin, TX: Pro-Ed.), 37–54.

Bondy, A., and Frost, L. A. (1998). The Picture Exchange Communication System. *Semin. Speech Lang.* 19, 373–389.

Bondy, A., and Frost, L. (2002). *A Picture's Worth: PECS and other Visual Communication Strategies in Autism. Topics in Autism.* Bethesda, MD: Woodbine House.

Bonvillian, J. D., and Blackburn, D. W. (1991). "Manual communication and autism: factors relating to sign language acquisition," in *Theoretical Issues in Sign Language and Research.* Vol. 2, Psychology, eds P. Siple and S. D. Fischer (Chicago, IL: University of Chicago), 255–257.

Bonvillian, J. D., and Nelson, K. E. (1976). Sign language acquisition in a mute autistic boy. *J. Speech Hear. Disord.* 41, 339.

Brady, D. O., and Smouse, A. (1978). A simultaneous comparison of three methods for Language training *with anautistic* child: an experimental case analysis. *J. Autism Child. Schizophr.* 8, 271–279.

Brisson, J., Warreyn, P., Serres, J., Foussier, S., and Adrien-Louis, J. (2011). Motor anticipation failure in infants with autism: a retrospective analysis of feeding situations. *Autism* 16, 420–429.

Brown, S., Martinez, M. J., Hodges, D. A., Fox, P. T., and Parsons, L. M. (2004). The song system of the human brain. *Brain Res. Cogn. Brain Res.* 20, 363–375.

Campos, J. J., Anderson, D. I., Barbu-Roth, M. A., Hubbard, E. M., Hertenstein, M. J., and Witherington, D. (2002). Travel broadens the mind. *Infancy* 1, 149–219.

Cardon, T. A., and Wilcox, M. J. (2011). Promoting imitation in young children with autism: a comparison of reciprocal imitation training and video modeling. *J. Autism Dev. Disord.* 41, 654–666.

Carpenter, M., Nagell, K., and Tomasello, M. (1998). Social cognition, joint attention, and communicative competence from 9 to 15 months of age. *Monogr. Soc. Res. Child Dev.* 63, 1–143.

Carr, D., and Felce, J. (2007a). Brief report: increase in production of spoken words in some children with autism after PECS teaching to phase III. *J. Autism Dev. Disord.* 37, 780–787.

Carr, D., and Felce, J. (2007b). The effects of PECS teaching to phase iii on the communicative interactions between children with autism and their teachers. *J. Autism Dev. Disord.* 37, 724–737.

Carr, E. G. (1979). Teaching autistic children to use sign language: some research issues. *J. Autism Dev. Disord.* 9, 345–359.

Carr, E. G., Binkoff, J. A., Kologinsky, E., and Eddy, M. (1978). Acquisition of sign language by autistic children. 1: expressive labelling. *J. Appl. Behav. Anal.* 11, 489–501.

Carr, E. G., Kologinsky, E., and Leff-Simon, S. (1987). Acquisition of sign language by autistic children. III: generalized descriptive phrases. *J. Autism Dev. Disord.* 17, 217–229.

Carré, A. J., Le Grice, B., Blampied, N. M., and Walker, D. (2009). Picture Exchange Communication (PECS) training for young children: does training transfer at school and to home? *Behav. Change* 26, 54–65.

Carter, M., and Wheldall, K. (2008). Why can't a teacher be more like a scientist? Science, pseudoscience and the art of teaching. *Australas. J. Spec. Educ.* 32, 5–21.

Casey, L. O. (1978). Development of communicative behavior in autistic children: a parent program using manual signs. *J. Autism Child. Schizophr.* 8, 45–59.

Catmur, C., Walsh, V., and Heyes, C. (2007). Sensorimotor learning configures the mirror neuron system. *Curr. Biol.* 17, 1527–1531.

Charlop-Christy, M. H., Carpenter, M., Le, L., LeBlanc, L. A., and Kellet, K. (2002). Using the picture exchange communication system (PECS) with children with autism: assessment of pecs acquisition, speech, social-communicative behavior, and problem behavior. *J. Appl. Behav. Anal.* 35, 213–231.

Charman, T. (2003). Why is joint attention a pivotal skill in autism? *Philos. Trans. R. Soc. Lond. B Biol. Sci.* 358, 315–324.

Charman, T., Baron-Cohen, A., Swettenham, J., Baird, G., Cox, A., and Auriol, D. (2000). Testing joint attention, imitation, and play as infancy precursors to language and theory of mind. *Cogn. Dev.* 15, 481–498.

Charman, T., Drew, A., Baird, C., and Baird, G. (2003). Measuring early language development in preschool children with autism spectrum disorder using the MacArthur Communicative Development Inventory (Infant Form). *J. Child Lang.* 30, 213–236.

Chumpelik, D. (1984). The PROMPT system of therapy: theoretical framework and applications for developmental apraxia of speech. *Semin. Speech Lang.* 5, 139–156.

Cobo-Lewis, A. B., Oller, D. K., Lynch, M. P., and Levine, S. L. (1996). Relations of motor and vocal milestones in typically developing infants and infants with Down syndrome. *Am. J. Ment. Retard.* 100, 456.

Cohen, M. (1979). "The development of language behavior in an autistic child using a total communication approach," in *A Paper Presented at the Annual International Convention, The Council for Exceptional Children* (Dallas, TX).

Colonnesi, C., Zijlstra, B. J., van der Zande, A., and Bögels, S. M. (2012). Coordination of gaze, facial expressions and vocalizations of early infant communication with mother and father. *Infant Behav. Dev.* 35, 523–532.

Curcio, F. (1978). Sensorimotor functioning in mute autistic children. *J. Autism Child. Schizophr.* 8, 281–292.

Dawson, G., and Adams, A. (1984). Imitation and social responsiveness in autistic children. *J. Abnorm. Child Psychol.* 12, 209–225.

Dawson, G., Carver, L., Meltzoff, A. N., Panagiotides, H., McPartland, J., and Webb, S. J. (2002). Neural correlates of face and object recognition in young children with autism spectrum disorder, developmental delay, and typical development. *Child Dev.* 73, 700–717.

Dawson, G., Jones, E. J., Merkle, K., Venema, K., Lowy, R., Faja, S., et al. (2012). Early behavioral intervention is associated with normalized brain activity in young children with autism. *J. Am. Acad. Child Adolesc. Psychiatry* 51, 1150–1159.

Dawson, G., Rogers, S., Munson, J., Smith, M., Winter, J., Greenson, J., et al. (2010). Randomized, controlled trial of an intervention with toddlers with autism: the early start denver model. *Pediatrics* 125, 17–23.

di Pellegrino, G., Fadiga, L., Fogassi, L., Gallese, V., and Rizzolatti, G. (1992). Understanding motor events: a neurophysiological study. *Exp. Brain Res.* 91, 176–180.

Dodd, B., and Bradford, A. (2000). A comparison of three therapy methods for children with different types of developmental phonological disorders. *Int. J. Lang. Commun. Disord.* 35, 189–209.

Dowell, L. R., Mahone, E. M., and Mostofsky, S. H. (2009). Associations of postural knowledge and basic motor skill with dyspraxia in autism: implication for abnormalities in distributed connectivity and motor learning. *Neuropsychology* 23, 563.

Dziuk, M. A., Larson, J. C., Apostu, A., Mahone, E. M., Denckla, M. B., and Mostofsky, S. H. (2007). Dyspraxia in autism: association with motor, social, and communicative deficits. *Dev. Med. Child Neurol.* 49, 734–739.

Eilers, R., Oller, D. K., Levine, S., Basinger, D., Lynch, M. P., and Urbano, R. (1993). The role of prematurity and socioeconomic status in the onset of canonical babbling in infants. *Infant Behav. Dev.* 16, 297–315.

Enticott, P. G., Kennedy, H. A., Rinehart, N. J., Tonge, B. J., Bradshaw, J. L., Taffe, J. R., et al. (2012). Mirror neuron activity associated with social impairments but not age in autism spectrum disorder. *Biol. Psychiatry* 71, 427–433.

Fatemi, S. H., Aldinger, K. A., Ashwood, P., Bauman, M. L., Blaha, C. D., Blatt, G. J., et al. (2012). Consensus paper: pathological role of the cerebellum in autism. *Cerebellum* 11, 777–807.

Fecteau, S., Agosta, S., Oberman, L., and Pascual-Leone, A. (2011). Brain stimulation over Broca's area differentially modulates naming skills in neurotypical adults and individuals with Asperger's syndrome. *Eur. J. Neurosci.* 34, 158–164.

Feldman, R., Greenbaum, W. C., Yirmiya, N., and Mayes, L. C. (1996). Relations between cyclicity and regulation in mother–infant interaction at 3 and 9 months and cognition at 2 years. *J. Appl. Dev. Psychol.* 17, 347–365.

Fiese, B. H. (1990). Playful relationships: a contextual analysis of mother-toddler interaction and symbolic play. *Child Dev.* 61, 1648–1656.

Flom, R., Deak, G. O., Phill, C. G., and Pick, A. (2004). Nine-month-olds' shared visual attention as a function of gesture and object location. *Infant Behav. Dev.* 27, 181–194.

Folstein, S., and Rutter, M. (1977). Infantile autism: a genetic study of 21 twin pairs. *J. Child Psychol. Psychiatry* 18, 297–321.

Folstein, S. E., Santangelo, S. L., Gilman, S. E., Piven, J., Landa, R., Lainhart, J., et al. (1999). Predictors of cognitive test patterns in autism families. *J. Child Psychol. Psychiatry* 40, 1117–1128.

Fournier, K. A., Hass, C. J., Naik, S. K., Lodha, N., and Cauraugh, J. H. (2010). Motor coordination in autism spectrum disorders: a synthesis and meta-analysis. *J. Autism Dev. Disord.* 40, 1227–1240.

Fox, S. E., Levitt, P., and Nelson, C. A. 3rd. (2010). How the timing and quality of early experiences influence the development of brain architecture. *Child Dev.* 81, 28–40.

Freed, D. B., Marshall, R. C., and Frazier, K. E. (1997). Long-term effectiveness of PROMPT treatment in a severely apractic-aphasic speaker. *Aphas* 11, 365–372.

Fregni, F., Otachi, P. T. M., Do Valle, A., Boggio, P. S., Thut, G., Rigonatti, S. P., et al. (2006). A randomized clinical trial of repetitive transcranial magnetic stimulation in patients with refractory epilepsy. *Ann. Neurol.* 60, 447–455.

Frost, L., and Bondy, A. (2002). *PECS: The Picture Exchange Communication System Training Manual.* 2nd Edn. Cherry Hill, NJ: Pyramid Educational Consultants.

Frye, R. E., Rotenberg, A., Ousley, M., and Pascual-Leone, A. (2008). Transcranial magnetic stimulation in child neurology: current and future directions. *J. Child Neurol.* 23, 79–96.

Fulwiler, R. L., and Fouts, R. S. (1976). Acquisition of american sign language by a non-communicating autistic child. *J. Autism Child. Schizophr.* 6, 43–51.

Gandiga, P. C., Hummel, F. C., and Cohen, L. G. (2006). Transcranial DC stimulation (tDCS): a tool for double-blind sham-controlled clinical studies in brain stimulation. *Clin. Neurophysiol.* 117, 845–850.

Ganz, J. B., and Simpson, R. L. (2004). Effects on communicative requesting and speech development of the Picture Exchange Communication System in children with characteristics of autism. *J. Autism Dev. Disord.* 34, 395–409.

Gazzola, V., Aziz-Zadeh, L., and Keysers, C. (2006). Empathy and the somatotopic auditory mirror system in humans. *Curr. Biol.* 16, 1824–1829.

Gernsbacher, M. A., Sauer, E. A., Geye, H. M., Schweigert, E. K., and Hill Goldsmith, H. (2008). Infant and toddler oral- and manual-motor skills predict later speech fluency in autism. *J. Child Psychol. Psychiatry* 49, 43–50.

Gillespie-Lynch, K., Sepeta, L., Wang, Y., Marshall, S., Gomez, L., Sigman, M., et al. (2012). Early childhood predictors of the social competence of adults with autism. *J. Autism Dev. Disord.* 42, 161–174.

Goldberg, W. A., Jarvis, K. L., Osann, K., Laulhere, T. M., Straud, C., Thomas, E., et al. (2005). Brief report: early social communication behaviors in the younger siblings of children with autism. *J. Autism Dev. Disord.* 35, 657–664.

Gordon, K., Pasco, G., McElduff, F., Wade, A., Howlin, P., and Charman, T. (2011). A communication-based intervention for nonverbal children with autism: what changes? Who benefits? *J. Consult. Clin. Psychol.* 79, 447–457.

Gowen, E., and Hamilton, A. (2013). Motor abilities in autism: a review using a computational context. *J. Autism Dev. Disord.* 43, 323–344.

Gowen, E., Stanley, J., and Miall, R. C. (2008). Movement interference in autism spectrum disorder. *Neuropsychologia* 46, 1060–1068.

Greenberg, A. L., Tomaino, M. A. E., and Charlop, M. H. (2012).

Assessing generalization of the Picture Exchange Communication System in children with autism. *J. Dev. Phys. Disabil.* 24, 539–558.

Grigos, M. I., Hayden, D., and Eigen, J. (2010). Perceptual and articulatory changes in speech production following PROMPT treatment. *J. Med. Speech Lang. Pathol.* 18, 46–53.

Hallett, M., Lebiedowska, M. K., Thomas, S. L., Stanhope, S. J., Denckla, M. B., and Rumsey, J. (1993). Locomotion of autistic adults. *Arch. Neurol.* 50, 1304–1308.

Hallmayer, J., Cleveland, S., Torres, A., Phillips, J., Cohen, B., Torigoe, T., et al. (2011). Genetic heritability and shared environmental factors among twin pairs with autism. *Arch. Gen. Psychiatry* 68, 1095–1102.

Hamilton, A. F. D. C. (2009). Research review: goals, intentions and mental states: challenges for theories of autism. *J. Child Psychol. Psychiatry* 50, 881–892.

Hayden, D. (2002). *Introduction to PROMPT: Technique Manual Revised.* Sante Fe, NM: The PROMPT Institute.

Hayden, D. (2006). The PROMPT model: use and application for children with mixed phonological-motor impairment. *Int. J. Speech Lang. Pathol.* 8, 265–281.

Hayden, D. A., and Square, P. A. (1994). Motor speech treatment hierarchy: a systems approach. *Clin. Commun. Disord.* 4, 162–174.

Howlin, P., Gordon, R. K., Pasco, G., Wade, A., and Charman, T. (2007). The effectiveness of Picture Exchange Communication System (PECS) training for teachers of children with autism: a pragmatic, group randomised controlled trial. *J. Child Psychol. Psychiatry* 48, 473–481.

Hughes, C., Leboyer, M., and Bouvard, M. (1997). Executive function in parents of children with autism. *Psychol. Med.* 27, 209–220.

Hummel, F., and Cohen, L. G. (2005). Improvement of motor function with noninvasive cortical stimulation in a patient with chronic stroke. *Neurorehabil. Neural Repair* 19, 14–19.

Iacoboni, M., and Dapretto, M. (2006). The mirror neuron system and the consequences of its dysfunction. *Nat. Rev. Neurosci.* 7, 942–951.

Iacoboni, M., Woods, R. P., Brass, M., Bekkering, H., Mazziotta, J. C., and Rizzolatti, G. (1999). Cortical mechanisms of human imitation. *Science* 286, 2526–2528.

Ingersoll, B. (2010). Brief report: pilot randomized controlled trial of reciprocal imitation training for teaching elicited and spontaneous imitation to children with autism. *J. Autism Dev. Disord.* 40, 1154–1160.

Ingersoll, B., and Gergans, S. (2007). The effect of a parent-implemented imitation intervention on spontaneous imitation skills in young children with autism. *Res. Dev. Disabil.* 28, 163–175.

Ingersoll, B., Lewis, E., and Kroman, E. (2007). Teaching the imitation and spontaneous use of descriptive gestures in young children with autism using a naturalistic behavioral intervention. *J. Autism Dev. Disord.* 37, 1446–1456.

Ingersoll, B., and Schreibman, L. (2006). Teaching reciprocal imitation skills to young children with autism using a naturalistic behavioral approach: effects on language, pretend play, and joint attention. *J. Autism Dev. Dis.* 36, 487–505.

Iverson, J. M. (2010). Multimodality in infancy: vocal-motor and speech-gesture coordination's in typical and atypical development. *Enfance* 2010, 357–274.

Iverson, J. M., and Fagan, M. K. (2004). Infant vocal–motor coordination: precursor to the gesture–speech system? *Child Dev.* 75, 1053–1066.

Iverson, J. M., Hall, A. J., Nickel, L., and Wozniak, R. H. (2007). The relationship between reduplicated babble onset and laterality biases in infant rhythmic arm movements. *Brain Lang.* 101, 198–207.

Iverson, J. M., and Wozniak, R. H. (2007). Variation in vocal-motor development in infant siblings of children with autism. *J. Autism Dev. Disord.* 37, 158–170.

Jansiewicz, E. M., Goldberg, M. C., Newschaffer, C. J., Denckla, M. B., Landa, R., and Mostofsky, S. H. (2006). Motor signs distinguish children with high functioning autism and Asperger's syndrome from controls. *J. Autism Dev. Disord.* 36, 613–621.

Jurgens, A., Anderson, A., and Moore, D. W. (2009). The effect of teaching PECS to a child with autism on verbal behaviour, play, and social functioning. *Behav. Change* 26, 66–81.

Kirton, A., deVeber, G., Gunraj, C., and Chen, R. (2010). Cortical excitability and interhemispheric inhibition after subcortical pediatric stroke: plastic organization and effects of rTMS. *Clin. Neurophysiol.* 121, 1922–1929.

Koegel, L. K. (2000). Interventions to facilitate communication in autism: treatments for people with autism and other pervasive developmental disorders: research perspectives [Special issue]. *J. Autism Dev. Disord.* 35, 383–391.

Koegel, R. L., and Koegel, L. K. (2006). *Pivotal Response Treatments for Autism: Communication, Social, and Academic Development.* Baltimore, MD: Paul, H. Brookes Publishing Co.

Koegel, L. K., Koegel, R. L., and Brookman, L. I. (2005). "Child-initiated interactions that are pivotal in intervention for children with autism," in *Psychosocial Treatments for Child and Adolescent Disorders: Empirically Based Strategies for Clinical Practice,* 2nd Edn., eds E. D. Hibbs and P. S. Jensen (Washington, DC: American Psychological Association), 633–657.

Koegel, L. K., Singh, A. K., and Koegel, R. L. (2010). Improving motivation foracademics in children with autism. *J. Autism Dev. Disord.* 40, 1057–1066.

Kohler, E., Keysers, C., Umiltà, M. A., Fogassi, L., Gallese, V., and Rizzolatti, G. (2002). Hearing sounds, understanding actions: action representation in mirror neurons. *Science* 297, 846–848.

Konstantareas, M. M. (1984). Sign language as a communication prosthesis with language-impaired children. *J. Autism Dev. Disord.* 14, 9–25.

Kopp, S., Beckung, E., and Gillberg, C. (2010). Developmental coordination disorder and other motor control problems in girls with autism spectrum disorder and/or attention-deficit/hyperactivity disorder. *Res. Dev. Disabil.* 31, 350–361.

Kravits, T. R., Kamps, D. M., Kemmerer, K., and Potucek, J. (2002). Brief report: increasing communication skills for an elementary-aged student with autism using the Picture Exchange Communication System. *J. Autism Dev. Disord.* 32, 225–230.

Lahab, A., Saltzman, E., and Schlaug, G. (2007). Action representation of sound: audiomotor recognition network while listening to newly acquired actions. *J. Neurosci.* 27, 208–214.

Landa, R., Folstein, S. E., and Isaacs, C. (1991). Spontaneous narrative-discourse performance of parents of autistic individuals. *J. Speech Hear. Res.* 34, 1339–1345.

Landa, R., Holman, K. C., O'Neill, A. H., and Stuart, E. A. (2010). Intervention targeting development of socially synchronous engagement in toddlers with autism spectrum disorder: a randomized controlled trial. *J. Child Psychol. Psychiatry* 52, 13–21.

Layton, T. (1988). Language training with autistic children using four different modes of presentation. *J. Commun. Disord.* 21, 333–350.

Layton, T., and Baker, P. (1981). Description of semantic-syntactic relations in an autistic child. *J. Autism Dev. Disord.* 11, 385–399.

Layton, T. L., and Watson, L. R. (1995). "Enhancing communication in nonverbal children with autism," in *Teaching Children with Autism: Strategies to Enhance Communication and Socialization,* ed K. A. Quill (New York, NY: Delmar), 73–103.

Lerna, A., Esposito, D., Conson, M., Russo, L., and Massagli, A. (2012). Social-communicative effects of the Picture Exchange Communication System (PECS) in autism spectrum disorders. *Int. J. Lang. Commun. Disord.* 47, 609–617.

Lerna, A., Esposito, D., Russo, L., and Massagli, A. (2009). P02-254 The efficacy of the PECS for improving the communicative, relational and social skills in children with autistic disorder: preliminary results. *Eur. Psychiatry* 24, S944.

Liddle, K. (2001). Implementing the Picture Exchange Communication System (PECS). *Int. J. Lang. Commun. Disord.* 36, 391–395.

Linkenauger, S. A., Lerner, M. D., Ramenzoni, V. C., and Proffitt. (2012). A perceptual-motor deficit predicts social and communicative impairment in individuals with autism spectrum disorders. *Autism Res.* 5, 352–362.

Lisanby, S. H., Kinnunen, L. H., and Crupain, M. J. (2002). Applications of TMS to therapy in psychiatry. *J. Clin. Neurophysiol.* 19, 344–360.

Locke, J. L., Bekken, K. E., McMinnlarson, L., and Wein, D. (1995). Emergent control of manual and vocal-motor activity in relation to the development of speech. *Brain Lang.* 51, 498–508.

Loftin, R. L., Odom, S. L., and Lantz, J. F. (2008). Social interaction and repetitive motor behaviors. *J. Autism Dev. Disord.* 38, 1124–1135.

Loo, C. K., McFarquhar, T. F., and Mitchell, P. B. (2008). A review of the safety of repetitive transcranial magnetic stimulation as a clinical treatment for depression. *Int. J. Neuropsychopharmacol.* 11, 131.

Lord, C., and Jones, R. M. (2012). Annual research review: rethinking the classification of autism spectrum disorders. *J. Child Psychol. Psychiatry* 53, 490–509.

Lord, C., Risi, S., Lambrecht, L., Cook, E. H., Leventhal, B. L., DiLavore, P. C., et al. (2000). The autism diagnostic observation schedule—generic: a standard measure of social and communication deficits associated with the spectrum of autism. *J. Autism Dev. Disord.* 30, 205–223.

Lord, C., Rutter, M., and Le Couteur, A. (1994). Autism diagnostic interview-revised: a version of diagnostic interview for care-givers of individuals with pervasive developmental disorders. *J. Autism Dev. Disord.* 24, 659–685.

Magiati, I., and Howlin, P. (2003). A pilot evaluation study of the Picture Exchange Communication System (PECS) for children with autistic spectrum disorders. *Autism* 7, 297–320.

Malandraki, G. A., and Okalidou, A. (2007). The application of PECS in a deaf child with autism: a case study. *Focus Autism Other Dev. Disabil.* 22, 23–32.

Martin, P. I., Naeser, M. A., Theoret, H., MariaTormos, J., Nicholas, M., Kurland, J. M., et al. (2009). Transcranial magnetic stimulation as a complementary treatment for aphasia. *Curr. Neurol. Neurosci. Rep.* 9, 451–458.

Masataka, N. (2001). Why early linguistic milestones are delayed in children with Williams syndrome: late onset of hand banging as a possible rate–limiting constraint on the emergence of canonical babbling. *Dev. Sci.* 4, 158–164.

Maski, K. P., Jeste, S. S., and Spence, S. J. (2011). Common neurological co-morbidities in autism spectrum disorders. *Curr. Opin. Pediatr.* 23, 609–615.

Meister, I. G., Boroojerdi, B., Foltys, H., Sparing, R., Huber, W., and Topper, R. (2003). Motor cortex hand area and speech: implications for the development of language. *Neuropsychologia* 41, 401–406.

Meister, I. G., Buelte, D., Staedtgen, M., Borooierdi, B., and Sparing, R. (2009). The dorsal premotor cortex orchestrates concurrent speech and fingertapping movements. *Eur. J. Neurosci.* 29, 2074–2084.

Meltzoff, A. N., and Moore, M. K. (1977). Imitation of facial and manual gestures by human neonates. *Science* 198, 75–78.

Millar, D., Light, J., and Schlosser, R. (2000). "The impact of AAC on natural speech development: a meta-analysis," in *Proceedings of the 9th biennial conference of the International Society for Augmentative and Alternative Communication,* (Washington, DC: ISAAC), 740–741.

Miller, A., and Miller, E. E. (1973). Cognitive developmental training with elevated boards and sign language. *J. Autism Child. Schizophr.* 3, 65–85.

Mimura, M., Kato, M., Kato, M., Sano, Y., Kojima, T., Naeser, M., et al. (1998). Prospective and retrospective studies of recovery in aphasia. Changes in cerebral blood flow and language functions. *Brain* 121, 2083–2094.

Minshew, N. J., Sung, K., Jones, B. L., and Furman, J. M. (2004). Underdevelopment of the postural control system in autism. *Neurology* 63, 2056–2061.

Mirenda, P., and Erickson, K. (2000). "Augmentative communication and literacy," in *Autism Spectrum Disorders: A Transactional Developmental Perspective,* eds A. Wetherby and B. Prizant (Baltimore, MD: Paul, H. Brookes), 333–367.

Mostofsky, S. H., Dubey, P., Jerath, V. K., Jansiewicz, E. M., Goldberg, M. C., and Denckla, M. B. (2006). Developmental dyspraxia is not limited to imitation in children with autism spectrum disorders. *J. Int. Neuropsychol. Soc.* 12, 314–326.

Murphy, M., Bolton, P. F., Pickles, A., Fombonne, E., Piven, J., and Rutter, M. (2000). Personality traits of the relatives of autistic probands. *Psychol. Med.* 30, 1411–1424.

Myers, S. M., and Johnson, C. P. (2007). Management of children with autism spectrum disorders. *Pediatrics* 120, 1162–1182.

Nahmias, A. S., Kase, C., and Mandell, D. S. (2012). Comparing cognitive outcomes among children with autism spectrum disorders receiving community-based early intervention in one of three placements. *Autism.* doi: 10.1177/1362361312467865. [Epub ahead of print].

National Research Council. (2001). *Educating Children with Autism.* Washington, DC: National Academy Press.

Nitsche, M. A., Cohen, L. G., Wassermann, E. M., Priori, A., Lang, N., Antal, A., et al. (2008). Transcranial direct current stimulation: state of the art. *Brain Stimul.* 1, 206–223.

Nobile, M., Perego, P., Piccilini, L., Mani, E., Rossi, A., Bellina, M., et al. (2011). Further evidence of complex motor dysfunction in drug naïve children with autism using automatic motion analysis of gait. *Autism* 15, 263–283.

Oberman, L. M., Hubbard, E. M., McCleery, J. P., Altschuler, E. L., Ramachandran, V. S., and Pineda, J. A. (2005). EEG evidence for mirror neuron dysfunction in autism spectrum disorders. *Brain Res. Cogn. Brain Res.* 24, 190–198.

Oberman, L. M., McCleery, J. P., Hubbard, E. M., Bernier, R., Wiersema, J. R., Raymaekers, R., et al. (2012). Developmental changes in mu suppression to observed and executed actions in autism spectrum disorders. *Soc. Cogn. Affect. Neurosci.* 8, 300–304.

Oberman, L. M., and Ramachandran, V. S. (2007). The simulating social mind: the role of the mirror neuron system and simulation in the social and communicative deficits of autism spectrum disorders. *Psychol. Bull.* 133, 310–327.

Oberman, L. M., Ramachandran, V. S., and Pineda, J. A. (2008). Modulation of mu suppression in children with autism spectrum disorders in response to familiar or unfamiliar stimuli: the mirror neuron hypothesis. *Neuropsychologia* 46, 1558–1565.

Oliveri, M., Rossini, P. M., Traversa, R., Cicinelli, P., Filippi, M. M., Pasqualetti, P., et al. (1999). Left frontal transcranial magnetic stimulation reduces contralesional extinction in patients with unilateral right brain damage. *Brain* 122, 1731–1739.

Oller, D. K., Eilers, R. E., Neal, A. R., and Cobo-Lewis, A. B. (1998). Late onset canonical babbling: a possible early marker of abnormal development. *Am. J. Ment. Retard.* 103, 249–263.

Ozdemir, E., Norton, A., and Schlaug, G. (2006). Shared and distinct neural correlates of singing and speaking. *Neuroimage* 33, 628–635.

Pascual-Leone, A., and Walsh, V. (2002). "Transcranial magnetic stimulation," in *Brain Mapping: The Methods,* eds A. Toga and J. Mazziotta (San Diego, CA: Academic Press), 255–290.

Petitto, L. A., Holowka, S., Sergio, L. E., Levy, B., and Ostry, D. J. (2004). Baby hands that move to the rhythm of language: hearing babies acquiring sign languages babble silently on the hands. *Cognition* 93, 43–73.

Petitto, L. A., and Marentette, P. F. (1991). Babbling in the manual mode: evidence for the ontogeny of language. *Science* 251, 1493–1496.

Pickles, A., Starr, E., Kazak, S., Bolton, P., Papanikolaou, K., Bailey, A., et al. (2000). Variable expression of the autism broader phenotype: findings from extended pedigrees. *J. Child Psychol. Psychiatry* 41, 491–502.

Pierce, K., and Redcay, E. (2008). Fusiform function in children with an ASD is a matter of "who". *Biol. Psychiatry* 64, 552.

Pierce, K., and Schreibman, L. (1995). Increasing complex social behaviours in children with autism: effects of peer-implemented pivotal response training. *J. Appl. Behav. Anal.* 28, 285–295.

Piven, J., and Palmer, P. (1997). Cognitive deficits in parents from multiple-incidence autism families. *J. Child Psychol. Psychiatry* 38, 1011–1021.

Piven, J., Palmer, P., Landa, R., Santangelo, S., Jacobi, D., and Childress, D. (1997). Personality and language characteristics in parents from multiple-incidence autism families. *Am. J. Med. Genet.* 74, 398–411.

Preston, D., and Carter, M. (2009). A review of the efficacy of the picture exchange communication system intervention. *J. Autism Dev. Disord.* 39, 1471–1486.

Provost, B., Lopez, B. R., and Heimerl, S. (2007). A comparison of motor delays in young children: autism spectrum disorder, developmental delay, and developmental concerns. *J. Autism Dev. Disord.* 37, 321–328.

Pugh, K. R., Mencl, W. E., Jenner, A. R., Katz, L., Frost, S. J., Lee, J. R., et al. (2001). Neurobiological studies of reading and reading disability. *J. Commun. Disord.* 34, 479–492.

Ritvo, E. R., Jorde, L. B., Mason-Brothers, A., Freeman, B. J., Pingree, C., Jones, M. B., et al. (1989). The UCLA-University of Utah epidemiologic survey of autism: recurrence risk estimates and genetic counselling. *Am. J. Psychiatry* 146, 1032–1036.

Rizzolatti, G., and Craighero, L. (2004). The mirror-neuron system. *Annu. Rev. Neurosci.* 27, 169–192.

Rizzolatti, G., Fadiga, L., Fogassi, L., and Gallese, V. (1996). Premotor cortex and the recognition of motor actions. *Cogn. Brain Res.* 3, 131–141.

Rogers, S. J. (2009). What are infant siblings teaching us about autism in infancy? *Autism Res.* 2, 125–137.

Rogers, S. J., Bennetto, L., McEvoy, R., and Pennington, B. F. (1996). Imitation and pantomime in high-functioning adolescents with autism spectrum disorders. *Child Dev.* 67, 2060–2073.

Rogers, S. J., and Dawson, G. (2009a). *Play and Engagement in Early Autism: Early Start Denver Model.*

Vol. I, The treatment. New York, NY: Guilford Press.

Rogers, S. J., and Dawson, G. (2009b). *Play and Engagement in Early Autism. Early Start Denver Model.* Vol. II, The curriculum. New York, NY: Guilford Press.

Rogers, S. J., Estes, A., Lord, C., Vismara, L., Winter, J., Fitzpatrick, A., et al. (2012). Effects of a brief Early Start Denver Model (ESDM)–based parent intervention on toddlers at risk for autism spectrum disorders: a randomized controlled trial. *J. Am. Acad. Child Adolesc. Psychiatry* 51, 1052–1065.

Rogers, S. J., Hall, T., Osaki, D., Reaven, J., and Herbison, J. (2000). "A comprehensive, integrated, educational approach to young children with autism and their families," in *Preschool Education Programs for Children with Autism,* 2nd Edn., eds S. L. Harris and J. S. Handleman (Austin, TX: Pro-Ed), 95–134.

Rogers, S. J., Hayden, D., Hepburn, S., Charlifue-Smith, R., Hall, T., and Hayes, A. (2006). Teaching young nonverbal children with autism useful speech: a pilot study of the Denver Model and PROMPT interventions. *J. Autism Dev. Disord.* 36, 1007–1024.

Rogers, S. J., Hepburn, S. L., Stackhouse, T., and Wehner, E. (2003). Imitation performance in toddlers with autism and those with other developmental disorders. *J. Child Psychol. Psychiatry* 44, 763–781.

Rossi, S., Hallett, M., Rossini, P. M., and Pascual-Leone, A. (2009). Safety, ethical considerations, and application guidelines for the use of transcranial magnetic stimulation in clinical practice and research. *Clin. Neurophysiol.* 120, 2008–2039.

Sanchez, C. E., Richards, J. E., and Almli, C. R. (2012). Age-specific MRI templates for pediatric neuroimaging. *Dev. Neuropsychol.* 37, 379–399.

Schepis, M. M., Reid, D. H., Fitzgerald, J. R., Faw, G. D., van den Pol, R. A., and Welty, P. A. (1982). A program for increasing manual signing by autistic and profoundly retarded youth within the daily environment. *J. Appl. Behav. Anal.* 15, 363–379.

Schneider, H. D., and Hopp, J. P. (2011). The use of the Bilingual Aphasia Test for assessment and transcranial direct current stimulation to modulate language acquisition in minimally verbal children with autism. *Clin. Linguist. Phon.* 25, 640–654.

Schwartz, I. S., Garfinkle, A. N., and Bauer, J. (1998). The picture exchange communication system: communicative outcomes for young children with disabilities. *Top. Early Child. Spec. Educ.* 18, 144–159.

Schwartz, J. B., and Nye, C. (2006). A systematic review, synthesis, and evaluation of the evidence for teaching sign language to children with autism. *EBP Briefs* 1, 1–17.

Seal, B. C., and Bonvillian, J. D. (1997). Sign language and motor functioning in students with autistic disorder. *J. Autism Dev. Disord.* 27, 437–466.

Shore, C., Bates, E., Bretherton, I., Beeghly, M., and O'Connell, B. (1990). "Vocal and gestural symbols: similarities and differences from 13 to 28 months," in *From Gesture to Language in Hearing and Deaf Children,* eds V. Volterra and C. Erting (New York, NY: Springer-Verlag), 79–91.

Smith, C. J., Lang, C. M., Kryzak, L., Reichenberg, A., Hollander, E., and Silverman, J. M. (2009). Familial associations of intense preoccupations, an empirical factor of the restricted, repetitive behaviors and interests domain of autism. *J. Child Psychol. Psychiatry* 50, 982–990.

Sokhadze, E. M., El-Baz, A., Baruth, J., Mathai, G., Sears, L., and Casanova, M. F. (2009). Effects of low frequency repetitive transcranial magnetic stimulation (rTMS) on gamma frequency oscillations and event-related potentials during processing of illusory figures in autism. *J. Autism Dev. Disord.* 39, 619–634.

Southgate, V., and Hamilton, A. F. D. C. (2008). Unbroken mirrors: challenging a theory of autism. *Trends Cogn. Sci.* 12, 225–229.

Sowa, M., and Meulenbroek, R. (2012). Effects of physical exercise on autism spectrum disorders: a meta-analysis. *Res. Autism Spectr. Disord.* 6, 46–57.

Square, P. A., Chumpelik (Hayden), D. A., Morningstar, D., and Adams, S. G. (1986). "Efficacy of the PROMPT system of therapy for the treatment of apraxia of speech: a follow-up investigation," in *Clinical Aphasiology: Conference Proceedings,* ed R. H. Brookshire (Minneapolis, MN: BBK Publishers), 221–226.

Square, P. A., Goshulak, D., Bose, A., and Hayden, D., (2000). "The effects of articulatory subsystem treatment for developmental neuromotor speech disorders," in *Paper Presented at the Tenth Biennial Conference on Motor Speech Disorders and Speech Motor Control* (San Antonio, TX).

Stahmer, A. C. (1995). Teaching symbolic play skills to children with autism using pivotal response training. *J. Autism Dev. Disord.* 25, 123–141.

Stahmer, A. C., Collings, N. M., and Palinkas, L. A. (2005). Early intervention practices for children with autism: descriptions from community providers. *Focus Autism Other Dev. Disabil.* 20, 66–79.

Stahmer, A. C., Schreibman, L., and Cunningham, A. B. (2011). Toward a technology of treatment individualization for young children with autism spectrum disorders. *Brain Res.* 1380, 229–239.

Stieglitz Ham, H., Corley, M., Rajendran, G., Carletta, J., and Swanson, S. (2008). Brief report: imitation of meaningless gestures in individuals with Asperger syndrome and High-Functioning Autism. *J. Autism Dev. Disord.* 38, 569–573.

Stone, W. L., Ousley, O. Y., and Littleford, C. D. (1997). Motor imitation in young children with autism: what's the object? *J. Abnorm. Child Psychol.* 25, 475–485.

Stone, W. L., and Yoder, P. J. (2001). Predicting spoken language level in children with autism spectrum disorders. *Autism* 5, 341–361.

Stull, S., Edkins, E. C., Krause, M., McGavin, G., Brand, L. H., and Webster, C. D. (1980). "Individual differences in the acquisition of sign language by severely communicatively-impaired children," in *Autism: New Directions in Research and Education* eds C. D. Webster, M. M., Konstantareas, J. Oxman, and J. E. Mack (Oxford: Pergamon Press), 202–211.

Sulzer-Azaroff, B., Hoffman, A. O., Horton, C. B., Bondy, A., and Front, L. (2009). The Picture Exchange Communication System (PECS): what do the data say? *Focus Autism Other Dev. Disabil.* 24, 89–103.

Sundberg, M. L., Endicott, K., and Eigenheer, P. (2000). Using intraverbal prompts to establish tacts for children with autism. *Anal Verbal Behav.* 17, 89.

Tomasello, M., and Farrar, M. J. (1986). Joint attention and early language. *Child Dev.* 57, 1454–1463.

Travis, J., and Geiger, M. (2010). The effectiveness of the Picture Exchange Communication System (PECS) for children with autism spectrum disorder (ASD): a South African pilot study. *Child Lang. Teach. Ther.* 26, 39–59.

Uzgiris, I. C. (1991). "The social context of infant imitation," in *Social Influences and Socialization in Infancy,* eds M. Lewis and S. Feinman (New York, NY: Plenum Press), 215–251.

Vanvuchelen, M., Roeyers, H., and De Weerdt, W. (2007). Nature of motor imitation problems in school-aged males with autism: how congruent are the error types? *Dev. Med. Child Neurol.* 49, 6–12.

Vanvuchelen, M., Roeyers, H., and De Weerdt, W. (2010). Imitation assessment and its utility to the diagnosis of autism: evidence from consecutive clinical preschool referrals for suspected autism. *J. Autism Dev. Disord.* 41, 484–496.

Vismara, L. A., Colombi, C., and Rogers, S. J. (2009). Can one hour per week of therapy lead to lasting changes in young children with autism? *Autism* 13, 93–115.

Vismara, L. A., and Lyons, G. L. (2007). Using perseverative interests to elicit joint attention behaviors in young children with autism: theoretical and clinical implications to understanding motivation. *J. Pos. Beh. Interv* 9, 214–228.

Vismara, L. A., and Rogers, S. J. (2008). The early start denver model a case study of an innovative practice. *J. Early Interv.* 31, 91–108.

Volterra, V., Bates, E., Benigni, L., Bretherton, I., and Camaioni, L., (1979). "First words in language and action: a qualitative look," in *The Emergence of Symbols: Cognition and Communication in Infancy,* eds E. Bates, L. Benigni, I. Bretherton, L. Camaioni, and V. Volterra (New York, NY: Academic Press), 141–222.

Voos, A. C., Pelphrey, K. A., Tirrell, J., Bolling, D. Z., Vander Wyk, B. C., Kaiser, M. D., et al. (2012). Neural mechanisms of improvements in social motivation after pivotal response treatment: two case studies. *J. Autism Dev. Disord.* 43, 1–10.

Walter, G., Tormos, J. M., Israel, J. A., and Pascual-Leone, A. (2001). Transcranial magnetic stimulation in young persons: a review of known cases. *J. Child Adolesc. Psychopharmacol.* 11, 69–75.

Wan, C. Y., Bazen, L., Baars, R., Libenson, A., Zipse, L., Zuk, J., et al. (2011). Auditory-motor mapping training as an intervention to facilitate speech output in nonverbal children with autism: a proof of concept study. *PLoS ONE* 6:e25505. doi: 10.1371/journal.pone.0025505

Wan, C. Y., Demaine, K., Zipse, L., Norton, A., and Schlaug, G. (2010a). From music making to speaking: engaging the mirror neuron system in autism. *Brain Res. Bull.* 82, 161–168.

Wan, C. Y., Rüber, T., Hohmann, A., and Schlaug, G. (2010b). The therapeutic effects of singing in neurological disorders. *Music Percept.* 27, 287–295.

Wan, C. Y., Zipse, L., Norton, A., Demaine, K., Baars, R., Zuk, J., et al. (2009). "Using an auditory-motor mapping therapy to improve expressive language abilities in nonverbal children with autism," in *Poster Session Presented at the 8th Annual Auditory Perception, Cognition, and Action Meeting* (Boston, MA).

Ward, R., Leitao, S., and Strauss, G. (2009a). The effectiveness of prompt therapy for children with cerebral palsy. *Dev. Med. Child Neurol.* 51, 76.

Ward, R., Leitao, S., and Strauss, G. (2009b). "The effectiveness of prompt therapy for children with cerebral palsy," in *As presented at AACPDM: American Academy of Cerebral Palsy and Developmental Medicine Annual Meeting* (Scottsdale, AZ).

Warren, Z., McPheeters, M. L., Sathe, N., Foss-Feig, J. H., Glasser, A., and Veenstra-VanderWeele, J. (2011). A systematic review of early intensive intervention for autism spectrum disorders. *Pediatrics* 127, e1303–e1311.

Wassermann, E. M. (1998). Risk and safety of repetitive transcranial magnetic stimulation: report and suggested guidelines from the International Workshop on the Safety of Repetitive Transcranial Magnetic Stimulation, June 5–7, 1996. *Electroencephalogr. Clin. Neurophysiol.* 108, 1–16.

Webb, T. (2000). Can children with autism and severe learning disabilities be taught to communicate spontaneously and effectively using the picture exchange communication system? *Good Autism Pract.* 1, 29–42.

Webster, C., McPherson, H., Sloman, L., Evans, M., and Kuchar, E. (1973). Communication with an autistic boy by gestures. *J. Autism Child. Schizophr.* 3, 337–346.

Williams, J. H. G., Whiten, A., and Singh, T. (2004). A systematic review of action imitation in autistic spectrum disorder. *J. Autism Dev. Disord.* 34, 285–299.

Williams, J. H. G., Whiten, A., Suddendorf, T., and Perrett, D. I. (2001). Imitation, mirror neurons and autism. *Neurosci. Biobehav. Rev.* 25, 287–295.

Windsor, J., Benigno, J. P., Wing, C. A., Carroll, P. J., Koga, S. F., Nelson, C. A., et al. (2011). Effect of foster care on young children's language learning. *Child Dev.* 82, 1040–1046.

Winhuisen, L., Thiel, A., Schumacher, B., Kessler, J., Rudolf, J., Haupt, W. F., et al. (2007). The right inferior frontal gyrus and poststroke aphasia: a follow-up investigation. *Stroke* 38, 1286–1292.

Yirmiya, N., and Charman, T. (2010). The prodrome of autism: early behavioural and biological signs, regression, peri- and post-natal development and genetics. *J. Child Psychol. Psychiatry* 51, 432–458.

Yirmiya, N., Gamliel, I., Pilowsky, T., Feldman, R., Baron-Cohen, S., and Sigman, M. (2006). The development of siblings of children with autism at 4 and 14 months: social engagement, communication, and cognition. *J. Child Psychol. Psychiatry* 47, 511–523.

Yoder, P., and Layton, T. (1988). Speech following sign language training in autistic children with minimal verbal language. *J. Autism Dev. Disord.* 18, 217–229.

Yoder, P. J., and Lieberman, R. G. (2010). Brief report: randomized test of the efficacy of Picture Exchange Communication System on highly generalized picture exchanges in children with ASD. *J. Autism Dev. Disord.* 40, 629–632.

Yoder, P., and Stone, W. L. (2006a). A randomized comparison of the effect of two prelinguistic communication interventions on the acquisition of spoken communication in preschoolers with ASD. *J. Speech Lang. Hear. Res.* 49, 698–711.

Yoder, P., and Stone, W. L. (2006b). Randomized comparison of two communication interventions for preschoolers with autism spectrum disorders. *J. Consult. Clin. Psychol.* 74, 426–435.

Yoder, P., Stone, W. L., Walden, T., and Malesa, E. (2009). Predicting social impairment and ASD diagnosis in younger siblings of children with autism spectrum disorder. *J. Autism Dev. Disord.* 39, 1381–1391.

Conflict of Interest Statement: The authors declare that the research was conducted in the absence of any commercial or financial relationships that could be construed as a potential conflict of interest.

3

An exploration of sensory and movement differences from the perspective of individuals with autism

Jodi Robledo[1]*, Anne M. Donnellan[2] and Karen Strandt-Conroy[3]

[1] School of Education, California State University San Marcos, San Marcos, CA, USA
[2] School of Leadership and Education Sciences, University of San Diego, San Diego, CA, USA
[3] Parkview School District, Orfordville, WI, USA

Edited by:
Elizabeth B. Torres, Rutgers University, USA

Reviewed by:
Antonio Pereira, Federal University of Rio Grande do Norte, Brazil
Gary W. LaVigna, Institute for Applied Behavior Analysis, USA
Trevor McDonald, Education Associates Inc., USA

***Correspondence:**
Jodi Robledo, School of Education, California State University San Marcos, 333 S. Twin Oaks Valley Road, San Marcos, CA 92096-0001, USA.
e-mail: jrobledo@csusm.edu

Parents, teachers, and people who themselves experience sensory and movement differences have consistently reported disturbances of sensation and movement associated with autism. Our review of the literature has revealed both historical and recent references to and research about sensory and movement difference characteristics and symptoms for individuals with autism. What is notably infrequent in this literature, however, is research that highlights the perspective of the individual with autism. If we wish to truly understand the experience of sensory and movement differences for individuals with autism, we must explore their experiences and perspectives. This study presents a qualitative analysis of more than 40 h in-depth inquiry into the lives of five individuals with the autism label. Data were sorted into six categories: perception, action, posture, emotion, communication, and cognition. The insights into sensory and movement differences and autism offered by these individuals was illuminating. We found that the data strongly supported the presence of disruption of organization and regulation of sensory and movement differences in the lived experience of these participants with autism. The present data suggests that in autism this disruption of organization and regulation is amplified in terms of quantity, quality, intensity, and may affect everyday life. These data contribute to a more expansive view of autism that incorporates the possibility that autism is a disorder that affects motor planning, behavior, communication, the sensory motor system, and the dynamic interaction of all of these.

Keywords: autism, sensory and movement differences, first-person accounts

INTRODUCTION

The history of autism reflects the prevailing understandings and misunderstandings about human development and communication that characterized professional writings in psychology, psychiatry, and special education over the past 60 years. In the absence of a clear understanding of cause or symptoms, many definitions and theories about autism have been developed. Most often the descriptions offered by the professionals pay little attention to the experience of people who live with autism.

Seventy years after Leo Kanner's original paper on autism (1943), the orthodox "scientific" thinking is that autism is a separate psychiatric disorder, reliably distinguishable from other human conditions, likely the result of absence or error in or affecting the social brain. Moreover, the abilities of the person with autism can be reliably and validly determined through our psychological and behavioral assessments (e.g., *DSM-IV-TR*, American Psychiatric Association, 2000). This view draws on a dualistic tradition in psychology and psychiatry that separates mind and body (seeRogers, 1990; Damasio, 1994). It leaves out a long and rich history of writing and research which suggests that individuals with a variety of disabilities or disorders may, in fact, be experiencing differences in their sensory, motor, perceptual, and other systems, which confound and confuse the picture (e.g., Kahlbaum, 1874/1973; Bleuler, 1911/1950). A series of papers by Donnellan, Leary, and Hill spells out in detail the effect this dichotomy has had on our understanding of autism (Hill and Leary, 1993; Donnellan and Leary, 1995; Leary and Hill, 1996; Leary and Donnellan, 2012). They posit that assuming mind can be studied separately from body ignores the importance of felt experience on the development of social interaction, communication, and behavior. Even in the more recent research that studies the body (motor differences) and autism, there is little understanding of the potential affect of these differences on social, communication, and behavioral functioning (see Leary and Donnellan, 2012[1]).

Leary et al. (1999, as cited in Donnellan, 2006) have defined a sensory and movement difference as a difference, interference or shift in the efficient, effective utilization and integration of movement; a disruption in the organization and regulation of perception, action, posture, language, speech, thought, emotion, and/or memory. Typically, the word "movement" refers to observable actions, such as posture, muscle tone, head and eye movements, facial expression, vocalization, speech, whole body movements, reaching, gesturing, running, and walking. Here, the

[1] For additional references of sensory and movement literature see Leary and Hill, 2012, pp.101–115

use of the word movement is consistent with research that considers internal mental processes of sensory perceptions (touch, taste, smell, vision, hearing, and proprioception), language, thoughts, and emotions as aspects of human movement.

A review of published first-hand accounts of autism and research studies with participants with autism revealed numerous references to sensory and movement differences in the areas of perception, action, emotion, communication, and cognition. Each area will be briefly described below.

Perceptual differences, such as differences in hearing, vision, smell, taste, proprioception, and synesthesia were all noted in numerous published first-hand accounts (e.g., White and White, 1987; Cesaroni, 1990; Barron and Barron, 1992; Grandin, 1992, 1995; Williams, 1992, 1994; McKean, 1994; Blackman, 1999; Mukhopadhyay, 2000; Rubin, in Biklen, 2005). Tito Mukhopadhyay described his perceptual experiences as a *"fragmented world perceived through isolated sense organs"* (2000, p. 74). Jim, a research participant in a study conducted by Cesaroni indicated, *"Sometimes I know that something is coming in somewhere, but I can't tell right away what sense it's coming through"* (Cesaroni, 1990, p. 74).

First-hand accounts of autism also revealed challenges with controlling, executing, and combining action or movements (Volkmar and Cohen, 1985; Cesaroni, 1990; Grandin, 1992; Williams, 1992, 1994; McKean, 1994; Hale and Hale, 1999; Mukhopadhyay, 2000; Frugone, in Biklen, 2005; Mukhopadhyay, in Biklen, 2005; Goddard and Goddard, 2012). Alberto Frugone described his challenges with action and movements: *"Right from the beginning of an action, I was conscious of my inability to access motor planning and I was lost in an unacceptable motor silence"* (Frugone, in Biklen, 2005, p. 190). Charles Hale described his difficulty with actions and movements:

> *I think my movement disorder is most apparent in the fact that I am unable to respond to someone or something, when my intelligence would tell me to respond in an appropriate manner. For instance, when I should be smiling, sometimes I know that I am not smiling but may be even frowning. This causes me a great deal of pain and makes me look as though I am not comprehending when, in fact, I am crying to respond in an appropriate manner. (Hale and Hale, 1999, p. 32)*

First-hand accounts of autism described challenges with regulating emotions (e.g., Cesaroni, 1990; Barron and Barron, 1992; Jolliffe et al., 1992; Williams, 1992, 1994). Sean Barron described that he could not control his emotions and he was terrified of his "feelings and temperament" (Barron and Barron, 1992, p. 118). Many first-hand accounts described stressful feelings and anxiety as predominant emotions. Another individual with autism, Therese Jolliffe commented: *"It [stress] occurs at any time, but always when I know I have to go somewhere stressful. Sometimes the pain is so bad that my whole body becomes stiff and then I am unable to move."* (Jolliffe et al., 1992, p. 14)

Communication challenges were also noted in numerous first-hand accounts of autism (e.g., Cesaroni, 1990; Barron and Barron, 1992; Jolliffe et al., 1992; Williams, 1992, 1994; Grandin, 1995; Blackman, 1999; Mukhopadhyay, 2000; Rubin, in Biklen, 2005; Goddard and Goddard, 2012). Sue Rubin, a non-verbal individual with autism who independently uses augmentative and alternative communication described her difficulty with initiating speech: *"I rarely find the strength in my autistic capabilities to initiate a conversation. There may be times where something pertinent eats away at me until either I find a moment where my body and mind coincide and I am able to go get a device to converse with."* (Rubin, in Biklen, 2005, p. 85)

Individuals with autism in first-hand accounts also described differences in cognition (e.g., Jolliffe et al., 1992; Williams, 1994; Grandin, 1995). Temple Grandin (1995) outlined her thought process in her book entitled "*Thinking in Pictures*." She explained that she translates spoken and written words into *"full-color movies, complete with sound, which run like a VCR tape"* (p. 19) in her head. She labeled this technique as visual thinking. To create new images, she takes parts of *"video memories"* (p. 21). To recall a memory she replays various video memory tapes until she finds the information she is searching for. Her videos, however, sometimes trigger a series of free associations. Sometimes certain words can also trigger the incorrect association and she can look for an incorrect video, which she says leads to misunderstandings.

It is essential that the exploration of autism include sensory and movement differences and involve the people who experience autism first-hand for a number of reasons: (1) professionals investigating autism from a perspective that separates mind and body may have overlooked sensory and movement differences, and/or their possible effect on behavior; (2) published first-hand accounts of autism suggest that this is a fruitful area for investigation; (3) in studying autism we need to elicit information from one of the most valuable resources—people with the label of autism.

Most of the disciplines studying autism have investigated autism through clinical research looking at significant group differences. This pursuit has brought valuable information but, in addition, has brought about confusing, confounding, and contradictory results. Researchers are beginning to explore the experience of autism through a critical disability perspective by including the perspective and experience of people with autism (e.g., Strandt-Conroy, 1999; Broderick and Kasa-Hendrickson, 2001; Biklen, 2005; Robledo and Donnellan, 2008). Biklen (2005) summarized the importance of qualitative methodologies in a field that has been dominated by positivist research:

> *In one central way, their accounts diverge dramatically from the prevailing clinical literature ... Their richness suggests the danger of privileging other forms of research about autism as more deserving of authority or as being in some way uncontestable. Their forcefulness and consistency should signal clinical researchers to question every assumption brought to the topic of autism. (p. 281)*

MATERIALS AND METHODS

A qualitative research design was utilized in this study to gather data aimed at describing the experience of sensory and movement differences in individuals with autism. Qualitative designs foster interpretations and descriptions that allow understanding of the concept being studied (Ferguson et al., 1992). Further, qualitative research attempts to create a naturalistic paradigm in which the researcher is able to understand an individual's experiences.

PARTICIPANTS

Five people with the diagnosis of autism participated in this study. It was anticipated that obtaining data from this population would be challenging due to the well-documented social, communication, and behavioral challenges experienced by many people with this diagnosis. For that reason, the researchers used a variety of methods to obtain meaningful data. These methods included in-depth interviews, questionnaires, and participant observations. All aspects of this study conformed to the Institutional Review procedures of the School of Education, University of Wisconsin-Madison.

There were five-independently communicating participants in this study. Each person was sought through a number of associations involving people with autism. They were each contacted regarding the research and depending on their personal preferences, were provided with background information regarding their involvement. Subsequent to this, informed consent was sought. At the outset of the study, participants were asked to provide information regarding his or her autism, including Asperger's syndrome or autism spectrum disorder. Confirmation of diagnosis was obtained from a review of past records, interviews with family or involved staff members, and/or direct observation of the individual. Although we intended to use pseudonyms, all participants asked that their real names be used. For purposes of this paper, only the participant's first names were used. A brief description of each participant at the time of data collection follows.

Geneva was a 57-years-old female. At age six, Geneva was diagnosed with encephalitis. Early in Geneva's educational experience she received little to no help in school despite the fact that, she was having difficulties. In third grade, school staff investigated Geneva's learning problems. Testing was done but no assistance was given to her. It was not until junior college that the discrepancy between Geneva's receptive and expressive language skills was discovered. She was tested and given a list of her learning disabilities. Subsequent diagnostic labels include: Aphasia, Dyslexia, Sequential Learning Deficit, and Epstein Barr Syndrome. Later in life she went to doctors including Dr. B. J. Freeman at the University of California Los Angeles's Neuropsychiatric Institute, and was diagnosed with a form of high functioning autism known as Asperger's syndrome.

Jean Paul was a 29-years-old male. He was diagnosed with autism and mental retardation at age 3. Professionals recommended to his mother that he be placed in an institution while she underwent psychotherapy. During his early days in school, an attempt was made to place Jean Paul in a program designed for the cognitively disabled. Jean Paul's mother did not listen to the medical or school personal. Instead she worked very hard to provide her son with the needed resources. As a result of Jean Paul's and his mother's hard work, Jean Paul has two college degrees.

Kathy-Xania was a 33-years-old female. Kathy-Xania remembered experiencing information and her surroundings differently from an early age. In her early childhood, her father, a physician, sought out advice but disregarded many of the explanations of autism given to him during the late 1960s and early 1970s. Kathy-Xania was appreciative of that fact and said that as a result of her father's actions, she was educated with her non-disabled peers. Kathy-Xania attended college and earned her bachelor's degree. She is divorced from her husband and lives independently.

Barbara was a 40-years-old female. At an early age Barbara was placed in a psychiatric institution. At age 17 she became an outpatient of the institution and lived with a foster family for 10 years. During that time she attended 1 year of college. She decided to leave college and began working in the kitchen of a nursing home. She held the job for 22 years despite her dislike of the job. She lives independently receiving support from her siblings, especially her sister, Ruth.

Matt was a 19-years-old male. Matt's parents were given a diagnosis of autism when Matt was 18 months old. His mother was very supportive of Matt and advocated for his inclusion in school and the community. Matt received special education support throughout his school years. During high school, Matt attended all regular education classes. Matt is extremely skilled in mathematics and subsequent to his participation in this study he received a bachelor's degree in mathematics from a major university.

INSTRUMENTATION AND DATA COLLECTION

Each participant was asked to identify their preferred method(s) for data collection (i.e., face-to-face or phone interviews, completion of written questionnaire, and/or participant observation). In order to optimize their participation in the interview process, those interested in completing interviews were given a choice as to how, where and when they would like to be interviewed. Additionally, any accommodations an individual needed to make the interview more productive were provided. One such example included the option to respond to oral questions in writing.

Depending on individual preference and the extent to which individuals were able to participate in extended interviews, multiple interviews of varying length and format were completed. While no set number of interviews was required of participants, the total time taken to complete interviews was in the vicinity of 40-h. Prior to beginning each interview, the researcher conducting the interview talked informally with the participants to create rapport.

If the participant wished to complete a questionnaire packet, he/she was asked to select a method of sharing information (e.g., E-mail, U.S. Mail or telephone). Also, any accommodations needed to make the questionnaire more productive were provided and included the option for further oral explanation of questionnaires or the completion of portions of the questionnaire during telephone conversations.

In addition to the use of interviews and questionnaires, participant-produced data (e.g., drawings, writings) were reviewed and observations of four of the five participants who selected face-to-face interviews were completed.

The researchers approached the interviews from a primary principle of qualitative interviewing by providing "a framework within which respondents can express their own understandings in their own terms" (Patton, 2002, p. 205). In order to provide a framework, a minimally structured interview format was used.

A variety of predetermined questions were derived from the professional literature and published first-hand accounts of autism. These questions were used as a guide rather than a script during the interview. Possible interview questions were sorted into nine categories: hearing, vision, touch, action, posture, emotion, communication, cognition, and general. Examples of interview questions included requests for information on the extent to which elements in the environment provoked an adverse response in the individual, whether movement or control of the body was problematic, and what accommodations assisted the individual in these situations. Upon completion of questions in a specific topic area, participants were asked if they had any additional information or examples they wished to add. Information provided by the participants was reviewed after each interview and was used to develop structured questions for subsequent interviews.

Four of the five participants stated that the phone interview was a better format because it allowed them to be more active in the dialog. One participant described that they were best able to respond to questions during a phone interview if they were also taking a bath. To ensure adequate information from the participants they were asked to think about certain topics ahead of time and additional response time was offered.

A questionnaire written at approximately the 6th grade level was created using the professional literature and published first-hand accounts of autism. Vignettes incorporating the themes introduced earlier were presented in the questionnaire packet and participants were asked about the extent to which their own experiences were similar to or different from those in the vignettes. After each vignette additional questions were asked. Questionnaires included short answers, multiple choice, and fill-in the blank answers.

Along with the audiotaping of each of the interviews, memos and field notes during and after each interview were completed (Lincoln and Guba, 1985). Memos involved the researchers in writing ideas, thoughts, assumptions, concepts, and relationships between concepts that emerged while interviewing, coding the data, consulting with others, or contemplating what had occurred during data collection (Strauss, 1987).

The researchers reviewed portions of dairies, newspaper articles, drawings, poems, and photographs from three of the five participants. Any artifact or documentation (i.e., diaries, drawings) that the participant wished to share with the researchers was used for document and artifact review. Memos were written up about each document. These artifacts assisted the researchers with gaining an in-depth and more complete understanding of the participant.

DATA ANALYSIS

Data analysis occurred throughout the data collection phase using the constant comparative approach (Charmaz, 2000, 2006). This allowed the researchers to collect data, analyze it, and then collect additional data. Information was shared with participants to confirm interpretations of the data. As the participant data was collected, all the interview transcripts were analyzed and themes or categories were changed or expanded upon. For example, the themes "memory" and "thoughts" were combined into the category of "cognition." Initially, data were coded using two descriptors that were typed before each excerpt. The first descriptor was the area (e.g., perception/vision). The second descriptor was a specific attribute (e.g., difficulty integrating visual stimuli). After these two descriptors had been assigned, data were sorted into categories. These excerpts were again read and changes were made to the categories and codes. After all the data were collected from the participants, all interview transcripts, questionnaires, coded data, and researcher notes including notes from the document review, and notes from listening to the audio tapes were re-analyzed to confirm themes/categories and codes.

RESULTS

For clarity of presentation data will be presented in six categories: perception, action, posture, emotion, communication, and cognition. It is important for the reader to note that there is a dynamic interaction among these areas as no category operates in isolation.

PERCEPTION

Sensory and perceptual differences related to hearing, vision, and touch were common in the experiences of participants. Challenges with proprioception were also described; however, these findings will be presented in the "posture" category. Some participants indicated differences in smell and taste, but they will not be reported here as differences in hearing, vision, and touch yielded the greatest amount of data.

Hearing

Auditory differences were noted in the experiences of participants. For some, certain sounds evoked physical pain and anxiety. For others, sounds elicited emotions not necessarily related to the present context. Some participants indicated differences in their ability to selectively focus on auditory input.

Jean Paul indicated that ambulances, airplanes taking off, and loud screechy noises are problematic, creating a sense of "*having the jitters.*" Similarly, Matt explained his painful reaction to certain sounds:

> *Especially things like gunshots, loud motors, and brass bands. My mom took me through a drive-thru car wash once when I was in grade school and I was terrified. The brushes sounded to me like the sound of intense machine gun fire, but I could not communicate well enough to explain why I got so upset.*

Barbara discussed how sounds triggered her emotions. She said, "*It seems like there is something in my brain that certain noises trigger my emotions the way pain does.*" She described how the sound of a crying baby could "*agitate and anger*" her. Barbara further explained:

> *Some sounds make me feel really bad in the pit of my stomach. I feel angry and aggressive and out of control; feeling aggressive towards someone who doesn't deserve it makes me feel guilty. I get very agitated. I may yell at people. My behavior gets out of control. It can*

ruin my mood sometimes for days. The effects of the noise last much longer than the noise itself.

She expressed concerns during a phone interview as the researcher conducting the interview had recently had a baby. Barbara was very fearful that she would hear the baby over the phone. She explained, "*If you really understand how I feel about babies, you'd move heaven and earth to keep that baby away from me.*"

Through her questionnaire she indicated that these emotional reactions caused her problems including:

a) I complain a lot and then get criticized a lot; b) If I know I can't get away from bad sounds I get irritated and depressed; c) If I anticipate a situation where there may be bad sounds, I get depressed, feel helpless; d) sometimes a loud sound will provoke me to tears.

Whenever Barbara is in public she wears earplugs and a radio headset. She said, "*this can provide competing sound which may be distracting so I won't focus so much on the bad sounds.*" She also indicated that she was appreciative for those who allow her to leave noisy situations: "*It really helps when other people understand. I feel guilty mostly because of others' reactions. It's painful to be criticized.*"

Kathy-Xania noted that she experienced times when sounds faded in and out making it difficult at times to focus on auditory input. She hypothesized that when there was too much "*static*" in the sound it was more likely to fade in and out. Kathy-Xania, noted:

It is hard to hear when a person has static in their voice. I don't like it when babies cry. I don't like static. I don't like high-pitched noise. I don't like hearing gunshots. I do hear gunshots. I don't like gunshots, I don't like kids screaming. I don't like staticky voices. I don't like some of those old women who have those horrible voices.

Vision

Participants described several different types of visual differences: unique interactions with colors, stimulation or pain caused by visual stimuli, different responses to lighting, and challenges with eye contact.

Primarily, participants spoke about negative reactions to visual stimuli. Barbara, however, described that at times she greatly enjoyed bright lights and certain combination of colors. For example she described enjoying looking at traffic lights, "*if they are put together right; modern ones disappoint me.*" Barbara also indicated she had a strong need for visual stimulation:

In other words, I crave light and colors. I always feel my best on a bright, sunny day. I like rooms to be brightly lit and if you saw my apartment, you'd see that I papered the walls with all kinds of pictures. I turned an art gallery out of it.

Kathy-Xania also spoke about her need for bright light. She indicated that she has been told that she experiences seasonal-affective disorder. She described that a few days of cloudy weather affects her adversely, leaving her feeling sad and depressed. She explained, "*I can feel my body chemistry change when there is sun.*"

Jean Paul, Matt, and Geneva spoke about negative and painful reactions to certain visual stimuli. Geneva said, "*There are certain types of light I cannot tolerate—they make me nervous. If I am in a hall and it is too bright, I can't handle it, I have to put a sun hat on.*" She also said she was not able to handle fluttering fluorescent lights because that type of light "*absolutely turns my stomach into knots. It does a trip on my nervous system.*" Even the sun can be problematic. Geneva explained that when she walks out the door on a bright day her eyes take up to 3 min to adjust:

Because it hits my head like a lightening bolt. I have to stand there with my eyes closed and hold on to something so I don't fall over because a lightening bolt goes through my head when the sun hits my head. Then I have to wait a minute and then slowly open my eyes.

Other lighting, such as strobe lights, wreak havoc on Geneva's emotions, nervous system, and perception which may lead her to feeling nauseous, dizzy and provoke panic attacks.

Challenges with eye contact also emerged from the data. Matt explained, "*It is painful for me to look people in the eye ... This lack of "eye contact" sometimes make people (especially teachers) think I'm not paying attention to them.*" Barbara explained that she avoided eye contact as well:

I can hear a person better if I don't look at their face. When somebody talks, I tend to turn my ear towards them, because I want to hear what they're saying.... Well, what I mean if I'm looking at them, it's kind of a mild distraction, because you know, if somebody is talking, I concentrate more on listening more than looking. So when I'm making an effort to listen, I'm not making an effort to look, so sometimes when I'm listening to somebody, I might look away from them, but I might turn my ear towards them.

At times, Barbara was able to make eye contact, yet it was atypical:

I feel that looking into someone's eyes is intrusive, like I'm staring at them. I have been criticized in the past for how I've looked at other people and about my facial expressions. I can do the right thing in the wrong way and not even know what it is that I'm doing wrong. If someone was doing something I was interested in, I might stare at them.

Touch

Participants described challenges with tactile input. Both hypo- and hyper- reactions to touch were described. Barbara described her hypersensitivity to fabric, sweat, and touch. She indicated that she does not wear any clothes that feel sticky or make her sweat. She only wears loose fitting clothes such as cotton or cotton polyester combinations. She also described having a sensitive scalp. Barbara recalled when she had long hair:

Hair was a big battle for me when I was growing up because you know how when your hair's long enough—it gets in the way, and even if you tied it back, the little fuzzies will work their way out

> *and tickle your face. But I'm talking about if there were tangles in it, and I pulled it. That would drive me nuts... I over react to painful stimuli.*

This reaction to painful stimuli was extremely problematic when it came to touching during medical procedures. As a child Barbara was very scared, over-sensitive and over-anxious about anything medical. She shared a story she had written about the experience.

Kathy-Xania explained her sense of touch as more hyposensitive. She said, *"I have a high pain tolerance, except around my mouth... I have a very high pain tolerance... I like deep pressure... I prefer deep pressure over light pressure."* Like Barbara, Kathy-Xania also had an aversion to sweat. She stated:

> *I just don't like sweat. It's like disgusting. It's wet and sticky... But my neck—especially the back of my neck where my hairline is. Yeah, I just don't like it and I don't usually get as hot as easily as other people. But I don't like sweat. I think it's because I don't like wet feeling and sweat is wet.*

Geneva explained that her sense of touch and pain is much different than others. She described that sometimes when she cut herself she most likely would not feel pain. She stated, *"I didn't feel the skin being pierced because I don't have normal feeling in my skin. I don't have normal sensitivity in my skin."* She further explained how some of her body was unresponsive to some touch while other parts of her body (e.g., the back of her neck) were very sensitive. She said that in *"some areas my sensory system I have deficits, in other areas I have super sensitivity. That goes back and forth."*

Geneva described avoiding touch from people she did not know well. She explained that if a person that, she had not seen touched her she would get *"scared out of my heebie jeebies—I will jump a foot in the air... Startled, heart pounding, panic attack."* Geneva said that there were certain clothes that she was not able to wear mostly because of the material used in making the garment. For example, she needed to wear cotton underwear rather than synthetic underwear. If she did not wear the cotton underwear she would sweat, itch, and break out in a rash.

ACTION

Participants revealed difficulties with controlling, executing, and combining movements. Most participants discussed difficulties controlling movements. Jean Paul described difficulty with holding his body still, particularly when he was nervous. Matthew spoke about difficulty controlling his actions, even basic day-to-day motor actions.

Barbara also discussed challenges with controlling her movements during times when she felt nervous, excited, or overloaded. She described, *"I had an automatic urge to touch my body—rub my thighs or my stomach and chest."* Barbara expressed that she became upset and felt criticized when others did not understand her challenges related to controlling her actions:

> *I want to stop doing anything that doesn't look normal. But if I am feeling really bad inside, I want people to see the distress signals for what they are. I want people to understand I don't want to hide the urges if I'm feeling really bad. I want people to let me be. I've had all kinds of people who thought they were helping me stop doing things. I have been endlessly criticized about how different I looked, criticized about all kinds of tiny differences in my behavior. There's a point where you say to hell with it, its impossible to please you people.... No one ever tried to really understand what it was like to be me.... I wish they had accepted some of my behaviors I didn't have any control over. You don't criticize people with cerebral palsy.*

Participants expressed challenges with execution of movement. Differences could result in problems with starting or stopping movements. Barbara discussed how she wished she had better coordination. Her difficulty and lack of coordination caused her frustration. Balance was also difficult for Barbara. Motor coordination was difficult for other participants.

Kathy-Xania had been told her movements were different. As she said, *"I was sitting on the floor and when I got up after looking at a couple of books, my friend said I got up like an animal does."* She said that she was aware that her movements were different, but she was not quite sure how her movements differed from others. One observation she made was that her lack of depth perception had a dramatic affect on her movements. She said sometimes when she needed to go up the steps she got down on all fours. She said she was able to execute the movement of walking up the stairs on two feet, but it was very challenging. For that reason when she was at home or was unable to execute the movement she might need to *"crawl"* up the steps.

Participants mentioned challenges around combining two or more movements or actions. Geneva said that she was able to combine two tasks but she would easily *"lose the rhythm."* She recalled the example of learning to dance:

> *I tried to learn a very simple line dance. I could not learn my footsteps and my hand movements at the same time. I had to teach my feet how to do it then stand still. I had to hold on to a rail, teach my feet their steps then lean against the wall with my feet out balancing me and learn my arm steps. Then hold on to the bar and learn my torso steps and then from there you learn what to do with the hips. Slowly, I turn the music on slow and I very, very, very slowly start the feet and very slowly add the hands then very, very slowly add the torso, etc. Everything has to be thought out, that is what is so annoying. There are just a very few things that I do two things at the same time without thinking them through as I am going.*

At times, Geneva needed to separate tasks out while other times combining was necessary. For example, *"If I am running and I look away from the sidewalk, I'll trip on the next thing on the sidewalk."*

POSTURES

The trouble that some individuals with autism have with action may be due in part to differences in postures. A few experiences from participants as they related to posture are briefly noted.

As a teenager, Barbara was told that she grinned and that others *"... didn't like my posture or how I sat at the dinner table. My body just never seemed to be in a position that was acceptable."* She explained that she did not choose her body postures rather than her postures were a result of the way her body positioned itself in space.

Other participants noted difficulties with proprioception and posture. Geneva, illustrated the difficulty in knowing where her body was in space. Geneva said not only was this *"a frustrating annoyance"* it could be life threatening as in the time *"where I almost died because I was drowning in a pool because I couldn't find up."* Geneva said that she was best able to focus on the task at hand when she had some body awareness. For example she was better able to think and communicate during the interview because she was sitting with her body supported in a recliner or the bathtub. This accommodation of the recliner or bathtub assisted her both physically and emotionally.

EMOTIONS

Participants discussed challenges with expressing, controlling, identifying, and/or changing emotions. In addition, many participants spoke about specific accommodations that allowed them to manage their emotions more effectively.

Participants varied in how they described their challenges with emotions. Most felt they had the most trouble with expressing emotions. Barbara described challenges with both expressing and controlling emotions:

> *I think I've had times where I wasn't able to express how I was feeling and sometimes it was hard to experience my feelings directly. And one of the biggest problems was that I tried to express how I felt and people just didn't understand, my feelings were just so much different than another person that they just simply disregarded it.*

She went on to say:

> *I had a problem with controlling my behavior. I did a lot of crying and a lot of complaining and I tried real hard to express my feelings to them, but people just didn't understand my feelings. I didn't have the same kind of feelings other people had.*

Kathy-Xania described a different experience with expressing emotions. She stated:

> *I don't cry easily. I feel it inside, but I don't always show it on the outside. I think I get affected by things very easily... With me, it's all in my face. Usually if anything happens, emotionally, it's usually—my head gets affected first.... Expressing it and with me, expression tends to be hard... The emotions with people like me are much more intense. We have them, they're just intense and expressed differently... It's how we express it. I think it's there, but the expression is maybe different.*

Participants discussed challenges with controlling and modulating their emotions. A few participants described their emotions as a *"roller coaster."* Barbara described her emotional roller coaster connected by extreme depression and intense excitement: *"I could get very upset very easily, but I couldn't get over it."* On the other hand, Barbara indicated, *"there have been lots of times that I wasn't really able to feel my feelings directly and there were some things I couldn't deal with directly because it was too painful."* Kathy-Xania indicated that she, too, felt like she was on an emotional roller coaster. She explained:

> *There is a lot of rage in me and I think that is due to a lot of experiences that I have had. When I get rageful it is usually an event or an emotion or something that I have to be to work. Dealing with, like I am going to be going to the Social Security office on Tuesday with my social worker and just, well, I am trying to get health benefits and it just pisses me off to no end. If I read about the economy and read things like that—I start raging.*

Challenges with identifying their own emotions were also discussed by participants. Geneva spoke extensively of this. She provided herself with a mental checklist that assisted her with identifying her own emotions. For example, she said:

> *I go into a room and I see somebody I knew in school. I don't fully remember the relationship because I didn't really know them that well. But an intense emotion comes inside of me... I have to stop and think are my hands sweating, is my stomach in a knot, is my face turning red or white, am I shaking or frozen in my steps, is my breathing fast or slow, do I feel a panic reaction or do I feel magnetically drawn. I have to go through this checklist until I get enough guesses to identify—Oh, I must have liked him.*

Embarrassment would involve a different checklist. Geneva said, *"I wouldn't want to look but I did want to look. There would be a polarity between looking and not looking. My face would be warm and I would want to run in both directions...."* Panic *"poses a breathing off, makes us feel like we are in a straight jacket that is slowly being tightened....To us a panic attack is more like an attack of horror."* The checklist for happy would be:

> *Somebody gives me something that I have never seen before, but I have never wanted one but it would be useful. I have to put it into a scenario to make it make sense. When I discover my hands are trembling ever so slightly and I have got this giggle inside my stomach and when I look at my face on the inside I have got this smile, this itty bitty smile, and I am looking around at other people, especially the gigglers, and I try to pick up on what they might be thinking or what they are saying and I would go through this and the last thing that would go make up my mind would be do I want to put it under the table or do I want to take it home? Do I want to accidentally leave it under the table or take it home?*

Participants also talked about difficulty identifying or understanding the emotions of other people. Kathy-Xania explained that she could identify and understand anger, friendship, loyalty, and dishonesty. She expressed that she has difficulty understanding sexuality and jealousy. As she explained:

> *I mean all the sexuality stuff I have really very little understanding of. I acknowledge it. I know it exists, the emotions people have about that area—I just don't understand. I have envy and jealousy myself but not over things of other people.... It's hard for me understand why they would have those feelings.*

Although Kathy-Xania and other participants stated that they have difficulty identifying the emotions of others, all participants disagreed with the assumption that individuals with autism lack a theory of mind or are unable to take the perspective of others. Participants expressed feelings they experienced and also spoke about relating to another person's feelings. It was apparent that for these participants there was a difference in understanding emotions, not an absence.

Participants talked extensively about accommodations they have used to manage their emotions. Barbara described often hiding her emotions and isolating herself, however, this made her feel miserable. She explained that when she personified objects and projected her feeling to that object, she felt better:

> *It seemed in order for me to have any happiness, I had to personify objects and treat them like they were human....Well, lots of times I would project my feelings onto something, rather than being able to feel them directly.... I don't know how to explain it. Lots of times I would say the feelings that I had I wasn't able to feel was like maybe feelings of pleasure—like for me to enjoy something—I'd have to sense that one of my fantasy objects enjoyed it too.*

Barbara further explained:

> *When I could interact with a personified object I felt content. For example, I personified the building where I went to high school and called it Troy. When I could talk to the building or interact with it, I felt content. At that time I got no good feelings from being around people. There was always tension when I was around people because I never fit in and I had nothing in common with people and there was no sense of connection, objects were my only source of comfort.*

Two other participants also described personifying objects. Geneva personified a large stuffed rabbit. This personification provided Geneva with a comforting feeling. Kathy-Xania found the feeling of security when holding wooden puzzle pieces of California, Texas, Montana, and Africa.

Participants talked about the impact of stress on both their emotions and their behavior. Barbara explained that she tried to *"stay out of a situation where I am stressed. Otherwise, there is no controlling my emotions."* She described feeling stress, nervousness, and depression caused by criticism from others regarding her behavior. Barbara added:

> *The more people that criticized me—what it did was made me angry and want to rebel. When people criticized me a lot I just didn't like being around them and I got angry a lot and I cried a lot. And it just simply—it caused more tension. In fact it just took a bad situation and made it worse. There were times when I was in a situation where I sometimes had to act a little bit silly to keep myself from getting upset because if I would have had that defense mechanism I would have just fallen apart.... Well sometimes I felt so nervous that sometimes I would have to act silly. In order to keep from getting upset.... If I got upset I stayed that way. I had to really do everything I could to try and avoid getting that way....because I have been hurt so much. I have so much bitterness. And I have to deal with forgiving a lot of people.*

Barbara further explained that, she felt isolated and that no one understood how hard things were for her; instead they only focused on her outward behavior. As she stated, *"No one cared about how terrible I felt from the inside."* Barbara wanted others to understand, help her understand, and to support her. Jean Paul agreed. He said that connecting with and providing feedback to a person with autism on his/her level without criticism was extremely helpful.

Matt described a variety of strategies to deal with stress. He explained that some books, pictures, and electronic equipment (e.g., computers, Game Boy) reminded him of home. This memory of a quiet, safe place created a calming feeling and allowed him to better deal with stress. While these and other strategies were helpful, he explained that other people often did not understand his strategies. He explained others' reactions to his strategies:

> *Some of these things upset my teachers because they don't understand why I do them. And I couldn't communicate well enough to explain things, even to myself. For example, my parents said I banged my head a lot when I got frustrated when I was young. But I usually banged it on soft things so it didn't hurt much. Sometimes when I am mad now I still swing my head through the air. But I don't hit anything with my head. Head banging motions help me deal with my nervousness.*

COMMUNICATION

Participants described challenges with both verbal and nonverbal communication. Specifically participants described challenges with speech execution and control, rhythm in conversation, and using and understanding nonverbal communication. Many described the dynamic interaction between speech and emotions.

Barbara described difficulty with speech execution and control. She described how emotional reactions caused changes in her ability to control her speech:

> *I know my voice is loud now—but when I talk about emotional things, it just bursts out of me—there's just so much pressure. In fact, lots of times my voice sounds bad—it's only part of the emotion—you know—it's sort of like be thankful it's only a whine—I'm holding in a scream.... But if an autistic person's voice is loud, it's not because they're trying to be loud, it's because there's tension there. An autistic person is sitting on a powder keg of emotions. And it's gotta go somewhere—and perhaps talking loud is the only way they can get any relief from that tension. It's the only outlet that I had that worked. If I was angry, I could exercise, I could do anything but it wouldn't do any good. Talking or yelling or something was the only thing that gave me any relief at all.... My voice was the only emotional release. It was the only safety valve on that pressure. But the funny thing about it—was the more people nagged me, the more it aggravated what it was they were nagging me about.*

Kathy-Xania also described difficulty controlling her speech and vocal outbursts when she was emotional, even if the emotion was excitement. She described often making *"uncontrollable sounds"* when she heard the name of a geographic location.

Kathy-Xania also commented on how difficult it was for her to understand the rhythm or pattern in conversations. She explained that this was exacerbated when the subject matter was *"historical or talking about something I really like. I want to jump in there you know. But I never know when to jump in and often get it wrong."*

Participants also described challenges with becoming stuck in words or phrases and/or sounds. Jean Paul described repeating words and phrases over and over again. As he said, *"I could not stop, even when I wanted to."* Geneva described similar challenges with speech execution:

> *There would be a lot of times that I would stop in mid-word and maybe repeat a syllable and go into verbal perseverations. I would start to say things, I would use the wrong words. Like I would say: 'let's go into that store' in my mind, but the words would come out 'let's go in that box'.... I would lose my train of thought constantly.*

Participants also described challenges with using and understanding nonverbal communication. Barbara said, *"As a child growing up, as an autistic person, I could not read body language.... because all that was too abstract."* She further explained:

> *I don't understand body language. And I had very little body language. My face tended to have a blank expression on it a lot. And I did not have body language or understand body language but they put all the burden of that on me. As if I was suppose to change it. It was neurological but they didn't recognize anything as neurological. I think eventually I started to develop more body language. But it was just something that took a long time to develop. But one of the things that happened is that I had a very high level of nervous tension so I just looked and acted very nervous. And a lot of times I grinned a lot because of tension. And lots of times I laughed so I wouldn't cry because I knew if I didn't act silly that I would get upset and I really had to struggle just to keep myself together.*

Barbara further explained:

> *I'd sometimes look like I wasn't paying attention because I'd be preoccupied or I'd grin, or I'd grimace, or I'd frown. I got criticized for my facial expressions. I got criticized for things that happened automatically. I got criticized for things I had no control over. Things other people don't think about. Normal people's faces look like they're supposed to look—when you're autistic—your face does not look like you're supposed to look. Different things go on inside you. Different things show on the outside. It's automatic. Nobody sits around and says I'll move this muscle here—I'll move this muscle there—I'll put this muscle there—they don't stare in a mirror and think—move this muscle, move that muscle, yeah that's the look and practice that. Nobody does that. But my facial expressions I got criticized for.*

COGNITION

Data from the categories "memory" and "thought" were combined into the category of "cognition." Thought processes of the individuals from this study proved unique and distinctive.

Geneva had been told that she was born mentally gifted. She described her IQ scores:

> *What they didn't know was that I may have been as high as 150 to begin with. I am about 135 now, but I may have been as high as 150, but I used everything over 100 to pass in society. So I brought it down, down, down to where now it is 135 where it should be 150 but I have to pass in society.*

She described that *"passing in society or keeping your outward appearance looking typical"* required a *"huge portion"* of her mental energy. As a result she created a variety of accommodations to reduce the amount of energy or thinking needed to complete a cognitive task. She summarized some of her thinking and the accommodations she had created for herself to be a more effective thinker. For example, Geneva described her optimal studying experience in college:

> *I would go in the bathroom and start the bath water, right? Then I would get this desk I had made to go across the bathtub, then I would put the notebooks on there and my textbook and then I would put the tape recorder with the taped book from books for the blind on the commode seat and I would read the text, hear the tape and take notes at the same time and if at any point something happened to my concentration that it stopped or something, I could just stop the tape and go back.*

This atmosphere seemed to organize her system. Geneva explained further using a computer analogy:

> *Now, comparing my mind to a computer, it is like I have the input card but the output card is all jumbled up. There is no alphabetical order and half of them are missing but the input is there. But I can't get to the output.... I have no idea why. Somebody will ask me a question and I will say I will have to get back to you and I just have to forget about it and walk around till the stuff pops up and it pops up eventually or sometimes it doesn't.*

Geneva also described that one of the major difficulties she experienced was because:

> *People don't realize the major problem that nobody ever sees or realizes is how much conscious thinking we have to do just to function. Walking takes thinking. So if I am walking and you ask me a question I could trip or I could mess up the sentence and put the wrong word in. Or have to stop and say, 'what did you say?' I can walk with my girl friend down the street and carry on a conversation as long as she is right there but I have to look down at the sidewalk. I have to keep track of where the sidewalk is and where any obstacles are and all that stuff and sometimes if I have to keep walking and I feel like I am going to blow any second I make sure the path is clear ahead of me and close my eyes and continue walking.*

Kathy-Xania described herself as an *"entirely visual thinker."* She said that the way she thought was:

> *Similar to Temple Grandin—and that's why I like countries and states so much. Because it is all visual to me. History is movement. It is movement. Economy moves and countries move. People, countries and their governments have their ups and downs and I like looking at pictures and maps and flags. It is all visual to me. It is like a story. I can just visualize it all.*

Kathy-Xania's mind also connected many ideas and words. For example, she enjoyed hearing where people were from. When she heard one of the researchers was from Wisconsin she said that the first thoughts that came to her mind were *"University of Wisconsin, Madison, Cheese, History, my name is Yon Yonson and I come from Wisconsin."* In fact, she voiced some of these thoughts during the interview. She said:

> *I always have to know what city people come from but there are times I don't always ask, especially if I am dealing with a business situation or whatever. I usually deal with business at hand. But usually I am very compelled to know what city people are from or places they have been to, you know.*

Barbara's thought process also involved such connections. These connections however, often lead to intrusive thoughts. She stated:

> *I think in some situations it's just harder for me not to have intrusive thoughts. Some autistic people, they say, block things out or they shut things down or whatever. My mind doesn't think—I'm not able to stop an intrusive thought or block something out unless it's something really, really, really mild—but if it's severe, it all comes in and there's no way I can stop it. I'm not able to tune out anything.... Intrusive thoughts would be nonsense syllables or something. I don't understand why this is—but if I was trying to study a foreign language or if I tried to study anything with odd-sounding words, I'd get nonsense syllables and stuff would pop in my mind and anxiety. It doesn't make a bit of sense. I don't know why it happens.*

As a result, *"it takes a lot of concentration and I'm not able to process that much information at one time."* Barbara stated that when she does not put forth a great deal of conscious effort she has a hard time staying focused. She explained:

> *Like if I was in the music room and I saw a musical instrument or the record player was turned off, I would have intrusive thoughts about songs in my mind. Or if I was trying to read my geography assignment, a whole bunch of nonsense syllables would pop into my mind and would be triggered by funny-sounding names. Just stupid things like that—that wouldn't amount to a hill of beans, but I would just get this terrible anxiety and boy, I would just scream.*

Matt explained that, excessive stress could be problematic for his processing of thoughts. He described how some people pressure him by yelling at him to respond. He explained, *"This type of pressure causes my thought processes to 'crash' like an overworked computer disk. It's like my thoughts are trying to get out of my head at once and I can't deal with it."*

Barbara and Kathy-Xania each explained that sometimes they had *"cognitive overload."* This might happen when either of them had difficulty integrating different areas such as thought, perception and action. Both gave the example of driving. Barbara explained her experience of driving:

> *When you're driving you have about 20 different things you have to keep track of—traffic going in all different directions—you have to watch the traffic, the light's red, then it's green, then it's red, then it's green—you have to pay attention to whether the light's red and green and go to the corner—pay attention to the speed limit and the signs and staying in your lane and watching all the other cars at the same time—I could pay attention and not see something else. I might avoid hitting a car only to hit another one.*

DISCUSSION

We started this project with the conceptual model of sensory and movement differences and a conviction that it is important to listen to people with autism. This model was based on that offered by Hill and Leary (1993), Donnellan and Leary (1995), Leary and Hill (1996), and Leary and Donnellan (2012). Sensory and movement differences is a disruption in the organization and regulation of perception, action, posture, language, speech, thought, emotion, and/or memory. This definition guided data collection and analysis. We found that the data strongly supported the presence of disruption of organization and regulation of sensory and movement differences in the lived experience of these participants with autism. Typically developing people experience sensory and movement differences as well, of course. However, the present data suggests that in autism this disruption of organization and regulation is amplified in terms of quantity, quality, intensity, and may affect everyday life. For example, recall how Barbara found it almost impossible to let go of an intrusive thought, how she was often not able to move past a negative emotion, or how the effects of an unpleasant noise lasted much longer than the noise itself.

The professional literature on autism, from Kanner (1943) to the present relies heavily on the "etic" or outsider view (Pike, 1950; Berreman, 1966). The assumption, unstated but generally operationalized, is that our experience of these individuals is essentially the same as their own. Here, we have attempted to offer the "emic" view, i.e., at least some of their experience, in their own voices. With this information, we might begin to understand that when Barbara looks away in a conversation it could be her best accommodation in order to understand our words. And perhaps we could see her behavior as less a social inadequacy that fits our definition of autism than an individual's best attempt to overcome a sensory problem that otherwise would interfere with her attempt to interact. And, this information might inform teachers and therapists who have been taught that they must get eye contact before providing instruction. In another example, recall that Geneva described her need to think about how to walk in order to walk. For most non-autistic individuals, this is automatic, smooth, and fluid. She described further challenges when combining walking and speech. Geneva explained that she had to look down at the sidewalk while having a conversation with a friend so that she could continue to talk and walk. Without knowing this was an accommodation used by Geneva one might assume her behavior indicated a social deficit.

Additionally, these data suggest that sensory and movement differences are not the same for all people with the autism label, nor always the same for any given person. Moreover, those of us who support people with autism should be mindful that:

> *Movement disturbance can clearly have a profound effect on a person's ability to regulate movement in order to effectively communicate, relate, and participate with others. Once this possibility is acknowledged, it becomes necessary to suspend absolute trust in one's intuitive interpretation of actions and intent. Behaviors may not be what they seem. (Leary and Hill, 1996, p.44)*

Our understanding of each individual requires awareness of the dynamic, multi-layered, contextually determined aspects of organization and regulation. It is a tall order, worthy of our attention.

For the purpose of this study, it was necessary to describe various areas separately, it is important to remember that perception, action, emotion, communication, cognition, and posture operates in an interactive dynamic fashion (see Thelen and Smith, 1994; Thelen, 1995). Continual interaction occurs across the areas in a dynamic process. These connections seem to be dependent on context. Context includes a wide variety of factors not limited to overt, observable stimuli. Context also includes emotional status, environmental stimuli, memory triggers, etc. Recall that many participants discussed the effect of stress on their ability to organize and regulate their perceptions and movements. In other words, a person's ability to function is highly dependent on context, which is ever shifting, and the unique and intimate interconnections of the various areas may contribute to sensory and movement difference for an individual with autism at any moment in time.

One obvious implication is that "interventions," medical, behavioral or educational, ought not be pre-packaged nor assumed to work for all people with autism. They must be personalized accommodations (Luria, 1932/1976; Sacks, 1990) and personalization requires that we "learn to listen" (Lovett, 1996) to the individual rather than rely on our preconceived notions of our own expertise on the topic. Moreover, it must be said that each of the participants (and many others with the autism label to whom we have spoken) expressed gratitude for the information about sensory and movement differences. While they knew their own experience, and could talk about it, they did not know that others had similar experiences. Moreover, they thought they were to "blame" for their challenges, because they had so often been blamed by others and subjected to so much behavioral modification with the goal of eliminating behavior beyond their own volition. The separation of mind from body noted earlier (Damasio, 1994) has contributed to this situation where the literature concentrates on "mind," leaving most autistic people to deal with problems of their bodies on their own. Their experience described here and in first-hand accounts suggests that a change on our part as professionals is essential. With sensitivity and humility about how little we actually know compared to what we think we know; this more personalized path could have significant effect in some lives affected by autism (Donnellan, 1999).

We are not saying sensory and movement differences are the cause of autism; in fact, occasional challenges or differences in perception, action, emotion, communication, cognition, posture are part of our shared human experience. We all occasionally forget why we went into a particular room and have to return to the original context to remember. We sometimes have trouble with a sound or a touch under the "wrong" circumstances, for example. For people with the autism label, however, these differences may have at least the following effects: (1) that sensory and movement differences may be more problematic for people with autism because of the magnitude of differences they experience with intensity, duration, rhythm, rate, frequency and /or timing of movement they experience; (2) events, stimuli and experiences in the world seem to elicit different response in some people with autism than the typical patterned response of other non-labeled people; and (3) areas may affect these individuals in an unusual and dynamic fashion which is highly dependent upon external and internal context.

Interviewing individuals with autism about sensory and movement differences was challenging. At times, despite their interest in the topic, it was difficult to know the "right" questions to elicit information in some areas, such as posture and cognition. Though the vignettes helped, it was not always clear if the participant actually experienced differences but was unable to articulate the information or if the person did not experience challenges in a particular area. Each of the categories discussed in this study warrant further investigation.

These individuals are considered "high functioning," and yet live with challenges that are poorly understood by their community, colleagues and peers and seldom reflected in professional descriptions and studies. Despite the occasional difficulties, qualitative research that seeks the perspectives and experiences of people with autism is essential if we seek to understand how sensory and movement differences impact these individuals. In particular, we need to explore whether and to what extent these sensory movement difficulties create or contribute to the difficulties that we experience as impairments in social interaction, communication and behavior. We must listen carefully to individuals with autism and be willing to incorporate their perspectives into our learning.

Many experts in the field of autism, especially and specifically people with autism (Kathy-Xania, interview; Barbara, interview; Geneva, interview; Ne'eman and Kapp, personal communication, July 29, 2012), disagree with much of the explanation of autism currently available in the autism literature. Kathy-Xania (interview) and others (Mackay, 2003; Biklen, 2005) suggest that there be more qualitative studies to gain the perspective of people with autism. This study supports the notion that more qualitative research, including in-depth interviews, case studies and first-hand accounts, that elicit the experiences and perspectives of individuals with autism would be prudent. These data would contribute to a more expansive view that incorporates the possibility that autism is a disorder that affects motor planning, behavior, communication, the sensory motor system, and the dynamic interaction of all of these (Herbert, 2012). Current definitions may fail to communicate the depth, breadth, and infinite variability in the experience of autism.

Five participants identified with the label of autism provided data for this study. People with autism have well documented social and communication difficulties. For that reason, a variety of methods were used to obtain meaningful data.

For in-depth interviews, we selected only verbal people with autism who were able to articulate at least a portion of their experiences. All research participants were able to communicate independently. This may have limited the generalizability to individuals with autism who are not able to articulate in the conventional manner or through augmentative or alternative forms of communication. Furthermore, all the participants in the study were white middle to upper-middle class. In addition, the ratio of females to males in this study (3:2) is not representative of the ratio of females to males in the literature, which is one to four/five.

Certainly further inquiry is needed that explores the experiences of less articulate verbal and nonverbal men and women with autism as well as exploring the experiences of individuals with autism from various socioeconomic backgrounds. There is sufficient information in the first-hand accounts of autism to suggest that such inquiry would be a contribution to our understanding of all people with the autism label (Barron and Barron, 1992; Grandin, 1992, 1995; Williams, 1992, 1994; McKean, 1994; Blackman, 1999; Hale and Hale, 1999; Mukhopadhyay, 2000; Biklen, 2005; Goddard and Goddard, 2012).

Finally, this research raises new questions that, when answered, may further expand current definitions and understanding of autism. How do differences in magnitude of intensity, duration, rhythm, rate, frequency and /or timing of movement create challenges for people with autism? Do differences in intensity, duration, rhythm, rate, frequency and /or timing of movement occur more frequently in people with autism? Why do different type of events, stimuli and experiences in the world elicit different responses in some people with autism? For example, how does pain tolerance and internal auto-regulation of temperature impact individuals with autism? What is it about the areas of perception, action, posture, emotion, communication, and cognition that affect these individuals in an unusual and interdependent fashion? What is the role of external and internal context on the experiences of individuals with autism? How might current treatments and teaching strategies be modified to include the possibility of sensory and movement difference in autism? What types of personalized accommodations are helpful to individuals with autism?

We hope this research will serve as a catalyst for additional studies that explore the experience of sensory and movement differences in autism. This will encourage the collaboration of individuals with autism and professionals in fields such as neurology, psychiatry, neuroscience, education, psychology as well as basic biological sciences so that autism is explored through the lens of more recent relevant research on how the brain and body work.

REFERENCES

American Psychiatric Association. (2000). *Diagnostic and Statistical Manual of Mental Disorders, 4th Edn.*, text revision. Washington, DC: Author.

Barron, J., and Barron, S. (1992). *There's a Boy in Here*. New York, NY: Simon and Schuster.

Berreman, G. (1966). Anemic and emetic analyses in social anthropology. *Am. Anthropol.* 68, 346–354.

Biklen, D. (2005). *Autism and the Myth of the Person Alone*. New York, NY: New York University Press.

Blackman, L. (1999). *Lucy's Story: Autism and Other Adventures*. Brisbane, QLD: Book in Hand.

Bleuler, E. (1911/1950). *Dementia Praecox or the Group of Schizophrenias*. Trans. J. Zinkin New York, NY: International Universities Press.

Broderick, A., and Kasa-Hendrickson, C. (2001). "Say just one word at first": the emergence of reliable speech in a student labeled with autism. *Res. Pract. Pers. Sev. Disabil.* 26, 13–24.

Cesaroni, L. (1990). *Exploring the Autistic Experience Through First-Hand Accounts from High-Functioning Individuals with Autism*. Unpublished document, University of Toronto.

Charmaz, K. (2000). "Grounded theory: objectivist and constructivist methods," in *Handbook of Qualitative Research, 2nd Edn*, eds N. Denzin and Y. Lincoln (Thousand Oaks, CA: Sage Publications), 509–535.

Charmaz, K. (2006). *Constructing Grounded Theory: A Practical Guide Through Qualitative Analysis*. London: Sage Publications.

Damasio, A. R. (1994). *Descartes Error: Emotion, Reason, and the Human Brain*. New York, NY: G.P. Putnam.

Donnellan, A. M., and Leary, M. R. (1995). *Movement Differences and Diversity in Autism/Mental Retardation*. Madison, WI: DRI Press.

Donnellan, A. M., Leary, M. R., and Robledo, J. (2006). "I can't get started: stress and the role of movement differences for individuals with the autism label," in *Stress and Coping in Autism*, eds G. Baron, J. Groden, G. Groden, and L. Lipsitt (Oxford: Oxford University Press), 205–245.

Donnellan, A. M. (1999). Invented knowledge and autism: highlighting our strengths and expanding the conversation, *JASH* 24, 230–236.

Ferguson, P., Ferguson, D., and Taylor, S. (1992). *Interpreting Disability: A Qualitative Reader*. New York, NY: Teachers College Press.

Goddard, P., and Goddard, D. (2012). *I Am Intelligent: From Heartbreak to Healing – A Mother and Daughter's Journey Through Autism*. Guiford, CT: Globe Pequot Press.

Grandin, T. (1992). "An inside view of autism," in *High-Functioning Individuals with Autism*, eds E. Schopler and G. B. Mesibov (New York, NY: Plenum), 105–126.

Grandin, T. (1995). *Thinking in Pictures and Other Reports from My Life with Autism*. New York, NY: Doubleday.

Hale, M., and Hale, C. (1999). *I Had No Means to Shout!* Bloomington, IN: 1st Books.

Herbert, M. (2012). *The Autism Revolution: Whole-Body Strategies*. New York, NY: Ballantine Books.

Hill, D., and Leary, M. (1993). *Movement Disturbance: A Clue to Hidden Competencies in Persons Diagnosed with Autism and Other Developmental Disabilities*. Madison, WI: DRI Press.

Jolliffe, T., Lansdown, R., and Robinson, C. (1992). Autism: a personal account. *Communication* 26, 12–19.

Kahlbaum, K. (1874/1973). *Catatonia*. Trans. Y. Levij and T. Pridan. Baltimore, MD: Johns Hopkins University Press.

Kanner, L. (1943). Autistic disturbances of affective contact. *Nerv. Child* 2, 217–250.

Leary, M. R., and Donnellan, A. M. (2012). *Autism: Sensory-Movement Differences and Diversity*. Cambridge, WI: Cambridge Book Review Press.

Leary, M. R., and Hill, D. (1996). Moving on: autism and movement disturbance. *Ment. Retard.* 34, 39–53.

Leary, M. R., Hill, D., and Donnellan, (1999). *Autism: Myths and Misunderstandings*. Presented to the School of Psychology, University of Michigan, Ann Arbor.

Lincoln, Y. S., and Guba, E. G. (1985). *Naturalistic Inquiry*. Beverly Hills, CA: Sage.

Lovett, H. (1996). *Learning to Listen: Positive Approaches and People with Difficult Behavior*. Baltimore, MD: Paul, H. Brookes.

Luria, A. R. (1932/1976). *The Nature of Human Conflicts: Or Emotion, Conflict and Will*. New York, NY: Liveright.

Mackay, R. (2003). "Tell them who I was": the social construction of aphasia. *Disabil. Soc.* 16, 811–826.

McKean, T. A. (1994). *Soon Will Come the Light*. Arlington, TX: Future Education.

Mukhopadhyay, T. R. (2000). *Beyond the Silence*. London: National Autistic Society.

Patton, M. Q. (2002). *Qualitative Research and Evaluation Methods, 3rd Edn*. Thousand Oaks, CA: Sage.

Pike, K. L. (1950). *Axioms and Procedures for Reconstructions in Comparative Linguistics: An Experimental Syllabus*. Glendale, CA: Summer Institute of Linguistics.

Robledo, J., and Donnellan, A. M. (2008). Properties of supportive relationships from the perspective of academically successful individuals with autism. *Intellect. Dev. Disabil.* 46, 299–310.

Rogers, D. (1990). Psychiatric consequences of basal ganglia disease. *Semin. Neurol.* 10, 262–266.

Sacks, O. (1990). *Awakenings, 6th Edn*. New York, NY: Harper Perennial.

Strandt-Conroy, K. (1999). *Exploring Movement Differences in Autism Through First-Hand Accounts*. Doctoral Dissertation, University of Wisconsin, Madison.

Strauss, A. L. (1987). *Qualitative Analysis for Social Scientists.* Cambridge, UK: Cambridge University Press.

Thelen, E., and Smith, L. B. (1994). *A Dynamic Systems Approach to Development and Cognition.* London: MIT Press.

Thelen, E. (1995). Motor development: a new synthesis. *Am. Psychol.* 50, 79–95.

Volkmar, F. R., and Cohen, D. J. (1985). The experience of infantile autism: a first-person account by Tony, W. *J. Autism Dev. Disord.* 15, 47–54.

White, G. B., and White, M. S. (1987). Autism from the inside. *Med. Hypothesis* 24, 223–229.

Williams, D. (1992). *Nobody Nowhere.* London: Doubleday.

Williams, D. (1994). *Somebody Somewhere.* New York, NY: Times Books.

Conflict of Interest Statement: The authors declare that the research was conducted in the absence of any commercial or financial relationships that could be construed as a potential conflict of interest.

4

Rethinking autism: implications of sensory and movement differences for understanding and support

Anne M. Donnellan[1*†], David A. Hill[2†] and Martha R. Leary[3†]

[1] School of Leadership and Education Sciences, University of San Diego, San Diego, CA, USA
[2] Tri-County Regional School Board, Yarmouth, NS, Canada
[3] Private Practice, Halifax, NS, Canada

Edited by:
Elizabeth B. Torres, Rutgers University, USA

Reviewed by:
Trevor McDonald, Education Associates Inc, USA
Ralph J. Savarese, Duke University, USA

***Correspondence:**
Anne M. Donnellan, School of Leadership and Education Sciences, Autism Institute, University of San Diego, 5998 Alcala Park, San Diego, CA 92110, USA.
e-mail: anned@sandiego.edu

† These authors equally contributed to this work.

For decades autism has been defined as a triad of deficits in social interaction, communication, and imaginative play. Though there is now broad acknowledgment of the neurological basis of autism, there is little attention paid to the contribution of such neurological differences to a person's development and functioning. Communication, relationship, and participation require neurological systems to coordinate and synchronize the organization and regulation of sensory information and movement. Developmental differences in these abilities are likely to result in differences in the way a person behaves and expresses intention and meaning. The present paper shares our emerging awareness that people may struggle with difficulties that are not immediately evident to an outsider. This paper explores the symptoms of sensory and movement differences and the possible implications for autistic people. It provides a review of the history and literature that describes the neurological basis for many of the socalled behavioral differences that people experience. The paper emphasizes the importance of our acknowledgment that a social interpretation of differences in behavior, relationship, and communication can lead us far away from the lived experience of individuals with the autism label and those who support them. We suggest alternative ways to address the challenges faced by people with autism.

Keywords: autism, autism: sensory-movement differences, autism: sensory-motor difficulties, autism: neurological implications, autism: movement perspective

INTRODUCTION

> *I was intensely preoccupied with the movement of the spinning coin or lid and I saw nothing and heard nothing. I did it because it shut out sound that hurt my ears. No sound intruded on my fixation. It was like being deaf. Even a sudden noise didn't startle me out of my world.* (Grandin, 1992a,b,c)

People with autism often move their bodies in ways that are unfamiliar to us. Some people rock, repeatedly touch an object, jump, and finger posture while other people come to a standstill in a doorway, sit until cued to move or turn away when someone beckons. As professionals trained to see these as *autistic behaviors*, most of us have interpreted such movements as both volitional and meaningless; or as communicative acts signaling avoidance of interaction and evidence of diminished cognitive capacity; or as some combination of these, often to be targeted for reduction. We have taken a socially constructed interpretation of what we see and have built a "theory" of autism.

This paper challenges the traditional definitions of autism that give primacy to a triad of deficits in social interaction, communication, and imaginative play (Wing, 1981; *DSM-IV- TR* American Psychiatric Association, 2000). The approach is both widely known and essentially unchallenged despite broad acknowledgment that autism is a condition that reflects some differences in a person's neurology. Typically, the neurological implications have not become part of the description. Over the past two decades, however, researchers and self-advocates have begun to rethink this socially defined focus. They express concern that children and adults with the autism label may be challenged by unrecognized and significant sensory and movement differences (e.g., (Williams, 1992; Hill and Leary, 1993; Donnellan and Leary, 1995; Bristol et al., 1996; Leary and Hill, 1996; Donnellan, 1999; Filipek et al., 2000; Sullivan, 2002; Dhossche, 2004; Bluestone, 2005; Nayate et al., 2005; Endow, 2006; Jansiewicz et al., 2006; Mostofsky et al., 2006; Leekam et al., 2007; Markram et al., 2007; Tomchek and Dunn, 2007; Gernsbacher et al., 2008; Goldman et al., 2009).

Researchers and others describe these differences using a variety of terms such as: motor problems, sensory-integration problems, inertia, sensory overload, apraxia, dyspraxia, echolalia, mutism, behavior disorder, catatonia, or clumsiness. To reflect the range and complexity of sensory perception and movement related phenomena, we use the term "sensory and movement differences" as it encompasses the dynamic interaction of sensation and movement (Gibson, 1979; Thelen and Smith, 1994) while acknowledging that many differences are merely part of the richness of human diversity.

Behavior is highly interpretable. Some behaviors may be communicative; some may be volitional (Donnellan et al., 1984).

Some behaviors, however, may not be intentional. Rather, observed behaviors may be artifacts of the difficulties a person may be having in organizing and regulating sensation and movement. Still others may be subtle signals of the desire for relationship or expressions of meaning. Therapeutic and intervention-based approaches, designed to address perceived and identified challenging and problematic behaviors of individuals with autism, tend to oversimplify the complex nature of human interactions in an attempt to delineate and manipulate variables contributing to and sustaining particular behaviors.

As we have *professionalized* interactions with people with autism, we have trained professionals, parents, and others to interpret what happens in terms of simple, binary views of behavior (i.e., good/bad or positive/negative), and to see behaviors as controlled by immediate, situational antecedents, and consequences. When we focus on these socially constructed expectations for behavior and communication in our fast-paced, super-technological world, we miss opportunities to know and understand people who may experience their existence and interactions in very different ways. Behaviors may not be what they seem (Donnellan et al., 2006; Robledo et al., 2012).

Our interest in the topic of sensory and movement differences has grown from reports by many self-advocates with the autism label and their caregivers that disturbances of sensation and movement are a constant concern, frequently constraining ability to communicate, relate to others and participate in life (e.g., Barron and Barron, 1992; Strandt-Conroy, 1999; Rubin et al., 2001; Robledo et al., 2012). Organizing and regulating sensory information and movement in order to participate in social relationships may be frustrating for people with such differences. These differences can involve difficulties initiating and executing movements or difficulties with stopping, combining, and switching sensation and movement including speech, thought and emotion, (Hill and Leary, 1993; Donnellan and Leary, 1995; Donnellan et al., 2006) making social relationships and many other activities very challenging, even overwhelming.

Self-advocates also report that they lack sensation or feedback from their bodies and may feel physically unaware of their facial expressions, position in space and movements (e.g., Williams, 1996a,b, 2003; Blackman, 1999; Hale and Hale, 1999). Some experience the sights and sounds of their world as being painfully intense (Condon, 1985; Williams, 1992, 1996b; Markram et al., 2007). Extreme emotions can cause the individual to become stuck, unable to cease repetition of a movement. Self-confidence and reputation often suffer when others assume a person is repeating an action "on purpose." Sean Barron (Barron and Barron, 1992, p. 181) wrote: "All I wanted was to be like the other kids my age. It felt as if I was weird and strange on the outside, but inside I was not like that. The inside person wanted to get out and break free of all the behaviors that I was a slave to and could not stop." For many people, as for Sean, simple movements can lead to repetitions or perseveration, even when they want to stop the movement.

Our concern here is not to discard useful information already accumulated via a primarily socially defined approach to autism. Nor are we interested in enhancing a deficit-based approach to understanding autism, or in creating a new disability category. We do not propose to specify a cause of autism or a site of lesion or dysfunction within the central nervous system. Rather, we write to share our emerging awareness that people may struggle with difficulties that are not immediately evident to an outsider. That is, our experience of individuals with autism ought no longer to be assumed the same as their experience. Individuals with the autism label often describe experiences which are not immediately obvious to the rest of us but which may well-affect our understanding of their behavior. These experiences frequently fit the definition of sensory and movement differences. Sue Rubin (pers. communication, August 4, 2007) described her dilemma with intention and action: "When you said we could stay and asked dad to do the shopping for the Asperger's barbeque, my body relaxed and autism let me eat the melon." And two other autistic adults had the following interaction about sensory and movement differences. Judy Endow (pers. communication via Facebook, January 25, 2009) described her experiences in relation to sensory and movement differences:

> *I think the fluidity of access to various places in the brain is dependent upon neurological movement between places. I'm no scientist, but have always been able to "see" this inside of me. Sometimes my speaking is hindered, other times my thinking and sometimes my physical movement. The hardest is when thinking is not working smoothly. When that happens I have to line up one thought at a time, like train cars. I like it much better when my thoughts do not have to be methodically lined up, but are more fluid with colors coming in and out and swirling into unique and beautiful patterns. (My thoughts are in pictures and sometimes moving colors.)*

Phil Schwarz (pers. communication via Facebook, January 25, 2009) commented on Judy's description by using another analogy:

> *I think that processing bandwidth—what Judy calls "neurological movement between places"—is a critical factor in autism. I think that those of us who do learn to cope develop adaptations that allow more parsimonious use of the bandwidth available to us: love of sameness, or of patterns, or of predictability (so that we can apply the bandwidth we do have to "deviations" from the predicted or from the patterns). There is a coherent autistic aesthetic sensibility that is informed by this search for parsimony of bandwidth use, and for titration of excesses.*

This paper explores some of the implications of sensory and movement differences in the development and experiences of individuals with the autism label. We note, of course, that some researchers and clinicians completely deny the possibility that individuals with autism might experience any problems with movement. Rimland (1993, p. 3), a psychologist long a proponent of a biological approach to autism, wrote:

> *It has been widely recognized for many decades that the vast majority of autistic persons are quite unimpaired with regard to their finger dexterity and gross motor capabilities. They have in fact often been described as especially dexterous and coordinated. The literature abounds with stories of young autistic children who can take apart and reassemble small mechanical devices, build towers of blocks and dominos higher than a normal adult can, assemble jigsaw puzzles*

> *and climb to dangerously high places without falling. The files of the Autism Research Institute contain over 17,000 questionnaires completed by the parents of autistic children. Finger dexterity is one question we've asked about since 1965. Most parents indicate that their children are average or above in the use of their hands. The idea that autism is, or typically involves, a "movement disorder" is simply ludicrous.*

Likewise, Mulick et al. (1993), behavioral psychologists, stated unequivocally that clinical experience argues against any motor/movement difficulties, particularly voluntary control of movement in apraxia:

> *Scientific evidence for developmental apraxia in autism is lacking. Autistic youngsters are often characterized by better-developed [emphasis in original] motor skills than verbal skills, even real nonverbal problem solving talent ... There is no research evidence at all to support the position that people with autism experience such global problems. The usual clinical finding, familiar to any psychologist who routinely works in this area, is that motor impairment and delay is much less common than communication disorder and delay.* (p. 274)

The common approach in autism pays scant attention to possible somatic difficulties resulting from neurological differences. Perhaps, this is a function of the dominance of psychology and psychiatry for the first 50 or more years of the autism story. Yet, some psychologists and psychiatrists did report movement differences and even catatonic symptoms in autism long before Rimland or Mulick et al. and others denied the existence of such evidence (e.g., Damasio and Maurer, 1978; Wing and Attwood, 1987). More recently, many researchers have noted the presence of impairments in basic motor skills: gait, posture, balance, speed, coordination (e.g., Ghaziuddin and Butler, 1998; Noterdaeme et al., 2002; Jansiewicz et al., 2006; Rinehart et al., 2006; Green et al., 2009; Mostofsky et al., 2009; Fournier et al., 2010). Fournier et al. (2010) in their meta-analysis of claims of motor differences in autism since 1981 write:

> *Based on our synthesis of the existing literature and comprehensive meta-analytic techniques, we conclude that ASD is associated with significant and widespread alterations in motor performance. Recent neuroanatomical and neurophysiologic studies implicate cortical and subcortical areas including the motor context, supplementary motor deficits in motor planning, sensorimotor integration, and motor execution .... Our current findings serve as the basis for tentatively arguing that motor deficits are a potential core feature of ASD, and that treatment of ASD should consider including interventions aimed at improving motor performances involved with motor coordination (i.e., gait and balance, arm functions, and movement planning).* (p. 1237)

Many neuroscientists now are stressing the significance and implications of motor and sensory difficulties in the development of children with autism. For example, Sutera et al. (2007) looked at 4-years-old who had been diagnosed at age two and received early intervention of various amounts and types. Of particular interest were the children who "lost" the diagnosis of autism by age four. Sutera et al., found that the best predictor of this outcome for very young children with autism is motor skill at age two. Mostofsky et al. (2007) noted this finding and addressed concerns about the exclusion of motor problems from the "core" features of autism in the *Diagnostic and Statistical Manual of Mental Disorders* (*DSM-IV-TR*; American Psychiatric Association, 2000) "... despite [an] abundance of literature suggesting otherwise." A growing number of researchers and clinicians in a broad range of disciplines continue to stress the importance of studying motor function in autism because, as Rogers et al. (2003) reported, "Simple imitation skills were differentially impaired in young children with autism, and lack of social cooperation did not account for their poor performance p. 763). Mostofsky et al. (2007) reported, "Motor signs are highly quantifiable and reproducible and can serve as markers for deficits in parallel systems important for socialization and communication" (p. 2117). For example, children with autism are often described as lacking reciprocity. Esther Thelen (1941–2004), an innovative researcher of infant development, upon reviewing the issue of motor development in autism, asked: "How can you talk about "reciprocity" or lack thereof as a psychological phenomenon if the child has motor problems?" (pers. communication, 1997). In the course of development, if individuals move and respond in idiosyncratic ways from infancy, they will experience all interactions within a unique frame that most certainly differs from that which is called typical. The cumulative effect of such interactions will be one in which all aspects of relationships, including how to establish and maintain them, may be markedly skewed from the broader cultural consensus and expected rules of how relationships work [1]. Our experience and self-advocate reports have taught us that individuals with autism often are aware of their idiosyncrasies, may not be able to control them but do want communication, participation and relationship. In order to make this possible, we need to acknowledge and accommodate the differences so that communication, relationship, and participation can happen.

DYNAMIC INTERACTIONS OF NERVOUS SYSTEM, BODY, AND ENVIRONMENT

As we have noted elsewhere (Donnellan et al., 2006), the writings of many authors interested in movement describe a unity of perception, action, emotion, and thought. Feldenkrais, a physicist, martial artist, and renowned movement innovator noted: "Our self-image consists of four components that are involved in every action: movement, sensation, feeling and thought" (Feldenkrais, 1972, p. 10). Likewise, in his fascinating book, *Awakenings*, Sacks (1990) wrote of the self-reports of his patients with post-encephalitic Parkinson's disease who temporarily "awoke" through the use of the drug L-Dopa. They all had been sick from the same disease, *Encephalitis lethargica*. The area of damage in their brains from the disease was clearly established. Nonetheless, each developed his or her own personalized version of movement disorder and many of their difficulties were unknown to the medical staff until they were able to speak. The variety of manifestations of symptoms encompassed difficulties with many

[1] For reviews of the complex and dynamic interrelationship of movement, perception, relationship, and cognitive development, see: (Gibson, 1979; Thelen and Smith, 1994; Stern, 2000).

hidden aspects of human experience: perception of the passing of time, interest in normal activities, fatigue, memory, and recurring thoughts. These complex phenomenon related to organization and regulation, now commonly recognized in other neurological disorders, require us to think about movement disorders beyond observable motor difficulties.

Thelen incorporated dynamic systems models in her innovative research on movement in child development (Thelen and Smith, 1994; Thelen, 1995). In this view, perceptions, movement, thoughts, and emotions can be linked together by having coincidentally (and possibly routinely) co-occurred. Experience may selectively reinforce them as a bundle. They can be unbundled or softly assembled as required by the context. The individual is always operating within an environment or context and, as the context changes, systems scan, adjust, and shift as necessary to meet new demands. These contextual shifts play a vital role in movement. Context comes together with in such a way as to allow the movement to emerge or not; a movement and, indeed, the person or persons are part of the context (Thelen and Smith, 1994). As Bateson (1972) told us years ago, context is far more than what is left when we take out the part we wish to study.

No single component is causal in determining the movement. As these are dynamic systems, the components are the context that determine the product. Thelen and Smith (1994, p. 73) further explained that "... even behaviors that look wired in or program-driven can be seen as dynamically emergent: behavior is assembled by the nature of the task, and opportunistically recruits the necessary and available organic components (which themselves have dynamic histories) and environmental support." These may be actions, thoughts, words, memories, or sense experiences. Recall Proust, where the taste of a cookie released the hundreds of pages of *Remembrance of Things Past*.

Thelen's approach offers new ways to understand the inconsistent abilities and disabilities of individuals with the autism label. Speech is an example of dynamic behavior. Speech is not lost or gained; it emerges when all necessary components, recruited and appropriately regulated and organized, allow its production. Stress often makes speech difficult or even impossible. And stress need not be negative; excitement may also cause difficulties. Paradoxically, for some people with sensory and movement differences, stress also may help produce speech. While presenting with the authors at an Autism Society of America conference in July 1996, Arthur Shawlow, Nobel laureate and father of an adult son with autism, reported that his son could say a complete, and original, context-appropriate sentence about once every 8–10 years. He asked the audience, how many parents had similar experiences and at least 18 sets of parents raised their hands. They met and compared notes. Most of the labeled children of these individuals were able to speak under extreme, often negative, circumstances. Some had only spoken once or twice in a lifetime.

Reports of this kind are not unusual in the sensory and movement differences literature, among the autism community or our own 100+ years of combined experience with children and adults with the autism label. More common are phenomena such as echolalia, mutism, speech uttered only under unique circumstances, e.g., speaking what they have written. In the dynamic system model the notion of emergence begins to give us a way to understand and perhaps support people with these differences. Robledo et al. (2012) report on 40 h of interviews with adults with autism who experienced such symptoms and more. The interviews had to be adjusted to the specialized needs of the interviewees. Several could only answer written questions sent in advance; others if they were on the phone and in a warm bath. Likewise, the autistic people in Robledo and Donnellan (2008) each had personalized supports to enable them to participate in the interviews. We refer to these specialized arrangements as accommodations after Luria (1932) and Sacks (1990). We define accommodations as adjustments or adaptations of an interaction, a task, situation, or the environment that assist a person to temporarily get around difficulties organizing and regulating sensory information or movement (for example, see Donnellan et al., 2006).

LEARNING FROM NEUROLOGICAL SYMPTOMS IN OTHER SENSORY AND MOVEMENT DISORDERS

In our review of the history of movement differences we found early descriptions of catatonia in the work of Kahlbaum (1874/1973) which seemed startlingly familiar (see Hill and Leary, 1993; Donnellan and Leary, 1995; Starkstein et al., 1995; Leary and Hill, 1996). In the nineteenth century there was no clear distinction between neurological and psychiatric symptoms. As the two fields diverged in the early twentieth century, however, some conditions gravitated into one or the other. Catatonia is presently defined as a characteristic of certain kinds of schizophrenia, though many have argued over the years for a more neurological view of the disorder (Abrams and Taylor, 1976; Rogers, 1992). The discussion of where to place catatonia and catatonic symptoms is once again topical because of the plan to update the *Diagnostic and Statistical Manual* of the APA. Some, in fact, are arguing for the inclusion of catatonia as a separate diagnostic category or under "movement disturbances" (Taylor and Fink, 2003; Fink and Taylor, 2006; Penland et al., 2006; Caroff and Ungvari, 2007). Irrespective of that discussion, it is useful to look at the symptoms described by Kahlbaum and other early and recent authors as these may illuminate the symptoms seen in individuals with autism and other developmental disabilities.

In **Table 1**, the characteristic features and symptoms on the left side of the table are borrowed from descriptors specific to several kinds of movement disorders (Kahlbaum, 1874/1973; Fink and Taylor, 2003, 2006; Taylor et al., 2005; Caroff and Ungvari, 2007; The Movement Disorder Society, 2010). The list of movement disorders symptoms is not in any particular order or hierarchy; rather, symptoms are listed randomly as taken from the above literature sources. The intent here is to show the scope of symptoms by feature that may account for certain behaviors seen in autism. Examples of behaviors listed on the right side of **Table 1** appear there because they have been discussed in a previously published review of the autism literature and movement disturbances (Leary and Hill, 1996). The majority of these have also been documented and observed throughout many years of clinical practice with a large number of individuals with autism across the life span.

Leary and Hill (1996) analyzed the literature on symptoms associated with established movement disorders and those

Table 1 | Characteristic features of substantial movement disturbances and evidence of possible overlap of symptoms in autism.

Movement disturbance feature	Symptoms evidence in autism
Repetitive motor actions	e.g., Tapping, touching, grimacing
Rhythmical, cyclical movements	e.g., Rocking, shrugging, squinting, pouting
Lack of initiation	Requires prompts and cues to perform
Difficulty imitating others' actions	Both immediate and delayed motor imitation difficulties
Echophenomena	Mimesis; elaborate copying of others' actions—verbal and/or motor
Immobility	Remains fixed and inert in position and posture for extended time periods
Withdrawal	Isolates self away from focal activity and others
Grimacing	Facial/oral-motor movements
Stereotypies	Repetitive movements of the hands, limbs, extemities, and whole body
Aversion	Of eye gaze and attention to others
Negativism	Oppositional actions elicited with passive movement and overall behavior
Automatic obedience; suggestibility	Extreme compliance in response to verbal suggestion and environmental cues
Rigidity	Muscles rigid to passive movement
Bradykinesia	Slowness of movements, feebleness
Tremor	Essential, intentional, rest, postural, etc.
Forced grasping	Of another's hands, wrists, etc., or items in the environment
Akinesia	Marked absence of action and movements
Akathisia	Motor restlessness, moves about but not goal-directed
Ataxia	Loss of coordination in motor action execution
Perseveration	Motor or other repeated behavior after being elicited an initial stimulus
Ambitendency	Appears "stuck" in indecisive, hesitant movements
Tics	Motor and/or verbal
Obstruction; blocking	Incomplete movement toward a goal—"gets stuck" en route to goal
Difficulty with stopping, cessation of movement	Will continue movements unless redirected or stopped by an external means
Mannerisms	Uses intact and entire motor action sequences out of context, e.g., salutes
Waxy flexibility	Automatic ease and compliance with assuming unusual postures for extended time
Ballismus	Violent, rapid and apparently involuntary actions and movements
Choreiform movements	Rapid and apparently involuntary traveling and "dancing" ripples of movement
Catalepsy (posturing)	Maintains seemingly uncomfortable and imposed postures for extended time
Atheloid movements	Slow, writhing movements and actions
Spasms	Muscular spasms of varying durations affecting muscle groups
Dystonias	Sustained torsion due to muscle contractions in varied muscle groups
Impulsivity	Actions and movements triggered suddenly
Self-injury, mutilation	Disturbing and persistent attempts to inflict pain on self
Excitement; frenzy	Marked episodes of extreme amounts of activity for extended time
Aggression, destruction	Unprecipitated violent actions directed to others and the environment
Stupor	Prolonged period of total immobility, lack of responsiveness and mutism
Rituals	Object-related actions on objects as part of a routine, repeated event
Motility changes	e.g., Toe walking, skipping, hopping
Changes in speech behavior	e.g., Mutism; question repetition; echolalia; verbigeration; logorrhoea; foreign accent; changes in prosody; difficulty modulating volume
Automatic changes	Changes in typical autonomic functions, e.g., heart rate, perspiration, breathing, core body temperature

associated with autism. The greatest difference among these disabilities was the interpretation of the symptoms. In Tourette syndrome, Parkinson's disorder and catatonia, there was a neurological interpretation of symptoms. A social rather than a neurological interpretation was applied if the person had a label of autism. That which is called a "tic" in a person with Tourette syndrome is most often assumed to be a "behavior" (and often a conscious choice) in a person with autism. For symptoms interpreted through a neurological lens, individuals tend to be appropriately supported. In autism, symptoms are viewed frequently as behaviors to be reduced or eliminated often with a negative intervention and results. **Table 2** illustrates descriptions given to similar behaviors dependent on a person's diagnosis.

The sensory and movement differences reported by and observed in individuals with autism may have a significant impact on their and our ability to relate and participate in social interactions. A neurological view of symptoms possibly affecting autistic individuals will help us to understand further the

Table 2 | Differences in descriptions of behavior.

Neurological terms	Social interpretation of behavior
Akinesia	Non-compliance, social indifference
Festination	Behavior excess, careless
Bradykinesia	Lazy, slow
Bradyphrenia	Mental retardation
Tics	Aberrant behavior
Obsessional/adventitious behaviors	Autistic behavior, "stims"

nature of differences experienced by these individuals. While the psychological impact is very real as experienced first-hand by participants in such interactions, it is useful to suspend social interpretations of the symptoms so as not to mistakenly ascribe intent and volition to individuals whose behavior may be contrary to what really is intended and able to be communicated.

Detailed personal descriptions of movement and sensory differences found in other disabilities have given us some additional insight as to what it may be like for a person to deal with various symptoms such as compelling impulses, a loss of conscious control, lack of initiation, akinetic moments, and unusual ways of being in the world (e.g., McGoon, 1994). Frequently, the person has both the challenge of the movement difference and burden of blame and misunderstanding. In the Robledo et al. (2012) research it was often necessary to use vignettes from people with other sensory movement differences to enable the autistic interviewees to recognize their own experience. Most expressed gratitude for the opportunity to learn about movement differences as they often had blamed themselves for their behavior and all thought they were alone in having these difficulties.

IMPLICATIONS OF SENSORY AND MOVEMENT DIFFERENCES FOR UNDERSTANDING PEOPLE LABELED WITH AUTISM

A different kind of science.

> *Woe to that science whose methods are developed in advance of its problems, so that the experimenter can see only those phases of a problem for which a method is already at hand.*
>
> (Murphy, 1939, p. 114)

We have stressed the neurological aspects of what are commonly thought of as autistic characteristics and behavior problems. We do not intend, however, to either suggest a whole new category of disabilities in autism or to eliminate the psychological aspects. The issues here are similar to the challenges faced by those interested in Tourette syndrome. The syndrome was elucidated before the fields of neurology and psychiatry diverged (Gilles de la Tourette, 1885). For many years, psychiatry dominated the discussion and the treatment. In the past few decades, there has been a far greater emphasis on the neurology of the disorder. Yet, it is clear that it is not possible to separate the neurological from the psychological in a living human being. As Sacks (1989) suggests, there is need for a different kind of science that views the individual as a whole person, mind and body. This shift has begun in Tourette syndrome. In addition, dynamic systems models of development suggest an emphasis on the unique history and the critical importance of context on the manifestations of the symptoms. Perhaps the present emphasis on discrete "autistic" behaviors tied to specific interventions should be seen in terms of more circumscribed value and utility.

DEVELOPMENTAL vs. ACQUIRED SYMPTOMS

In addition to the personalized nature of the characteristics and the dynamic nature of the manifestations of a movement difference mentioned above, it is impossible to overemphasize the importance of the developmental aspects of movement differences in autism vs. adult acquired disorders. For example, bradykinesia, or very slow movements, might have a wide range of effects on adults with acquired disorders such as Parkinsonism. In an infant or a toddler, the possible effects of slow responding or delayed initiating would surely have an effect on the entire trajectory of development even if the difference were intermittent or barely perceptible to the parents or professionals. Of course, we are not suggesting that these autistic people have Parkinson's syndrome; rather that they report sensory and movement differences which are not obvious to their caregivers, particularly parents of young children. Yet, the potential changes to the "dance of relationships" (Stern, 2000) alone would be worthy of many dissertations in child development. But the complexity of the task ought not deter us from attempting such inquiry because it could have enormous implications for our understanding of human development and diversity.

INTERPRETATION OF SYMPTOMS AS VOLITIONAL

Many of us have accepted without question the implicit message that unusual movements presented by people with autism are always volitional and often pleasurable. Sensory and movement difference symptoms in autism are consistently interpreted by others as *autistic behaviors*. Neurological symptoms such as sudden, loud vocalizations; being in constant motion; extreme response to minor changes; unusual mannerisms and gait; and "unmotivated" laughter are examples of behaviors commonly thought to be performed "on purpose" and targeted for behavioral intervention. A social interpretation of these symptoms often leaves people with the assumption that they occur as a matter of choice, apathy, or learned behavior. Aggression during an episode of catatonic frenzy is viewed differently if the neurological aspects of the person's experience are considered. Typically, reprimands or contingent praise would not be used to change a recognized neurological symptom. As noted, the non-volitional aspects of behavior are rarely considered for people with autism. For example, the authors have all too often heard criticism and disparaging descriptions such as *lazy* or *non-compliant* applied to a person with autism who is in a non-responsive state. Frequently, the difficulty is related to stress, even the stress of excitement. An all too typical example is staff or family reporting that the child or adult *refused* to get out of the car or van to go to a place; he or she seems to like. Intervention or support that is based on our social interpretations of symptoms may not always be helpful. Returning the *non-compliant* person to home, school, or program usually results in additional trouble. We need a clearer understanding of people's experiences if we are to provide appropriate care and support that boosts self-confidence and is the product of collaboration rather than control. Donnellan et al. (2006) offer many suggestions for accommodations that may help people with autism deal with these situations.

INTERPRETATION OF SYMPTOMS AS MEANINGLESS

Our assumptions about a person's intention or meaning directly influence the way we respond moment to moment, the relationships we form and the support we give to people. When we label aspects of a person's behavior as meaningless, we may miss opportunities to extend learning and develop our relationships. Echolalia serves as well as an illustration. In the early years of behavioral intervention for people with autism (e.g., 1960–1980), professionals assessing a child's communication abilities were trained to assume that echolalia was the "meaningless repetition of a word or word group just spoken by another person" (Fay, 1969, p. 39), a non-functional, undesirable and "sick" behavior of autism (Lovaas, 1966; Lovaas et al., 1974), and a communication disorder in itself to be extinguished through behavior modification (Lovaas, 1977). The fine and detailed work of researchers such as Baltaxe and Simmons (1977), Prizant and Duchan (1981), and Prizant and Rydell (1984) began to influence our assumptions about the intentions of autistic speakers. Many people now understand that echolalia is neither always meaningless nor always meaningful. Although sometimes not intentional, many who lack other strategies for communicating may use echolalia intentionally to maintain relationships, improve their comprehension of spoken language and to express meaning (see Kanner, 1946). Acknowledgment of a person's efforts to accommodate, improvise, and create meaning is a cause for celebration and an opportunity to improve communication and boost self-esteem.

INTERPRETATION OF SYMPTOMS AS "NOT INTERESTED" IN RELATING OR COMMUNICATING

People with autism often communicate, behave and participate in unique, very personal, perhaps idiosyncratic ways, that require their partners to be more flexible and open than usual in interpreting meaning and intention. Differences in the way people are able to use their bodies and focus their attention lead many to assume that a person does not care to participate or communicate and does not desire relationships. These assumptions affect our expectations, the way we speak with them and the educational and social opportunities we offer to them. Under the "criterion of the least dangerous assumption" (Donnellan, 1984) it is safest to assume that relationships are critical to human beings for learning and development even if, and perhaps especially if, they have difficulties in these areas (Fogel, 1993; Robledo and Donnellan, 2008).

THE CRITICAL IMPORTANCE OF RELATIONSHIP IN LEARNING AND DEVELOPMENT

The past 40 years have witnessed the growth of a body of knowledge, approaches, and intervention methodologies designed to address the needs of individuals with autism. Often the kinds of intervention strategies at our disposal are based on ideas and theories that conflict with each other. The content of interventions may be highly prescriptive or more loosely defined. Research can be cited in support of the efficacy of any kind of approach for at least some individuals in some situations. We struggle as well as to explain and describe that quality within any intervention that works and leads to growth and development between the partners involved. Perhaps, the essential factor underlying any successful intervention has been overlooked or at least not credited in the research. We propose, along with a growing number of investigators, that the undefined element is the presence and nature of the relationship between persons in any interaction (Maurer, 1993; Hill and Leary, 2009).

The role of relationship in learning is the centerpiece of socio-cultural psychology. While most of us believe that learning is enhanced by a facilitative relationship with a *more mature thinker*, western psychology has only recently directed attention to the nature of that relationship. Lev Vygotsky (1896–1934) was a Russian psychologist whose work described and defined the role of relationship in human development. His work emphasized the notion that *cognitive and specific skill development* is the result of *internalizing* interactions with others within a *relationship* (Bedrova and Leong, 1996). Ylvisker and Feeney (1998) have translated Vygotskian theory into a support model that focuses on apprenticeship and collaboration between the person and another with more expertise in the areas where support is needed. The "tutor" provides collaborative mediation that is fine-tuned to the learner's changing needs for support to enable participation in meaningful, project-oriented work: "The roots of cognitive, executive and communication functions, as well as behavioral self-regulation, are everyday social interaction routines" (Ylvisker and Feeney, 1998, p. 15–16). In the socio-cultural models of development, relationship with others serves as the springboard for learning. Learning happens within a social context, within a dialogue with others. We acquire cognitive skills, knowledge and *behavior regulation*, not simply through memorization of facts or actions, but through our interactions in the social world where this knowledge has function and meaning.

INCONSISTENCY IN ABILITIES

People report sensory and movement inconsistencies such as: fluctuations in speed and clarity of sensory perception; unreliable ability to maintain or release body postures; delays in speed and accuracy of movement and speech; unpredictable changes in muscle tone; and unwanted vocal, verbal, and physical tics and extraneous non-functional movement (e.g., Mirenda and Donnellan, 1986; Williams, 1996a; Harp, 2008; Robledo et al., 2012). A sensory and movement difference is characterized by this inconsistency, causing stress for the most common of movements (Baggs, 2007). A person struggling with these performance characteristics may not be able to predict, plan for or sustain effective participation. For example, a person with a 14-s delay in her ability to respond to others (e.g., Mirenda and Donnellan, 1986) is likely to be misinterpreted and misunderstood and unlikely to be offered time to respond. This is illustrated by **Figure 1**, Harp (2008) on her blog *Asperger's Square 8* (used with permission).

SUPPORTING SELF-ESTEEM

Humans carry inside themselves an image that includes reasons for and the possibility of change. We need to know that we are

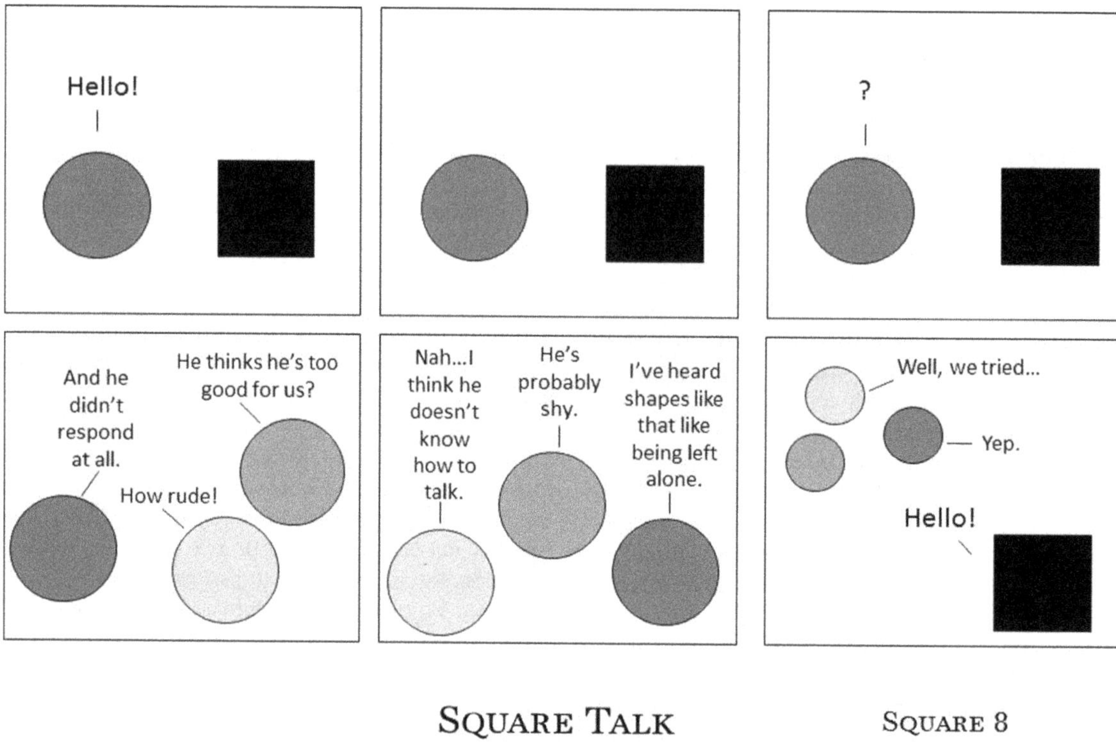

FIGURE 1 | Square Talk. Harp (2008), reprinted with permission.

OK just as we are, even though there are things we may want to learn or to do better.

A current trend in early intervention for young children with autism is to provide guidance in massive quantities (e.g., 40 h a week of one-to-one instruction). This guidance is naturally accompanied by frequent corrections and redirection. Given the intensity of this intervention, special care is needed to promote children's self-esteem at any age.

Equally important is the need for positive, optimistic, respectful support for adults with autism. The paucity of quality programs, diminished opportunity for interesting lives, effects of medication and chemical restraint are just a few of the additional burdens on these individuals and their families. Issues of collaboration, personalization, and comfort are also essential for children and particularly pressing for the adult population with the autism label. McGinnity and Negri (2005) offer helpful suggestions on how students and staff can learn to be more sensitive to the differences in those on the autism spectrum.

COLLABORATION, PERSONALIZATION, AND COMFORT

The growth of the autism industry over the past two decades has spawned no end of books, interventions, programs and products. Yet, the diagnosis of autism is not prescriptive of the type of supports needed for assisting any particular person to participate, relate, and communicate. Supports for people with autism should be personalized, reflect the respect and dignity due to all people and address the challenges with which people struggle to organize and regulate themselves in response to the sensory environment and their movement differences. Appropriate supports require a deep and local knowledge of the individual. This can be gained from those who know and appreciate them, but often such information is not available. Then it is even more essential to spend significant time with the person in a variety of activities and settings and with people who respect and admire him or her. We need to learn to listen with all of our senses and compassion (e.g., Lovett, 1996; Savarese, 2007) and to "presume competence" (Biklen and Cardinal, 1997) in all interactions. We do not put people in jeopardy by overestimating their experience. We do look for competence instead of deficits and talk to people in age-appropriate ways. And we model such interactions for all those who are, or may become, willing to know them better.

Moreover, we need to remember that in our journey of change, we all need allies who will collaborate with us to find the most comfortable and effective ways for us to learn to participate in our families, with our friends and as contributing members of our communities (Schwarz, 2004; Robledo and Donnellan, 2008). This is particularly critical for those persons who are challenged by the movement differences that often make such comfort temporary, personhood elusive, and collaboration a mystery. There is much to be learned from self-advocates with autism as well as from individuals who share some of the symptoms of movement differences such as Tourette syndrome, Parkinson's disorder and from their supporters (e.g., Williams, 1992; McGoon, 1994). For example, individuals with Tourette syndrome have taught us that calling attention to a behavior might make it much more difficult for a person to inhibit that behavior. It is roughly analogous to telling a stutterer not to stutter. Anyone familiar with classrooms and programs that have people with autism will recognize the value of that cautionary comment.

CONCLUSION

> *When I was growing up, speaking was so frustrating. I could see the words in my brain, but then I realized that making my mouth move would get those letters to come alive, they died as soon as they were born. What made me feel angry was to know that I knew exactly what I was to say and my brain was retreating in defeat . . .*
>
> (Burke, 2005, p. 250)

Jamie Burke is a college student who now is able to speak the words he types with two fingers on his Augmentative and Alternative Communication (AAC) device. We have proposed that many other individuals with the autism label may be challenged by sensory movement differences in starting, stopping, executing, combining, and/or switching actions, thoughts, emotions and speech. These symptoms have been described in the literature for many years but generally not integrated into our descriptions or understanding of *autistic behaviors*.

Sensory and movement differences often escape the notice of those of us who do not typically experience them but have been well-described by autistic self-advocates and persons interested in individuals with autism and other disability labels. Ignoring these differences (or redefining them as *autistic behaviors* to be controlled) has made life unnecessarily more difficult for individuals with autism and those who care about and for them. Many of the assumptive errors we have made are based on our own social history. In the absence of clarity about the nature of these movement differences, we will continue to be forced into the default position of seeing all unfamiliar behaviors as intentional, deliberate evidence of intellectual impairments and even pleasurable. We have not proposed another list of deficits but a greater understanding of the complexity of what we call *autistic behaviors* and the necessity to rethink our assumptions about them. The task is not going to be easy. Such sensory movement differences are manifest in autism and many other disorders in strikingly unique, personalized and dynamic ways that test present research strategies that rely heavily on a positivist-reductionist philosophy. Yet, some of the brightest scientific lights of the twentieth century reminded us that the best way to approach objectivity in science is to view the phenomenon from as many perspectives as possible (Luria, 1932; Edelman, 1992; Arthur Schawlow, pers. communication, 1996). As Einstein shared: "Not everything that counts can be counted and not everything that is counted, counts" (Einstein, 2004 as quoted in Cunningham and Scott, 2004, p. 208).

There is a long, continual path of misunderstanding in the field of autism. People have been thought of, and referred to, as "non-persons," "behavior problems," and "sub-normal" in every imaginable way. If they cannot speak, we assume they have little to say and offer only the most limited of communication options. Irrespective of the precision and intensity of our interventions, more often than not they experience isolation, segregation, homogeneous grouping, loneliness, pain, and boredom as part of their customary care across the life span. Often their sensory and movement differences contribute to such outcomes as these leave the rest of us unaware of the true nature of their challenges.

Any view of autism at this time needs to reflect the experience of self-advocates with autism and others who describe sensory and movement differences, as well as the latest in the neuroscience and child development literature. We need a research agenda that focuses on understanding and supporting autistic people and others in more respectful, personalized, and successful ways. It is the least dangerous assumption (Donnellan, 1984) to see all as full human beings who may have formidable and unfamiliar challenges to overcome and who, of course, desire social interaction, communication and participation.

Too often autistic children are raised to believe they are broken and need to be fixed. Adults with autism too often live lives of isolation and poverty. Understanding people's experiences may lead to acceptance, accommodation and appropriate support. To continue down the same paths, well-worn for 65 years, when all these data impel us to *re*think our assumptions and broaden our path is *un*thinkable.

ACKNOWLEDGMENTS

A version of this paper was originally published in *Disabilities Studies Quarterly (2010) Vol 30, 1.* and is included here with permission. The authors wish to thank Gail I. Evra, Ph.D. for her assistance with this manuscript.

REFERENCES

Abrams, R., and Taylor, M. A. (1976). Catatonia: a prospective clinical study. *Arch. Gen. Psychiatry* 33, 579–581.

American Psychiatric Association. (2000). *Diagnostic and Statistical Manual of Mental Disorders: Text Revision*. 4th Edn. Washington, DC: Author.

Baggs, A. (2007). *I knew moving took effort, but . . . .* Retrieved January 15, 2009, from Ballastexistenz. Available online at: http://ballastexistenz.autistics.org/?p=379

Baltaxe, C., and Simmons, J. (1977). Bedtime soliloquies and linguistic competence in autism. *J. Speech Hear. Disord.* 42, 376–393.

Barron, J., and Barron, S. (1992). *There's a Boy in Here*. New York, NY: Simon and Schuster.

Bateson, G. (1972). *Steps to an Ecology of Mind*. New York, NY: Ballantine.

Bedrova, E., and Leong, D. (1996). *Tools of the Mind: The Vygotskian Approach to Childhood Education*. Englewood Cliffs, NJ: Prentice-Hall.

Biklen, D., and Cardinal, D. (1997). *Contested Words, Contested Science: Unraveling the Facilitated Communication Controversy*. New York, NY: Teachers College Press.

Blackman, L. (1999). *Lucy's Story: Autism and Other Adventures*. Brisbane, QLD: Book in Hand.

Bluestone, J. (2005). *The Fabric of Autism: Weaving the Threads into a Cogent Theory*. Seattle, Washington: Sapphire Enterprises.

Bristol, M. M., Cohen, D. J., Costello, E. J., Denkla, M., Eckberg, T. J., Kallen, R., et al. (1996). State of the science in autism: report to the National Institutes of Health. *J. Autism Dev. Disord.* 26, 121–154.

Burke, J. (2005). "The world as I'd like it to be," in *Autism and the Myth of the Person Alone*, ed D. Biklen (New York, NY: NYU Press), 250.

Caroff, S., and Ungvari, G. (2007). Expanding horizons in catatonic research. Guest Editorial. *Psychiatr. Ann.* 37, 7–9.

Condon, W. S. (1985). "Sound-film microanalysis: a means for correlating brain and behavior," in *Dyslexia: A Neuroscientific Approach to Clinical Evaluation*, eds F. Duffy and N. Geschwind (Boston, MA: Little-Brown Co), 123–156.

Cunningham, H., and Scott, D. (2004). Software architecture for language engineering. *Nat. Lang. Eng.* 10, 205–209.

Damasio, A. R., and Maurer, R. G. (1978). A neurological model for childhood autism. *Arch. Neurol.* 35, 777–786.

Dhossche, D. M. (2004). Autism as early expression of catatonia. *Med. Sci. Monit.* 10, RA31–RA39.

Donnellan, A. M. (1984). The criterion of the least dangerous assumption. *Behav. Disord.* 9, 141–150.

Donnellan, A. M. (1999). Invented knowledge and autism: highlighting our strengths and expanding the conversation. *J. Assoc. Pers. Sev. Handicaps* 24, 230–236.

Donnellan, A. M., and Leary, M. R. (1995). *Movement Differences and Diversity in Autism/Mental Retardation.* Madison, WI: DRI Press.

Donnellan, A. M., Leary, M., and Robledo, J. (2006). "I can't get started: stress and the role of movement differences for individuals with the autism label," in *Stress and Coping in Autism,* eds G. Baron, J. Groden, G. Groden, and L. Lipsitt (Oxford: Oxford University Press), 205–245.

Donnellan, A. M., Mirenda, P., Mesaros, R. A., and Fassbender, L. (1984). A strategy for analyzing the communicative functions of behavior. *J. Assoc. Pers. Sev. Handicaps* 2, 201–212.

Edelman, G. M. (1992). *Bright Air, Brilliant Fire.* New York, NY: Basic Books.

Einstein, A. (2004). Software architecture for language engineering. *Nat. Lang. Eng.* 10, 205–209.

Endow, J. (2006). *Making Lemonade: Hints for Autism's Helpers.* Cambridge, WI: Cambridge Book Review Press.

Fay, W. (1969). On the basis of autistic echolalia. *J. Commun. Disord.* 2, 38–47.

Feldenkrais, M. (1972). *Awareness Through Movement.* New York, NY: HarperCollins.

Filipek, P., Accardo, P., Ashwal, S., Baranek, G., Cook, E. Jr., Dawson, G., et al. (2000). Practice parameter: screening and diagnosis of autism. *Neurology* 55, 468–479.

Fink, M., and Taylor, M. A. (2003). *Catatonia: A Clinician's Guide to Diagnosis and Treatment.* Cambridge: Cambridge University Press.

Fink, M., and Taylor, M. A. (2006). Catatonia: subtype or syndrome in DSM? *Am. J. Psychiatry* 163, 1875–1876.

Fogel, A. (1993). *Developing Through Relationships.* Chicago, IL: The University of Chicago Press.

Fournier, C. A., Hass, C. J., Naik, S. K., Lodha, N., and Cauraugh, J. H. (2010). Motor coordination in autism spectrum disorders. *J. Autism Dev. Disord.* 40, 1227–1240.

Gernsbacher, M. A., Sauer, E. A., Geye, H. M., Schweigert, E. K., and Goldsmith, H. H. (2008). Infant and toddler oral- and manual- motor skills predict later speech fluency in autism. *J. Child Psychol. Psychiatry* 49, 43–50.

Ghaziuddin, M., and Butler, E. (1998). Clumsiness in autism and asperger syndrome: a further report. *J. Intellect. Disabil. Res.* 42, 43–48.

Gibson, J. J. (1979). *The Ecological Approach to Perception.* Boston, MA: Houghton Mifflin.

Gilles de la Tourette, G. (1885). Etude sur nerveus caracteristee par de l'incoordination motrice accompagnee d'echolalie et de copralic. *Arch. Neurol.* 9, 19–42; 158–200.

Goldman, S., Wang, C., Salgado, M. W., Greene, P. E., Kim, M., and Rapin, I. (2009). Motor stereotypies in children with autism and other developmental disorders. *Dev. Med. Child Neurol.* 51, 30–38.

Grandin, T. in A is For Autism. British Film Institute. (1992a). *Fine Take Production for Channel 4.* Available online at: http://filmstore.bfi.org.uk.

Grandin, T. (1992b). A is for autism. *Chanel 4 TV,* UK.

Grandin, T. (1992c). "An insider view of autism," in *High Functioning Individuals with Autism,* eds E. Schopler and G. B. Mesibov (New York, NY: Springer), 105–124.

Green, D., Charman, T., Pickles, A., Chandler, S., Loucas, T., Simonoff, E., et al. (2009). Impairment of movement skills of children with autistic spectrum disorders. *Dev. Med. Child Neurol.* 51, 311–316.

Hale, M., and Hale, C. (1999). *I Had No Means to Shout!* Bloomington, IN: 1stBooks.

Harp, B. (2008). *Square Talk: Processing. Asperger Square 8,* online blog, Available online at: http://aspergersquare8.blogspot.com/.

Hill, D. A., and Leary, M. R. (1993). *Movement Disturbance: A Clue to Hidden Competencies in Persons Diagnosed with Autism and Other Developmental Disabilities.* Madison, WI: DRI Press.

Hill, D. A., and Leary, M. R. (2009). Casting call for a supporting role. *J. Intellect. Dev. Disabil.* 47, 469–472.

Jansiewicz, E., Goldberg, M., Newschaffer, C., Denckla, M., Landa, R., and Mostofsky, S. (2006). Motor signs distinguish children with high functioning autism and Asperger's syndrome from controls. *J. Autism Dev. Disord.* 36, 613–621.

Kahlbaum, K. (1973). *Catatonia* (Y. Levij and T., Pridan, Trans.). Baltimore, MD: Johns Hopkins University Press. (Original work published in 1874).

Kanner, L. (1946). Irrelevant and metaphorical language in early infantile autism. *Am. J. Psychiatry* 103, 242–246.

Leary, M., and Hill, D. (1996). Moving on: autism and movement disturbance. *Ment. Retard.* 34, 39–53.

Leekam, S. R., Nieto, C., Libby, S. J., Wing, L., and Gould, J. (2007). Describing the sensory abnormalities of children and adults with autism. *J. Autism Dev. Disord.* 37, 894–910.

Lovaas, O. I. (1966). "A program for the establishment of speech in psychotic children," in *Childhood Autism,* ed J. Wing (London: Pergamon Press), 115–144.

Lovaas, O. I. (1977). *The Autistic Child: Language Development Through Behavior Modification.* New York, NY: Halstead Press.

Lovaas, O. I., Schreibman, L., and Koegel, R. L. (1974). A behavior modification approach to the treatment of autistic children. *J. Autism Child. Schizophr.* 4, 111–129.

Lovett, H. (1996). *Learning to Listen: Positive Approaches and People with Difficult Behavior.* Baltimore, MD: Paul, H. Brookes.

Luria, A. R. (1932). *The Nature of Human Conflicts or Emotion, Conflict and Will.* New York, NY: Liveright, Inc.

Markram, H., Rinaldi, T., and Markram, K. (2007). The intense world syndrome–an alternative hypothesis for autism. *Front. Neurosci.* 1, 77–96.

Maurer, R. G. (1993). *What Autism and Facilitated Communication Have to Teach Us About the Neurology of Relationship (Audiotape from Lecture).* Toronto, ON: MacKenzie Group International.

McGinnity, K., and Negri, N. (2005). *Walk Awhile in My Autism.* Cambridge, WI: Cambridge Book Review Press.

McGoon, D. C. (1994). *The Parkinson's Handbook.* New York, NY: W.W. Norton.

Mirenda, P., and Donnellan, A. (1986). Effects of adult interaction style on conversational behavior in students with severe communication problems. *Lang. Speech Hear. Serv. Sch.* 17, 126–141.

Mostofsky, S., Dubey, P., Jerath, V., Jansiewicz, E., Goldberg, M., and Denckla, M. (2006). Developmental dyspraxia is not limited to imitation in children with autism spectrum disorders. *J. Int. Neuropsychol. Soc.* 12, 314–326.

Mostofsky, S. H., Burgess, M. P., and Larson, J. C. G. (2007). Increased motor cortex white matter volume predicts motor impairment in Autism. *Brain* 130(Pt 8), 2117–2122.

Mostofsky, S. H., Powell, S. K., Simmonds, D. J., Goldberg, M. C., Caffo, B., and Pekar, J. J. (2009). Decreased connectivity and cerebellar activity in autism during motor task performance. *Brain* 132, 2413–2425.

Movement Society. (2010). Available online at: http://www.movementdisorders.org. [Accessed on line, January, 2010].

Mulick, J. A., Jacobson, J. W., and Kobe, F. H. (1993). Anguished silence and helping hands: autism and facilitated communication. *Skeptical Inquirer* 17, 270–280.

Murphy, G. (1939). The research task of social psychology. *J. Soc. Psychol. SPSSI Bull.* 10, 107–120.

Nayate, A., Bradshaw, J., and Rinehart, N. (2005). Autism and asperger's disorder: are they movement disorders involving the cerebellum and/or basal ganglia? *Brain Res. Bull.* 67, 327–334.

Noterdaeme, M., Mildenberger, K., Minow, F., and Amorosa, H. (2002). Evaluation of neuromotor deficits in children with autism and children with a specific speech and language disorder. *Eur. Child Adolesc. Psychiatry* 11, 219–225.

Penland, H. R., Weder, N., and Tampi, R. R. (2006). The catatonic dilemma expanded. *Ann. Gen. Psychiatry* 5, 1–9.

Prizant, B., and Duchan, J. (1981). The functions of immediate echolalia in autistic children. *J. Speech Hear. Disord.* 46, 241–249.

Prizant, B., and Rydell, P. (1984). Analysis of functions of delayed echolalia in autistic children. *J. Speech Hear. Res.* 27, 183–192.

Rimland, B. (1993). Editor's notebook. *Autism Res. Rev. Int.* 7, 3.

Rinehart, N., Tonge, B., Iansek, R., McGinley, J., Brereton, A., Enticott, P., et al. (2006). Gait function in newly diagnosed children with autism: cerebellar and basal ganglia related motor disorder. *Dev. Med. Child Neurol.* 48, 819–824.

Robledo, J., and Donnellan, A. (2008). Properties of supportive relationships from the perspective of academically successful individuals with autism. *Intellect. Dev. Disabil.* 46, 299–310.

Robledo, J., Donnellan, A., and Strandt-Conroy, K. (2012). An exploration of sensory and movement differences from the perspective of individuals with autism. *Front. Integr. Neurosci.* 6:107. doi: 10.3389/fnint.2012.00107

Rogers, D. (1992). *Motor Disorder in Psychiatry: Towards a Neurological Psychiatry.* Chichester, England: John Wiley and Sons.

Rogers, S. J., Hepburn, S. L., Stackhouse, T., and Wehner,E. (2003). Imitation performance in toddlers with autism and those with other developmental disorders. *J. Child Psychol. Psychiatry* 44, 763–781.

Rubin, S., Biklen, D., Kasa-Hendrickson, C., Kluth, P., Cardinal, D., and Broderick, A. (2001). Independence, participation, and the meaning of intellectual ability. *Disabil. Soc.* 16, 415–429.

Sacks, O. (1990). *Awakenings.* New York, NY: Harper Perennial.

Sacks, O. W. (1989). "Neuropsychiatry and tourette's," in *Neurology and Psychiatry: A Meeting of Minds,* ed J. Mueller (Basel: Karger), 156–174.

Savarese, R. (2007). *Reasonable People: Autism and Adoption.* New York, NY: Other Press.

Schwarz, P. (2004). "Building alliances: community identity and the role of allies in autistic self-advocacy," in *Ask and Tell: Self-Advocacy and Disclosure for People on the Autisms Spectrum,* ed S. S. Shore (Shawnee Mission, KS: Autism Asperger Publishing Co.), 143–176.

Starkstein, S. E., Goldar, J. C., and Hodgkiss, A. (1995). Karl Ludwig Kahlbaum's concept of catatonia. *Hist. Psychiatry* 6(22 Pt 2), 201–207.

Stern, D. N. (2000). *The Interpersonal World of the Infant.* New York, NY: Basic Books.

Strandt-Conroy, K. (1999). *Exploring Movement Differences in Autism Through First-Hand Accounts,* Doctoral Dissertation, University of Wisconsin, Madison.

Sullivan, A. (2002). *Inertia: From Theory to Praxis.* Available online at: http://www.autistics.org/library/inertia.html

Sutera, S., Pandey, J., Esser, E., Rosenthal, M., Wilson, L., Barton, M., et al. (2007). Predictors of optimal outcome in toddlers diagnosed with autism spectrum disorders. *J. Autism Dev. Disord.* 37, 98–107.

Taylor, B. A., Hoch, H., Weissman, M. (2005). The analysis and treatment of vocal stereotypy in a child with autism. *Behav. Interv.* 20, 239–253.

Taylor, M., and Fink, M. (2003). Catatonia in psychiatric classification: a home of its own. *Am. J. Psychiatry* 160, 1233–1241.

Thelen, E. (1995). Motor development: a new synthesis. *Am. Psychol.* 50, 79–95.

Thelen, E., and Smith, L. B. (1994). *A Dynamic Systems Approach to the Development of Cognition and Action.* Cambridge, MA: MIT Press.

Tomchek, S. D., and Dunn, W. (2007). Sensory processing in children with and without autism: a comparative study using the short sensory profile. *Am. J. Occup. Ther.* 61, 190–200.

Williams, D. (1992). *Nobody Nowhere.* New York, NY: Avon.

Williams, D. (1996a). *Like Color to the Blind.* New York, NY: Times Books.

Williams, D. (1996b). *Autism: An Inside-Out Approach.* London: Jessica Kingsley.

Williams, D. (2003). *Exposure Anxiety – The Invisible Cage: An Exploration of Self-Protection Responses in the Autism Spectrum Disorders.* London: Jessica Kingsley.

Wing, L. (1981). Language, social and cognitive impairments in autism and severe mental retardation. *J. Autism Dev. Disord.* 11, 31–44.

Wing, L., and Attwood, A. (1987). "Syndromes of autism and atypical development," in *Handbook of Autism and Pervasive Developmental Disorders,* eds D. Cohen and A. Donnellan (New York, NY: Wiley), 3–19.

Ylvisker, M., and Feeney, T. J. (1998). *Collaborative Brain Injury Intervention: Positive Everyday Routines.* San Diego, CA: Singular Publishing Group, Inc.

Conflict of Interest Statement: The authors declare that the research was conducted in the absence of any commercial or financial relationships that could be construed as a potential conflict of interest.

5

Rhythm, movement, and autism: using rhythmic rehabilitation research as a model for autism

Michelle W. Hardy and A. Blythe LaGasse*

Center for Biomedical Research in Music, Colorado State University, Fort Collins, CO, USA

Edited by:
Anne M. Donnellan, University of Wisconsin-Madison, Uzbekistan

Reviewed by:
Adrian Rodriguez-Contreras, City College of New York, USA
Nienke Van Atteveldt, Netherlands Insititute for Neuroscience, Netherlands

***Correspondence:**
A. Blythe LaGasse, Center for Biomedical Research in Music, Colorado State University, 1778 Campus Delivery, Fort Collins, CO 80523, USA.
e-mail: blagasse@colostate.edu

Recently, there has been increased focus on movement and sensory abnormalities in autism spectrum disorders (ASD). This has come from research demonstrating cortical and cerebellar differences in autism, with suggestion of early cerebellar dysfunction. As evidence for an extended profile of ASD grows, there are vast implications for treatment and therapy for individuals with autism. Persons with autism are often provided behavioral or cognitive strategies for navigating their environment; however, these strategies do not consider differences in motor functioning. One accommodation that has not yet been explored in the literature is the use of auditory rhythmic cueing to improve motor functioning in ASD. The purpose of this paper is to illustrate the potential impact of auditory rhythmic cueing for motor functioning in persons with ASD. To this effect, we review research on rhythm in motor rehabilitation, draw parallels to motor dysfunction in ASD, and propose a rationale for how rhythmic input can improve sensorimotor functioning, thereby allowing individuals with autism to demonstrate their full cognitive, behavioral, social, and communicative potential.

Keywords: autism spectrum disorders, synchronization, movement regulation, neurologic music therapy, rhythm

INTRODUCTION

Autism Spectrum Disorder (ASD) is traditionally characterized by deficits in social interaction, communication, and restricted repetitive and stereotyped patterns of behaviors, interests, and activities (American Psychiatric Association, 2000). Although there will be changes to the diagnostic criteria with the DSM-V, the proposed criteria maintain focus on social/communicative symptoms and restricted/repetitive behaviors (Wing et al., 2011; Nishawala, 2012). This focus is maintained despite research demonstrating an extended profile of ASD that includes movement impairments (Staples and Reid, 2010; MacNeil and Mostofsky, 2012; Whyatt and Craig, 2012). Movement research has vast implications for treatment and therapy for individuals with autism, as the coordination and regulation of sensory and movement information is required for social interaction, speech communication, and participation in the environment (Donnellan et al., 2012). Since movement is a new area of consideration in ASD, there are few research studies focused on accommodations or treatments to improve movement in children with ASD. One accommodation that has not yet been explored is the use of rhythmic cueing to improve sensorimotor functioning in ASD.

Recent comprehensive research reviews have established that auditory rhythmic cueing is an effective tool for gross motor rehabilitation in populations including stroke (Bradt et al., 2010) and Parkinson's disease (de Dreu et al., 2012). Success observed with these populations has been attributed to processing of rhythm in the brain, motor synchronization to an auditory stimulus, and the intact motor synchronization ability of persons with neurological disease and disorder. Furthermore, rhythmic cueing is proposed to activate motor neurons via reticulospinal pathways, effectively priming the motor system (Rossignol and Melvill Jones, 1976; Thaut, 2005). Based on this rehabilitation research, we propose that rhythm may also be used in the treatment of movement differences in individuals with ASD. The purpose of this paper is to illustrate the potential impact of rhythmic cueing for sensorimotor regulation in persons with ASD. To this effect, we review research on rhythm in motor rehabilitation, draw parallels to motor dysfunction in autism resulting primarily from differences in the cerebellum, and propose a rationale for how rhythmic input can improve motor functioning, based on initial research indicating that rhythmic synchronization is intact despite cerebellar deficits. Furthermore, the potential benefits of rhythm for social/communicative behaviors will be explored.

RHYTHM IN REHABILITATION

Over the past two decades, researchers have begun to understand the neurological basis of music in the brain. Researchers have demonstrated that music processing and production are distributed throughout the cortex, subcortex, and cerebellum (Peretz and Zatorre, 2005). Areas engaged with music perception and production are not unique to music; rather, they overlap with non-musical networks (Thaut, 2005; Patel, 2011). Furthermore, the distributed nature of music in the brain allows preservation of musical functions despite the loss of a related non-musical function. For example, in persons with non-fluent aphasia, the ability to sing is unimpaired despite loss of speech production (Özdemir et al., 2006; Schlaug et al., 2009b). Research findings in music neuroscience have led to the development of neurologic music therapy techniques that drive cortical plasticity for rehabilitative gain.

Elements of music have been used effectively in therapy in collaboration as well as in isolation for various therapeutic needs. These elements include melody, harmony, tempo, dynamics, timbre, form, and rhythm. The organizing factor in all music is rhythm; therefore, rhythm serves as a timekeeper in the therapeutic application of music for motor rehabilitation goals and is foundational to auditory-motor synchronization. Auditory rhythmic cueing refers to an auditory sound stimulus with a fixed inter stimulus interval (such as the output from a metronome). As rhythmic cueing is well-documented to facilitate motor improvements in persons with neurological impairments, this paper will hypothesize the role of auditory rhythmic cueing in motor improvement in autism.

Bengtsson et al. (2009) demonstrated that auditory rhythm activates motor areas of the brain including the pre-motor cortex, supplementary motor areas, pre-supplementary motor area, and the lateral cerebellum. Rhythm not only activates motor areas of the brain, there is evidence of rapid motor synchronization to an external rhythmic cue in persons with and without neurological disability (Thaut et al., 1999a). Initial evidence of auditory-motor synchronization led to investigation of the auditory-motor pathway, with suggested involvement of the reticulospinal connections (Rossignol and Melvill Jones, 1976), cerebellum, brainstem, and the basal ganglia (Thaut and Abiru, 2010). This unique relationship between rhythm and motor function has been studied extensively in the rehabilitation sciences, where auditory rhythmic cueing has been utilized as an effective treatment in motor rehabilitation for over a decade (Thaut, 2005). There are two primary factors that contribute to the success of auditory rhythm in rehabilitation (1) rhythmic synchronization and (2) evidence that rhythmic cueing used systematically can facilitate cortical plasticity.

RHYTHMIC SYNCHRONIZATION

Rhythm refers to the division of time through distinguishable order and patterns of events, objects, symbols, or signs. It is one of the most important organizational aspects of music (Thaut et al., 1999a). Rhythmicity plays a critical part in learning, development, and performance, as timing of movement is essential in many motor control and cognitive functions (Thaut et al., 1999a, 2009; Molinari et al., 2005). Rhythm formation can integrate basic levels of sensory perception and motor entrainment into complex cognitive processes and motor adaptations (Thaut et al., 1999a). Findings in rhythmicity and brain research provide evidence that interaction between auditory rhythm and motor responses can be effectively employed for rehabilitation in movement disorders (Thaut et al., 1999a).

The role of rhythm in movement rehabilitation has been well-established through studies focused on persons with neurological disease and disorder. Thaut and colleagues found that rhythmic auditory cueing facilitated immediate improvement in gait parameters of persons with neurological injury, specifically cadence, velocity, and stride length (McIntosh et al., 1997; Thaut et al., 1997, 2001; Hurt et al., 1998). They concluded that the motor system is physiologically very sensitive to arousal by the auditory system and that rhythm facilitated positive change in motor output. Rhythm not only affected the timing of movement, but the total movement pattern. Specific findings indicate that auditory rhythmic cues add stability in motor control immediately (within two or three stimuli) rather than through a gradual learning process (Kenyon and Thaut, 2000). Rhythmic entrainment of neural auditory and motor impulses is based on motor synchronization to auditory signal frequency. This suggests that rhythm provides time information across the duration of the movement and not just the endpoints of movement when a response is matched to the period of the rhythmic signal.

The concept of frequency entrainment or period matching can happen at subliminal levels of sensory perception and allows "the brain to map and scale smoother time parameters of position change" due to the precise reference interval (Thaut et al., 1999a, p. 105). This research provides evidence of auditory-motor coupling, where the auditory external cue acts as a "forcing function" that optimizes the efficiency of kinematic movement parameters (Thaut et al., 1999a). Several studies have demonstrated that rhythmic synchronization is an effective tool for rehabilitation of gait in persons with Parkinson's disease (Miller et al., 1996; Thaut et al., 1996; McIntosh et al., 1997; Prassas et al., 1997; Howe et al., 2003; Arias and Cudeiro, 2008; Rochester et al., 2009), traumatic brain injury (Hurt et al., 1998; Kenyon and Thaut, 2000), spinal cord injury (de l'Etoile, 2008), stroke (Thaut et al., 1997; Roerdink et al., 2007, 2009; Hayden et al., 2009), Huntington's disease (Thaut et al., 1999b), and in patients with cerebellar ataxia (Abiru et al., 2008). Results of one study indicated that gait gains with 6 weeks of rhythmic auditory stimulation lasted 4 weeks after cessation of the treatment intervention in persons with Parkinson's disease (Kadivar et al., 2011). Researchers have also demonstrated success with rhythmic cueing for upper body rehabilitation goals for arm hemiparesis. Results of upper limb studies indicated decreased movement variability, increased speed of movement, smoothing of the movement trajectory (Thaut et al., 2002), and a decrease of compensatory trunk movements that often accompany arm movements in persons with stroke (Malcolm et al., 2009). These results are due to the neurobiological basis of timing in motor control and the impact of auditory-motor cueing.

The profound impact of rhythm on the motor system strongly suggests that the vital element linking music to motor behavior is time. Although the exact neurobiological process of rhythmic synchronization remains unclear; researchers have demonstrated that different aspects of processing time information are attributed to the neocortex, basal ganglia, cerebellum (Thaut et al., 2009) and thalamus (Krause et al., 2010). Regarding the cerebellum, researchers have shown that the cerebellar cortex and vermis contribute to the production of a timed motor response, particularly if it is complex and/or novel (Penhune et al., 1998; Thaut et al., 2009). From these analyses, the cerebellum makes a specific contribution to movement timing, aiding in computing the temporal parameters of incoming sensory stimuli and outgoing movements as well as in novel, temporally precise motor responses (Penhune et al., 1998; Thaut et al., 2008). Other data using auditory rhythmic cues evidenced contrasting cerebellar activation patterns associated with motor vs. perceptual and cognitive functions and that activation was neuroanatomically distinct based on function (Thaut et al., 2009). Because tasks of daily living require sensory input for successful completion, the cerebellum is likely necessary for the successful timing of these functions and the complex exchange between sensory and motor brain circuits (Molinari et al., 2007).

Individuals with cerebellar impairment show deficits in motor planning (Fisher et al., 2006) and adaptation (Block and Bastian, 2012); however, are relatively unimpaired in sensory adaptation (Block and Bastian, 2012). An intact sensory adaptation may be utilized to impact motor networks. Molinari et al. (2005) found that patients with cerebellar impairment demonstrated unimpaired motor synchronization to an external auditory cue. These findings suggest a direct drive between auditory and motor structures that may be pertinent for rehabilitation strategies in movement disorders (Molinari et al., 2005). Intact synchronization ability also demonstrates that even in the presence of cerebellar damage, temporal information could be available for the motor system through the auditory system to elicit functional change (Molinari et al., 2007).

The tight relationship between auditory rhythmic stimuli and motor responses has been demonstrated across many studies (Malcolm et al., 2008; Thaut et al., 2008, 2009). The evidence demonstrates that auditory-motor synchronization occurs rapidly and is maintained with tempo changes below conscious perception (Kenyon and Thaut, 2000; Tecchio et al., 2000). This subconscious adaptation is maintained in patients with cerebellar damage (Molinari et al., 2005), suggesting that the distributed nature of rhythm in the brain and underlying networks can function despite damage. This has further been demonstrated in gait rehabilitation of a person with cerebellar ataxia (Abiru et al., 2008). Observation of intact synchronization ability in persons with cerebellar differences suggests that rhythm could be utilized with other disabilities that show indication of cerebellar differences, including ASD.

RHYTHM AND CORTICAL PLASTICITY

Researchers have demonstrated cortical changes in persons who engage in music over time. Compared to non-musicians, adult musicians have differences in auditory areas, sensorimotor areas, and areas involved in multisensory integration (Gaser and Schlaug, 2003; Bermudez and Zatorre, 2005; Imfeld et al., 2009; Luo et al., 2012). Since it is expected that a life-long musician would have differences in the brain, researchers have sought to determine if short-term training could change neural connections. Hyde et al. (2009) demonstrated that 15 months of musical training changed motor, auditory, frontal, and occipital regions in the brains of children with no formal musical training. Schlaug et al. (2009a) demonstrated changes in the anterior corpus callosum after 29 months of instrument training. Evidence of cortical plasticity has also been demonstrated in adults. Pascual-Leone (2001) showed increased connectivity of the hand area of the sensorimotor cortex after only a few weeks of training on the piano. Furthermore, musical training has been shown to increase responses of motor and pre-motor areas of the brain.

Listening to rhythmic sequences engages cortical areas for movement, even in the absence of the movement or planning to complete the movement (Bangert et al., 2006; Bengtsson et al., 2009). Furthermore, Lahav et al. (2007) demonstrated that non-musicians who received a short period of musical training increased activations in the motor areas of the brain when listening to the same music. Cortical plasticity has also been documented in persons with neurological disability following rhythmic interventions. Luft et al. (2004) and Whitall et al. (2011) demonstrated greater activation of motor areas including the precentral gyrus, supplementary motor area (Whitall et al., 2011), and the cerebellum (Luft et al., 2004) following a 6-week bilateral arm training intervention paired with auditory rhythmic cueing. This intervention was compared to a dose-matched intervention without rhythmic cueing. This research demonstrates that short periods of engagement with rhythmic cueing can drive cortical plasticity, promoting structural and functional connectivity changes in the brain.

The above research demonstrates that auditory-motor coupling is not only possible, but occurs in persons who have neurological disease and disability. Although auditory rhythms have been applied widely in rehabilitation sciences, rhythm for synchronization has not yet been used to improve motor outcomes in individuals with ASD. Current neuroscience and motor research suggests that children with ASD have motor differences, which may benefit from the application of rhythmic cueing.

MOTOR CONTROL IN AUTISM SPECTRUM DISORDERS

Motor disturbances are not part of proposed DSM-V diagnostic criteria of autism; however, growing evidence indicates that neurological dysfunction may be associated with abnormal movements seen in individuals with autism. In a study of 67 children with ASD, Hilton et al. (2012) found that 83% of children with ASD presented motor scores at least one standard deviation below the general population, with greater impairments seen in children with more severe autism. This was compared to 6% of children from the same families without ASD showing a similar deficit. Other studies have estimated that between 80 and 90% of children with ASD demonstrate some degree of motor abnormality (Ghaziuddin and Butler, 1998; Dziuk et al., 2007; Ming et al., 2007; David et al., 2009). Although studies focused on incidence of motor abnormality are relatively recent, the earliest description of ASD included motor differences.

In Kanner's earliest paper describing autism (1943), he acknowledged a variety of motor differences in the individuals with autism he observed. He noticed that while all of the children demonstrated skilled fine muscle coordination, several of the children exhibited clumsiness in gait and gross motor performances. He observed individuals with autism failing to assume an anticipatory posture as well as passive positioning like "a sack of flour" (p. 243). In some cases, the individuals he studied lacked the ability to adjust their body to the person holding them. Kanner also noted that the children's verbal utterances and motor performances were monotonous and repetitive, "resulting in marked limitation in the variety of spontaneous activity" (p. 245). He proposed that if the slightest element of a given action was modified, altered, or removed, it was not considered the same or accepted as such by the child (Kanner, 1943).

Since these earliest reports, researchers documented motor impairments in ASD including clumsiness and poor coordination (Hallett et al., 1993; Teitelbaum et al., 1998; Vernazza-Martin et al., 2005), gait abnormalities (Hallett et al., 1993; Vernazza-Martin et al., 2005; Rinehart et al., 2006), impaired performance of skilled motor tasks (Dewey, 1995; Mostofsky et al., 2006; Dziuk et al., 2007), and motor planning deficits (Rinehart et al., 2001; Schmitz et al., 2003; Gidley Larson et al., 2008; Fabbri-Destro et al., 2009). Motor deficits could have vast implications for communicative and social functioning, as these skills rely on the organization of sensory and motor responses (Donnellan et al., 2012). Teitelbaum et al. (1998, 2002) indicated that motor differences were apparent in infancy, including differences in the development of infantile reflexes, which may be indicative of a neurological difference in early childhood. Although researchers have documented abnormalities in nearly every brain system in persons with ASD (Minshew, 1994; Ciaranello and Ciaranello, 1995; Courchesne and Allen, 1997), MRI, and autopsy studies have consistently reported that the cerebellum is a common site of neuroanatomic abnormality.

Differences observed in the cerebellum of persons with ASD have included hyperplasia or hypoplasia of cerebellar hemispheres (Murakami et al., 1989; Hardan et al., 2001; Pierce and Courchesne, 2001) and one or more regions of cerebellar vermis (Pierce and Courchesne, 2001; Sparks et al., 2002; Allen and Courchesne, 2003), and differences in the presence of Purkinje neurons (Kemper and Bauman, 1998; Allen and Courchesne, 2003). Fatemi et al. (2012) recently reviewed literature on the cerebellum in ASD and found points of consensus including abnormal anatomy, abnormal neurotransmitter systems, deficits in cerebellar motor and cognition, and neuroinflammation. The authors of this consensus paper presented evidence of a clear difference in cerebellar anatomy and function; however, the exact implications of these differences and treatment options are not yet understood (Fatemi et al., 2012).

Allen and Courchesne (1998) suggested that, based on connectivity, the cerebellum must function in both a general and highly integrative manner. These researchers suggested that the cerebellum may be responsible for purposes within multiple domains inclusive of cognitive, sensory, affective, and motor functions (Allen and Courchesne, 2003). Due to this widespread connectivity, Schmahmann and Pandya (2008) proposed that the cerebellum is involved with automatizing and optimizing functions around a "homeostatic baseline"; indicating that the cerebellum coordinates cognitive and emotional functions in the same way that it regulates and controls motor activity. Just as the cerebellum predicts the neural systems needed for a particular motor action, researchers suggest that it also predicts neural systems needed for a motor operation and then prepares for the operation at hand (Akshoomoff et al., 1997; Courchesne and Allen, 1997; Allen and Courchesne, 1998).

If the fundamental role of the cerebellum were to predict the neural systems needed to plan, adjust, and execute movements, then cerebellar damage or disease would likely affect the optimal functioning of a given neural system (Allen et al., 2004). Furthermore, the cerebellum's role in planning and coordinating movement would result in a lack of coordination in a person with cerebellar damage (Holmes, 1939). Persons with cerebellar damage maintain the ability to move; however, the quality and efficiency of movements is altered (Robinson, 1995). Although other neural systems continue to perform, they will do so sub-optimally without the preparatory role of the cerebellum to aid in performance (Allen et al., 2004). It is clear that individuals with ASD have the ability to move; however, Allen et al. (2004) proposed that they lack coordination due to a preparatory deficit. This preparatory deficit may account for the overall intact gross motor system that manifests differences in coordination and motor planning.

CAN AUDITORY RHYTHM ENHANCE MOTOR REGULATION IN ASD

The findings that rhythmic synchronization behavior is intact in patients with both atrophic and focal cerebellar lesions suggests the possibility that rhythm could be utilized in motor differences in ASD despite the presence of cerebellar abnormalities. One of the findings in the cerebellum in autism is abnormal development of vermal lobules VI and VII (Carper and Courchesne, 2000). These areas are known to process auditory information on a more arousal-oriented level and activation of lobule VI revealed a time sensitive response to modifications of the rhythmic tempo (Thaut et al., 2009). In rhythmic synchronization tasks, Stephan et al. (2002) showed different cerebellar circuit involvement in varying aspects of the presented tasks. Activation in vermal regions ipsilateral to the movement was consistent in novel and/or complex tasks and resulted in activation that was incrementally larger in these areas (Stephan et al., 2002; Molinari et al., 2007). Rhythmic auditory cues may therefore facilitate activations in these areas to elicit shared networks for motor performance, or if needed, may provide compensatory accommodations to activate other areas. Further research in this area is needed in order to assess the impact of rhythmic auditory-motor cues in therapy in this population.

One proposed function of the cerebellum as "comparator" is to adjust motor output related to planned actions (Penhune et al., 1998; Zatorre et al., 2007). The cerebellum predicts the timing of an upcoming movement, utilizes sensory feedback from the current movement, compares ongoing performance to an internal model, and then adapts responses such as force and/or trajectory (Penhune et al., 1998; Zatorre et al., 2007). Schmitz et al. (2003) observed that children with ASD exhibited latency of movement events, indicating over reliance on proprioceptive feedback to maintain postural stability. Bower (1996) suggested that the posterior cerebellar vermis coordinates proprioceptive input from muscle stretch receptors to optimize motor control. If there are cerebellar differences in ASD, the integration and response to feedback may be challenged or require additional accommodation. Since auditory feedback has been utilized to aid in proprioceptive muscular control (Thaut et al., 1999a; González and Yu, 2009; González et al., 2010), rhythmic auditory stimuli may create a feed-forward interaction directly influencing motor output in a predictive way (Zatorre et al., 2007). This would provide the person with ASD an accommodation facilitating more efficient and fluid movement without over-reliance on proprioceptive feedback.

The application of rhythm may serve to facilitate sensorimotor synchronization in autism, but based on other implicated deficits, it may contribute not only to gross motor functioning, but also related perceptual motor responses. One such perceptual motor skill is anticipatory preparation of movement. Gerloff et al. (1998) demonstrated that internal pacing of movement poses higher demands on the motor system than external pacing. Since individuals with autism exhibit deficits in anticipation (Rinehart et al., 2001) and appear to lack sufficient internal cueing, an external auditory rhythmic cue could provide a temporal template for organization of motor output while simultaneously decreasing the demand and increasing efficiency of movement. Auditory rhythmic stimuli can serve as predictable timing cues that influence motor anticipation resulting in the response pattern gradually becoming automatized (Thaut et al., 1999a).

Adams and Chambers (1962) and Schmidt (1968) investigated the automatization process of motor patterns and suggested that anticipation appeared to be "variable depending on the predictability of external response cues," and temporal and spatial predictability of those cues was most influential on anticipation. Because rhythmic tracking requires predictability of the stimulus, typical participants demonstrated anticipation as their motor responses were slightly ahead of the beat [as cited in Thaut et al. (1999a)]. Patients with cerebellar impairment showed intact rhythmic synchronization and evidenced similar anticipatory responses (Molinari et al., 2007); therefore, an auditory-motor stimulus of rhythm would likely impact anticipatory preparation in movement in persons with autism. Treatment geared toward building an anticipatory means of motor control in autism might then facilitate the development of internal models for motor planning.

Motor planning or praxis is an essential skill for motor function. Studies have shown that persons with autism exhibit a generalized praxis deficit (Mostofsky et al., 2006; Dewey et al., 2007; Dziuk et al., 2007) and that this may be attributed to perceptual motor elements (Vanvuchelen et al., 2007). It has been found that children with autism are not able to translate their motor intention into a global action, but that they program single acts independently from each other (Fabbri-Destro et al., 2009). External cueing of rhythm might lessen the internal demands placed on an individual with autism by providing precise reference intervals at each stage of the movement. This might allow for an increase in fluency and accuracy of movement parameters, as well as organization of the overall movement sequence.

Although rhythm has not yet been studied in this context with persons who have ASD, the above evidence suggests that motor differences observed including planning and coordination of movement might benefit from auditory rhythmic cueing. It is important to note that this is not simply listening to rhythms; rather, interventions involve the application of rhythm at a tempo appropriate for facilitating a movement pattern or increasing motor stability. The development of interventions using rhythm for motor skills may also include other musical elements such as pitch, structure, and dynamics. These elements can further emphasize motor patterns and engage the client in the therapeutic process. Clinical music therapy interventions often involve music with a strong or embedded rhythm. The emphasis is on the temporal aspect; however, melody, lyrics, structure, and style are incorporated for motivation.

NEUROLOGIC MUSIC THERAPY

Neurologic music therapy is the therapeutic application of music to cognitive, sensory, and motor dysfunctions due to neurologic disease or disability. Neurologic music therapy is a particular method of music therapy that was developed from neuroscience models of music perception and production (Thaut, 2005). Treatment in neurologic music therapy is focused on the use of rhythm and music stimuli to drive cortical plasticity. Traditionally, music therapy has been utilized to address social, communicative, and cognitive needs of children with ASD (e.g., Kern and Humpal, 2012). There are no systematic studies investigating the use of neurologic music therapy for movement disturbances in autism, likely due to the focus of social and communication skills in the diagnostic criteria. However, based on the above findings of movement differences in autism and the use of rhythm for other gross motor deficits, rhythm may be an appropriate accommodation for motor skill acquisition in ASD. Evidence that rhythm can be used for motor gains in a person with cerebellar ataxia can be used as a theoretical basis for using rhythm and music for movement in ASD.

Thaut (1988) derived a clinical motor rehabilitation model based on auditory-motor research. Within this model, auditory rhythmic signals as external stimuli can facilitate temporal muscular control of movement patterns by: (1) influencing timing and potentiation of motor neuron discharge, (2) decreasing muscular fatigue sensation, (3) facilitating automatized movement performance through the temporal predictability of its timing cues, (4) improving reaction time and response quality through facilitated response anticipation, and (5) providing auditory feedback for proprioceptive control mechanisms (p. 130). These elements have more recently been translated into neurologic music therapy techniques to address range of motion, muscle strength and endurance, muscle control and coordination, motor planning, and functional motor skills (Thaut, 2005). For example, music instrument playing has been utilized to improve functional reach in persons who have had a stroke (Sutton, 1984; Neugebauer et al., 2008; Altenmüller et al., 2009). Given motor deficits due to neurological differences in ASD, it is reasonable to apply these techniques to persons with ASD to address motor skills. Furthermore, the use of music may be especially effective due to unique responses to music in the brain.

There have been several reports that persons with ASD have enhanced pitch and/or melodic perception (Bonnel et al., 2003, 2010; Ouimet et al., 2012; Stanutz et al., 2012) Recently, Lai et al. (2012) demonstrated that low functioning children with ASD had stronger activations of the inferior frontal gyrus and superior temporal gyrus in song than in speech, exceeding cortical responses of typical children in the song condition. Furthermore, a greater activation of frontal-posterior networks was observed within the song condition, suggesting that children with ASD may be more effectively engaged in musical stimuli. Similar studies investigating rhythmic processing have not yet been conducted and research on perceptual timing in ASD is inconclusive (Falter et al., 2012). However, if music processing is enhanced or similar to that seen in typical children, the overall evidence provides a basis for using music embedded with a strong auditory rhythmic cue for greater global awareness within a task.

Neurologic music therapy interventions would use rhythm as an accommodation, providing a temporal template for the completion of complex motor tasks that require chaining of motor acts through activation of compensatory neural networks.

The predictability of musical stimuli and the use of stimuli to improve motor planning may have additional effects on cognitive, communicative, and social functioning. Although the research presented thus far has been focused on sensorimotor deficits, evaluations of movement might serve as effective comparisons for deficits in parallel systems important for socialization and communication (Mostofsky et al., 2007). This may be observed in the timing involved in speech production or the ability to predict and respond to social cues in the moment. Motor regulation is required for postural control, gesture, facial expression, speech production, social interaction; all processes that are documented as impaired in ASD (Robledo et al., 2012). There may even be cases where motor deficit or difficulty appears as behavior; for example, the individual throwing an object or falling on the floor. In some cases, the individual may understand the necessary action, but fail to complete the action due to motor planning deficits. Therefore, improvements in motor functioning due to predictability and anticipation of rhythmic and musical stimuli may facilitate or improve functioning in other areas including social and communication skills.

The impact of auditory rhythms utilized to promote functional skills in therapy may also benefit other skill areas, due to the highly predicable nature of rhythmic stimuli. One study demonstrated that musical stimuli with a strong rhythmic foundation increased synchronized alpha and gamma bandwidths, as measured by Electroencephalogram, which corresponded to improved memory (Thaut et al., 2005). If systematically applied rhythmic stimuli can increase the timing of networks beyond movement, interventions may yield greater impact. This may be one reason that studies on music therapy and ASD have demonstrated improved social (Brownell, 2002; Kern and Aldridge, 2006; Kim et al., 2008; Finnigan and Starr, 2010) and communication skills (Lim, 2010; Wan et al., 2011). Changes documented in these studies may even be in part due to improved ability to regulate motor patterns and interact with the environment. Improvement in motor functioning would allow individuals with autism to demonstrate their full cognitive, social, and communicative potential as demands in these domains typically require a movement to respond such as a gesture or initiation.

CONCLUSION

Autism is primarily defined with social and communication deficits; however, current literature suggests that movement differences play a part in autism and that this component warrants further investigation. If clinical treatment of autism addressed motor deficits, appropriate therapeutic goals to impact functional change might include motor coordination, motor planning, and functional motor skill development. Rhythmic auditory cueing could be an appropriate technique to provide a predictable structure to stabilize variability in the movement pattern and facilitate a motor plan. Given the current evidence, this is an area where further research is required to better understand the potential impact of rhythm on movement in persons with ASD.

REFERENCES

Abiru, M., Kikuchi, Y., Tokita, K., Mihara, Y., Fujimoto, M., and Mihara, B. (2008). The effects of neurologic music therapy on gait disturbance in a cerebellar ataxia: a case study. *Gunma Med. J.* 87, 213–218.

Adams, J. A., and Chambers, R. W. (1962). Response to simultaneous stimulation with two sense modalities. *J. Exp. Psychol.* 63, 198–206.

Akshoomoff, N. A., Courchesne, E., and Townsend, J. (1997). Attention coordination and anticipatory control. *Int. Rev. Neurobiol.* 41, 575–598.

Allen, G., and Courchesne, E. (1998). The cerebellum and non-motor function: clinical implications. *Mol. Psychiatry* 3, 207–210.

Allen, G., and Courchesne, E. (2003). Differential effects of developmental cerebellar abnormality on cognitive and motor functions in the cerebellum: an fMRI study of autism. *Am. J. Psychiatry* 160, 262–273.

Allen, G., Müller, R. A., and Courchesne, E. (2004). Cerebellar function in autism: functional magnetic resonance image activation during a simple motor task. *Biol. Psychiatry* 56, 269–278.

Altenmüller, E., Marco-Pallares, J., Münte, T. F., and Schneider, S. (2009). Neural reorganization underlies improvement in stroke-induced motor dysfunction by music-supported therapy. *Ann. N.Y. Acad. Sci.* 1169, 395–405.

American Psychiatric Association. (2000). *Diagnostic and Statistical Manual Of Mental Disorders, 4th Edn., Text Revision*. Washington, DC: American Psychiatric Association.

Arias, P., and Cudeiro, J. (2008). Effects of rhythmic sensory stimulation (auditory, visual) on gait in Parkinson's disease patients. *Exp. Brain Res.* 186, 589–601.

Bangert, M., Peschel, T., Schlaug, G., Rotte, M., Drescher, D., Hinrichs, H., et al. (2006). Shared networks for auditory and motor processing in professional pianists: evidence from fMRI conjunction. *Neuroimage* 30, 917–926.

Bengtsson, S. L., Ullén, F., Ehrsson, H. H., Hashimoto, T., Kito, T., Naito, E., et al. (2009). Listening to rhythms activates motor and premotor cortices. *Cortex* 45, 62–71.

Bermudez, P., and Zatorre, R. J. (2005). Differences in gray matter between musicians and nonmusicians. *Ann. N.Y. Acad. Sci.* 1060, 395–399.

Block, H. J., and Bastian, A. J. (2012). Cerebellar involvement in motor but not sensory adaptation. *Neuropsychologia* 50, 1766–1775.

Bonnel, A., McAdams, S., Smith, B., Berthiaume, C., Bertone, A., Ciocca, V., et al. (2010). Enhanced pure-tone pitch discrimination among persons with autism but not Asperger syndrome. *Neuropsychologia* 48, 2465–2475.

Bonnel, A., Mottron, L., Peretz, I., Trudel, M., Gallun, E., and Bonnel, A. M. (2003). Enhanced pitch sensitivity in individuals with autism: a signal detection analysis. *J. Cogn. Neurosci.* 15, 226–235.

Bower, J. (1996). Perhaps it's time to completely rethink cerebellar function. *Behav. Brain Sci.* 19, 438–439.

Bradt, J., Magee, W. L., Dileo, C., Wheeler, B. L., and McGilloway, E. (2010). Music therapy for acquired brain injury. *Cochrane Database Syst. Rev.* 7:CD006787. doi: 10.1002/14651858.CD006787

Brownell, M. (2002). Musically adapted social stories to modify behaviors in students with autism: four case studies. *J. Music Ther.* 39, 117–144.

Carper, R. A., and Courchesne, E. (2000). Inverse correlation between frontal lobe and cerebellum sizes in children with autism. *Brain* 123, 836–844.

Ciaranello, A. L., and Ciaranello, R. D. (1995). The neurobiology of infantile autism. *Ann. Rev. Neurosci.* 18, 101–128.

Courchesne, E., and Allen, G. (1997). Prediction and preparation, fundamental functions of the cerebellum. *Learn. Mem.* 4, 1–35.

David, F. J., Baranek, G. T., Giuliani, C. A., Mercer, V. S., Poe, M. D., and Thorpe, D. E. (2009). A pilot study: coordination of precision grip in children and adolescents with high functioning autism. *Pediatr. Phys. Ther.* 21, 205–211.

de Dreu, M. J., van der Wilk, A. S., Poppe, E., Kwakkel, G., and van Wegen, E. E. (2012). Rehabilitation, exercise therapy and music in patients with Parkinson's disease: a meta-analysis of the effects of music-based movement therapy on walking ability, balance and quality of life. *Parkinsonism Relat. Disord.* 18, S114–S119.

de l'Etoile, S. K. (2008). The effect of rhythmic auditory stimulation on the gait parameters of patients with incomplete spinal cord injury: an exploratory pilot study. *Int. J. Rehabil. Res.* 31, 155.

Dewey, D. (1995). What is developmental dyspraxia? [Review]. *Brain Cogn.* 29, 254–274.

Dewey, D., Cantell, M., and Crawford, S. G. (2007). Motor and gestural performance in children with autism spectrum disorders, developmental coordination disorder, and/or attention deficit hyperactivity disorder. *J. Int. Neuropsychol. Soc.* 13, 246–256.

Donnellan, A. M., Hill, D. A., and Leary, M. R. (2012). Rethinking autism: implication of sensory and movement differences for understanding and support. *Front. Integr. Neurosci.* 6:124. doi: 10.3389/fnint.2012.00124

Dziuk, M. A., Larson, J. C., Apostu, A., Mahone, E. M., Denckla, M. B., and Mostofsky, S. H. (2007). Dyspraxia in autism: association with motor, social, and communicative deficits. *Dev. Med. Child Neurol.* 49, 734–739.

Fabbri-Destro, M., Cattaneo, L., Boria, S., and Rizzolatti, G. (2009). Planning actions in autism. *Exp. Brain Res.* 192, 521–525.

Falter, C. M., Noreika, V., Wearden, J. H., and Bailey, A. J. (2012). More consistent, yet less sensitive: interval timing in autism spectrum disorders. *Q. J. Exp. Psychol.* 65, 2093–2107.

Fatemi, S. H., Aldinger, K. A., Ashwood, P., Bauman, M. L., Blaha, C. D., Blatt, G. J., et al. (2012). Consensus paper: pathological role of the cerebellum in autism. *Cerebellum* 11, 777–807.

Finnigan, E., and Starr, E. (2010). Increasing social responsiveness in a child with autism: a comparison of music and non-music interventions. *Autism* 14, 321–348.

Fisher, B. E., Boyd, L., and Winstein, C. J. (2006). Contralateral cerebellar damage impairs imperative planning but not updating of aimed arm movements in humans. *Exp. Brain Res.* 174, 453–466.

Gaser, C., and Schlaug, G. (2003). Gray matter differences between musicians and nonmusicians. *Ann. N.Y. Acad. Sci.* 999, 514–517.

Gerloff, C., Richard, J., Hadley, J., Schulman, A. E., Honda, M., and Hallett, M. (1998). Functional coupling and regional activation of human cortical motor areas during simple, internally paced and externally paced finger movements. *Brain* 121, 1513–1531.

Ghaziuddin, M., and Butler, E. (1998). Clumsiness in autism and AS: a further report. *J. Intellect. Disabil. Res.* 42, 43–48.

Gidley Larson, J., Bastian, A., Donchin, O., Shadmehr, R., and Mostofsky, S. H. (2008). Acquisition of internal models of motor tasks in children with autism. *Brain* 131, 2894–2903.

González, J., and Yu, W. (2009). "Multichannel audio aided dynamical perception for prosthetic hand biofeedback," in *Rehabilitation Robot International Conference on Rehabilitation Robotics CORR'09* (Kyoto), 240–245.

González, J., Yu, W., and Arieta, A. H. (2010). Multichannel audio biofeedback for dynamical coupling between prosthetic hands and their users. *Ind. Rob.* 37, 148–156.

Hallett, M., Lebiedowska, M. K., Thomas, S. L., Stanhope, S. J., Denckla, M. B., and Rumsey, J. (1993). Locomotion of autistic adults. *Arch. Neurol.* 50, 1304–1308.

Hardan, A. Y., Minshew, N. J., Harenski, K., and Keshavan, M. (2001). Posterior fossa magnetic resonance imaging in autism. *J. Am. Acad. Child Adolesc. Psychiatry* 40, 666–672.

Hayden, R., Clair, A. A., Johnson, G., and Otto, D. (2009). The effect of rhythmic auditory stimulation (RAS) on physical therapy outcomes for patients in gait training following stroke: a feasibility study. *Int. J. Neurosci.* 119, 2183–2195.

Hilton, C. L., Zhang, Y., Whilte, M. R., Klohr, C. L., and Constantino, J. (2012). Motor impairment in sibling pairs concordant and discordant for autism spectrum disorders. *Autism* 16, 430–441.

Holmes, G. (1939). The cerebellum of man. *Brain* 30, 466–488.

Howe, T. E., Lovgreen, B., Cody, F. W., Ashton, V. J., and Oldham, J. A. (2003). Auditory cues can modify the gait of persons with early-stage Parkinson's disease: a method for enhancing Parkinsonian walking performance? *Clin. Rehabil.* 17, 363–367.

Hurt, C. P., Rice, R. R., McIntosh, G. C., and Thaut, M. H. (1998). Rhythmic auditory stimulation in gait training for patients with traumatic brain injury. *J. Music Ther.* 35, 228–241.

Hyde, K. L., Lerch, J., Norton, A., Forgeard, M., Winner, E., Evans, A. C., et al. (2009). Musical training shapes structural brain development. *J. Neurosci.* 29, 3019–3025.

Imfeld, A., Oechslin, M. S., Meyer, M., Loenneker, T., and Jancke, L. (2009). White matter plasticity in the corticospinal tract of musicians: a diffusion tensor imaging study, *Neuroimage* 46, 600–607.

Kadivar, Z., Corcos, D. M., Foto, J., and Hondzinski, J. M. (2011). Effect of step training and rhythmic auditory stimulation on functional performance in Parkinson patients. *Neurorehabil. Neural Repair* 25, 626–635.

Kanner, L. (1943). Autistic disturbances of affective contact. *Nerv. Child* 2, 217–250.

Kemper, T. L., and Bauman, M. L. (1998). Neuropathology of infantile autism. *J. Neuropathol. Exp. Neurol.* 57, 645–652.

Kenyon, G. P., and Thaut, M. H. (2000). A measure of kinematic limb instability modulation by rhythmic auditory stimulation. *J. Biomech.* 33, 1319–1323.

Kern, P., and Aldridge, D. (2006). Using embedded music therapy interventions to support outdoor play of young children with autism in an inclusive community-based child care program. *J. Music Ther.* 43, 270–294.

Kern, P., and Humpal, M. (2012). *Early Childhood Music Therapy and Autism Spectrum Disorders: Developing Potential in Young Children and Their Families.* Philadelphia, PA: Jessica Kingsley.

Kim, J., Wigram, T., and Gold, C. (2008). The effects of improvisational music therapy on joint attention behaviors in autistic children: a randomized control trial. *J. Autism Dev. Disord.* 38, 1758–1766.

Krause, V., Schnitzler, A., and Pollok, B. (2010). Functional network interactions during sensorimotor synchronization in musicians and non-musicians. *Neuroimage* 52, 245–251.

Lahav, A., Saltzman, E., and Schlaug, G. (2007). Action representation of sound: audiomotor recognition network while listening to newly acquired actions. *J. Neurosci.* 27, 308–314.

Lai, G., Pantazatos, S., Schneider, H., and Hirsch, J. (2012). Neural systems for speech and song in autism. *Brain* 135(Pt 3), 961–975.

Lim, H. A. (2010). Effects of "Developmental Speech and Language Training through Music" on speech production in children with autism spectrum disorders. *J. Music Ther.* 47, 2–26.

Luft, A. R., McCombe-Waller, S., Whitall, J., Forrester, L. W., Macko, R., Sorkin, J. D., et al. (2004). Repetitive bilateral arm training and motor cortex activation in chronic stroke: a randomized controlled trial. *JAMA* 292, 1853–1861.

Luo, C., Guo, Z. W., Lai, Y. X., Liao, W., Liu, Q., Kendrick, K. M., et al.. (2012). Musical training induces functional plasticity in perceptual and motor networks: insights from resting-state FMRI. *PLoS ONE* 7:e36568. doi: 10.1371/journal.pone.0036568

MacNeil, L. K., and Mostofsky, S. H. (2012). Specificity of dyspraxia in children with autism. *Neuropsychology* 26, 165–171.

Malcolm, M. P., Lavine, A., Kenyon, G., Massie, C., and Thaut, M. (2008). Repetitive transcranial magnetic stimulation interrupts phase synchronization during rhythmic motor entrainment. *Neurosci. Lett.* 435, 240–245.

Malcolm, M. P., Massie, C., and Thaut, M. (2009). Rhythmic auditory-motor entrainment improves hemiparetic arm kinematics during reaching movements: a pilot study. *Top. Stroke Rehabil.* 16, 69–79.

McIntosh, G. C., Brown, S. H., Rice, R. R., and Thaut, M. H. (1997). Rhythmic auditory-motor facilitation of gait patterns in patients with Parkinson's disease. *J. Neurol. Neurosurg. Psychiatry* 62, 22–26.

Miller, R. A., Thaut, M. H., McIntosh, G. C., and Rice, R. R. (1996). Components of EMG symmetry and variability in parkinsonian and healthy elderly gait. *Electroencephalogr. Clin. Neurophysiol.* 101, 1–7.

Ming, X., Brimacombe, M., and Wagner, G. C. (2007). Prevalence of motor impairment in autism spectrum disorders. *Brain Dev.* 29, 563–570.

Minshew, N. J., (1994). "*In vivo* neuroanatomy of autism: neuroimaging studies," in *The Neurobiology of Autism*, eds M. L. Bauman and T. L. Kemper (Baltimore, MD: Johns Hopkins University Press), 66–85.

Molinari, M., Leggio, M. H., Cerasa, A., and Thaut, M. H. (2005). Sensorimotor transduction of time information is preserved in subjects with cerebellar damage. *Brain Res. Bull.* 67, 448–458.

Molinari, M., Leggio, M. G., and Thaut, M. H. (2007). The cerebellum and neural networks for rhythmic sensorimotor synchronization in the human brain. *Cerebellum* 6, 18–23.

Mostofsky, S. H., Burgess, M. P., and Gidley Larson, J. C. (2007). Increased motor cortex white matter volume predicts motor impairment in autism. *Brain* 130, 2117–2122.

Mostofsky, S. H., Dubey, P., Jerath, V. K., Jansiewicz, E. M., Goldberg, M. C., and Denckla, M. B. (2006). Developmental dyspraxia is not limited to imitation in children with autism spectrum disorders. *J. Int. Neuropsychol. Soc.* 12, 314–326.

Murakami, J. W., Courchesne, E., Press, G. A., Yeung-Courchesne, R., and Hesselink, J. R. (1989). Reduced cerebellar hemisphere size and its relationship to vermal hypoplasia in autism. *Arch. Neurol.* 46, 689–694.

Neugebauer, C. T., Serghiou, M., Herndon, D. N., and Suman, O. E. (2008). Effects of a 12-week rehabilitation program with music and exercise groups on range of motion in young children with severe burns. *J. Burn Care Res.* 29, 939–948.

Nishawala, M. (2012). *Autism Changes in the DSM V: A Step Toward Clarifying a Confusing Diagnosis.* Available online at: http://www.aboutourkids.org/articles/autism_changes_in_dsm_v_step_toward_clarifying_confusing_diagnosis

Ouimet, T., Foster, N. E., Tryfon, A., and Hyde, K. L. (2012). Auditory-musical processing in autism spectrum disorders: a review of behavioral and brain imaging studies. *Ann. N.Y. Acad. Sci.* 1252, 325–331.

Özdemir, E., Norton, A., and Schlaug, G. (2006). Shared and distinct neural correlates of singing and speaking. *Neuroimage* 33, 628–635.

Pascual-Leone, A. (2001). The brain that plays music and is changed by it. *Ann. N.Y. Acad. Sci.* 930, 315–329.

Patel, A. D. (2011). Why would musical training benefit the neural encoding of speech? The OPERA hypothesis. *Front. Psychol.* 2:142. doi: 10.3389/fpsyg.2011.00142

Penhune, V. B., Zatorre, R. J., and Evans, A. C. (1998). Cerebellar contributions to motor timing: a PET study of auditory and visual rhythm reproduction. *J. Cogn. Neurosci.* 10, 752–765.

Peretz, I., and Zatorre, R. J. (2005). Brain organization for music processing. *Ann. Rev. Psychol.* 56, 89–114.

Pierce, K., and Courchesne, E. (2001). Evidence for a cerebellar role in reduced exploration and stereotyped behavior in autism. *Biol. Psychiatry* 49, 655–664.

Prassas, S. G., Thaut, M. H., McIntosh, G. C., and Rice, R. R. (1997). Effect of auditory rhythmic cuing on gait kinematic parameters in stroke patients. *Gait Posture* 6, 218–223.

Rinehart, N. J., Bradshaw, J. L., Brereton, A. V., and Tonge, B. J. (2001). Movement preparation in high-functioning autism and Asperger disorder: a serial choice reaction time task involving motor reprogramming. *J. Autism Dev. Disord.* 31, 79–88.

Rinehart, N. J., Tonge, B. J., Iansek, R., McGinley, J., Brereton, A., Enticott, P., et al. (2006). Gait function in newly diagnosed children with autism: cerebellar and basal ganglia related motor disorder. *Dev. Med. Child Neurol.* 48, 819–824.

Robinson, F. R. (1995). Role of the cerebellum in movement control and adaptation. *Curr. Opin. Neurobiol.* 5, 755–762.

Robledo, J., Donnellan, A. M., and Strandt-Conroy, K. (2012). An exploration of sensory and movement differences from the perspective of individuals with autism. *Front. Integr. Neurosci.* 6:107. doi: 10.3389/fnint.2012.00107

Rochester, L., Burn, D. J., Woods, G., Godwin, J., and Nieuwboer, A. (2009). Does auditory rhythmical cueing improve gait in people with Parkinson's disease and cognitive impairment? A feasibility study. *Mov. Disord.* 24, 839–845.

Roerdink, M., Lamoth, C. J. C., Kwakkel, G., van Wieringen, P. C. W., and Beek, P. J. (2007). Gait coordination after stroke: benefits of acoustically paced treadmill walking. *Phys. Ther.* 87, 1009–1022.

Roerdink, M., Lamoth, C. J. C., van Kordelaar, J., Elich, P., Konijnenbelt, M., Kwakkel, G., et al. (2009). Rhythm perturbations in acoustically paced treadmill walking after stroke. *Neurorehabil. Neural Repair* 23, 668–678.

Rossignol, S., and Melvill Jones, G. (1976). Audiospinal influences in man studied by the h-reflex and its possible role in rhythmic movement synchronized to sound. *Electroencephalogr. Clin. Neurophysiol.* 41, 203–208.

Schlaug, G., Forgeard, M., Zhu, L., Norton, A., Norton, A., and Winner, E. (2009a). Training-induced neuroplasticity in young children. *Ann. N.Y. Acad. Sci.* 1169, 205–208.

Schlaug, G., Marchina, S., and Norton, A. (2009b). Evidence for plasticity in white-matter tracts of patients with chronic Broca's aphasia undergoing intense intonation-based speech therapy. *Ann. N.Y. Acad. Sci.* 1169, 385–394.

Schmahmann, J. D., and Pandya, D. N. (2008). Disconnection syndromes of basal ganglia, thalamus, and cerebrocerebellar systems. *Cortex* 44, 1037–1066.

Schmidt, R. (1968). Anticipation and timing in human motor performance. *Psychol. Bull.* 70, 631–646.

Schmitz, C., Martineau, J., Barthelemy, C., and Assaiante, C. (2003). Motor control and children with autism: deficit of anticipatory function? *Neurosci. Lett.* 348, 17–20.

Sparks, B. F., Friedman, S. D., Shaw, D. W., Aylward, E. H., Echelard, D., Artru, A. A., et al. (2002). Brain structural abnormalities in young children with autism spectrum disorder. *Neurology* 59, 184–192.

Stanutz, S., Wapnick, J., and Burack, J. (2012). Pitch discrimination and melodic memory in children with autism spectrum disorder. *Autism.* doi: 10.1177/1362361312462905. [Epub ahead of print].

Staples, K. L., and Reid, G. (2010). Fundamental movement skills and autism spectrum disorders. *J. Autism Dev. Disord.* 40, 209–217.

Stephan, K. M., Thaut, M. H., Wunderlich, G., Schicks, W., Tian, B., Tellmann, L., et al. (2002). Conscious and subconscious sensorimotor synchronization–prefrontal cortex and the influence of awareness. *Neuroimage* 15, 345–352.

Sutton, K. (1984). The development and implementation of a music therapy physiological measures test. *J. Music Ther.* 21, 160–169.

Tecchio, F., Salustri, C., Thaut, M. H., Pasqualetti, P., and Rossini, P. M. (2000). Conscious and preconscious adaptation to rhythmic auditory stimuli: a magnetoencephalographic study of human brain responses. *Exp. Brain Res.* 135, 222–230.

Teitelbaum, P., Teitelbaum, O., Fryman, J., and Maurer, R. (2002). Infantile reflexes gone astray in autism. *J. Dev. Learn Disord.* 6, 15–22.

Teitelbaum, P., Teitelbaum, O., Nye, J., Fryman, J., and Maurer, R. (1998). Movement analysis in infancy may be useful for early diagnosis of autism. *Proc. Natl. Acad. Sci. U.S.A.* 95, 13982–13987.

Thaut, M. H. (1988). Rhythmic intervention techniques in music therapy with gross motor dysfunction. *Arts Psychother.* 15, 127–137.

Thaut, M. H. (2005). *Rhythm, Music, and the Brain.* London: Taylor and Francis.

Thaut, M. H., and Abiru, M. (2010). Rhythmic auditory stimulation in rehabilitation of movement disorders: a review of current research. *Music Percept.* 27, 263–269.

Thaut, M. H., DeMartin, M., and Sanes, J. N. (2008). Brain networks for integrative rhythm formation. *PLoS ONE* 3:e2312. doi: 10.1371/journal.pone.0002312

Thaut, M. H., Kenyon, G. P., Hurt, C. P., McIntosh, G. C., and Hoemberg, V. (2002). Kinematic optimization of spatiotemporal patterns in paretic arm training with stroke patients. *Neuropsychologia* 40, 1073–1081.

Thaut, M. H., Kenyon, G. P., Schauer, M. L., and McIntosh, G. C. (1999a). The connection between rhythmicity and brain function: implications for therapy of movement disorders. *Eng. Med. Biol. Mag.* 18, 101–108.

Thaut, M. H., Miltner, R., Lange, H. W., Hurt, C. P., and Hoemberg, V. (1999b). Velocity modulation and rhythmic synchronization of gait in Huntington's disease. *Mov. Disord.* 14, 808–819.

Thaut, M. H., McIntosh, K. H., McIntosh, G. C., and Hoemberg, V. (2001). Auditory rhythmicity enhances movement and speech motor control in patients with Parkinson's disease. *Funct. Neurol.* 16, 163–172.

Thaut, M. H., McIntosh, G. C., and Rice, R. R. (1997). Rhythmic facilitation of gait training in hemiparetic stroke rehabilitation. *J. Neurol. Sci.* 151, 207–212.

Thaut, M. H., McIntosh, G. C., Rice, R. R., Miller, R. A., Rathbun, J., and Brault, J. M. (1996). Rhythmic auditory stimulation in gait training for Parkinson's disease patients. *Mov. Disord.* 11, 193–200.

Thaut, M. H., Peterson, D. A., and McIntosh, G. C. (2005). Temporal entrainment of cognitive functions: musical mnemonics induce brain plasticity and oscillatory synchrony in neural networks underlying memory. *Ann. N.Y. Acad. Sci.* 1060, 243–254.

Thaut, M. H., Stephan, K. M., Wunderlich, G., Schicks, W., Tellmann, L., Herzog, H., et al. (2009). Distinct cortico-cerebellar activations in rhythmic auditory motor synchronization. *Cortex* 45, 44–53

Vanvuchelen, M., Roeyers, H., and De Weerdt, W. (2007). Nature of motor imitation problems in school-aged boys with autism: a motor or a cognitive problem? *Autism* 11, 225–240.

Vernazza-Martin, S., Martin, N., Vernazza, A., Lepellec-Muller, A., Rufo, M., Massion, J., et al. (2005).

Goal directed locomotion and balance control in autistic children. *J. Autism Dev. Disord.* 35, 91–102.

Wan, C. Y., Bazen, L., Baars, R., Libenson, A., Zipse, L., Zuk, J., et al. (2011). Auditory-motor mapping training as an intervention to facilitate speech output in non-verbal children with autism: a proof of concept study. *PLoS ONE* 6:e25505. doi: 10.1371/journal.pone.0025505

Whitall, J., Waller, S. M., Sorkin, J. D., Forrester, L. W., Macko, R. F., Hanley, D. F., et al. (2011). Bilateral and unilateral arm training improve motor function through differing neuroplastic mechanisms: a single-blinded randomized controlled trial. *Neurorehabil. Neural Repair* 25, 118–129.

Whyatt, C. P., and Craig, C. M. (2012). Motor skills in children aged 7-10 years, diagnosed with autism spectrum disorder. *J. Autism Dev. Disord.* 42, 1799–1809.

Wing, L., Gould, J., and Gillberg, C. (2011). Autism spectrum disorders in the DSM-V: better or worse than the DSM-IV? *Res. Dev. Disabil.* 32, 768–773.

Zatorre, R. J., Chen, J. L., and Penhune, V. B. (2007). When the brain plays music: auditory-motor interactions in music perception and production. *Nat. Rev. Neurosci.* 8, 547–558.

Conflict of Interest Statement: The authors declare that the research was conducted in the absence of any commercial or financial relationships that could be construed as a potential conflict of interest.

6

A review of "music and movement" therapies for children with autism: embodied interventions for multisystem development

Sudha M. Srinivasan[1,2] and Anjana N. Bhat[1,2,3*]

[1] Department of Kinesiology, Neag School of Education, University of Connecticut, Storrs, CT, USA
[2] Center for Health, Intervention, and Prevention, University of Connecticut, Storrs, CT, USA
[3] Center for the Ecological Study of Perception and Action, University of Connecticut, Storrs, CT, USA

Edited by:
Elizabeth B. Torres, Rutgers University, USA

Reviewed by:
Jessica Phillips-Silver, International Laboratory for Brain, Music and Sound, Canada
Jafri M. Abdullah, Universiti Sains Malaysia, Malaysia

***Correspondence:**
Anjana N. Bhat, Assistant Professor in Kinesiology, U2101, University of Connecticut, 358 Mansfield Road, Storrs, CT 06269, USA.
e-mail: anjana.bhat@uconn.edu

The rising incidence of Autism Spectrum Disorders (ASDs) has led to a surge in the number of children needing autism interventions. This paper is a call to clinicians to diversify autism interventions and to promote the use of embodied music-based approaches to facilitate multisystem development. Approximately 12% of all autism interventions and 45% of all alternative treatment strategies in schools involve music-based activities. Musical training impacts various forms of development including communication, social-emotional, and motor development in children with ASDs and other developmental disorders as well as typically developing children. In this review, we will highlight the multisystem impairments of ASDs, explain why music and movement therapies are a powerful clinical tool, as well as describe mechanisms and offer evidence in support of music therapies for children with ASDs. We will support our claims by reviewing results from brain imaging studies reporting on music therapy effects in children with autism. We will also discuss the critical elements and the different types of music therapy approaches commonly used in pediatric neurological populations including autism. We provide strong arguments for the use of music and movement interventions as a multisystem treatment tool for children with ASDs. Finally, we also make recommendations for assessment and treatment of children with ASDs, and provide directions for future research.

Keywords: music, movement, motor, social, communication, autism, children

INTRODUCTION

Autism Spectrum Disorders (ASDs) are a group of neurological disorders characterized by social communication impairments as well as the presence of stereotyped and repetitive behaviors and interests (American Psychiatric Association, 2000). Children with ASDs demonstrate social impairments such as poor social and emotional reciprocity or turn taking and reduced eye contact during social exchanges (Mundy and Crowson, 1997; Dawson et al., 2004). Communication impairments in autism typically involve the lack of or a delay in the acquisition of language, difficulties in initiating and sustaining conversations with social partners, and the idiosyncratic use of language (Tager-Flusberg, 1999). In addition, the presence of repetitive and stereotypical behaviors is a hallmark of autism; children with ASDs demonstrate repetitive manipulations of objects, stereotypical behaviors such as flapping of hands, twisting of the body, and compulsive behaviors such as inflexible adherence to fixed routines and rituals (Bodfish et al., 2000; Boyd et al., 2012). In addition to these core impairments, children with ASDs may demonstrate several secondary impairments or comorbidities including significant behavioral and emotional problems as well as perceptuo-motor impairments. Behavioral and emotional problems include anxiety, aggression, depression, hyperactivity, temper tantrums, and/or self-injurious behaviors (Bodfish et al., 2000; Lecavalier, 2006; Loh et al., 2007; Mazefsky et al., 2012). A growing body of evidence suggests that perceptuo-motor impairments are frequently present in children with ASDs (Fournier et al., 2010; Bhat et al., 2011). Specifically, children with autism have difficulty modulating sensory inputs (Baranek, 1999; Baranek et al., 2005; Tomchek and Dunn, 2007) which may manifest as enhanced perception of auditory and visual stimuli (Bonnel et al., 2003; Heaton, 2003; Gernsbacher et al., 2008). Furthermore, they have significant and pervasive motor impairments such as problems with dual and multi-limb coordination (Green et al., 2009; Fournier et al., 2010), postural control (Minshew et al., 2004), gait (Vilensky et al., 1981; Hallett et al., 1993), as well as imitation and praxis (Mostofsky et al., 2006; Dewey et al., 2007). Comorbidities in perceptuo-motor performance could contribute to the social communication impairments of ASDs. Specifically, limited movement exploration and motor clumsiness may lead to missed opportunities to develop social connections with peers and caregivers (Leary and Hill, 1996; Jansiewicz et al., 2006; Bhat et al., 2011). Taken together, ASDs are multisystem disorders with both primary social communication impairments and secondary perceptuo-motor and behavioral comorbidities.

The current standard of care for ASDs includes the use of Applied Behavioral Analysis (ABA) (Lovaas, 1987), Picture Exchange Communication Systems (PECS) (Bondy and Frost, 2003), Teaching and Education of Autistic and Related Communication Handicapped Children (TEACHH) (Mesibov et al., 2004) as well as developmental, skill-based approaches (Pierce and Schreibman, 1995; Kasari et al., 2008). ABA, PECS, and TEACHH approaches recommend specific strategies for social interaction and environmental structure to promote positive behaviors and communication in children with ASDs (Lovaas, 1987; Bondy and Frost, 2003; Mesibov et al., 2004). The developmental approaches promote specific early social communication skills such as joint attention and imitation. While these approaches have significant evidence to support their use, they are primarily used to promote social communication and academic skills (Landa, 2007). Few approaches such as Sensory Integration therapy (Baranek, 2002) or Floortime (Greenspan and Wieder, 1999) promote perceptuo-motor development; however, there is limited evidence to support their use. Given the multisystem nature of the impairments in ASDs, there is a clear need to develop multisystem interventions that address their core social communication deficits as well as their perceptuo-motor and behavioral comorbidities. In this review, we highlight the multisystem effects of music therapies and how they might benefit children with ASDs.

Music-based therapies form about 12% of all autism interventions and 45% of all alternate treatment strategies used within school settings (Simpson et al., 2005; Hess et al., 2008). However, our review of published and unpublished research evaluating the efficacy of music therapies in autism revealed that the majority of the studies involved single-subject designs or small sample sizes (see **Table 1**). Moreover, these studies involved a pre-post comparison of outcomes in the treatment group and did not include a control group. The overall quality of studies was poor except for three published randomized controlled trials (Lundqvist et al., 2009; Lim, 2010; Gattino et al., 2011). The majority of the studies focused on addressing the communication impairments in autism. Few studies used musical experiences to facilitate social-emotional and behavioral outcomes in ASDs (see **Table 1** for details). Interestingly, the effects of music therapy on motor performance and motor stereotypies have never been examined. Given the current state of the music therapy literature, it is difficult to make definitive claims about the effects of music-based interventions in children with ASDs, except for the significant treatment effects in improving communication. In this review, we not only acknowledge the limitations of the music therapy literature, but also provide additional sources of evidence from the fields of music education, neuroscience, and special education to make a strong case for "music and movement" activities as multisystem interventions for children with ASDs. We believe that the multisystem nature of musical experiences warrants further systematic investigation as an effective treatment strategy to address both the core impairments and comorbidities of individuals with autism.

We propose that music-based interventions are effective treatment tools for individuals with ASDs because they harness the musical strengths of this population while alleviating their impairments. We are offering three different reasons that make

Table 1 | Music therapies in children with Autism Spectrum Disorders (ASDs).

Study	Sample size	Age of subjects in years	Therapy duration (number of days)	Therapy frequency (number of sessions per week)	Type of intervention (Active/Passive)	Type of music used (Live/Recorded)	Intervention design (Individual/Group)
STUDIES ASSESSING COMMUNICATION OUTCOMES							
Gattino et al., 2011	24	6.7–12.2	16	1	Active	Live	Individual
Wan et al., 2011	6	5.9–8.9	40	5	Active	Live	Individual
Lim, 2010	51	3–5	6	3	Passive	Recorded	Individual
Edgerton, 1994	11	6–9	10	1	Active	Live	Individual
Buday, 1995	10	4.4–9	8	4	Passive	Recorded	Individual
Lim and Draper, 2011	22	3–5	3	6	Active	Live	Individual
Corbett et al., 2008	11	3–7	38	7	Passive	Recorded	Individual
STUDIES ASSESSING SOCIAL OUTCOMES							
Kim et al., 2008	15	3–5	12	1	Active	Live	Individual
STUDIES ASSESSING EMOTIONAL OUTCOMES							
Katagiri, 2009	12	9–15	8	2	Active and Passive	Live and Recorded	Individual
Kim et al., 2009	15	3–5	12	1	Active	Live	Individual
STUDIES ASSESSING BEHAVIORAL OUTCOMES							
Lundqvist et al., 2009	20	22–57	10	2	Passive	Recorded	Individual
Boso et al., 2007	8	23–38	52	1	Active	Live	Group
Carnahan et al., 2009a,b	6	6–11	40	5	Active	Recorded	Group

Note: This table does not include case studies or unpublished theses and dissertations.

music-based interventions particularly attractive for individuals with ASDs. First, musical training may help address the various core autism impairments in joint attention, social reciprocity, and non-verbal and verbal communication, as well as comorbidities of atypical multisensory perception, poor motor performance, and behavioral problems. Second, children with ASDs find musical activities enjoyable, perhaps due to their enhanced musical understanding (Heaton, 2003). Children with autism have enhanced pitch perception abilities compared to typically developing children, for instance, enhanced pitch memory, labeling (Heaton, 2003), and discrimination (Bonnel et al., 2003). Therefore, clinicians and special educators often use music-based activities in school settings to engage children with ASDs (Hess et al., 2008). Third, music-based activities can be non-intimidating experiences wherein a child with ASD spontaneously explores various musical instruments, with the trainer joining in and copying the child's actions. Children with ASDs have difficulties with direct social engagement; hence, socially embedded group musical activities provide excellent opportunities to engage in predictable and comfortable interactions with social partners (Darrow and Armstrong, 1999; Allgood, 2003). In this review, we first provide evidence for the multisystem effects of musical experiences in facilitating various skills in children with autism, other neurological populations, and healthy individuals. Next, we discuss the critical elements of music-based activities and the popular music therapy approaches used in ASDs and other pediatric developmental disorders. Finally, based on the current literature, we provide recommendations for clinicians and clinical researchers working with children with autism including ideas for assessment and treatment.

MULTISYSTEM EFFECTS OF MUSICAL EXPERIENCES

In this section, we describe the supporting evidence for how embodied music therapies promote communication, social-emotional, perceptuo-motor, and behavioral skills in children with ASDs. In each sub-section, we will first explain the mechanism for positive effects of musical experiences and the evidence supporting the use of embodied music interventions in remediating the impairments in autism. Since the current research on music-based therapies in autism is limited, we will also rely on evidence from healthy individuals and pediatric populations with similar neurological impairments as autism. **Figure 1** shows the direct and indirect effects of musical experiences on the perceptuo-motor, communication, social-emotional, and behavioral domains of development. We will also offer recent neuroscientific evidence which suggests that musical experiences may shape the nervous system in healthy individuals and discuss its implications for individuals with ASDs.

EFFECT OF MUSICAL EXPERIENCES ON THE DEVELOPMENT OF LANGUAGE AND COMMUNICATION

Musical experiences involving singing, chanting, and playing of musical instruments clearly require communication between individuals. Music and language are closely related to each other

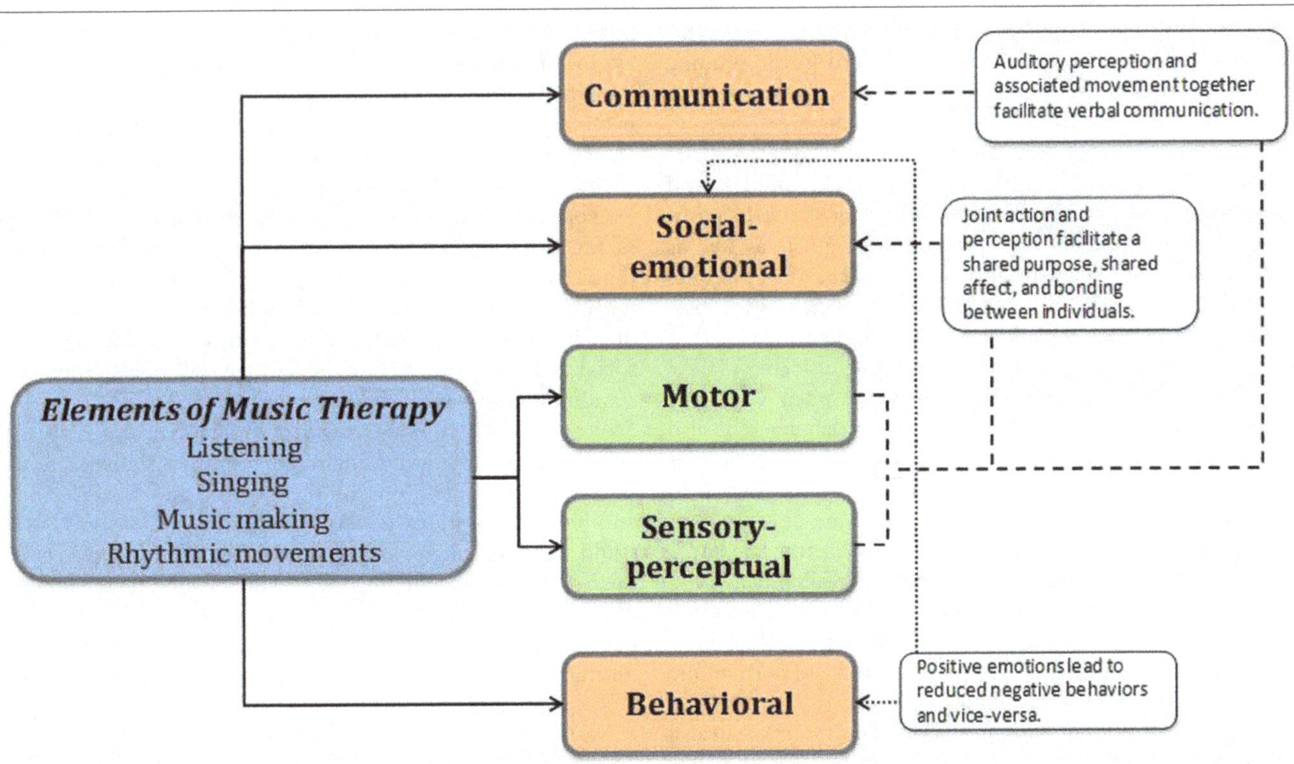

FIGURE 1 | Direct and indirect influences of musical experiences/therapies on the various domains of development.

in that both music and language are hierarchically arranged, with lower-level units such as notes/keys or letters/syllables integrated to form higher-level units such as chords/chord progressions or words/sentences (Molnar-Szakacs and Overy, 2006). Moreover, music and language are strikingly similar in the complexity of acoustic information, the use of spatial notation such as musical notation and the alphabet (Kraus and Chandrasekaran, 2010), as well as cognitive processes such as attention and memory (Patel et al., 1998; Foxton et al., 2003). These similarities allow easy transfer of learning between music and language (Tallal and Gaab, 2006). Children with ASDs have significant communication impairments despite relatively preserved musical skills (Bonnel et al., 2003; Heaton, 2003). Hence, music therapies have been used to facilitate verbal and gestural communication skills in children with ASDs (Edgerton, 1994; Buday, 1995; O'Loughlin, 2000; Farmer, 2003; Gold et al., 2006; Lim, 2010; Tindell, 2010; Gattino et al., 2011; Lim and Draper, 2011; Simpson and Keen, 2011; Wan et al., 2011) (see **Table 1**). A recent meta-analysis revealed that active music therapies involving singing and music-making led to significant improvements in verbal communication skills and non-verbal, gestural communication skills in children with ASDs (Gold et al., 2006). Effect sizes varied between 0.4 and 0.5 based on two randomized control trials involving 20 participants in the music therapy group compared to the control "placebo" therapy group (Buday, 1995; Farmer, 2003; Gold et al., 2006). Overall, there is some evidence from the autism literature supporting the links between music and language, thus justifying the use of music therapies to enhance communication skills in autism.

Literature from music education suggests strong links between musical training and enhanced communication skills in typically developing children and adults. Prolonged music training not only enhances musical perception but also speech perception/receptive language as well as expressive language (Butzlaff, 2000; Jakobson et al., 2003; Schlaug et al., 2005; Magne et al., 2006; Forgeard, 2008; Kraus and Chandrasekaran, 2010). Children and adults who received long-term musical training showed significant advances in basic auditory perception of music as well as speech, particularly, pitch perception (Schön et al., 2004; Marques et al., 2007; Moreno et al., 2009). Adult musicians were better able to detect weak violations/incongruities in pitch within both music and language compared to non-musicians (Schön et al., 2004). Moreover, the ability to detect pitch violations in language was not restricted to their native language; it also generalized to foreign languages (Marques et al., 2007). Similar enhancements in pitch perception were observed in children who had at least 4 years of musical training (Magne et al., 2006). Even children who received short-term musical training for a 6-month period were better able to detect weak pitch violations in both music and speech than children who received painting training (Moreno et al., 2009). Other perceptual skills that improve with prolonged musical training include rhythmic and auditory discrimination abilities (Jakobson et al., 2003) as well as melodic contour perception (Forgeard, 2008). Musical training not only enhances music and speech perception but also directly impacts expressive language. Musically trained children outperformed musically naïve children on tasks of verbal memory, verbal fluency, and non-verbal reasoning (Ho et al., 2003; Forgeard, 2008).

Lastly, music and movement therapies may enhance communication skills in children with other developmental disorders including children with dyslexia (Overy, 2003) and intellectual disabilities (Duffy and Fuller, 2000). Similar to children with autism, children with dyslexia have impairments in reading, phonological processing, and receptive vocabulary (Overy, 2000). Children with dyslexia significantly improved their spelling and phonological skills following a 15-week rhythm-based intervention involving singing and percussion games when compared to a control group receiving individual reading lessons (Overy, 2003). Engaging in timed rhythmic movement during singing may enhance the ability to parse words and give meaning to them during reading and verbalization (Sparks et al., 1974; Carroll, 1996; Overy, 2003, 2008; Roper, 2003; Overy and Molnar-Szakacs, 2009; Wan et al., 2011). This indirect linkage between perceptuo-motor and communication systems is shown in **Figure 1**. Children with moderate intellectual disability also showed improvements in verbal communication skills following an 8-week music therapy program (Duffy and Fuller, 2000). Overall, there is considerable evidence from music education, special education, and music therapies supporting linkages between musical experiences and communication development in children with autism, typically developing children, and children with other diagnoses.

EFFECT OF MUSICAL EXPERIENCES ON SOCIAL-EMOTIONAL DEVELOPMENT AND BEHAVIORAL SKILLS

Music-making or singing in dyadic or group settings create opportunities for developing social connections. Synchronous movements during rhythmic actions or music-making as well as unison singing creates a state of social cooperation, shared purpose, and a sense of togetherness which sparks a social connection between individuals, as highlighted in **Figure 1** (Marsh et al., 2009; Overy and Molnar-Szakacs, 2009; Kirschner and Tomasello, 2010). Moreover, group musical environments provide opportunities for learning social skills such as imitation, turn taking/social reciprocity, joint attention, shared affect, and empathy (Overy and Molnar-Szakacs, 2009), which are impaired in individuals with ASDs. While engaging in musical games, children will begin by imitating and synchronizing the actions of a social partner; however, gradually they will develop an understanding of their partner's intentions and emotions (Overy and Molnar-Szakacs, 2009). Overy and Molnar-Szakacs suggest that group music-making and singing conveys the affective state, physical state, and intentions of the partner and fosters empathy and positive emotions (Overy and Molnar-Szakacs, 2009). This could be particularly important in children with ASDs given their difficulties in empathizing and understanding the intentions of others (Koelsch, 2009). Moreover, different emotions such as happiness, sadness, fear, and anger can be effectively communicated to the listener through musical elements such as tempo and sound level of music as well as intonation and pauses in voice (Katagiri, 2009). Children with autism recognize affective signals conveyed through music, in spite of difficulties in recognizing emotions conveyed through speech (Heaton et al., 1999). Hence, we believe that socially embedded music and movement contexts involving listening, singing, moving, verbalizing, and playing, provide great opportunities to foster social connections and facilitate emotional understanding in children with ASDs. Further, the non-intimidating yet engaging nature of musical experiences and their ability to induce positive emotions while improving compliance may contribute to the behavioral effects of music therapies including a reduction in the frequency of negative behaviors. Conversely, the positive behavioral effects of music might in turn lead to enhanced social-emotional skills following musical training (see **Figure 1**).

Music-based interventions have been used to enhance social skills such as eye contact, engagement, and spontaneous initiation of social interactions in children with ASDs (Wimpory et al., 1995; Reitman, 2005; Kern and Aldridge, 2006; Kern et al., 2007; Stephens, 2008; Kim et al., 2009) (see **Table 1** for details). A 12-week intervention of improvisational music therapy led to significant increases in the frequency and duration of shared positive affect and joint attention with the therapist in the music group compared to the control group engaged in toy play (Kim et al., 2009). Similarly, a 7-month intervention involving different types of rhythmic movement games to music between a child with autism and his mother led to an increase in the frequency of eye contact episodes and spontaneous initiation of interactions by the child, post-intervention (Wimpory et al., 1995). Music has been used to promote emotional understanding in children with autism. Specifically, when children with autism were taught the four emotions of happiness, sadness, anger, and fear using verbal instructions or appropriate background music or specially composed songs, they improved their understanding of the selected emotions most in the background music condition (Katagiri, 2009). Further, music-based contexts have been used with success to reduce challenging behaviors such as self-injurious, aggressive, and stereotypical behaviors in children with autism (Wood, 1991; Gunter et al., 1993; Clauss, 1994; Orr et al., 1998; Brownell, 2002; Pasiali, 2004; Rapp, 2007; Devlin et al., 2008; Carnahan et al., 2009a,b; Lanovaz et al., 2009).

Studies in typically developing adults and children in the field of social psychology provide substantial evidence for how musical experiences facilitate the social and emotional development of individuals. Healthy adults and children tend to synchronize more with a human partner than with a recording or a drumming machine (Himberg, 2006; Kirschner and Tomasello, 2009). Joint rhythmic activities may intrinsically motivate adults and children to move in synchrony and engage in a cooperative effort (Tomasello and Carpenter, 2007). There is a developmental trajectory for joint action in that adult-adult pairs demonstrate greater interpersonal synchrony during drumming than child-child pairs suggesting that synchrony during joint action is a learned skill that improves over development (Kleinspehn-Ammerlahn et al., 2011). There is objective evidence for both adults and children to exhibit more cooperative and empathetic behaviors toward their social partner after engaging in a synchronized group musical experience (Anshel and Kipper, 1988; Wiltermuth and Heath, 2009; Kirschner and Tomasello, 2010). Adults who had previously engaged in synchronized singing or movement were more likely to be cooperative during a group economic game compared to those who had engaged in unsynchronized activities (Wiltermuth and Heath, 2009). Similarly, children who participated in an interactive musical game with adult partners were more likely to exhibit prosocial behaviors of helping and cooperating with their partners compared to a control group that engaged in a dyadic, non-musical, storytelling activity (Kirschner and Tomasello, 2010). The authors proposed that musical experiences may provide greater opportunities for fostering social connections than just verbal and non-verbal communication (Kirschner and Tomasello, 2010). Overall, there appears to be promising evidence for the potential use of socially embedded music and movement games to facilitate the social-emotional and behavioral skills in children with ASDs.

EFFECT OF MUSICAL EXPERIENCES ON THE REFINEMENT OF GROSS AND FINE MOTOR SKILLS

Whole body rhythmic actions such as clapping, marching, or walking to music provide significant opportunities to facilitate gross motor skills. Temporal patterning is inherently present in musical rhythms and an effort to synchronize arm and body movements to the rhythm of music could promote motor coordination in children. In addition, musical experiences that require fine motor skills of playing various musical instruments such as the piano, guitar, or drums have the potential to promote fine motor coordination and motor sequencing/praxis by providing numerous opportunities to practice, refine, and appropriately time finger, hand, and arm movements (Rodriguez-Fornells et al., 2012). It is also suggested that adding music through music-supported therapies can enhance patient motivation and compliance, provide opportunities for extensive practice, and offer continuous auditory feedback for online corrections (Schneider et al., 2007; Rodriguez-Fornells et al., 2012). Children with autism have significant impairments in gross motor skills such as bilateral motor coordination (Green et al., 2009; Fournier et al., 2010), balance (Minshew et al., 2004), and gait (Vilensky et al., 1981; Hallett et al., 1993) as well as significant fine motor delays (Provost et al., 2007; Downey and Rapport, 2012) that could be addressed using music and movement games targeted toward specific motor skills. As mentioned earlier, to the best of our knowledge there is no study that examined the effects of music and movement interventions on the gross and fine motor skills of children with ASDs. Hence, we will mainly draw upon evidence from typically developing children and individuals with other special needs to support the use of music and movement games in promoting motor skills in children with ASDs.

Several music education approaches including the Dalcroze and Kodaly methods of musical learning promote gross motor performance (Findlay, 1971; Hurwitz et al., 1975; Bachmann, 1991; Frego et al., 2004). These approaches promote the use of body movements to understand musical rhythms, but in the process facilitate gross motor coordination and movement timing (Findlay, 1971; Hurwitz et al., 1975; Bachmann, 1991; Frego et al., 2004). There is some evidence for the use of these approaches to improve gross motor performance in typically developing children. Four to six-year-old typically developing children who received a 2-month music and movement program showed significant improvements in their gross motor skills such as jumping and dynamic balance as measured by the Motor proficiency test (MOT 4–6) compared to children who engaged in a non-musical, physical education program (Zachopoulou et al., 2004). In another comparative study, 4 to 6-year-old typically developing children who received a 10-week, Dalcroze-based integrated music and physical education program outperformed children who received a general movement exploration program on various custom-developed, perceptuo-motor skills, and creative movement activities (Brown, 1981). These studies suggest that rhythmic accompaniment during motor practice enhances gross motor skill learning in typically developing children. In terms of fine motor skills, typically developing children who received 2 years of piano instruction showed significant improvements in fine motor skills as measured by the response speed, visuo-motor control, and upper limb speed and dexterity subtests of the Bruininks Osteresky Test of Motor Proficiency (BOTMP) compared to children who did not receive piano instruction (Costa-Giomi, 2005). The fine motor improvements observed in the children were directly related to the duration of musical training (Forgeard, 2008). Overall, there is considerable evidence from the field of early childhood music education to support the use of music and movement games for gross and fine motor development.

There is some evidence from special populations including children with dyslexia and adults with Parkinson's disease (PD) supporting the benefits of rhythmic movement and dance-based interventions. Specifically, rhythm training involving whole body actions such as clapping and percussion games has been used to promote movement timing in children with dyslexia (Overy, 2008). Overy proposed that poor movement timing may contribute to the poor phonological awareness and reading deficits observed in children with dyslexia (Overy, 2003). Moreover, children with dyslexia were more inaccurate and variable during multi-limb motions such as walking and clapping to a metronome beat compared to typically developing children (Getchell et al., 2010). However, a short-term auditory pacing program improved the multi-limb coordination of children with dyslexia suggesting that auditory feedback might supplement existing kinesthetic and visual feedback, and thereby facilitate motor coordination (Getchell et al., 2010). Along the same lines, dance has been used to promote balance, gait, and functional mobility in adults with PD (Hackney et al., 2007a,b; Duncan and Earhart, 2012). Adults with PD have significant motor impairments including impairments of gait as well as static and dynamic balance, similar to the motor deficits of individuals with ASDs (Bloem et al., 2001). A 12-month, bi-weekly, community-based tango dance program in patients with PD led to improvements in balance, gait patterns, and movement control in the treatment group compared to the control group that received no intervention (Duncan and Earhart, 2012). Dancing involves practice of precise movement sequences that demand dual and multi-limb coordination with varying balance requirements, thus providing an excellent alternative treatment tool for individuals with movement impairments such as PD as well as autism (Earhart, 2009). In summary, there is evidence for the potential use of music-based movement experiences to promote gross motor and fine motor performance in typically developing children as well as in individuals with special needs. Given this evidence from music education and neurorehabilitation literature and the nature of the motor impairments encountered in autism, we strongly believe that it is important to systematically explore the effects of embodied music therapies on the fine and gross motor skills of children with ASDs.

MUSICAL EXPERIENCES, PERCEPTION-ACTION LINKAGES, AND BRAIN DEVELOPMENT

Multiple brain regions, including motor, perceptual, language, and social-emotional systems are stimulated during musical experiences due to their multimodal, multisystem nature. For example, while playing a musical instrument the musician reads the complex musical notation and translates it into highly time-locked, synchronized, sequential, and precise finger and hand movements. In addition, the musician will use the auditory feedback produced by his/her music to adjust the timing, spatial organization, and sequence of future movements (Zatorre et al., 2007). The very nature of this task demands a strong coupling between the auditory, visual, somatosensory, and motor cortices (Schlaug et al., 2010). In this section, we provide evidence for neural substrates that contribute to perceptuo-motor, communication, and social-emotional enhancement following musical training and their implications for individuals with autism.

Music produced during music making is a multimodal perceptual experience produced by the integration of sensory and motor systems involved in the experience (Phillips-Silver, 2009). During a musical activity, the movements produced by adults are intimately linked to the sounds perceived: what one hears depends on how one moves and vice-versa (Phillips-Silver and Trainor, 2007). Neuroanatomical evidence for a perception-action linkage during musical activities comes from brain imaging studies in trained musicians (Haueisen and Knösche, 2001; Gaser and Schlaug, 2003; Bangert et al., 2006; Habib and Besson, 2009). Musicians showed activity in the premotor areas while simply listening to piano melodies, whereas non-musicians did not show such activity (Haueisen and Knösche, 2001). However, non-musicians trained over 5 days to play a melody, demonstrated premotor cortical activity while simply listening to the trained melody; they did not demonstrate similar premotor activity on listening to an untrained melody suggesting the important role that perceptuo-motor mapping plays during the initial stages of learning (Lahav et al., 2007). Similar premotor activation is seen during both simple listening and covert/overt singing (Callan et al., 2006). Musical tasks involving only auditory, only visual, or only motor components led to co-activation of the auditory, visual, and motor areas suggestive of strong visuo-motor and audio-motor integration following musical training (Bangert et al., 2006). Similarly, presentation of musical notation alone led to co-activation in the visual and motor cortices following training in reading music and playing the keyboard (Stewart et al., 2003). Thus, there is considerable evidence for the ability of musical experiences to recruit multiple areas of the brain and promote multimodal integration.

The multimodal nature of musical experiences is especially important for individuals with autism due to their known deficits in multimodal integration (Minshew and Williams, 2007). According to the connectivity hypothesis, brains of individuals with autism are characterized by short-range over-connectivity and long-range under-connectivity (Belmonte et al., 2004; Courchesne et al., 2007). To be clear, there is an increase in the short-range cortico-cortical connections and an under-development of long-range connections between different brain regions including the frontal, temporal, parietal, and subcortical areas (Belmonte et al., 2004; Courchesne et al., 2007). The impaired functions of long-range networks are thought to underlie the social-emotional and communication impairments of autism (Courchesne et al., 2007). Based on the evidence presented earlier, the ability of music to recruit multiple brain areas simultaneously might help address some of the multimodal integration deficits in autism. As an example, there is some evidence for a reversal in the left-right asymmetry in the arcuate fasciculus of non-verbal children with autism (Wan et al., 2012). The arcuate fasciculus is a long-distance white-matter tract that connects temporo-parietal areas with the frontal areas of the brain and is important for audio-motor integration of speech and language skills (Hickok and Poeppel, 2004; Glaser and Rilling, 2008). In healthy individuals, there is a left-right asymmetry in this tract with greater volumes in the left hemisphere than in the right hemisphere; in children with autism this asymmetry is reversed (Herbert et al., 2002; De Fossé et al., 2004; Wan et al., 2012) and is thought to underlie some of the language deficits in this population (Wan et al., 2012). However, there is promising evidence suggesting that novel music and movement interventions such as Auditory Motor Mapping Technique (AMMT) focused on promoting multimodal integration may in fact recruit these dysfunctional networks in children with ASDs (Wan et al., 2012, see **Table 2** and within music therapy approach section).

Music and language systems also share common neural substrates. Specifically, the Heschl's gyrus, planum temporale, secondary auditory cortex, and the corpus callosum are all involved in both music and language processing (Meyer et al., 2002). Musical training leads to structural changes in the planum temporale, primary and secondary auditory cortices, and the Heschl's gyrus, all of which are important for auditory processing (Wan and Schlaug, 2010). Further, the magnitude of these changes is greater in musicians who begin training early in life (Gaser and Schlaug, 2003). Six-year old children who received musical training for 15 months demonstrated structural changes in the precentral gyrus, the corpus callosum, and the Heschl's gyrus (Hyde et al., 2009). Similarly, 9–11 year old instrumentalists with 4 years of musical training showed larger gray matter volumes in the sensorimotor and occipital cortices as well as greater activation of the mirror neuron systems (MNS) during rhythm and melody discrimination tasks compared to non-instrumentalists (Schlaug et al., 2005). Hence, in typically developing individuals, neuroanatomical evidence suggests strong links between musical training and activation of substrates common to both music and language processing.

There is clear evidence for the relatively unimpaired musical skills despite significant language impairments in individuals with autism (Bonnel et al., 2003; Heaton, 2003). There is also mounting evidence for abnormalities in neural networks

Table 2 | Music therapy approaches: critical elements, domains of development, targeted skills, and populations.

Music therapy approach	Type of music therapy	Critical elements	Domains of development	Targeted skills and populations
Auditory motor mapping technique	Active	Listening Singing Music-making	Communication	Speech sounds and word approximations in non-verbal children with autism (Wan et al., 2011)
Melodic intonation therapy	Active	Singing Gross-motor tapping	Communication	Phonation and speech production in children with apraxia (Roper, 2003)
Rhythm therapy	Active	Singing Music-making Rhythmic actions like clapping	Social communication	Movement timing, phonologic skills, auditory processing, and spelling in children with dyslexia (Overy, 2003)
Improvisational music therapy	Active	Music-making	Social communication Emotional	Eye contact, turn taking, spontaneous joint attention, behavioral compliance, and positive affect in children with autism (Kim et al., 2008, 2009)
Sound therapies such as Auditory Integration Therapy, Tomatis Method, and Samonas Therapy	Passive	Listening to music that has been modified by filtering and modulation	Sensory Behavioral Communication	Sound sensitivity, behavioral compliance, listening and comprehension. Majority of the studies found non-significant results for these outcomes (Rimland and Edelson, 1995; Bettison, 1996; Zollweg, 1997; Edelson et al., 1999; Mudford et al., 2000; Corbett et al., 2008)

underlying speech in autism (Hesling et al., 2010; Lai et al., 2012; Wan et al., 2012). A comparison of neural systems sensitive to both speech and music in low-functioning children with autism and age-matched healthy controls using functional magnetic resonance imaging and diffusion tensor imaging revealed that the activation in the inferior frontal gyrus in children with autism was lower than in controls during speech stimulation but higher than controls during song stimulation. This study argues for the potential utility of music-based therapies in remediating the core language impairments in autism (Lai et al., 2012). Some mechanisms have been proposed to explain the positive effects of musical training on speech impairments in autism. For instance, the OPERA hypothesis proposes that speech-related impairments could benefit from musical training due to its following characteristics—(1) *O*verlap exists in the brain regions processing speech and music (Patel, 2003), (2) *P*recision of processing required during musical activities is more intense than that needed for speech processing, (3) *E*motions invoked by musical activities are strong and positive, (4) *R*epetition and practice are the integral elements of all musical experiences, and lastly, (5) Focused *A*ttention is required for accurate musical performance (Patel, 2011). Taken together, these factors associated with musical training can drive experience-dependent plasticity in speech processing in individuals with autism (Patel, 2011).

Socially synchronous movements and unison singing during group music activities evoke the MNS activity in the brain. MNS has been postulated as the neural basis for social abilities of shared attention, affect, and empathy (Molnar-Szakacs and Overy, 2006; Cattaneo and Rizzolatti, 2009). The MNS includes a group of neurons thought to be present in the inferior frontal cortex, inferior parietal lobule, and superior temporal sulcus of the human brain (Buccino et al., 2004; Cattaneo and Rizzolatti, 2009). These neurons are activated both during action production and during observation of actions performed by others (Buccino et al., 2004; Cattaneo and Rizzolatti, 2009; Rizzolatti et al., 2009). An additional subset of premotor "mirror" neurons have been postulated to possess audio-motor properties so that they are activated just by listening to someone else singing or making music (Molnar-Szakacs and Overy, 2006). This may allow students to learn not just by playing the instrument on their own but also by listening to the sounds and watching the movements produced by their teacher (Schlaug et al., 2005). The shared and temporally synchronous activation of the MNS in individuals involved in a group music-making experience provides a neural basis for the shared experiences and social connections within the group (Molnar-Szakacs and Overy, 2006). There is mounting evidence that individuals with autism have a dysfunctional MNS which might underlie some of the social-emotional and motor imitation deficits observed in this population (Williams et al., 2001; Dapretto et al., 2005; Wan et al., 2010a,b). Hence, music-based activities involving imitation and rhythmic synchronization within socially embedded contexts may engage the dysfunctional MNS of children with ASDs (Wan et al., 2010a,b). Taken together, the neuroanatomical evidence presented in this section suggests that music and movement activities within social contexts can serve as a powerful medium to induce a range of plastic changes in brain structure and connectivity in individuals with ASDs.

PROPOSITIONS FOR USING MUSICAL EXPERIENCES IN CHILDREN WITH AUTISM

Having reviewed strong behavioral and neuroanatomical evidence in favor of music and movement therapies for children with ASDs, we will now discuss the critical elements of musical experiences and their potential benefits for remediating the core impairments and comorbidities in autism. We will also review in detail the critical elements and potential benefits of three active music-based therapies that are currently utilized in the treatment of children with special needs.

CRITICAL ELEMENTS OF MUSICAL EXPERIENCES FOR CHILDREN WITH AUTISM

Musical experiences can vary depending on the activities involved, but the four most critical elements are listening, singing, music-making, and rhythmic actions synchronized to music, experienced in individual or socially embedded, dyadic, and group activities (Edelson et al., 1999; Pellitteri, 2000; Schlaug et al., 2005; Overy, 2008; Wan et al., 2010a,b, 2011). Listening to music is predominantly a passive musical experience whereas singing, music-making, and rhythmic actions require active participation (Pellitteri, 2000). Each type of musical experience has its own applications. For example, passive listening techniques such as Auditory Integration Therapy (AIT) have been used to address behavioral problems and auditory hypersensitivity in children with ASDs (Rimland and Edelson, 1995; Bettison, 1996; Zollweg, 1997; Edelson et al., 1999; Mudford et al., 2000; Corbett et al., 2008); however, there is limited evidence to support their use (Sinha et al., 2011). Singing has been used as a communicative medium to compensate for language impairments as well as to promote language in individuals with various speech disorders including ASDs (Wan et al., 2010a,b). Music-making has been used extensively in music education to teach children concepts of rhythm, melody, and pitch as well as various spatio-temporal concepts such as slow-fast, soft-loud, moving on a count, etc. (Pellitteri, 2000). Specifically, improvisational music-making is an outlet for expression of creativity and individuality (Pellitteri, 2000). The last element of synchronized whole body rhythmic actions is often used to teach and internalize musical concepts such as rhythm. By grounding music in physical movements, eurhythmics provides an embodied musical experience (Findlay, 1971; Hurwitz et al., 1975; Bachmann, 1991; Frego et al., 2004). Structured and improvisational music-making as well as rhythmic whole body movements involve perception and action and promote fine and gross motor skills and bilateral and visuomotor coordination as discussed in the previous section (Phillips-Silver, 2009). Children can experience all the critical elements of music in individual as well as group settings. Individual experiences involve one-on-one interactions between the trainer and the child and are tailored to the individual needs of the child. Group sessions involve synchronous activities between members to ensure a meaningful and enjoyable musical experience and in turn facilitate social connections between members of the group (Pellitteri, 2000; Overy and Molnar-Szakacs, 2009). Moreover, careful additions of socially embedded, dyadic, and group activities would be important for children with ASDs to practice social communication skills.

CURRENT MUSIC THERAPY APPROACHES USED IN CHILDREN WITH AUTISM AND THOSE WITH OTHER SPECIAL NEEDS

Current music therapy approaches, their critical elements, domains of development, and targeted skills are highlighted in **Table 2**. In general, music therapies have been provided to children with ASDs (see **Table 1** for details), dyslexia (Overy, 2003), apraxia (Roper, 2003), and intellectual disabilities (Duffy and Fuller, 2000) (see **Table 2** for details).

1. *Auditory Motor Mapping Training (AMMT) and Melodic Intonation Therapy (MIT)* facilitate language production in non-verbal/low-verbal children by training an association between self-produced sounds (drum hit or finger tap) and articulatory movements or auditory-motor mapping (Sparks et al., 1974; Carroll, 1996; Roper, 2003; Norton et al., 2009; Wan et al., 2011) (see **Table 2**). AMMT combines critical elements of listening to the therapist's intonation and drum tapping, singing with the same intonation, and music-making by tapping on a pair of tuned drums. Therapists progress from sounding words and tapping the tuned drums alone to unison singing and music-making. It is proposed that ultimately the child produces the words on his/her own without any support from the therapist (Wan et al., 2011). Non-verbal children with ASDs demonstrated improvements in their ability to articulate words and phrases following an 8-week intervention of AMMT (Wan et al., 2011). Similarly, MIT which involves singing and associated gross motor tapping to mark the rhythm and stress of the intoned phrases was found to enhance phonation and speech production in children with apraxia (Roper, 2003; Norton et al., 2009).
2. *Rhythm training* has been used to address the timing deficits in language, motor control, perception, and cognition encountered in children with dyslexia (Overy, 2008) (see **Table 2**). Children with dyslexia significantly improved their phonological and spelling skills following a 15-week rhythm therapy intervention based on the critical elements of singing, joint music-making, and whole body rhythmic movements (Overy, 2008). The multisensory experience focused on rhythm and timing facilitated the temporal processing skills of children with dyslexia.
3. *Improvisational music therapy* is an individualized, patient-centered approach to facilitate social engagement and verbal and non-verbal communication skills in children with ASDs (Kim et al., 2009) (see **Table 2**). In this approach, the therapist uses improvised, shared music-making experiences to tune in to the patient's musical and non-musical non-verbal behaviors. Such moment-by-moment musical attunement of the therapist to the patient helps develop a medium of communication between the two, which in turn facilitates social skills such as turn taking, imitation, and joint attention as well as verbal communication skills (Kim et al., 2008). This approach has been used to improve social communication skills in children with autism (Kim et al., 2008, 2009).

Taken together, several attempts have been made to therapeutically utilize the various critical elements of musical experiences in the treatment of children with autism and other pediatric disorders.

RECOMMENDATIONS FOR CLINICIANS AND CLINICAL RESEARCHERS

In the above sections, we have reviewed vast evidence supporting the therapeutic use of embodied music interventions in addressing the multisystem impairments of children with autism and other similar developmental disorders. However, as outlined in the introduction, current research in this area has several limitations. In this section, we will provide recommendations for assessment and treatment of autism for clinicians and researchers working in this field. We hope that this discussion will provide guidelines for future systematic research on embodied music therapies and will bring multisystem music and movement interventions to the forefront in the treatment of autism.

RECOMMENDATIONS FOR ASSESSMENT OF CHILDREN WITH ASDs

In this review, we have offered substantial evidence on how musical experiences may impact the various forms of development in typically developing children and children with special needs. The majority of the evidence stems from literature in music education and special education and to some extent from the music therapy literature. Currently, there is limited evidence to support the use of music therapies in children with ASDs. Future research should consider using better study designs such as randomized controlled trials to examine the efficacy of music therapies on the various core deficits and comorbidities of children with ASDs. Standardized, reliable, and valid assessments should be routinely used to evaluate outcomes. In this section, we provide researchers with certain objective and subjective tools to better characterize their study populations and to assess the impact of music-based interventions on perceptuo-motor, communication, and social-emotional development. We strongly urge that whenever possible, researchers use a combination of subjective and objective tools to assess treatment effects.

To the best of our knowledge, no study to date has assessed the impact of music therapy on motor skills in ASDs. However, for future studies, we recommend that researchers consider the use of standardized tests such as the Bruininks Osteretsky Test of Motor Proficiency (BOTMP) (Bruininks, 1978), Sensory Integration and Praxis Tests (SIPT) (Ayres, 1996), Movement Assessment Battery for Children (MABC) (Henderson and Sugden, 1992), gross motor and fine motor subtests of the Mullen Scales of Early Learning (MSEL) (Mullen, 1995), and the Individualized Music Therapy Assessment Protocol (IMTAP) (Baxter, 2007) to assess for changes in motor function. In addition, context-specific changes in motor skills such as the accuracy of imitation or amount of time spent in synchrony can be examined using moment-to-moment video coding or quantitative measures such as relative phase analysis (Scholz and Kelso, 1989; Schmidt et al., 1991). Changes in sensory modulation could also be assessed using the Short Sensory Profile (Tomchek and Dunn, 2007), the sensory subtests of the IMTAP (Baxter, 2007), and the SIPT (Ayres, 1996).

Some common social communication measures for school-age children include the Assessment of Basic Language and Learning Skills-Revised (ABLLS-R) (Partington and Sundberg, 1998) and the Peabody Picture Vocabulary test (PPVT) (Dunn and Dunn, 1981). Non-verbal communication can be examined using the Early Social Communication Scale (ESCS) in young children (Mundy et al., 2003). In addition, researchers should also use video coding to measure socially directed verbal communication such as the frequency of spoken syllables/words, non-verbal communication such as social gaze, joint attention, and use of signs or gestures, as well as affective changes including durations or frequencies of positive, neutral, and negative affect.

For the assessment of changes in behavioral problems following intervention, several psychiatric measures, and parent/teacher questionnaires have been used. Some of the commonly used measures include the Brief Psychiatric Rating Scale (BPRS) (Lukoff et al., 1986), Repetitive Behaviors Scale-Revised (RBS-R) (Lam, 2004), Autism Behavior Checklist (ABC) (Krug et al., 1988), Pervasive Developmental Disorder Behavior Inventory (PDDBI) (Cohen and Sudhalter, 2005), Connor's Rating Scales (Conners, 1989), and the Aberrant Behavior Checklist (Aman and Singh, 1986). In addition, we recommend that researchers code for changes in the frequency of positive and negative behaviors within the music therapy sessions.

It would be important to characterize the study population given the diversity of impairments observed in ASDs. Group characterization measures include a confirmation of ASD diagnosis and its severity as well as a basic IQ measure. Autism-related impairments could be confirmed through medical records, screeners such as the Social Communication Questionnaire

Table 3 | Special considerations for music-based interventions for children with ASDs.

Domain	Special considerations
Structure of the environment	1. Predictability and familiarity is important. Follow a familiar activity schedule. Conduct sessions in the same physical space (Mesibov et al., 2004). 2. Use visual cues to indicate the child's spot and distinguish the space used. 3. Consider the needs of the child when setting up the environment. For example, avoid distractions, cover musical instruments until they are used, and avoid bright lights and loud sounds for hypersensitive children. 4. Use visual picture schedules to provide structure to the session (Bondy and Frost, 2003). This helps children with ASDs to understand the progression in the session and helps them anticipate transitions. 5. Allow time for the child to adapt to any new activity.
Instructions, prompts, and feedback	1. Be aware of the child's communication system in advance. 2. Avoid long verbal instructions. Be brief and precise in your instructions. 3. Whenever, possible, combine verbal and visual instructions. For example, use visual picture schedules and instructions such as "do this." 4. Make sure that the instructor is seated in front of the child to ensure that he/she is in the child's visual field. 5. Instructions can be provided through songs to ensure better comprehension. 6. A typically developing peer or adult could stand or be seated beside the child as a model for the child. 7. One of the adults could provide manual guidance during the motor activities. 8. Allow the child time to practice the activity independently (Shumway-Cook and Woollacott, 2007). 9. Use props whenever necessary to clarify the goals of the activity.
Repetition and reinforcement	1. Repetition is the key for learning (Lovaas, 1987). 2. Ask parents and caregivers to try out the activity in another environment to promote practice and generalization to other individuals and environments. 3. Various rewards such as stickers and small toys could also be provided (Lovaas, 1987; Landa, 2007). 4. Provide verbal and gestural reinforcement in the form of good jobs and hi-fives. 5. Provide breaks from activity to do favorite sensory activities. Edibles should be used as the last resort.
Nature of the interaction	1. During group sessions, be sensitive to the individual needs of the child. 2. Give sufficient breaks and avoid overwhelming the child. 3. Try to keep the child actively involved as much as possible. 4. Vary the level of task complexity. Use a mix of simple and complex activities to allow for success and engagement (Darrow, 2009). 5. Within activities, vary the verbal and motor complexity. 6. Allow time for free music-making and movements to sustain engagement. 7. Look out for negative behaviors such as tantrums, non-compliance, and self-injurious behaviors. If these are observed, then ask the child to communicate that the activity be stopped. Seek advice from caregivers on best ways to address negative behaviors (Lovaas, 1987; Landa, 2007).

(Berument et al., 1999) or the Social Responsiveness Scale (Constantino and Gruber, 2002) or through gold-standard assessments/interviews such as the Autism Diagnostic Observation Schedule (ADOS-2) (Lord et al., 2012a,b) and Autism Diagnostic Interview -Revised (ADI-R) (Lord et al., 1994). Autism severity can be determined through standardized tests such as the Childhood Autism Rating Scale (CARS) (Schopler et al., 1980). IQ could be measured using various measures such as the Kaufman Brief Intelligence Test (KBIT) (Kaufman, 1990), Wechsler Intelligence Scale (WISC) (Wechsler, 1949), Stanford-Binet Intelligence Test (SBIT), (Terman and Merrill, 1960), or Differential Abilities Scale (DAS) (Elliott, 1990). Given the evidence for the multisystem effects of music interventions discussed, we urge researchers to assess the multisystem effects of music-based therapies using various sensori-motor, communication, social-emotional, and behavioral measures.

RECOMMENDATIONS FOR TREATMENT OF CHILDREN WITH ASDs

There is a strong need to further develop comprehensive, multisystem, music interventions to facilitate the communication, social-emotional, behavioral, and perceptuo-motor skills of individuals with ASDs. In addition, we have various specific recommendations on the nature, intensity, and frequency of music interventions. First, active music interventions that emphasize participation through singing, music-making, and synchronized rhythmic actions must be promoted as opposed to passive listening. Second, given the positive effects of socially embedded activities it would be useful to consider dyadic, triadic, or group-based activities. However, we acknowledge that working with children with autism is very challenging and the needs of each child are unique. The other members in the group could be typically developing siblings, parents, or caregivers who will adjust to the needs of the child. Third, we recommend better content development as opposed to purely improvisational music-based activities. Fourth, there is a need for better reporting standards while disseminating the results. Fifth, there is a need to test for skill generalization to novel contexts or standardized tests and maintenance of learned skills through long-term follow-up. Sixth, interventions should be offered within natural settings such as home or school environments to ensure ecological validity and generalization. In terms of the intensity of interventions, music-based interventions have been provided at least 2–3 times per week with each session lasting for ~30 min (see **Table 1**). Repetition is of utmost importance to ensure learning in this population. Hence, we recommend involving parents and caregivers in the training activities to enhance skill learning, generalization, and maintenance. Some additional special considerations specific to training sessions and needs of children with ASDs are listed in **Table 3**. These considerations incorporate the ideas promoted by contemporary autism interventions such as ABA, PECS, and TEACHH. The recommendations provided in this section should be used as guidelines; however the training protocols will need to be tailored to the individual needs of the child. As mentioned earlier, various domains of development can be addressed through music-based activities; however, certain domains may require more training than others for an autistic child due to his or her individual impairments. Similarly, specific modifications may be needed for a child due to his or her unique behavioral or sensory modulation impairments.

CONCLUSIONS

In this review, we offered substantial evidence for the multisystem effects of musical experiences in children with ASDs, healthy individuals, as well as other pediatric neurological populations. We believe that novel, embodied rhythm-based, multisystem interventions grounded in singing, music-making, joint action, and social synchrony can be used to alleviate the core social communication deficits and perceptuo-motor and behavioral comorbidities of children with ASDs. Current evidence for the efficacy of music therapies in children with ASDs comes from a handful of studies that lack systematic study designs, assessments, and treatment protocols. There is an urgent need for systematic research in this field. Our research team has developed an intense, 8-week, novel, embodied musical intervention that will be tested within a pilot, randomized controlled trial to assess its effects on the multisystem performance of children with ASDs. If our hypotheses are upheld, we will be providing objective evidence to support the use of rhythm-based, music and movement intervention for children with ASDs. Future research should extend this work by examining multisystem effects of music therapies through larger clinical trials using larger sample sizes.

ACKNOWLEDGMENTS

We thank Autism Speaks for a pilot treatment award (#8137) to support our study on the effects of music and movement interventions in children with autism spectrum disorders.

REFERENCES

Allgood, N. (2003). Music and sensory integration for children with autism spectrum disorders. *Early Child. Connect.* 9, 21–27.

Aman, M. G., and Singh, N. N. (1986). *Aberrant Behavior Checklist: Manual.* East Aurora, NY: Slosson Educational Publications.

American Psychiatric Association. (2000). *Diagnostic and Statistical Manual of Mental Disorders (DSM-IV-TR).* 4th Edn. Washington, DC: American Psychiatric Publishing, Inc.

Anshel, A., and Kipper, D. A. (1988). The influence of group singing on trust and cooperation. *J. Music Ther.* 25, 145–155.

Ayres, J. (1996). *Sensory Integration and Praxis Tests (SIPT).* Los Angeles, CA: Western Psychological Services.

Bachmann, M. (ed.). (1991). *Dalcroze Today—An Education Through and into Music.* New York, NY: Oxford University Press.

Bangert, M., Peschel, T., Schlaug, G., Rotte, M., Drescher, D., Hinrichs, H., et al. (2006). Shared networks for auditory and motor processing in professional pianists: evidence from fMRI conjunction. *Neuroimage* 30, 917–926.

Baranek, G., Parham, L., and Bodfish, J. (2005). "Sensory and motor features in autism: assessment and intervention," in *Handbook of Autism and Pervasive Developmental Disorders,* eds F. P. R. Volkmar, A. Klin, and D. Cohen (Hoboken, NJ: Wiley), 831–857.

Baranek, G. T. (1999). Autism during infancy: a retrospective video analysis of sensory-motor and social behaviors at 9–12 months of age. *J. Autism Dev. Disord.* 29, 213–224.

Baranek, G. T. (2002). Efficacy of sensory and motor interventions for children with autism. *J. Autism Dev. Disord.* 32, 397–422.

Baxter, H. T. (2007). *The Individualized Music Therapy Assessment Profile: IMTAP.* Philadelphia, PA: Jessica Kingsley Pub.

Belmonte, M. K., Allen, G., Beckel-Mitchener, A., Boulanger, L. M., Carper, R. A., and Webb, S. J. (2004). Autism and abnormal development of brain connectivity. *J. Neurosci.* 24, 9228–9231.

Berument, S. K., Rutter, M., Lord, C., Pickles, A., and Bailey, A. (1999). Autism screening questionnaire: diagnostic validity. *Br. J. Psychiatry* 175, 444–451.

Bettison, S. (1996). The long-term effects of auditory training on children with autism. *J. Autism Dev. Disord.* 26, 361–374.

Bhat, A., Landa, R., and Galloway, J. C. (2011). Perspectives on motor problems in infants, children, and adults with autism spectrum disorders. *Phys. Ther.* 91, 1116–1129.

Bloem, B. R., van Vugt, J. P., and Beckley, D. J. (2001). Postural instability and falls in Parkinson's disease. *Adv. Neurol.* 87, 209–223.

Bodfish, J. W., Symons, F. J., Parker, D. E., and Lewis, M. H. (2000). Varieties of repetitive behavior in autism: comparisons to mental retardation. *J. Autism Dev. Disord.* 30, 237–243.

Bondy, A., and Frost, A. (2003). "Communication strategies for visual learners," in *Teaching Individuals with Developmental Delays: Basic Intervention Techniques*, ed O. I. Lovaas (Austin, TX: Pro-Ed), 291–304.

Bonnel, A., Mottron, L., Peretz, I., Trudel, M., and Gallun, E. (2003). Enhanced pitch sensitivity in individuals with autism: a signal detection analysis. *J. Cogn. Neurosci.* 15, 226–235.

Boso, M., Emanuele, E., Minazzi, V., Abbamonte, M., and Politi, P. (2007). Effect of long-term interactive music therapy on behavior profile and musical skills in young adults with severe autism. *J. Altern. Complement. Med.* 13, 709–712.

Boyd, B. A., McDonough, S. G., and Bodfish, J. W. (2012). Evidence-based behavioral interventions for repetitive behaviors in autism. *J. Autism Dev. Disord.* 42, 1236–1248.

Brown, J. (1981). Effects of an integrated physical education/music program in changing early childhood perceptual-motor performance. *Percept. Mot. Skills* 53, 151–154.

Brownell, M. D. (2002). Musically adapted social stories to modify behaviors in students with autism: four case studies. *J. Music Ther.* 39, 117–144.

Bruininks, R. (1978). *The Bruininks-Oseretsky Test of Motor Proficiency.* Circle Pines, MN: American Guidance Service.

Buccino, G., Binkofski, F., and Riggio, L. (2004). The mirror neuron system and action recognition. *Brain Lang.* 89, 370–376.

Buday, E. M. (1995). The effects of signed and spoken words taught with music on sign and speech imitation by children with autism. *J. Music Ther.* 32, 189–202.

Butzlaff, R. (2000). Can music be used to teach reading? *J. Aesthet. Educ.* 34, 167–178.

Callan, D. E., Tsytsarev, V., Hanakawa, T., Callan, A. M., Katsuhara, M., Fukuyama, H., et al. (2006). Song and speech: brain regions involved with perception and covert production. *Neuroimage* 31, 1327–1342.

Carnahan, C., Basham, J., and Musti-Rao, S. (2009a). A low-technology strategy for increasing engagement of students with autism and significant learning needs. *Exceptionality* 17, 76–87.

Carnahan, C., Musti-Rao, S., and Bailey, J. (2009b). Promoting active engagement in small group learning experiences for students with autism and significant learning needs. *Educ. Treat. Child.* 32, 37–61.

Carroll, D. (1996). *A Study of the Effectiveness of an Adaptation of Melodic Intonation Therapy in Increasing the Communicative Speech of Young Children with Down Syndrome.* Master's thesis, McGill University.

Cattaneo, L., and Rizzolatti, G. (2009). The mirror neuron system. *Arch. Neurol.* 66, 557.

Clauss, E. L. (1994). *Effects of Music on Attention and Self-Stimulatory Behaviors in Autistic People.* Doctoral thesis, Hofstra University.

Cohen, I. L., and Sudhalter, V. (2005). *PDD Behavior Inventory (PDDBI).* Lutz, FL: Psychological Assessment Resources.

Conners, C. K. (1989). *Manual for Conners' Rating Scales.* Toronto, ON: Multi-Health Systems.

Constantino, J. N., and Gruber, C. P. (2002). *The Social Responsiveness Scale.* Los Angeles, CA: Western Psychological Services.

Corbett, B. A., Shickman, K., and Ferrer, E. (2008). Brief report: the effects of tomatis sound therapy on language in children with autism. *J. Autism Dev. Disord.* 38, 562–566.

Costa-Giomi, E. (2005). Does music instruction improve fine motor abilities? *Ann. N.Y. Acad. Sci.* 1060, 262–264.

Courchesne, E., Pierce, K., Schumann, C. M., Redcay, E., Buckwalter, J. A., Kennedy, D. P., et al. (2007). Mapping early brain development in autism. *Neuron* 56, 399–413.

Dapretto, M., Davies, M. S., Pfeifer, J. H., Scott, A. A., Sigman, M., Bookheimer, S. Y., et al. (2005). Understanding emotions in others: mirror neuron dysfunction in children with autism spectrum disorders. *Nat. Neurosci.* 9, 28–30.

Darrow, A. A. (2009). Adapting for students with autism. *Gen. Music Today* 22, 24–26.

Darrow, A. A., and Armstrong, T. (1999). Research on music and autism: implications for music educators. *Update Appl. Res. Music Edu.* 18, 15–20.

Dawson, G., Toth, K., Abbott, R., Osterling, J., Munson, J., Estes, A., et al. (2004). Early social attention impairments in autism: social orienting, joint attention, and attention to distress. *Dev. Psychol.* 40, 271–283.

De Fossé, L., Hodge, S. M., Makris, N., Kennedy, D. N., Caviness, V. S., McGrath, L., et al. (2004). Language—association cortex asymmetry in autism and specific language impairment. *Ann. Neurol.* 56, 757–766.

Devlin, S., Healy, O., Leader, G., and Reed, P. (2008). The analysis and treatment of problem behavior evoked by auditory stimulation. *Res. Autism Spectr. Disord.* 2, 671–680.

Dewey, D., Cantell, M., and Crawford, S. G. (2007). Motor and gestural performance in children with autism spectrum disorders, developmental coordination disorder, and or attention deficit hyperactivity disorder. *J. Int. Neuropsychol. Soc.* 13, 246–256.

Downey, R., and Rapport, M. J. K. (2012). Motor activity in children with autism: a review of current literature. *Pediatr. Phys. Ther.* 24, 2–20.

Duffy, B., and Fuller, R. (2000). Role of music therapy in social skills development in children with moderate intellectual disability. *J. Appl. Res. Intellect. Disabil.* 13, 77–89.

Duncan, R. P., and Earhart, G. M. (2012). Randomized controlled trial of community-based dancing to modify disease progression in Parkinson disease. *Neurorehabil. Neural Repair* 26, 132–143.

Dunn, L. M., and Dunn, L. M. (1981). *Manual for the Peabody Picture Vocabulary Test-Revised.* Circle Pines, MN: American Guidance Service.

Earhart, G. M. (2009). Dance as therapy for individuals with Parkinson disease. *Eur. J. Phys. Rehabil. Med.* 45, 231.

Edelson, S. M., Arin, D., Bauman, M., Lukas, S. E., Rudy, J. H., Sholar, M., et al. (1999). Auditory integration training: a double-blind study of behavioral and electrophysiological effects in people with autism. *Focus Autism Other Dev. Disabil.* 14, 73–81.

Edgerton, C. L. (1994). The effect of improvisational music therapy on the communicative behaviors of autistic children. *J. Music Ther.* 31, 31.

Elliott, C. D. (1990). *The Differential Ability Scales.* San Antonio, TX: The Psychological Corporation.

Farmer, K. J. (2003). *The Effect of Music vs. Nonmusic Paired with Gestures on Spontaneous Verbal and Nonverbal Communication Skills of Children with Autism between the Ages 1-5.* Master's Thesis, Tallahassee, FL, Florida State University (School of Music).

Findlay, E. (1971). *Rhythm and Movement: Applications of Dalcroze Eurhythmics.* Evanston, IL: Summy-Birchard Inc.

Forgeard, M. (2008). Practicing a musical instrument in childhood is associated with enhanced verbal ability and nonverbal reasoning. *PLoS ONE* 3:e3566. doi: 10.1371/journal.pone.0003566

Fournier, K. A., Hass, C. J., Naik, S. K., Lodha, N., and Cauraugh, J. H. (2010). Motor coordination in autism spectrum disorders: a synthesis and meta-analysis. *J. Autism Dev. Disord.* 40, 1227–1240.

Foxton, J. M., Talcott, J. B., Witton, C., Hal, B., McIntyre, F., and Griffiths, T. D. (2003). Reading skills are related to global, but not local, acoustic pattern perception. *Nat. Neurosci.* 6, 343–344.

Frego, R. J. D., Gillmeister, G., Hama, M., and Liston, R. E. (2004). "The dalcroze approach to music therapy," in *Introduction to Approaches in Music Therapy*, ed A. Darrow (Silver Springs, MD: American Music Therapy Association), 15–24.

Gaser, C., and Schlaug, G. (2003). Brain structures differ between musicians and non-musicians. *J. Neurosci.* 23, 9240–9245.

Gattino, G. S., dos Santos Riesgo, R., Longob, D., Leite, J. C. L., and Faccini, L. S. (2011). Effects of relational music therapy on communication of children with autism: a randomized controlled study. *Nord. J. Music Ther.* 20, 142–154.

Gernsbacher, M. A., Stevenson, J. L., Khandakar, S., and Hill-Goldsmith, H. (2008). Why does joint attention look atypical in autism? *Child Dev. Perspect.* 2, 38–45.

Getchell, N., Mackenzie, S. J., and Marmon, A. R. (2010). Short term auditory pacing changes dual motor task coordination in children with and without dyslexia. *Adapt. Phys. Activ. Q.* 27, 32.

Glaser, M. F., and Rilling, J. K. (2008). DTI tractography of the human brain's language pathways. *Cereb. Cortex* 18, 2471–2482.

Gold, C., Wigram, T., and Elefant, C. (2006). Music therapy for autistic spectrum disorder. *Cochrane Database Syst. Rev.* CD004381. doi: 10.1002/14651858.CD004381.pub2

Green, D., Charman, T., Pickles, A., Chandler, S., Loucas, T., Simonoff, E., et al. (2009). Impairment in movement skills of children with autistic spectrum disorders. *Dev. Med. Child Neurol.* 51, 311–316.

Greenspan, S. I., and Wieder, S. (1999). A functional developmental approach to autism spectrum disorders. *Res. Pract. Pers. Sev. Disabil.* 24, 147–161.

Gunter, P. L., Fox, J. J., McEvoy, M. A., and Shores, R. E. (1993). A case study of the reduction of aberrant, repetitive responses of an adolescent with autism. *Educ. Treat. Child.* 16, 187–197.

Habib, M., and Besson, M. (2009). What do music training and musical experience teach us about brain plasticity? *Music Percept.* 26, 279–285.

Hackney, M. E., Kantorovich, S., and Earhart, G. M. (2007a). A study on the effects of argentine tango as a form of partnered dance for those with Parkinson disease and the healthy elderly. *Am. J. Dance Ther.* 29, 109–127.

Hackney, M. E., Kantorovich, S., Levin, R., and Earhart, G. M. (2007b). Effects of tango on functional mobility in Parkinson's disease: a preliminary study. *J. Neurol. Phys. Ther.* 31, 173.

Hallett, M., Lebiedowska, M. K., Thomas, S. L., Stanhope, S. J., Denckla, M. B., and Rumsey, J. (1993). Locomotion of autistic adults. *Arch. Neurol.* 50, 1304–1308.

Haueisen, J., and Knösche, T. R. (2001). Involuntary motor activity in pianists evoked by music perception. *J. Cogn. Neurosci.* 13, 786–792.

Heaton, P. (2003). Pitch memory, labelling and disembedding in autism. *J. Child Psychol. Psychiatry* 44, 543–551.

Heaton, P., Pring, L., and Hermelin, B. (1999). Can children with autistic spectrum disorders perceive affect in music? An experimental investigation. *Psychol. Med.* 29, 1405–1410.

Henderson, S. E., and Sugden, D. A. (1992). *Movement Assesment Battery for Children.* London: Psychological Corporation.

Herbert, M. R., Harris, G. J., Adrien, K. T., Ziegler, D. A., Makris, N., Kennedy, D. N., et al. (2002). Abnormal asymmetry in language association cortex in autism. *Ann. Neurol.* 52, 588–596.

Hesling, I., Dilharreguy, B., Peppé, S., Amirault, M., Bouvard, M., and Allard, M. (2010). The integration of prosodic speech in high functioning autism: a preliminary fMRI study. *PLoS ONE* 5:e11571. doi: 10.1371/journal.pone.0011571

Hess, K., Morrier, M., Heflin, L., and Ivey, M. (2008). Autism treatment survey: services received by children with autism spectrum disorders in public school classrooms. *J. Autism Dev. Disord.* 38, 961–971.

Hickok, G., and Poeppel, D. (2004). Dorsal and ventral streams: a framework for understanding aspects of the functional anatomy of language. *Cognition* 92, 67–99.

Himberg, T. (2006). "Co-operative tapping and collective time-keeping–differences of timing accuracy in duet performance with human or computer partner," in *Paper Presented at the 9th International Conference on Music Perception and Cognition* (Bologna, Italy).

Ho, Y. C., Cheung, M. C., and Chan, A. S. (2003). Music training improves verbal but not visual memory: cross-sectional and longitudinal explorations in children. *Neuropsychology* 17, 439.

Hurwitz, I., Wolff, P. H., Bortnick, B. D., and Kokas, K. (1975). Nonmusicol effects of the kodaly music curriculum in primary grade children. *J. Learn. Disabil.* 8, 167–174.

Hyde, K. L., Lerch, J., Norton, A., Forgeard, M., Winner, E., Evans, A. C., et al. (2009). Musical training shapes structural brain development. *J. Neurosci.* 29, 3019–3025.

Jakobson, L. S., Cuddy, L. L., and Kilgour, A. R. (2003). Time lagging: a key to musicians' superior memory. *Music Percept.* 20, 307–313.

Jansiewicz, E. M., Goldberg, M. C., Newschaffer, C. J., Denckla, M. B., Landa, R., and Mostofsky, S. H. (2006). Motor signs distinguish children with high functioning autism and asperger's syndrome from controls. *J. Autism Dev. Disord.* 36, 613–621.

Kasari, C., Paparella, T., Freeman, S., and Jahromi, L. B. (2008). Language outcome in autism: randomized comparison of joint attention and play interventions. *J. Consult. Clin. Psychol.* 76, 125–137.

Katagiri, J. (2009). The effect of background music and song texts on the emotional understanding of children with autism. *J. Music Ther.* 46, 15–31.

Kaufman, A. S. (1990). *Kaufman Brief Intelligence Test (KBIT).* Circle Pines, MN: American Guidance Service.

Kern, P., and Aldridge, D. (2006). Using embedded music therapy interventions to support outdoor play of young children with autism in an inclusive community-based child care program. *J. Music Ther.* 43, 270–294.

Kern, P., Wolery, M., and Aldridge, D. (2007). Use of songs to promote independence in morning greeting routines for young children with autism. *J. Autism Dev. Disord.* 37, 1264–1271.

Kim, J., Wigram, T., and Gold, C. (2008). The effects of improvisational music therapy on joint attention behaviors in autistic children: a randomized controlled study. *J. Autism Dev. Disord.* 38, 1758–1766.

Kim, J., Wigram, T., and Gold, C. (2009). Emotional, motivational and interpersonal responsiveness of children with autism in improvisational music therapy. *Autism* 13, 389–409.

Kirschner, S., and Tomasello, M. (2009). Joint drumming: social context facilitates syncrhonization in preschool children. *J. Exp. Child Psychol.* 102, 299–314.

Kirschner, S., and Tomasello, M. (2010). Joint music-making promotes prosocial behavior among four-yearolds. *Evol. Hum. Behav.* 31, 354–364.

Kleinspehn-Ammerlahn, A., Riediger, M., Schmiedek, F., von Oertzen, T., Li, S. C., and Lindenberger, U. (2011). Dyadic drumming across the lifespan reveals a zone of proximal development in children. *Dev. Psychol.* 47, 632–644.

Koelsch, S. (2009). A neuroscientific perspective on music therapy. *Ann. N.Y. Acad. Sci.* 1169, 374–384.

Kraus, N., and Chandrasekaran, B. (2010). Music training for the development of auditory skills. *Nat. Rev. Neurosci.* 11, 599–605.

Krug, D. A., Arick, J. R., and Almond, P. J. (1988). *Autism Behavior Checklist.* Portland, OR: ASIEP Education Company.

Lahav, A., Saltzman, E., and Schlaug, G. (2007). Action representation of sound: audiomotor recognition network while listening to newly acquired actions. *J. Neurosci.* 27, 308–314.

Lai, G., Pantazatos, S. P., Schneider, H., and Hirsch, J. (2012). Neural systems for speech and song in autism. *Brain* 135(Pt 3), 961–975.

Lam, K. (2004). *The Repetitive Behavior Scale–Revised: Independent Validation and the Effects of Subject Variables.* Doctoral Dissertation, Ohio State University.

Landa, R. (2007). Early communication development and intervention for children with autism. *Ment. Retard. Dev. Disabil. Res. Rev.* 13, 16–25.

Lanovaz, M. J., Fletcher, S. E., and Rapp, J. T. (2009). Identifying stimuli that alter immediate and subsequent levels of vocal stereotypy: a further analysis of functionally matched stimulation. *Behav. Modif.* 33, 682–704.

Leary, M. R., and Hill, D. A. (1996). Moving on: autism and movement disturbance. *Ment. Retard.* 34, 39–53.

Lecavalier, L. (2006). Behavioral and emotional problems in young people with pervasive developmental disorders: relative prevalence, effects of subject characteristics, and empirical classification. *J. Autism Dev. Disord.* 36, 1101–1114.

Lim, H. A. (2010). Effect of "Developmental Speech and Language Training through Music" on speech production in children with autism spectrum disorders. *J. Music Ther.* 47, 2–26.

Lim, H. A., and Draper, E. (2011). The effects of music therapy incorporated with applied behavior analysis verbal behavior approach for children with autism spectrum disorders. *J. Music Ther.* 48, 532–550.

Loh, A., Soman, T., Brian, J., Bryson, S. E., Roberts, W., Szatmari, P., et al. (2007). Stereotyped motor behaviors associated with autism in high-risk infants: a pilot videotape analysis of a sibling sample. *J. Autism Dev. Disord.* 37, 25–36.

Lord, C., Luyster, R. J., Gotham, K., and Guthrie, W. (2012a). *Autism Diagnostic Observation Schedule, 2nd Edn., (ADOS-2) Manual (Part II): Toddler Module.* Torrance, CA: Western Psychological Services.

Lord, C., Rutter, M., DiLavore, P. C., Risi, S., Gotham, K., and Bishop, S. L. (2012b). *Autism Diagnostic Observation Schedule, 2nd Edn., (ADOS-2) Manual (Part 1): Modules 1–4.* Torrance, CA: Western Psychological Services.

Lord, C., Rutter, M., and Couteur, A. (1994). Autism diagnostic interview-revised: a revised version of a diagnostic interview for caregivers of individuals with possible pervasive developmental disorders. *J. Autism Dev. Disord.* 24, 659–685.

Lovaas, O. I. (1987). Behavioral treatment and normal educational and intellectual functioning in young autistic children. *J. Consult. Clin. Psychol.* 55, 3–9.

Lukoff, D., Nuechterlein, K. H., and Ventura, J. (1986). Manual for expanded brief psychiatric rating scale (BPRS). *Schizophr. Bull.* 12, 594–602.

Lundqvist, L. O., Andersson, G., and Viding, J. (2009). Effects of vibroacoustic music on challenging behaviors in individuals with autism and developmental disabilities. *Res. Autism Spectr. Disord.* 3, 390–400.

Magne, C., Schon, D., and Besson, M. (2006). Musician children detect pitch violations in both music and language better than nonmusician children: behavioral and electrophysiological approaches. *J. Cogn. Neurosci.* 18, 199–211.

Marques, C., Moreno, S., Castro, S. L., and Besson, M. (2007). Musicians detect pitch violation in a foreign language better than nonmusicians: behavioral and electrophysiological evidence. *J. Cogn. Neurosci.* 19, 1453–1463.

Marsh, K. L., Richardson, M., and Schmidt, R. C. (2009). Social connection through joint action and interpersonal coordination. *Top. Cogn. Sci.* 1, 320–339.

Mazefsky, C. A., Pelphrey, K. A., and Dahl, R. E. (2012). The need for a broader approach to emotion regulation research in autism. *Child Dev. Perspect.* 6, 92–97.

Mesibov, G. B., Shea, V., and Schopler, E. (2004). *The TEACCH Approach to Autism Spectrum Disorders.* New York, NY: Springer.

Meyer, M., Alter, K., Friederici, A. D., Lohmann, G., and Von Cramon, D. Y. (2002). FMRI reveals brain regions mediating slow prosodic modulations in spoken sentences. *Hum. Brain Mapp.* 17, 73–88.

Minshew, N. J., Sung, K. B., Jones, B. L., and Furman, J. M. (2004). Underdevelopment of the postural control system in autism. *Neurology* 63, 2056–2061.

Minshew, N. J., and Williams, D. L. (2007). The new neurobiology of autism: cortex, connectivity, and neuronal organization. *Arch. Neurol.* 64, 945.

Molnar-Szakacs, I., and Overy, K. (2006). Music and mirror neurons: from motion to 'e' motion. *Soc. Cogn. Affect. Neurosci.* 1, 235–241.

Moreno, S., Marques, C., Santos, A., Santos, M., Castro, S. L., and Besson, M. (2009). Musical training influences linguistic abilities in 8-year old children: more evidence for brain plasticity. *Cereb. Cortex* 19, 712–723.

Mostofsky, S. H., Dubey, P., Jerath, V. K., Jansiewicz, E. M., Goldberg, M. C., and Denckla, M. B. (2006). Developmental dyspraxia is not limited to imitation in children with autism spectrum disorders. *J. Int. Neuropsychol. Soc.* 12, 314–326.

Mudford, O. C., Cross, B. A., Breen, S., Cullen, C., Reeves, D., Gould, J., et al. (2000). Auditory integration training for children with autism: no behavioral benefits detected. *Am. J. Ment. Retard.* 105, 118–129.

Mullen, E. M. (1995). *Mullen Scales of Early Learning.* Circle Pines, MN: American Guidance Service.

Mundy, P., and Crowson, M. (1997). Joint attention and early social communication: implications for research on intervention with autism. *J. Autism Dev. Disord.* 27, 653–676.

Mundy, P., Delgado, C., Block, J., Venezia, M., Hogan, A., and Seibert, J. (2003). *Early Social Communication Scales (ESCS).* Coral Gables, FL: University of Miami.

Norton, A., Zipse, L., Marchina, S., and Schlaug, G. (2009). Melodic intonation therapy. *Ann. N.Y. Acad. Sci.* 1169, 431–436.

O'Loughlin, R. (2000). *Facilitating Prelinguistic Communication Skills of Attention by Integrating a Music Stimulus within Typical Language Intervention with Autistic Children.* Doctoral Thesis, University of Toledo.

Orr, T., Myles, B., and Carlson, J. (1998). The impact of rhythmic entrainment on a person with autism. *Focus Autism Other Dev. Disabil.* 13, 163–166.

Overy, K. (2000). Dyslexia, temporal processing and music: the potential of music as an early learning aid for dyslexic children. *Psychol. Music* 28, 218–229.

Overy, K. (2003). Dyslexia and music. from timing deficits to musical intervention. *Ann. N.Y. Acad. Sci.* 999, 497–505.

Overy, K. (2008). "Classroom rhythm games for literacy support," in *Music and Dyslexia: A Positive Approach,* eds J. Westcombe, T. Miles and D. Ditchfield (Chichester: John Wiley & Sons Ltd.), 26–44.

Overy, K., and Molnar-Szakacs, I. (2009). Being together in time: musical experience and the mirror neuron system. *Music Percept.* 26, 489–504.

Partington, J. W., and Sundberg, M. L. (1998). *The Assessment of Basic Language and Learning Skills (the ABLLS).* Pleasant Hill, CA: Behavior Analysts.

Pasiali, V. (2004). The use of prescriptive therapeutic songs in a home-based environment to promote social skills acquisition by children with autism: three case studies. *Music Ther. Perspect.* 22, 11–20.

Patel, A. D. (2003). Language, music, syntax and the brain. *Nat. Neurosci.* 6, 674–681.

Patel, A. D. (2011). Why would musical training benefit the neural encoding of speech? The OPERA hypothesis. *Front. Psychol.* 2:142. doi: 10.3389/fpsyg.2011.00142

Patel, A. D., Peretz, I., Tramo, M., and Labreque, R. (1998). Processing prosodic and musical patterns: a neuropsychological investigation. *Brain Lang.* 61, 123–144.

Pellitteri, J. (2000). THE CONSULTANT'S CORNER: music therapy in the special education setting. *J. Educ. Psychol. Consult.* 11, 379–391.

Phillips-Silver, J. (2009). On the meaning of movement in music, development and the brain. *Contemp. Music Rev.* 28, 293–314.

Phillips-Silver, J., and Trainor, L. J. (2007). Hearing what the body feels: auditory encoding of rhythmic movement. *Cognition* 105, 533–546.

Pierce, K., and Schreibman, L. (1995). Increasing complex social behaviors in children with autism: effects of peer-implemented pivotal response training. *J. Appl. Behav. Anal.* 28, 285.

Provost, B., Lopez, B. R., and Heimerl, S. (2007). A comparison of motor delays in young children: autism spectrum disorger, developmental delay, and developmental concerns. *J. Autism Dev. Disord.* 37, 321–328.

Rapp, J. T. (2007). Further evaluation of methods to identify matched stimulation. *J. Appl. Behav. Anal.* 40, 73–88.

Reitman, M. R. (2005). *Effectiveness of Music Therapy Interventions on Joint Attention in Children Diagnosed with Autism: A Pilot Study.* Doctoral Dissertation, Carlos Albizu University.

Rimland, B., and Edelson, S. M. (1995). Brief report: a pilot study of auditory integration training in autism. *J. Autism Dev. Disord.* 25, 61–70.

Rizzolatti, G., Fabbri-Destro, M., and Cattaneo, L. (2009). Mirror neurons and their clinical relevance. *Nat. Clin. Pract. Neurol.* 5, 24–34.

Rodriguez-Fornells, A., Rojo, N., Amengual, J. L., Ripolles, P., Altenmuller, E., and Munte, T. F. (2012). The involvement of audio-motor coupling in the music-supported therapy applied to stroke patients. *Ann. N.Y. Acad. Sci.* 1252, 282–293.

Roper, N. (2003). Melodic intonation therapy with young children with apraxia. *Bridges* 1, 1–7.

Schlaug, G., Altenmüller, E., and Thaut, M. (2010). Music listening and music making in the treatment of neurological disorders and impairments. *Music Percept.* 27, 249–250.

Schlaug, G., Norton, A., Overy, K., and Winner, E. (2005). Effects of music training on the child's brain and cognitive development. *Ann. N.Y. Acad. Sci.* 1060, 219–230.

Schmidt, R., Beek, P., Treffner, P., and Turvey, M. (1991). Dynamical substructure of coordinated rhythmic movements. *J. Exp. Psychol.* 17, 635–651.

Schneider, S., Schönle, P. W., Altenmüller, E., and Münte, T. F. (2007). Using musical instruments to improve motor skill recovery following a stroke. *J. Neurol.* 254, 1339–1346.

Scholz, J. P., and Kelso, J. A. (1989). *A Quantitative Approach to Understanding the Formation and Change of Coordinated Movement Patterns.* Vol. 21. Circle Pines, MN: American Guidance Service.

Schön, D., Cyrille, M., and Besson, M. (2004). The music of speech: music training facilitates pitch processing in both music and language. *Psychophysiology* 41, 341–349.

Schopler, E., Reichler, R. J., DeVillis, R. F., and Daly, K. (1980). Toward objective classification of childhood autism: childhood autism rating scale (CARS). *J. Autism Dev. Disord.* 10, 91–103.

Shumway-Cook, A., and Woollacott, M. H. (2007). *Motor Control: Translating Research in Clinical Practice.* 3rd Edn. Philadelphia, PA: Lippincott Williams and Wilkins.

Simpson, K., and Keen, D. (2011). Music interventions for children with autism: narrative review of the literature. *J. Autism Dev. Disord.* 41, 1507–1514.

Simpson, R., de Boer-Ott, S., Griswold, D., Myles, B., Byrd, S., and Ganz, J. (2005). *Autism Spectrum Disorders: Interventions and Treatments for Children and Youth.* Thousand Oaks, CA: Corwin Press.

Sinha, Y., Silove, N., Hayen, A., and Williams, K. (2011). Auditory integration training and other sound therapies for autism spectrum disorders (ASD). *Cochrane Database Syst. Rev.* CD003681. doi: 10.1002/14651858.CD003681.pub3

Sparks, R., Helm, N., and Albert, M. (1974). Aphasia rehabilitation resulting from melodic intonation therapy. *Cortex* 10, 303–316.

Stephens, C. E. (2008). Spontaneous imitation by children with autism during a repetitive musical play routine. *Autism* 12, 645–671.

Stewart, L., Henson, R., Kampe, K., Walsh, V., Turner, R., and Frith, U. (2003). Brain changes after learning to read and play music. *Neuroimage* 20, 71–83.

Tager-Flusberg, H. (1999). A psychological approach to understanding the social and language impairments in autism. *Int. Rev. Psychiatry* 11, 325–334.

Tallal, P., and Gaab, N. (2006). Dynamic auditory processing, musical experience and language development. *Trends Neurosci.* 29, 382–390.

Terman, L. M., and Merrill, M. A. (1960). *Stanford-Binet Intelligence Scale: Manual for the Third Revision, Form, L.-M.* Boston, MA: Houghton Mifflin Company.

Tindell, K. W. (2010). *Comparison of Music-Based Curriculum versus an Eclectic Curriculum for Speech Acquisition in Students with Autism Spectrum Disorder.* Doctoral Dissertation, Dallas Baptist University.

Tomasello, M., and Carpenter, M. (2007). Shared Intentionality. *Dev. Sci.* 10, 1–125.

Tomchek, S. D., and Dunn, W. (2007). Sensory processing in children with and without autism: a comparative study using the short sensory profile. *Am. J. Occup. Ther.* 61, 190–200.

Vilensky, J. A., Damasio, A. R., and Maurer, R. G. (1981). Gait disturbances in patients with autistic behavior: a preliminary study. *Arch. Neurol.* 38, 646–649.

Wan, C. Y., Bazen, L., Baars, R., Libenson, A., Zipse, L., Zuk, J., et al. (2011). Auditory-motor mapping training as an intervention to facilitate speech output in non-verbal children with autism: a proof of concept study. *PLoS ONE* 6:e25505. doi: 10.1371/journal.pone.0025505

Wan, C. Y., Demaine, K., Zipse, L., Norton, A., and Schlaug, G. (2010a). From music-making to speaking: engaging the mirror neuron system in autism. *Brain Res. Bull.* 82, 161.

Wan, C. Y., Rüber, T., Hohmann, A., and Schlaug, G. (2010b). The therapeutic effects of singing in neurological disorders. *Music Percept.* 27, 287–296.

Wan, C. Y., Marchina, S., Norton, A., and Schlaug, G. (2012). Atypical hemispheric asymmetry in the arcuate fasciculus of completely nonverbal children with autism. *Ann. N.Y. Acad. Sci.* 1252, 332–337.

Wan, C. Y., and Schlaug, G. (2010). Music-making as a tool for promoting brain plasticity across the life span. *Neuroscientist* 16, 566–577.

Wechsler, D. (1949). *Wechsler Intelligence Scale for Children.* New York, NY: Psychological Corporation.

Williams, J. H., Whiten, A., Suddendorf, T., and Perrett, D. I. (2001). Imitation, mirror neurons and autism. *Neurosci. Biobehav. Rev.* 25, 287–295.

Wiltermuth, S. S., and Heath, C. (2009). Synchrony and cooperation. *Psychol. Sci.* 20, 1–5.

Wimpory, D., Chadwick, P., and Nash, S. (1995). Brief report: musical interaction therapy for children with autism: an evaluative case study with two-year follow-up. *J. Autism Dev. Disord.* 25, 541–552.

Wood, S. R. (1991). *A Study of the Effects of Music on Attending Behavior of Children with Autistic-Like Syndrome.* Master's Thesis, San Jose State University.

Zachopoulou, E., Tsapakidou, A., and Derri, V. (2004). The effects of a developmentally appropriate music and movement program on motor performance. *Early Child. Res. Q.* 19, 631–642.

Zatorre, R. J., Chen, J. L., and Penhune, V. B. (2007). When the brain plays music: auditory–motor interactions in music perception and production. *Nat. Rev. Neurosci.* 8, 547–558.

Zollweg, W. (1997). The efficacy of auditory integration training: a double blind study. *Am. J. Audiol.* 6, 39.

Conflict of Interest Statement: The authors declare that the research was conducted in the absence of any commercial or financial relationships that could be construed as a potential conflict of interest.

7

Give spontaneity and self-discovery a chance in ASD: spontaneous peripheral limb variability as a proxy to evoke centrally driven intentional acts

Elizabeth B. Torres[1]*, Polina Yanovich[2] and Dimitris N. Metaxas[3]

[1] *Rutgers University Psychology Department, Computational Biomedicine Imaging and Medicine Center, Rutgers University Center for Cognitive Science, New Brunswick, NJ, USA*
[2] *Rutgers University Computer Science Department, Rutgers University Center for Cognitive Science Piscataway, NJ, USA*
[3] *Rutgers University Computer Science Department, Computational Biomedicine Imaging and Medicine Center, Rutgers University Center for Cognitive Science, Piscataway, NJ, USA*

Edited by:
Anne M. Donnellan, University of San Diego, USA

Reviewed by:
Lei Niu, Albert Einstein College of Medicine, USA
Jorge V. Jose, Indiana University, USA

***Correspondence:**
Elizabeth B. Torres, Rutgers University Psychology Department, Busch campus, 152 Frelinghuysen Rd., Piscataway, NJ 08854, USA
e-mail: ebtorres@rci.rutgers.edu

Autism can be conceived as an adaptive biological response to an early unexpected developmental change. Under such conceptualization one could think of emerging biological compensatory mechanisms with unique manifestations in each individual. Within a large group of affected people this would result in a highly heterogeneous spectral disorder where it would be difficult to tap into the hidden potentials of any given individual. A pressing question is how to treat the disorder while harnessing the capabilities and predispositions that the individual has already developed. It would indeed be ideal to use such strengths to accelerate the learning of self-sufficiency and independence, important as the person transitions into adulthood. In this report, we introduce a new concept for therapeutic interventions and basic research in autism. We use visuo-spatial and auditory stimuli to help augment the physical reality of the child and sensory-substitute corrupted kinesthetic information quantified in his/her movement patterns to help the person develop volitional control over the hand motions. We develop a co-adaptive child-computer interface that closes the sensory-motor feedback loops by alerting the child of a cause-effect relationship between the statistics of his/her real-time hand movement patterns and those of external media states. By co-adapting the statistics of the media states and those of the child's real-time hand movements, we found that without any food/token reward the children naturally remained engaged in the task. Even in the absence of practice, the learning gains were retained, transferred and improved 2–4 weeks later. This new concept demonstrates that individuals with autism do have spontaneous sensory-motor adaptive capabilities. When led to their self-discovery, these patterns of spontaneous behavioral variability (SBV) morph into more predictive and reliable intentional actions. These can unlock and enhance exploratory behavior and autonomy in the individual with autism spectrum disorders (ASD).

Keywords: autism spectrum disorders, proprioceptive feedback, kinesthetic perception, stochastic processes, stochasticity, predictive coding, reliability, motor learning and control, child development, interface

Each destiny-errored, differently-wired but "cares-to-learn"
child needs assurance they are not weeds
but fragrant flowers to be greeted as valuable.
There in either the tested room or the classroom,
best tell each cherub that they can lead.
Say that they are the guiders to test the best ways to heat their
versed, vested, vastly valuable, vellum varied, esteemed equated
equal, red news never viewed, volumed voices.

When children know their differences will be supported by you
saying you will never stop trying ways to help them find their very
best voice, their fears rest.
There, they are not awed by pity. There, esteem is greeted.
I'm in peace because someone saw all people are real and deserve
being supported to communicate their truths.

Peyton Goddard (Goddard et al., 2012), 65, 69

INTRODUCTION

How can a learner who does not know what there is to learn manage to learn anyway? (Thelen, 1994; Smith, 2006). As early as 3 months of age, before reaching or pointing fully matures, typically developing (TD) infants can learn to coordinate their legs and using their own physical movements self-discover coordination patterns that lead them to systematically attain a goal—a goal that has not been instructed or commanded (Thelen and Fisher, 1983a,b; Rovee-Collier, 1989).

Infants seem to have an inherent ability to self-discover goal-directness (Von Hofsten, 1982; Thelen et al., 1993, 1996; van der Meer et al., 1995; Von Hofsten, 2004; Heathcock et al., 2005; Bhat and Galloway, 2006, 2007; Bhat et al., 2007; Lee et al., 2008; van Wermeskerken et al., 2011). It is not known what underlies these abilities and whether they might also exist at a later stage of life in children with developmental delays or in those with behavioral manifestations that lead to a diagnosis of autism spectrum disorders (ASD). The very fact of surviving an early developmental glitch and being able to function in the world despite many developmental challenges, strongly suggests that these children are capable of creating -on their own- compensatory mechanisms that bypass corrupted sensory signals. Could we use adaptive capabilities already present in children and adolescents with a diagnosis of ASD to evoke the self-regulation of goal-directness and intentionality in their actions?

Not all physical movement segments in our actions are goal-directed or performed with the same level of intent (Torres, 2011). A large portion of our acts are spontaneous in nature, occurring beneath our full awareness. These action segments have spontaneous behavioral variability (SBV). This type of variability examined in isolation seems random and noisy, a kind of "nightmare" for researchers, who often try to get rid of it and conform to parametric models assuming a theoretical normal distribution, often without actually examining the statistical distributions inherently present in the experimental data. In order to study the structures inherent to SBV we have designed a new statistical platform for personalized behavioral analyses (SPBA) (Torres and Jose, 2012), which we use in this report to characterize limb motor variability from the periphery in a radically different way from current traditional methods (to be precisely explained in the Methods and Apparatus section of this report).

The SBV has not been widely explored in ASD motor research. The focus has rather been on goal-directed behaviors where the targets are explicitly defined, or where the child is explicitly instructed, often commanded to imitate a posture or action (Jones and Prior, 1985; Rogers et al., 1996; Rinehart et al., 2001; Williams et al., 2001; Noterdaeme et al., 2002; Minshew et al., 2004; Jansiewicz et al., 2006; Mostofsky et al., 2006; Gidley Larson et al., 2008; Gowen et al., 2008; Haswell et al., 2009; Fournier et al., 2010a,b; Izawa et al., 2012).

In contrast to the scarce ASD research regarding the potential roles of SBV in shaping the movement-based kinesthetic percept, an important body of knowledge has accumulated over the years in ASD with a focus on visual and auditory perception and their potential roles in cognitive specialization. Some of these spatial-processing capabilities can rather successfully lead to visuo-spatial or audio-spatial strengths, sometimes paired with complex visualization or auditory abilities (Samson et al., 2011, 2012). This literature examines differences in perceptual processing and over-reliance on complex specializations as successful adaptations of the autistic systems. These could possibly be self-discovered to bypass corrupted sensory input. From the therapeutic standpoint, this observation potentially opens new avenues where we could explore the possibility of sensory-substitution in ASD.

Sensory-substitution is germane to biological systems in general. When some of the sensory input is corrupted or lost in one modality, that missing information can be replaced with sensory input from another modality. Examples abound where a blind person learns to echolocate (Veraart et al., 1992; De Volder et al., 1999), or a person who loses his movement-based proprioception learns to control his body movements using vision (Cole, 1995; Riso, 1999). In all cases where there is cross-sensory transfer (Levy-Tzedek et al., 2012) the sensory-motor systems learn to close the sensory-motor feedback loops, to receive re-afferent sensory input in a compensatory manner that helps regulate the efferent motor output in anticipatory ways.

Anticipatory control of our actions is "the name of the game" in decision making. Decision-making is critical in all intentional aspects of our behaviors. In the words of Henry Markram "Decisions are the key things that support our perceptual bubble, that keep it alive. Without decisions you cannot see, you cannot think, you cannot feel ... " (TED talk, 2009/10/15 http://blog.ted.com/2009/10/15/supercomputing/). In the case of the affected nervous system, by closing the sensory-motor feedback loops the affected individual could regain predictive control of his/her actions and build motor expectations. This would enable the person to anticipate the consequences of immediate future actions and weigh the risks and benefits of impending decisions. That is, the person would regain or develop the ability to be thinking in the abstract, navigating a step ahead of the actual physical act; behaving without necessarily having to experience the physical external input during the action: without having to exclusively rely on "the here and now."

Given the often reported enhanced visual and auditory processing capabilities of individuals with autism (Mottron and Belleville, 1993, 1995; Mottron et al., 1998, 1999, 2000; Caron et al., 2004; Soulieres et al., 2009; Bonnel et al., 2010; Samson et al., 2012) and their statistical reliance on the "here and now" (Torres et al., 2013 in this issue), we asked if using sensory-substitution to bypass corrupted proprioception with visual and/or auditory feedback could help us connect their intentions to their actions. To this end we used SBV as a proxy to evoke and sharpen intentional behavioral variability (IBV). We then used precise statistical indexes to assess possible gains in volitional control over their own hand motions.

We present a new platform for *personalized intervention* where we close the sensory feedback loops by augmenting the physical external reality of the child with media. In this context we evoke the triggering and regulation of the temporal unfolding of the media using real time motions of their hand. In closed loop with the media, by co-adapting the statistics of his/her own physical micro-movements with those of the media states, the child spontaneously learns. Without instructions, each individual self-discovers where to move the hand to activate and eventually sustain the media.

We show that using this co-adaptive, closed loop interface is ideal to unveil the best form of sensory guidance (e.g., auditory, visual, or touch) that leads an individual toward a more predictive regime of behaviors. In this context the media-states' statistics and the statistics of the child's hand motions are interchangeably used as feedback to modify future performance. The use of our new SPBA enables us to dynamically track the rates of change of the hand-motions' stochastic signatures as the child explores and—through trial and error—self discovers the implicit goal of the task and solves it. We describe using precise statistical indexes how this general statistics driven co-adaptation concept, using sensory-substitution to close the sensory feedback loops, can lead to the development, retention, and improvement of intentional self-autonomy.

METHODS AND APPARATUS

MOTOR VARIABILITY REVISITED: A NECESSARY PREAMBLE TO OUR METHODS

Motor variability has come to play a relevant role in contemporary movement research, from infant development to adult performance. Inspired by the pioneering works of Esther Thelen (Thelen and Fisher, 1983a,b; Thelen and Smith, 1994) and Nikolai Bernstein (Bernstein, 1967) recent work has begun seriously considering behavioral variations and behavioral variability as useful quantitative research tools. An example specifically focusing on infant development can be appreciated in a special issue of Physical Therapy (2010 Volume 9) highlighting the important roles of motor variations and variability in childhood development as well as their potential use in diagnosis of early neurodevelopmental problems (Dusing and Harbourne, 2010; Fetters, 2010; Hadders-Algra, 2010; Vereijken, 2010).

It is important, however, to point out in our present report the fundamental differences between our new statistical approach to motor variability and the traditional approaches currently in use. To better appreciate such differences we quote Helders from the special issue (Helders, 2010): *"Intra-individual variability can be defined as differences in motor development or performance within individuals and between repeated measurements. The term 'fluctuations' is reserved for differences among consecutive points in a variable trajectory, whereas 'stability' indicates the counterpart of (or the lack of) variability."*

In the papers of that important special issue many forms of variability are defined, ranging from variations across the repertoire of tasks that an infant may develop to more specific statistical variability within a task. Statistical variability in the context of Dynamic Systems Theory used by these researchers and others, specifically refers to the "*Measure of how variable a specific, defined behavior is around a central value; typically measured using means and standard deviations and related to the amount of range of a movement or behavior*" [see Table 1 Definitions of Key Terminology in Dusing and Harbourne (2010) taken from (Stergiou et al., 2004)].

Our approach using variability as an objective quantitative tool is, in at least two important ways, fundamentally different from the aforementioned approaches. First and foremost, we do not define variability around a central mean value, quantified by the standard deviations from that mean value, taken across repeated trials. This definition would implicitly assume the existence of an underlying (theoretically justified) symmetric distribution. This is a dangerous assumption as normality in data obtained from naturally occurring phenomena is not always warranted (Limpert et al., 2001; Limpert and Stahel, 2011). For this reason, we do not assume a symmetric theoretical distribution and summarize the statistics of our data by the mean and the standard deviation ($\mu \pm \sigma$). Instead, we experimentally estimate the probability distribution governing the stochastic random process that gives rise to different statistical signatures in the movement data along with their rates of change specific to each individual (Torres, 2011, 2012, 2013; Torres et al., 2013).

Our recent research using the stochastic approach to assess the continuous flow of movements has revealed that our motions have non-stationary statistics. The probability distributions (experimentally estimated) governing our motions are highly skewed and the values of their parameters shift over time (even at the time scale of a very few minutes). We have found that the two-parameter continuous Gamma family of probability distributions describes with high confidence the human movement data across a wide range of behaviors (reach-to-grasp, pointing, gait, various sports routines, etc.). The degree of skewness and the reliability of the experimentally estimated probability distributions from the Gamma family undergo a maturation process (Torres et al., 2013), yet they change with context and sensory-guidance type at a rate that is unique to each person.

These recent experimental results suggest that it will be critical to personalize our assessments of behavior in compromised systems. Such systems are continually undergoing adaptive changes that observational inventories or metrics based on averaged quantities from discretely tallied scores could not detect. Besides potential confounds from fatigue and boredom of the observer, compounded at times with personal biases and lack of independent validation, such methods chop up the behavior. Behavior, however, continuously flows. The relevant parameters defining the probability distribution of movement kinematics variables at a given time change with the context of the task. They also change as a function of the sources of sensory guidance and as a function of many other developmental and neurodegenerative factors (Torres et al., 2010, 2011). Such dependencies make our proposed metrics ideal to dynamically and individually track the stochastic signatures of continuous behaviors in real time as well as to assess their longitudinal evolution. We not only use them to aid and identify important deviations from typical development and normal aging (Torres, under review; Torres et al., 2013; Yanovich et al., in press). We can also use them to track the rates of change of the stochastic trajectories of our movement variability during behavioral and drug-based therapies.

Unlike the previously cited literature, our approach does not look at fluctuations as "*differences among consecutive points in a variable trajectory*" (Helders, 2010). Rather, our approach (Torres and Jose, 2012) examines—in the context of stochastic processes—the accumulation of fluctuations over time for any given trajectory parameter as the person naturally moves. We have coined this type of fluctuation on the Gamma plane "*micro-movements*" to distinguish it from averaging a parameter across repeats of an action during some elapsed time period (e.g., the number of trials in an experimental session). Such averages are taken under the theoretical assumption of normality while measuring the standard deviations from the mean (Thelen and Smith, 1994; Stergiou et al., 2004; Helders, 2010).

Just as the notion of "fluctuation" that our stochastic approach uses is different from that currently in use by others (Stergiou et al., 2004; Dusing and Harbourne, 2010; Fetters, 2010; Hadders-Algra, 2010; Helders, 2010; Vereijken, 2010), the notion of "stability" is also different. In our approach stability of the sensory signal requires high predictability, high reliability and broad bandwidth in the range of values of the motion trajectory parameters of interest. Thus, across repeats of a movement, in our stochastic approach, lower variability in the patterns of velocity and acceleration does not imply higher stability of the system's motor output and motor kinesthetic re-afference. Take for example, **Figure 1A**

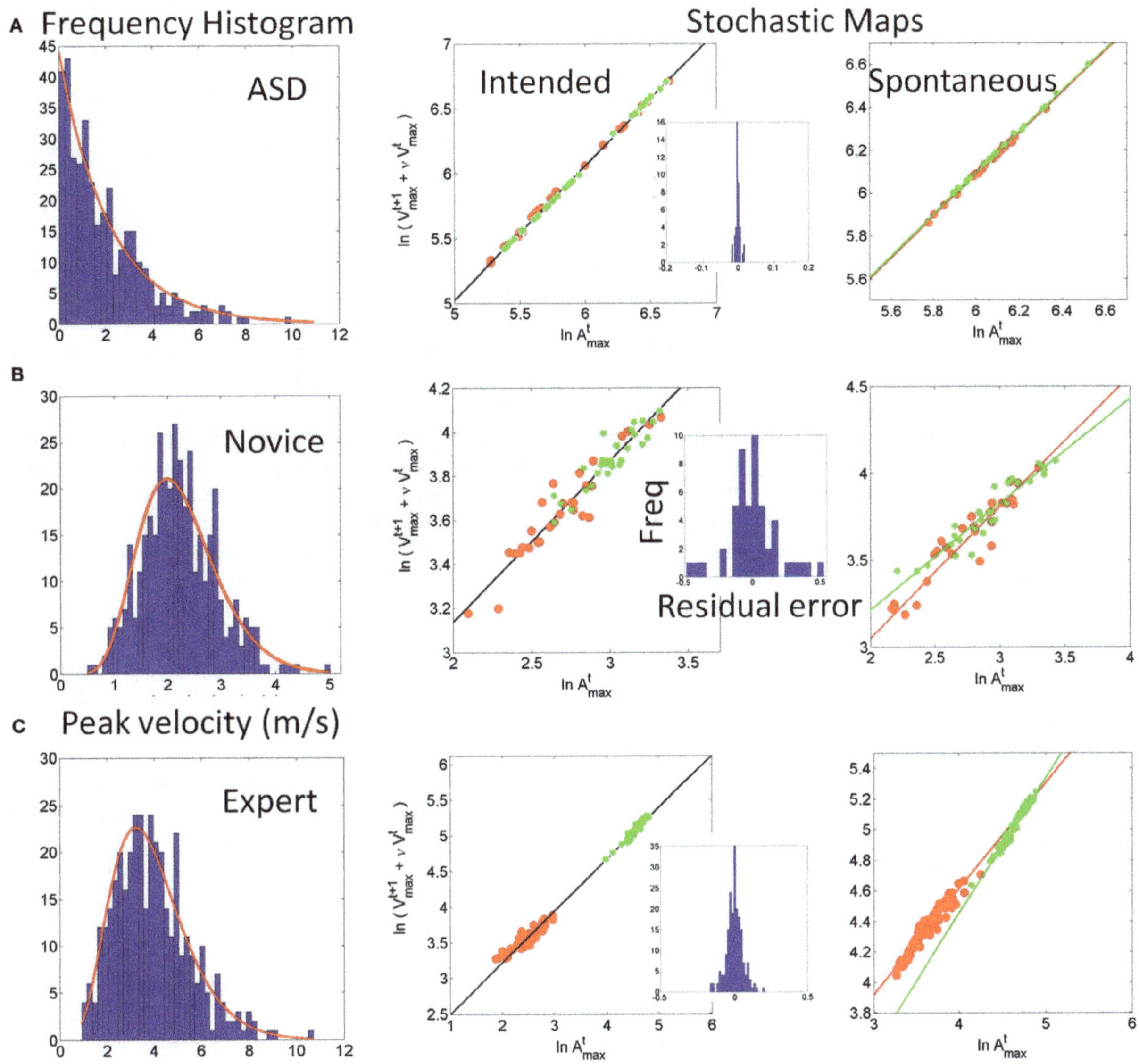

FIGURE 1 | The concept of motor variability revisited. An example that lower movement variability in our framework does not necessarily mean better performance. **(A)** Frequency histogram of the peak velocity from JAB boxing strikes performed by an individual with ASD are well-fit by the Exponential distribution (lowest bin centered at 0.16 m/s). Simple speed-acceleration dependent first-order stochastic map used to describe the noise of the performance and to characterize the anticipatory nature (or lack thereof) in speed variability across trials [explained in Torres (2013)]. Each dot represents a trial, red is slow and green is fast. Each speed in trial $n+1$ depends on the speed and acceleration from trial n. The decay parameters of the best fitting relation tend to be well-characterized by a power law and the exponent is generally similar for fast and slow speed when the motion is intended (as in the JAB's strike). The ASD participant had nearly zero noise in the residual error from the fitting and his motions did not group according to speed level as did those from the novice **(B)** and expert **(C)**. In his case the low variability made his motions non-anticipatory of impending speed. Furthermore, the performance was "memoryless" as past speeds did not contribute to the accurate prediction of present speeds and present events did not contribute to the accurate prediction of future speeds. In the panel of spontaneous retractions (reported by the subjects to be beneath their awareness) the ASD performance cannot distinguish speeds and the same slope fits the two scatters (fast and slow) unlike the controls requiring different slopes for a good fit of speed types. In the controls the intended and spontaneous segments of the JAB are different. Here stability is not defined as low variability. The distributions (which are experimentally determined) of the relevant motion parameters are skewed. The experimentally estimated shape and the scale parameters inform of the predictability and reliability of the random process underlying both the intended motion segments and the spontaneous ones that subjects perform without awareness. Rules such as this simple first order one can be informative of anticipatory strategies or lack thereof as the system learns. **(B)** Novice performance (a female spanning lower speed values) and learning the JAB has higher (and evolving) residual error than the participant with ASD whose noise is nearly absent and remains stationary throughout the sessions. Her speeds (randomly called by a computer program during the experiment) begin to group according to speed level unlike those from the participant with ASD. **(C)** Expert performance highly discriminates the randomly called speeds and has low noise (yet his noise level, despite over 20 years of training, is higher than that of the ASD nearly noiseless case). Notice his higher speed levels in the spontaneous segments than in the intended ones along with high discrimination between intended strikes (1 slope) and spontaneous retractions (2 slopes).

from a verbal participant with a diagnosis of ASD who performed a martial arts experiment in our laboratory (Torres, 2011, 2012, 2013). Compare his performance to that of a naïve typical participant in **Figure 1B** and to that of a typical expert in **Figure 1C**. According to a stochastic map relating velocity and acceleration maxima in the previous trial to the peak velocity of the impending trial [derived in Torres (2013)] the performance of the participant with ASD is nearly noiseless. This result suggests that his system was not exploring and using the information that is typically present in the natural variability of our actions. The lack of variability in his learning performance was accompanied by the Exponential distribution of his peak velocities. According to the "memoryless" Exponential distribution, past speeds did not contribute to present speeds in any predictive manner. His performance used the information in the "here and now" but did not keep a memory of it that enabled the anticipation of the impending peak velocities from prior velocities in the ways in which the naïve and the expert systems did. In those other systems the fluctuations of these parameters overtime gave rise to informative variability. This in turn led to a stable percept characterized by predictive and reliable statistics (Torres, 2011, 2013). Thus, in our model "stability" does not mean low variability or lack of fluctuations as it does in other approaches to movement variability (Thelen and Smith, 1994; Stergiou et al., 2004; Helders, 2010). On the contrary, movement variability stochastically defined in our approach is the most important part of the learning process. The relevant information lies in the statistical class of variability (rather than in the amounts of fluctuations of the standard deviations around a mean value taken under the assumption of normality). The class of variability reveals the individual rates of acquisition of anticipatory performance and expertise.

These distinctions between traditional approaches and ours are crucial as they open a completely new way of assessing *change* in the continuous flow of natural motions, both in real time and longitudinally. By itself, a micro-movement does not convey any meaningful information. It is the accumulation of these fluctuations over time that informs the system of expectations (or lack thereof). Consequently, in our new approach, the question is not whether a child has less or more variability in his/her motions. It is rather whether the rate of change of the *experimentally estimated parameters* describing the probability distribution underlying his/her motions' fluctuations describe a reliable and predictable random process with broad, explorative bandwidth of values (Torres et al., 2013). Those properties make the sensation of our motions emerge as a stable, predictive, verifiable, and anticipatory percept in a very precise statistical sense. Furthermore, in the context of the degrees of freedom (DoF) problem posed by Bernstein (Bernstein, 1967), we can assess stochastic patterns of variability along the dimensions of the space of body configurations that are relevant to the task at hand. These stand in contrast to the spontaneous variability of task-incidental dimensions (Torres and Zipser, 2002, 2004; Torres et al., 2011) so as to precisely examine in real-time the balance or lack thereof between the voluntary and spontaneous aspects of complex behaviors where multiple DoF continuously interact.

There is a second crucial difference between averaging across repeats of an action within a point-to-point given segment and tracking the stochastic signatures of micro-movements over time at the motor output. The former conceives movement as averaged efferent information within some elapsed time without informing us about non-stationary shifts of the efferent motor execution output in real time. This information, which we continuously track in our stochastic approach, is critical to gain a handle on the proprioceptive sensing of our real-time continuous flow of motions as re-afferent input, possibly sensed by kinesthetic transducers. Our definition of this type of sensory input can provide a precise metric of the emergence of a stable and reliable motor expectation (percept). Once that percept turns stable and tractable within the sensory-motor systems, it is also impinged by other forms of sensory guidance including the movement execution itself, all of which bring in new fluctuations.

We provide a way to measure the statistical anchors that the system self discovers in the "kinesthetic priors" that it builds and constantly adapts. This information contains a bundle of intermixed sensory and motor inputs. In the near future we need to deconstruct this bundle and develop new methods to separate various external from various internal influences. Yet at present, using this new personalized statistical platform, we can already track in real time the fluctuations and the acquired stability of this movement-based continuously flowing information on an individual basis. We can do so within the stochastic feedback control framework that others had previously introduced to the field of computational motor control (Todorov, 2005, 2009) but for which, up to now, no experimental estimation of the probability distributions underlying our continuous, unconstrained, natural behaviors had been provided during development and/or adulthood.

Esther Thelen proposed "...movement must itself be considered a perceptual system" (Thelen and Smith, 1994), p. 193. However, up to now no proper statistical framework had been suggested to provide a working definition to test this important proposition. Such a framework would have to enable the real-time and/or longitudinal tracking of the evolution of movement as a form of sensory input during infancy and adulthood. It would have to enable the assessment of the maturation process of our movement sensation as our sensory-motor systems learn to stabilize that sensation, turn it into a reliable signal and adapt that percept throughout our lives.

The new, stochastic notion of movement-based kinesthetic re-afference proposed by our group (Torres et al., 2013), the experimental assessment of motor-based kinesthetic sensations along with their emergence as a stable, reliable, and diversified percept permit the tracking of our continuous flow of movements over time as a form of sensory feedback. In our approach this information is tracked in tandem with basic cognitive processes involving decision-making and anticipatory estimation of the consequences of our actions (Torres, 2013; Torres et al., 2013).

For all the above mentioned reasons, the assessment of this form of proprioception and sensory feedback in our approach is radically different from what had been done in motor-related research in autism up to now, e.g., (Gidley Larson et al., 2008; Haswell et al., 2009; Izawa et al., 2012). Prior work had not provided a way to close the sensory-motor feedback loops and to quantify the continuous exchanges between decisions and actions *in real time*. They gave us a static snapshot of the system disconnected from basic cognitive decision making, and devoid of SBV. For a more in-depth review of the ASD motor literature we refer the reader to the introduction of Torres et al. (2013). In the present report we rather focus on the application of the new statistical framework to track kinesthetic motor re-afference in real-time and longitudinally within a new experimental therapeutic intervention concept.

PARTICIPANTS

A group of 25 individuals with ASD participated in this study, (17 males and 8 females) as well as 8 TD controls (6 males and 2 females). The ages ranged from 6–25 years of age for the individuals with ASD and 3–5 years of age for the TD controls. The IQ score of the individuals with ASD ranged between 40 and 107. Demographic information is presented in **Tables A1**, **A2**. Parents signed parental consent for the children and young adults provided their consent. The protocol was approved by the Institutional Review Boards at Rutgers University and at Indiana University in compliance with the Declaration of Helsinki.

SETUP

We designed an experimental setup that encourages intentional exploration of 3D space. The subjects were seated in front of a computer screen at a distance that often prevented them from touching the screen but that it encouraged them to point at the screen. They were wearing electromagnetic sensors (Polhemus Liberty, 240 Hz) attached to a vest and secured with Velcro strips to their hand, forearm, upper arm, and shoulder. The sensors and attaching Velcro were embedded in customs with different Disney themes of the children's liking. This assisted us in the processes of setting up and speeding up calibration.

Somewhere between the subject and the computer screen a virtual region of interest (vRoI) was defined by the experimenter, which the subject could not see (**Figure 2A**). This vRoI could be moved around and flexibly defined by the researcher as a local square, as a plane or as a 3D-volume of variable size. In this work we used a plane with volume. The goal of the task was implicitly designed so that the subject had to self-discover it. The implicit goal was to hold the hand inside the vRoI so as to trigger and continuously play external media. The subject could use both hands to explore the space but in this report we focus on the use of one hand at a time to transiently trigger the external media when crossing the vRoI and sustaining the media playing when holding the hand inside the vRoi. That is, only real time movements from one hand were tracked so as to register the entrance into the vRoI, the exit from it and the time period when the child was steadily keeping the hand inside the vRoI (see movie at http://www.youtube.com/watch?v=2DKc6aSgd20&feature=youtu.be). The external media could be:

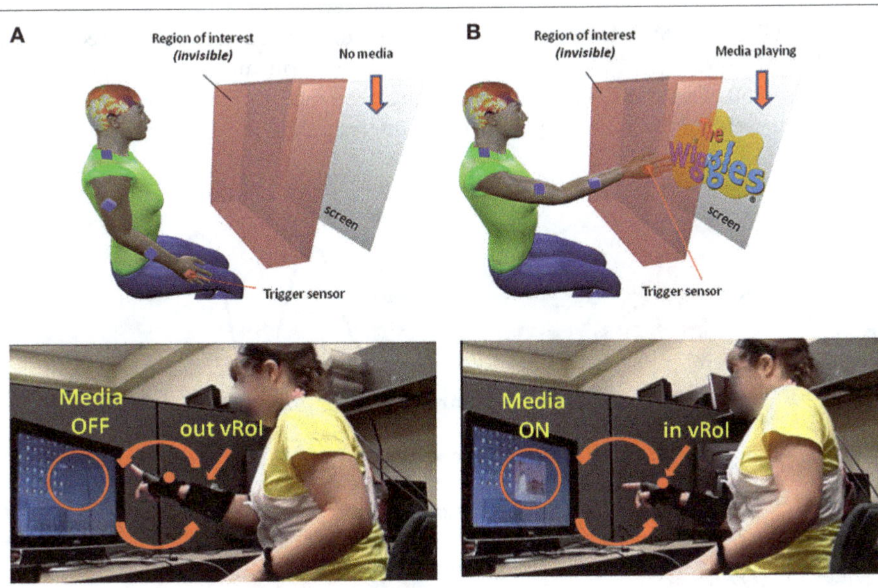

FIGURE 2 | Experimental Therapeutic Intervention: closing the noisy feedback loops by augmenting physical reality with external media. Co-adaptive, closed-feedback loop interface connecting the real time spontaneous movements of the hand and the audio-visual media through cause and effect so as to evoke goal-directed motions. **(A)** The set up consists of the person, media, and a way to capture the physical motions of the person's hand (electro-magnetic sensors in this case sampling at 240 Hz can also be replaced by video cameras). A virtual region of interest (vRoI) invisible and unknown to the subject is created in the peripersonal space. **(B)** Movements of the hand that cross that region will trigger the media ON and provide instantaneous explicit audio-visual feedback to the subject about his/her hand motions causing that effect. The vRoI can be a volume, a plane, a small area, or a grid of points. It can be moved around during the session or it can remain static in one place as in the present example. The child receives no instructions about the goal of the task or the way to accomplish the goal. She/he comes to uncover the goal which is to deliberately sustain the hand inside the vRoI in order to continuously play the media. Movements are registered and the shifts in their stochastic signatures tracked in real time to determine the media that drives the behavioral variability toward more predictive signatures conducive of anticipatory motor control.

1. Real-time video of the participant facing the monitor captured using a built-in camera facing the participant.
2. Cartoons with sounds (music, dialogues, etc.) of the participant's interest.
3. Cartoons with sounds (music, dialogues, etc.) that were not of the particular participant's interest.

The experimenter in coordination with the educators and therapists of the school (the Douglass Developmental Disability Center of Rutgers University, DDDC) compiled for each child the list of preferred and non-preferred media before the experiments began.

As the participant moved the hand around his/her peripersonal space the hand's changes in position and orientation in the 3D-space were tracked in real time so a computer interface could automatically detect entrance to and exit from the vRoI. This was based on the Euclidean metric tracking in real time the distances from the current hand position and orientation to the current position and orientation of the vRoI defined by the experimenter. Whenever the hand entered the vRoI (distance close to 0 with tolerance error set by the experimenter) the media was automatically triggered by the interface. If the hand remained at that spot, the video would continuously play (**Figure 2B**). If the hand moved out of the vRoI, the video would stop (**Figure 2A**). The subject had to realize these contingencies on his/her own. The motion was captured continuously and time-stamped as IN or OUT the vRoI. The stochastic patterns of the motion were analyzed using the SPBA that we describe next.

SENSING MOVEMENT FROM THE PERIPHERAL LIMBS: LIMB PROPRIOCEPTION-BASED MEDIA SELECTION

We used recording session lengths of 50 s and above. The majority of subjects had 2 or more sessions either the same day or on different dates (several weeks later). The sessions for the same subject involved different types of media which allowed us to evaluate movement-sensing (proprioceptive)-based media preferences. If the media made the motions statistically more predictable (in a very precise sense to be defined below), the media was considered as preferred. If the media made the motion patterns more random and noisier, the media was considered as non-preferred. The time-scales of these progressions were also automatically recorded to validate the notion of preference.

PARAMETERS OF INTEREST

We collected 3D position (**Figure 3A**) and orientation (**Figure 3B**) from all four sensors at the rate of 240 Hz as well as the hand sensor status (**Figures 3A,B,** red IN, blue OUT), which was based on the distance between the moving sensor at the hand and the plane defining the vRoI.

The velocity-dependent hand kinematics

The angular speed of the hand sensor was obtained from the changes in hand orientation tracked at 240 Hz. We parameterized these rotations using quaternions (a vector of four dimensions to represent points in the special group of rotations; Kuipers, 1999). A quaternion is a vector of 4 numbers. Three of them specify the unitary vector (axis) of rotation in 3D space and the fourth is the angular magnitude of the rotation of the rigid body (the sensor attached to the hand) around this vector. We defined angular speed as the Euclidean norm (the square root of the sum of squares, taken component wise) of the vector consisting of these 4 numbers. An example of the angular speed continuous sequence is shown in **Figure 3B** for one session and media type; the inset box zooms in the long sequence for just a few frames to show the parameters of interest.

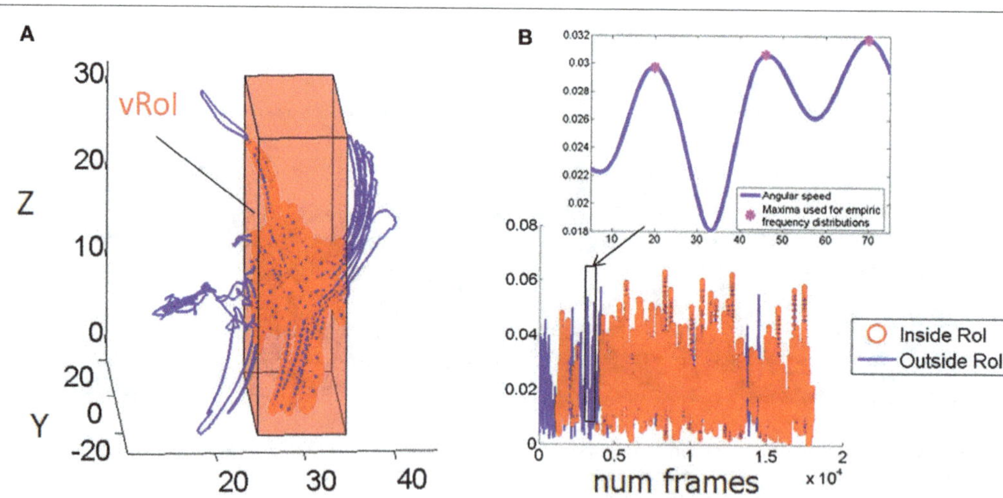

FIGURE 3 | Velocity dependent micro-rotations of the hand registered in real time while exploring the peripersonal space. (A) Virtual Region of Interest (vRoI) invisible to the subject marked as a cube colored in red. Hand positional trajectories captured at 240 Hz inside and outside the vRoI as the child continuously explores the space during 83.3 s. **(B)** Hand rotations displayed as angular speed (radians) obtained by parameterizing the rotations using the quaternion representation and computing the (Euclidean) norm of the angular velocity vector. Blue marks the rotations of the hand outside the vRoI and red marks them inside the vRoI. The peak angular velocity (marked by the magenta star) and the time (ms) to attain it from each minimum are the parameters of interest to track their micro-movements.

The main advantage of using the angular velocity is that it quantifies the changes in the hand posture (independent of the parameterization of the rotations). Moreover, the outcome of the rotation was neither instructed, nor restricted by the size and location of the region of interest (a goal of the task which the participant had to ultimately discover).

STATISTICAL PLATFORM FOR PERSONALIZED BEHAVIORAL ANALYSES (SPBA)

We estimate the probability distribution best characterizing the experimental frequency distribution of the hand's trajectories as it continuously crossed from the OUT to the IN vRoI. We use in this case angular velocity (**Figure 3B**) and read in a minimum of 100 points per estimation. The time scale of these readings will depend on the sampling resolution at the researcher's disposal. However, the rate of change of the stochastic trajectories generated by the person will be independent of this so long as the number of readings is large enough to have proper estimation with adequate goodness of fit tolerance values. For example the MATLAB algorithms for maximum likelihood estimation (MLE) of the parameters of the probability distributions will output the 95% confidence intervals for each estimated parameters and the goodness of fit values. In our case since the sampling resolution is 240 Hz we can obtain 100 readings of peak angular velocities in a few seconds and over minutes, sample densely the rotational motions of the wrist joint angles.

As previously explained by using the stochastic approach, we treat these fluctuations in the joint rotations as re-afferent sensory feedback continuously flowing between the peripheral and the central nervous system. As the actions continuously unfold, these micro-movements are sensed kinesthetically from the physical motions by joint and skin receptors and by muscle spindles.

The two parameters of the continuous Gamma probability distribution family, the shape and the scale, can be estimated from the experimental data using MLE algorithms and plotted in the Gamma (a,b)-plane (**Figure 4**) with 95% confidence intervals to label each individual during the baseline state, early in the task. As the system interacts with the statistics of the environment, the statistics of the continuous flow of hand motions change. These shifts can be captured over time as (a,b) points of the Gamma (shape, scale) plane, which span a trajectory (**Figure 4**). This trajectory will have different rates of change in direction and magnitude, which we can track as well. The latter uniquely define the person's compliance with or resistance to the manipulation of the sensory input that we use. In the **Figure 4** we provide an example in schematic form of the parallel learning process as the hand explores and moves IN and OUT of the vRoI.

We accumulate the minute fluctuations (micro-movements) on the Gamma plane and build a stochastic trajectory from the statistics of the hand's maximal angular speed, as the hand repeatedly enters or leaves the vRoI. In **Figure 4** we show in schematic form the stochastic trajectories in the Gamma plane for IN vRoI (red) and OUT vRoI (blue). The method applied to continuous human data has demonstrated that the continuous flow of movements in our behaviors has non-stationary statistics (Torres, 2013; Torres et al., 2013). The experimentally estimated parameters of the Gamma family of probability distributions shift values over time with the impinging external and internal sensory stimuli. This feature enables us to dynamically track the stochastic shifts in the Gamma plane in each person and for each individual assess the rates of change of the Gamma parameters caused by the impinging stimuli. This approach helps us establish a causal relationship between sensory input and motor output as it is the system itself that in the closed efferent-re-afferent loop controls the outcome. Thus, we can precisely parameterize the sensory input and readout in the motor output fluctuations the shifts in the stochastic signatures that the parameterized manipulation most likely will cause. Then we can use this feedback in effective ways to accelerate the learning progression toward anticipatory autonomous behaviors. More importantly, we can track these ***rates of change*** in the stochastic trajectories unique to each individual. They can inform us of the maximal shifts toward reliable and predictive signatures and can reveal the best source(s) of sensory guidance: e.g., the source(s) that will most likely turn decisions accurate and fast (Torres et al., 2013).

ASSESSING THE *CONTINUOUS* NATURAL FLOW OF BEHAVIOR

In the present work, since minimal to no instructions were given, the child's system had to learn both to self-discover the goal and find the solution to the "self-discovered" problem in order to get a reward (the triggering of the media) and eventually learn to sustain the continuous media-playing to maximize the reward time. The latter required deliberately holding the hand inside the vRoI once the target area was discovered and systematically visited.

The progression of building such expectations would evolve as follows:

1. Random motions of the hand transiently triggering the media ON and then OFF by chance;
2. Noticing external change in the media state(initially a flash of media);
3. Associating external change in media status to hand motion and space region;
4. Systematically exploring the peripersonal space in search of the "magic spot," the vRoI which would trigger the media;
5. Measurable shifts in the velocity-dependent stochastic patterns of the hand;
6. Development of intentional motions to keep the hand within the vRoI;
7. Deliberately holding the hand inside the region of interest to sustain the media playing continuously.

For the dynamic tracking analysis we register and separately analyze the periods inside the vRoI from the periods outside the vRoI (**Figures 3, 4**) for each session. We then take the maximal angular speeds (**Figure 3B**—zoomed in—inset) that are greater than 0.001 units as the significant rotation cut-off. Since we have participants from a variety of ages and body sizes we normalize these maxima to avoid allometric effects [i.e., we divide the peak angular velocity by the sum of the peak angular velocity and the averaged angular velocity in each rotation: this normalization is typically used in anthropological data (Mosimann, 1970;

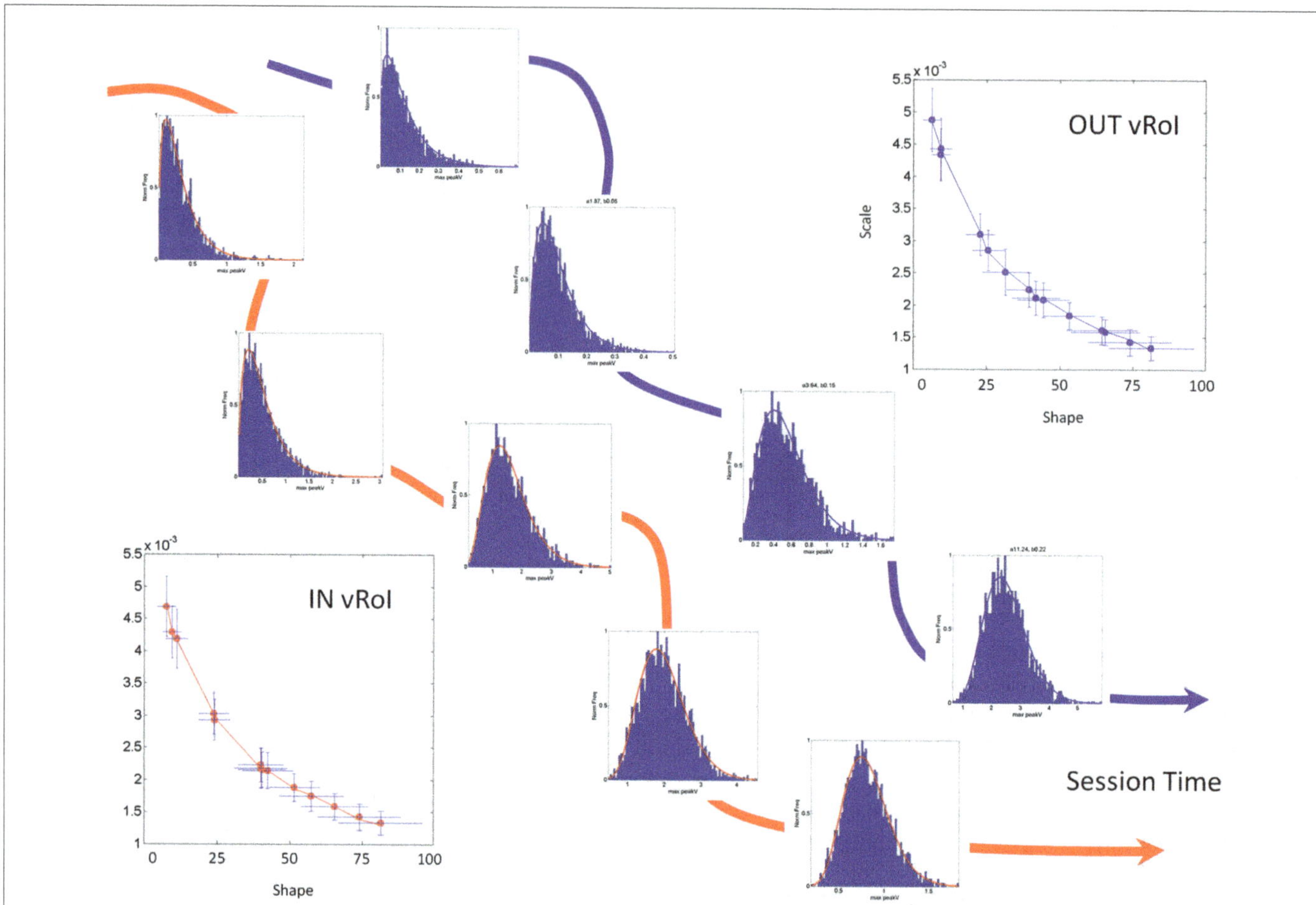

FIGURE 4 | Schematic explanation of the statistical platform for personalized behavioral analyses (SPBA) tracking the non-stationary statistics of continuous movements in real time. (The data sets in this schematic drawing were synthetically generated for explanation purposes using the actual Gamma estimates from a child's behavior as the seeds). The fluctuations in the peak angular velocity of the sensor at the hand are accumulated as the wrist rotates while the child explores the peripersonal space with his/her hand. The fluctuations occurring IN vRoI (red) are accumulated in parallel to those occurring OUT vRoI (blue) in the continuous flow of motions of the hand's behavior. Over time the behavior transitions from random to exploratory to systematic and goal directed, to intentional (as when the child deliberately holds the hand to sustain the media playing). In any given time period there can also be reversals toward a noisier random pattern as a function of the media. The faster the convergence toward anticipatory behavior (predictable, reliable and exploratory), the more preferred the media is by that child. Lower media preferences would thus be accompanied by stagnation in this process and reversals toward noisy and random patterns (up and to the left of the Gamma plane). The normalized frequencies histograms of the peak angular velocity represent selected times across one session as the stochastic trajectories IN and OUT vRoI evolve in time. The histograms are fit with members of the two parameter continuous Gamma family of probability distributions. The estimated (shape, scale) parameters are plotted as points in the Gamma plane with 95% confidence intervals. The stochastic trajectories from the orderly shifts are represented on the Gamma plane. Points to the right and down are predictive and reliable, thus marking anticipatory behavior. Points to the left and up are random and noisy. Notice that there are differences in the rate of change of the stochastic signatures. Underlying curves represent the flow of time in the session.

Lleonart et al., 2000)]. The empirical frequency histograms of the normalized angular speed maxima are then obtained for at least 100 points (as explained above the goodness of fit and 95% confidence intervals were adequate at 240 Hz) for the IN vRoI and the OUT vRoI. In each case (IN and OUT) the shape and the scale parameters (a,b) of the Gamma probability distribution are estimated with 95% confidence using MLE. The trajectory is tracked on the Gamma plane as suggested in schematic form on **Figure 4**. In the present report the points of this trajectory correspond to one recording session. And also, longitudinal assessment was done 2–4 weeks later during a different session with no training in between sessions.

QUANTIFYING PREDICTABILITY

The Gamma probability distribution describes a continuous family of skewed probability distributions smoothly ranging from Exponential to Gaussian.

The probability density of the Gamma distribution is governed by

$$y = f(x \mid a, b) = \frac{1}{b^a \Gamma(a)} x^{a-1} e^{-\frac{x}{b}} \tag{1}$$

where a is the shape of the Gamma and governs the degree of symmetry of the distribution; b is the scale and governs the height of the distribution. The Γ represents the Gamma function. The larger values of a (shape) correspond to more symmetric, therefore, closer to Gaussian distributions. The Exponential case is when $a = 1$.

The Exponential distribution is the only continuous memoryless distribution, whereby previous events do not contribute to the prediction of future events any more than current events do; while the Gaussian distribution has good predictive properties. Thus, a participant whose estimated probability distribution is a member of the Gamma family closer to the Gaussian range, s/he will have motions with more systematic (predictive) behavior than if the estimated probability distribution is closer to the Exponential range of the Gamma plane. **Figure 4** shows instances of (a,b) estimates corresponding to probability distribution curves, which fit the histograms in 4 with 95% confidence.

In our case the predictive ability (larger shape value) of a certain Gamma family member corresponds to the level of systematicity in the hand posture (orientation) changes. **Figure 4** illustrates the shift down and to the right along the trajectory. In general these fluctuations in the Gamma plane can vary in different directions and magnitude but for illustrative purposes they are shown in **Figure 4** as the ideal target stochastic behavior that one should aim for if predictability and reliability (low dispersion) are desired.

Our objective was indeed to achieve more predictive regimes once inside the vRoI by aiming for a shift in the (a,b) parameters toward the right, to the Gaussian limits of the Gamma plane. The media can be selected according to this objective so as to reinforce the predictive behavioral path to build a reliable motor expectation (a motor-kinesthetic prior) which can result in anticipatory behavior. Likewise, random and noisy statistical regimes shall be discouraged, so the external sensory input (media) that leads to such corrupted proprioceptive signal (toward the Exponential ranges) shall be downplayed.

QUANTIFYING RELIABILITY

The Fano Factor (Fano, 1947) is given by the noise to signal ratio. This is the dispersion of the experimentally estimated distribution, obtained by dividing the estimated variance by the estimated mean. This index can also be obtained for the estimated rates of change of the shifts in the non-stationary statistics of the behavior. In the case of the Gamma probability distribution, the mean is $a \times b$ and the variance is $a \times b^2$. This ties the scale b parameter to the dispersion because the Fano Factor = variance/mean = b. Thus, when the fitting is good these two estimated Gamma parameters provide information about the *predictability* and the *reliability* of the continuous flow of behavior—which we treat as a stochastic process. We specifically aim at systematically shifting the parameter values of the real-time estimated probability distribution *down and to the right of the Gamma plane.*

Using this framework and the new closed-loop co-adaptive paradigm we seek to:

1. Dynamically track the real time evolution of the non-stationary statistics of the velocity-dependent variability as the participants develop predictive statistics and transition from random to systematic to goal-directed, to intentional behaviors.
2. Longitudinally assess the retention of the changes in stochastic signatures: are these changes transient or are they retained and improved when presented with the same stimulus?
3. We seek to automatically and objectively extract from the statistics of the physical movements which media type makes the child's hand motions more predictive so as to reinforce that media type. Likewise we seek to determine which media type makes the hand movements noisier and more random, so as to discount it.

IMPORTANT DISTINCTIONS FROM CURRENT BEHAVIORAL THERAPIES

This is an estimation process that experimentally obtains the statistical parameters from the behavior—as opposed to assuming a theoretical probability distribution such as the Gaussian distribution and summarizing the process by the mean and the variance parameters, $\mu \pm \sigma^2$. In current behavioral approaches these measurements are discretely rather than continuously obtained by tallying the *observed* responses over a certain number of trials and obtaining averages. It would be a mistake to do this. The behavior follows a continuous stream. Moreover, the frequency distributions of the kinematics motor parameters underlying the (observationally reported) behaviors have actually been experimentally determined. They do not follow a symmetric distribution. Their frequency distributions are skewed (Torres, 2011, 2012, 2013). It is known that under those statistical features it is incorrect to use the theoretical assumptions $\mu \pm \sigma$ or to use parametric models (such as Analyses of Variance, ANOVA, regression, etc.; Limpert et al., 2001; Limpert and Stahel, 2011). Current behavioral approaches do not consider these issues because physical movements present in all behaviors are not currently objectively registered and quantified (Cooper et al., 1987).

This approach is also different than reinforcing the movement itself so as to maximize the likelihood that a particular movement occurs in the future. Current behavioral therapies *command* the child to perform certain movement types. Such therapies try to reinforce a particular movement through repetitions, for example at different speeds, with different stimuli, etc. or to discourage the movement type corresponding to some stimulus set and so forth (Black et al., 1972; Cooper et al., 1987). These actions are driven by the therapist's opinion from tallying the discretized performance by some coding system. This is as opposed to other alternatives such as assessing the stochasticity of the continuous flow of motions—as we do here; or using the fractal dynamics of our motions (Hausdorff et al., 1999) and their metrics of stability [reviewed by Vereijken (2010)]; or using other non-invasive computational techniques to objectively quantify natural performance. Because we want to understand how the autistic system is coping with the corrupted sensory-motor feedback, we do not want to impose any biases in the assessments of their natural flow of movements. We do not seek to reinforce any movement type. Instead we let the child self-discover movement preferences.

Through the stochastic approach we can tell whether or not the motions are more reliable using the Fano Factor, the scale parameter in the case of the Gamma probability distribution. These indexes of predictability and reliability can be applied to any movement. We do not need to enforce or command any particular movement type (as it is routinely done in current behavioral therapies). If we were to enforce a movement type, such commanding would most likely interfere with the spontaneous self-discovery process that we are trying to evoke with our new approach.

The role of the experimenter in this proposed new concept is less active than in current approaches. That is, when following up each individual—through automatic computational tracking—as the system manifests real-time shifts in the stochastic signatures, the experimenter should not interfere with the self-discovery process. The child should lead.

This type of philosophy differs from that of the current behavioral therapies [e.g., Applied Behavioral Analyses (ABA) http://www.youtube.com/watch?v=SLBLnNxzftM], where the therapist would be the one determining which stimuli/behavior/letter would be the best to reinforce in any given session based on observation of the responses of the child. By objectively quantifying the continuous flow of expected behaviors in closed loop with actual physical behaviors driven by the child it will be possible to get at the implicit aspects of the learning process that the human eye will inevitably be missing when exclusively focusing on the discrete goal-directed segments embedded in the continuous flow of behavior.

The more traditional form of feedback-based correction tends to be rather centered on the experimenter's inferences. Yet, we aim here at shifting that focus from the experimenter's inferences to the statistical inferences based on the physical motor outcome of the child. Under these self-driven actions, we aim at using the SBV inherently present in the child's micro-movements as a proxy to spontaneously evoke intentionality in the child's actions. Intentionality in this case goes above and beyond attaining goal-directness. The objective is rather to have the child's self-discovered behaviors evolve toward statistical patterns with stochastic signatures that have precisely defined predictability and reliability ranges according to the statistical indexes (as defined above).

In the present experimental therapeutic intervention the statistics of the child's movements (rather than the experimenter's opinion) reveal the best source of sensory guidance: i.e., the media type that maximally shifts the probability distributions toward reliable and predictable regimes. This is done automatically, independent of the experimenter's inferences. It is through exploration and self-discovery that the child comes to find out what the problem is; solves it; and obtains the reward. The reward in this case is not food or a token, but the very solution of the problem: the media continuously playing, thus making the child acquire volitional control of his/her movements. This direct cause-effect realization and active use of intentionality by the child alone is at the core of this proposed intervention concept and the rewarding control of the child's own actions.

The non-stationary statistics of the natural flow of movements during the exploratory behavior and the analyses of the indexes of performance (reliability and predictability) permit real-time rapid and automatic personalized assessment of the child's preferences of self-video *vs.* cartoons, movies, music, dialogs, etc.

TIMES IN/OUT OF THE VIRTUAL REGION OF INTEREST

To establish the signatures of variability for motions IN and OUT of the vRoI indicating media preference we examined the time spent in random motions (or in goal-seeking) OUT of the vRoI; as well as the time spent goal-contacting IN the vRoI. The time in this case corresponds to the number of frames registered at 240 Hz resolution (which divided by 240 provides the number of seconds spanned by the frequency of visits to one region of space or another). Given a media type, the systematically higher % session time spent IN the vRoI simultaneously combined with faster rates of shift in stochastic signatures toward the more predictive and reliable statistical regimes of motion variability are the criteria for "preferred media."

We normalize the times by the session length to avoid the effect of varying session time lengths (**Figure 5A**) and express this parameter as a % of time. We also look at the sliding window progression of the fraction of time spent inside the region of interest within one session to get a sense of the exploratory progression within that session. We chose the sliding window size as 20% of session duration, as this was the minimum ideal window across all session lengths. And we can track, combining the Gamma parameter estimation and the temporal metric, the precise temporal progression of the stochastic evolution as a function of session time. The temporal metric for a session is depicted in **Figure 5B** where the session time is color-coded from darker (earlier in the session) to lighter (later in the session). The arrows highlight the order of the trajectory.

RESULTS AND DISCUSSION

THE TWO-PARAMETER CONTINUOUS GAMMA FAMILY OF PROBABILITY DISTRIBUTIONS CAPTURES BOTH TD AND ASD BEHAVIORAL VARIABILITY

The distributional analyses revealed that the Gamma family captured with high confidence the stochastic signatures and their shifts for each one of the TD and ASD participants. Each child's hand angular velocity peak inside the vRoI as well as outside the vRoI spanned a frequency histogram well-fit by one of probability distribution members of the Gamma family. The shape and scale parameters were plotted and tracked in the Gamma plane as they evolved with the search for the vRoI and the media type. **Figures 6A,C** show the scatters on the Gamma plane for each set of participants. **Figures 6B,D** show the estimated probability distributions of the normalized peak angular velocity corresponding to (**A** and **C**).

The evolution of the parameters revealed shifts in the stochastic signatures of each child with different step size and different directions (different rates of change). Shifts in the Gamma plane were sometimes to the left thus indicating a change in the shape of the distribution and more randomness in the variability. Other shifts were to the right indicating a change in the shape of the distribution to a more symmetric type, thus signaling acquired predictability in the variability. Likewise shifts up and down along the scale parameter helped determine the degree of dispersion in the distribution and informed of the reliability of the underlying random process. We report the values of the estimated parameters and the goodness of fit for each group on **Tables A2, A3**.

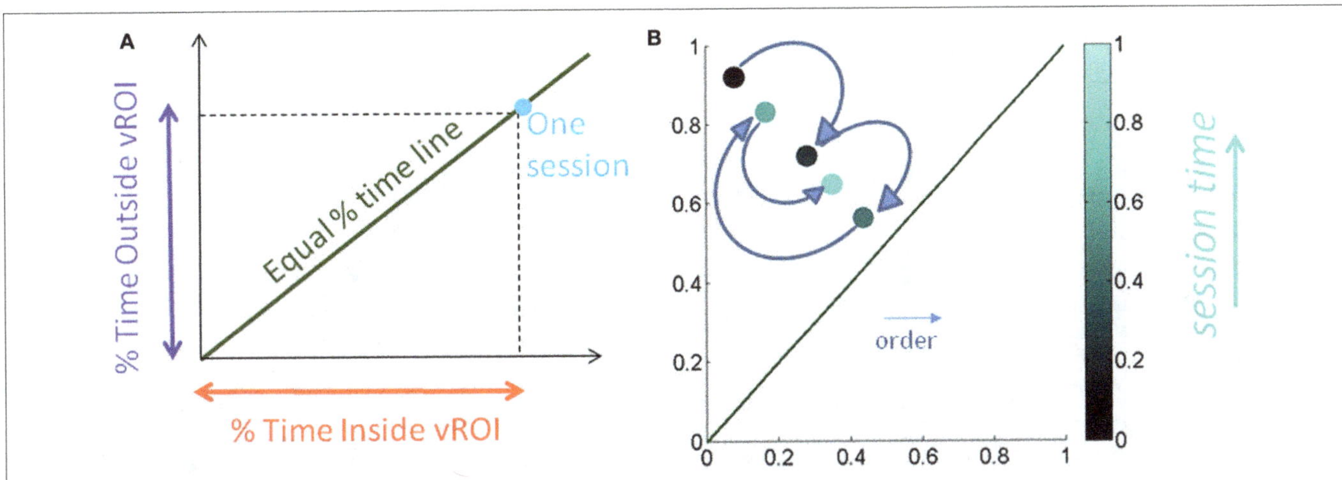

FIGURE 5 | Media preference metric validation for a session. (A) We used the percentage of time spent inside the vRoI *vs.* percent of time spent outside the vRoI to validate that more time inside the vRoI (lower right area, under the green line denoting equal percentage of time spent inside and outside vRoI) correspond to subject's stochastic signatures being in more predictive range. **(B)** We also looked at the time percentage inside the vRoI progression as the recording session goes on in a window of 20% of session time, to get a feeling of dynamics of the interest taken by the subject in media. As the recording session goes on, the colors get brighter. The ideal exploratory pattern would be when the dots shift toward lower right as the colors would become brighter.

MOTIONS OUTSIDE THE vRoI WERE LESS PREDICTIVE THAN THOSE INSIDE THE vRoI

We focused on two types of motions within the continuous flow of movements that the Gamma signatures revealed. The motions OUT vRoI turned out to be more random as their signatures were more often to the left of the Gamma plane than those of the IN vRoI cases. As the child's search became more systematic outside the vRoI, these motions also shifted the stochastic signatures to the right of the Gamma plane with consistency. **Figures 6A,B** show this trend in both the TD and the ASD groups.

THE RATE OF CHANGE OF STOCHASTIC SHIFTS AND THE TEMPORAL METRIC REVEAL THE MEDIA PREFERRED BY EACH CHILD

For each child the maximal step size of the shift of the stochastic signature given by the change over time of the (a,b) position in the Gamma plane was unique. **Figure 7** shows the evolution of the stochastic signatures of two TD children. The shift in the (a,b) points provide the rate of change of the stochastic signature over time. The maximal size in shift to the right (more predictive behavioral variability) among a set of media reveals the media that causes the shape of the probability distribution to turn more symmetric. Notice here that this is not just a correlation as it is the child who is in real-time, in closed loop with the media, causing the shifts in stochastic signatures from the hand motions to become more predictive.

This indicates that the goal-seeking movement patterns become more predictive and more reliable as the child searches for the "magic spot" and moves the hand outside the vRoI to try and trigger a particular media type. The largest shift in the stochastic signatures down and to the right of the Gamma plane reveals for each child the media type that would most likely maximally accelerate the acquisition of more predictive, reliable, and diversified movement patterns. Such media leads to the self-discovery of the primary implicit goal of the task (i.e., finding the vRoI) and in turn, to systematically accomplish the secondary implicit goal (sustaining the hand in that vRoI to continuously play that media).

These goals and sub-goals are implicit as they are not instructed but must be self-discovered. However, over time they shift priorities so the secondary goal becomes the goal of the task of playing the media continuously by holding the hand in a particular position of space (the vRoI). The relation of the change in distribution shape for each child and the Fano Factor quantifying the dispersion of the distribution is plotted in **Figure 11**. The **Figure 11** shows the worst and the best cases where the predictability and reliability of the INvRoI and the OUTvRoI cases are respectively quantified. Notice that the TD children separate the slopes of the power relations with faster rate of change for the INvRoI cases. **Table A2** provides examples of the evolution of the parameter for different media types.

A temporal metric revealing a systematic gain within a session is given by the frequency of the times during that session that the child's hand moved inside the vRoI *vs.* the frequency of the times that the child remained exploring the space outside the vRoI. This is quantified through the percent of time that the hand remained in each region (IN *vs.* OUT) which systematically coincided for each child with more predictive (IN vRoI) stochastic regimens or less predictive (OUT vRoI) stochastic regimes.

Figure 7 shows an example for a TD girl (A) and a TD boy (B) of the above metrics and quantifications. Notice that the patterns evoked by the "spongebob" cartoon shifted the stochastic signatures maximally for the girl (7A top black markers) during the 04-05-12 session as compared to the other videos. This can be appreciated in the shift in location down and toward the right of the Gamma plane from the OUT vRoI (black asterisk) to the IN vRoI (black dot). The step size caused by that media type was larger than that for all the other media played that day. Notice as

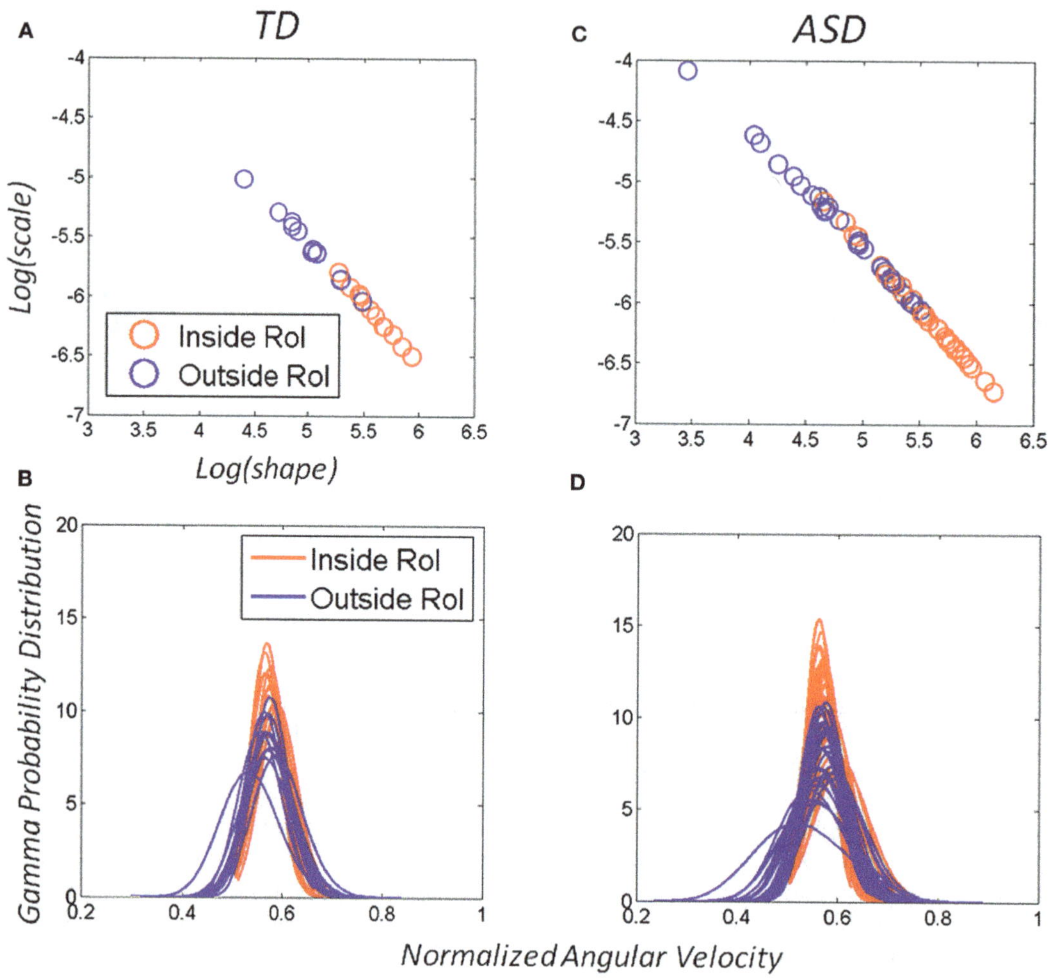

FIGURE 6 | Adaptive capabilities of participants with ASD: both TD children and children with ASD shifted the stochastic signatures of the angular-velocity dependent micro-movements. The orientations of their hand became more predictive as the hand deliberately remained in the vRoI to continuously play the external media. The estimated Gamma parameters for the normalized angular velocity [peak angular velocity/(peak angular velocity + averaged angular velocity)]. In this case a sliding window was used to track the stochastic value of the parameter every 100 peak velocity values as the hand explored the space in search for the vRoI and as it discovered it and the hand was held there continuously to sustain the media playing. **(A)** Patterns of a TD child. **(C)** Patterns of a child with ASD. **(B–D)** The Gamma probability distributions were estimated from the empirical data within the range of normalized angular velocity values for each child. Note that the child with ASD starts out with higher dispersion in the distribution (variance to mean ratio) but as the vRoI is discovered and the hand sustained inside it, the noise-to-signal ratio decreases, thus increasing the reliability of the probability distribution.

well that in the same session the red markers representing other media had a smaller shift from OUT to IN the vRoI. Overall in that session the hand was exploring more time outside the vRoI but the media represented by the black marker was already shifting toward a regime closer to spending more time inside the vRoI as the motions's variability became more predictive.

The gain experienced in the predictability of the stochastic signatures during the 04-05-12 session not only transferred 2 weeks later to the session of 04-19-12; it actually improved the gains in the percent of time that the child maintained the hand inside the vRoI (blue dot in bottom panel **A**). This indicates that consistently the "princess" video was preferred over the "spongebob" video in the very precise sense of an increase in the frequency of the visits of the hand to the space inside the vRoI and the shifts toward a more predictive location of the Gamma plane. Finally for the girl the video of the "mermaid" had the largest effect as the hand was deliberately spending more time inside the vRoI than with all other media during the second session.

Similar patterns can be seen for the sample data from a TD boy in **Figure 7B**. Here the real-time videos of himself triggered by placing the hand inside the vRoI shifted the stochastic patterns maximally (step from blue asterisk to blue dot in **7B** top panel is larger than step from cyan markers). Furthermore in the first visit 10-14-11 the child sustained the hand inside the vRoI for a longer % of time than in the second visit 04-05-12 indicating that despite the retained gains in predictability (shift to the right) during the second visit, it was the triggering of the real-time self-video that maintained his interest rather than the "spongebob." He visited

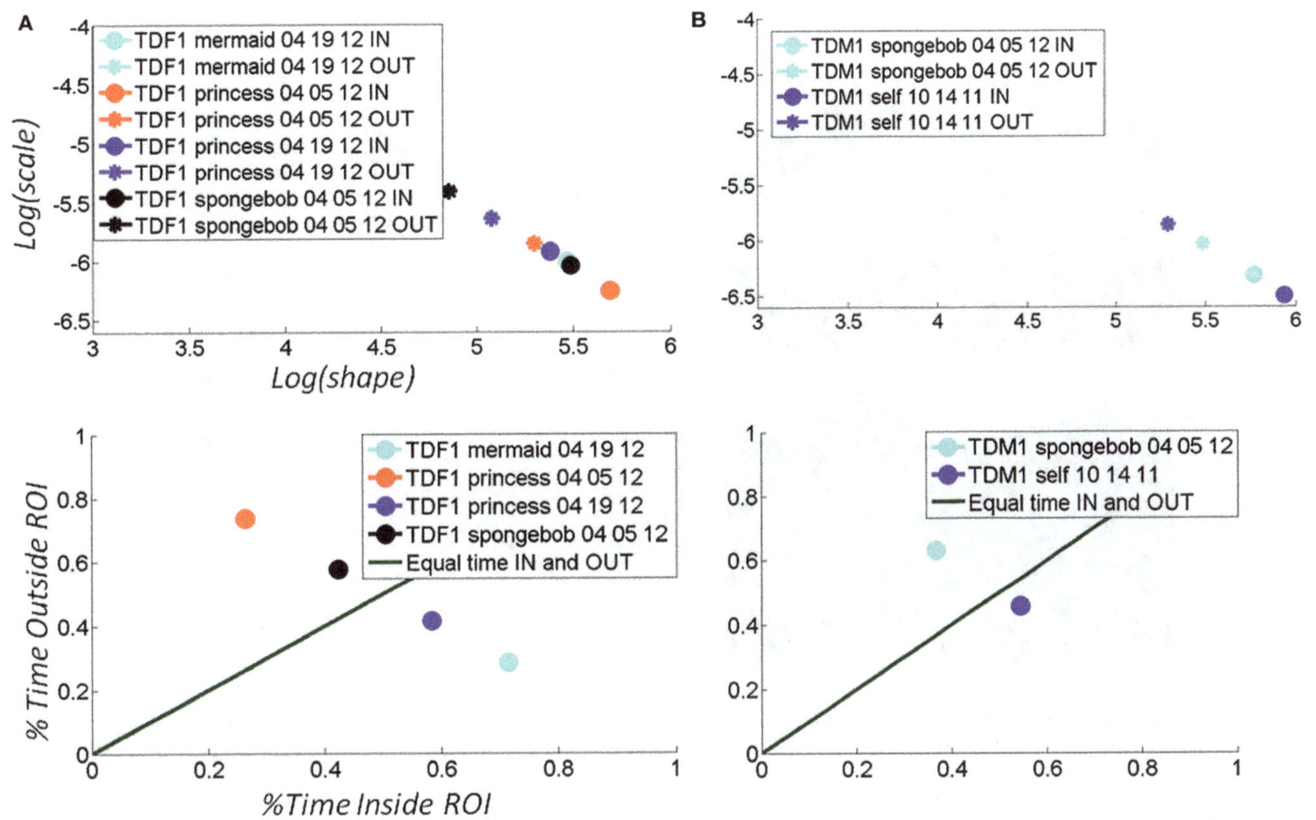

FIGURE 7 | Selectively finding and using the media type that shifts the stochastic signatures of the micro-movements of the TD child's hand toward the more predictive regime: building behavior that shifts the statistics of micro-movements toward spontaneous autonomous control. (A) The hand motions of a TD female were tracked longitudinally over the course of a week, shifting toward a region of more statistically predictive behavior as the hand spent more time in the vRoI (from red to black) when triggering a Disney cartoon involving "The Disney Princesses". Bottom panel shows the percent time spent inside (systematically exploring) the vRoI *vs.* that spent outside the vRoI (randomly exploring). This particular TD girl preferred "The Little Mermaid" video over the "SpongeBob SquarePants" video, demonstrated by the stochastic patterns of angular velocity micro-movements shifting to more systematic regimes for the former rather than the latter. Likewise, we longitudinally quantified improvements over the course of a week using the preferred media (from red to cyan). **(B)** A TD male prefers the real-time video of himself to the "SpongeBob SquarePants" videos. He spends over 50% of the time in the vRoI for the former media, deliberately holding his hand to watch himself, and over 60% of the time outside the vRoI exploring during SpongeBob. In the top panel, the patterns inside the vRoI can be seen to be consistently more predictive as they fall farther to the right of the Gamma plane than those outside the vRoI during random exploration.

the vRoI more frequently in the first visit (blue dot) than in the second (cyan dot) unambiguously informing us that he prefers video of the self over the cartoon.

Across ages the participants with ASD also showed adaptive capabilities as the TD children did. Remarkably, the non-verbal participants became as engaged as the TD participants and as their verbal ASD peers. As with the other participants the non-verbal participants with ASD spontaneously figured out the goal of the task and came to a correct solution without instructions. Examples of non-verbal children with ASD are shown in **Figure 8** (a girl) and **Figure 9** (a boy). Notice that the girl with ASD showed the largest shift for the "mermaid" (**Figure 8A** top) which also evoked the largest percentage of time deliberately exploring inside the vRoI. The video of the "princess" evoked a small shift in predictability during the first 04-05-12 session but in the following visit, during the 04-19-12 session the gain in predictability was higher and so was the % of time spent inside the vRoI. This reveals a gain that was not only retained but also enhanced 2 weeks later in the absence of additional practice sessions.

Consistent results are reported for a non-verbal boy with ASD in **Figure 9**. He, too, came to the realization on his own, without any verbal instructions, that (1) transient changes in media state were triggered by his hand; (2) by sustaining the hand inside the vRoI he could continuously watch the video of his preference. In his case, real-time self-videos were preferred according to the maximal step size in the Gamma plane of the stochastic signatures of the hand micro-rotations (from the brown asterisk representing the outside vRoI value to the brown dot representing the inside vRoI value). Likewise this is the media type that evokes the largest frequency of times that the hand visited inside the vRoI. Notice as well that as with the other participants in later sessions (e.g., from 03-23-12 to 04-13-12) there is a gain in predictability above and beyond its retention over time.

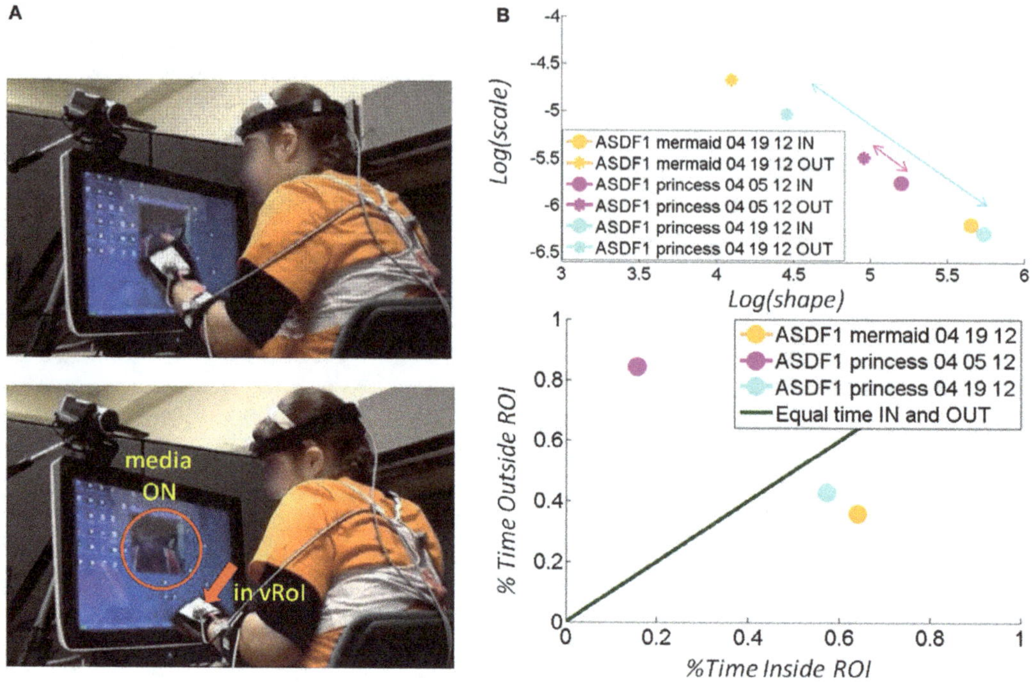

FIGURE 8 | Tracking the stochastic signatures of angular velocity-dependent hand's micro-movements in a child with ASD. **(A)** Non-verbal female child with ASD explores the vRoI and finds out how to trigger and maintain the media ON. **(B)** The real time shifts in the stochastic signatures of her hand movement's velocity-dependent variability are obtained for both the IN and OUT segments of her searching motions. Arrows highlight shifts toward the right (the predictive regimes) of the Gamma plane. The size of the arrow marks the rate of change which is larger (faster) for preferred media. The rate of change of the stochastic signatures speaks of their sensory preferences and adaptive capabilities. Longitudinally (from March to April) there is a shift for "The Disney Princesses" video (from magenta to cyan), but the shift in real time for "The Little Mermaid" is far more pronounced and occurs faster. This video was far more effective than "The Disney Princesses" video in shifting her stochastic patterns toward a more predictive behavioral regime. **(C)** Consistent with the largest shift toward the predictive regimes (preferred media) the child spends more time inside the vRoI with that media type.

TRANSIENT AND LONG-TERM EFFECTS REGISTERED IN ALL CHILDREN

Besides transient positive effects during a single session, the experimental results indicated in each child a long-lasting longitudinal effect after 2 weeks with marked improvements from the earlier session (despite no practice during the period between sessions). In **Figure 8** for example, the gains in predictability evoked by the "princess" video were retained from the 04-05-12 session to the 04-19-12 session. There was also a gain in predictability during the later 04-19-12 session as quantified by the shifts in the estimated parameters of the Gamma statistical distribution. On this later 04-19-12 session the "princess" video had a larger gain toward the Gaussian range of the Gamma plane (**Figure 8B** top) and the girl rotated her hand inside the vRoI for a larger percent of time than in the previous 04-05-12 session. This video without a doubt had a consistent positive longitudinal effect on the statistical signatures of the angular velocity-dependent variability of this participant.

In the example from the non-verbal boy with ASD, the real time self-video projected from the webcam facing him whenever the hand entered the vRoI had the largest shift (**Figure 9B** top) and led to the continuous and deliberate holding of the hand inside the vRoI. The "bluesclues" and "elmo" videos also shifted the stochastic signatures between OUT and IN the vRoI. The hand was exploring mostly outside the vRoI for the "bluesclues" and "elmo" videos (shown in **Figure 9B** bottom). This indicates that the search for the "magic spot" was not entirely random as indicated by the shifts in the stochastic signatures during this exploration outside the vRoI to more predictive ranges of the Gamma plane (**Figure 9B** top). As in the other children the second visit from 03-23-12 to 04-13-12 showed retention and improvement of the patterns, despite no practice sessions in the time between visits.

AUTOMATICALLY ASSESSING THE QUALITY OF THE SESSION OF THE EXPERIMENTAL INTERVENTION

The search patterns in real time for a given session were also informative of the quality of the session in terms of the learning stage. Goal-contacting sessions were those in which the search was conducive of intentionality, meaning that the goal was found and sustained the media playing most of the time. In this case the child deliberately held the hand inside the vRoI for the most part of the session in order to maximize the reward of continuously interacting with the media. Sessions that were mostly exploratory without success at figuring out the goal location were termed Goal-seeking sessions. The stochastic patterns could then reveal the level of randomness of predictability (systematicity) of the session and indicate if these were random motions or goal-seeking exploratory behaviors.

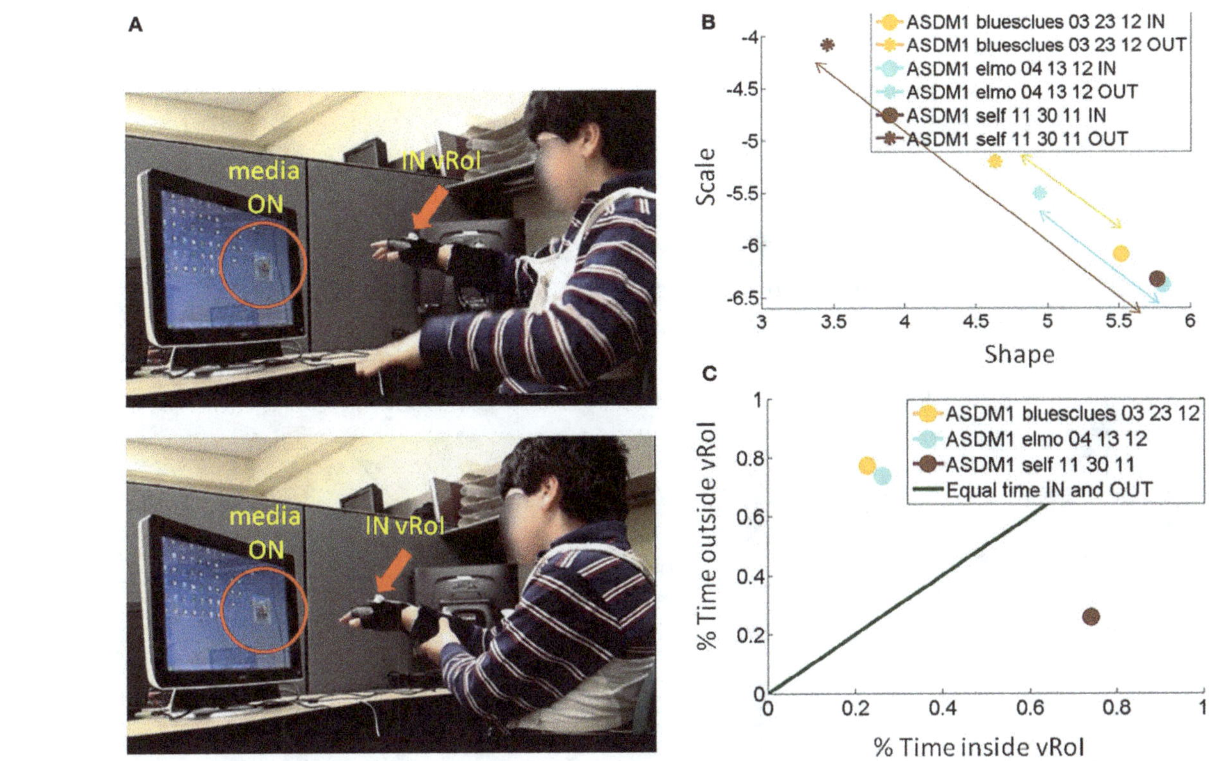

FIGURE 9 | Tracking the stochastic signatures of angular velocity-dependent hand's micro-movements in a child with ASD. (A) Non-verbal male child with ASD explores the peripersonal space in search for consistency of the cause and effect phenomena: i.e., the hand triggering the media, and then deliberately holds the hand to continuously play the media once it self-discovers the goal of the task and the solution to attain it. **(B)** Real-time shifts in the rates of change of the stochastic trajectories quantified from the non-stationary statistics of the hand micro-rotations. Largest shifts are due to viewing real time video of himself, while shifts quantified by triggering videos of "Elmo" and "Blue's Clues" are less pronounced. **(C)** The longitudinal measurement of the cartoons show improvements for "Elmo" in both the Gamma plane shifts and in the percent of session time spent exploring the vRoI, yet the percent of time spent deliberately holding the hand inside the vRoI and engaging the real-time video of himself is far larger. Notice as well-that transient predictive gains in 03-23-12 are retained weeks later and improved in 04-13-12 despite no practice of the task in between.

Examples of Goal-contacting sessions are shown on the top panels of the **Figure 10**. On the left panel the hand was maintained inside the vRoI the entire time while the right panel shows a transition from OUT to IN, as well as the intentional holding of the hand inside the vRoI as the session progresses in time (from darker to lighter colors). Examples of Goal-seeking sessions are shown on the bottom panels of **Figure 10** where the hand was mostly exploring outside the vRoI. At the start of this session (darker dots) the patterns are most of the time far from the vRoI but as time progresses within the session (lighter colors) the hand is closer to the line of unity where the child visits with equal frequency the areas of interest IN *vs.* OUT of the vRoI.

ADAPTIVE CAPABILITIES ARE PRESENT IN BOTH TD AND ASD CHILDREN

The most interesting result of this work is that all participants with ASD showed proficiency in this task. They were able to detect the change that their motions caused in the state of the media. This change-detection capability was sufficient to spontaneously, without instructions, trigger a search in peripersonal space that moved from random to systematic and eventually intentional, as when the hand was deliberately held inside the vRoI in order to continuously play the media.

This progression was captured in the evolution of their stochastic signatures of movement variability according to the statistical patterns of the angular rotations of the hand. This form of movement-based proprioceptive sensory input reshaped their behaviors and sustained their interest in the task. The **Figure 6** shows that both TD and ASD participants improved their motion patterns by making them more reliable and predictable (shifted them down and to the right of the Gamma plane). Both groups came to discover on their own the goal(s) of the task and developed predictable and reliable statistics in their hand micro-movements. Their spontaneously emerging self-control resulted in motions with lower dispersion of the estimated probability distributions (**Figures 6B,D**) according to the Fano Factor which decreased in both the TD and the ASD participants when comparing the inside to the outside vRoI states and also when examining the gains over time (**Figure 11** and **Table A3**).

An important result here which confirmed our previous findings in a larger group of ASD participants and under different experimental conditions (using open loop reaches; Torres et al., 2013), was that the subjects with ASD showed less discrimination

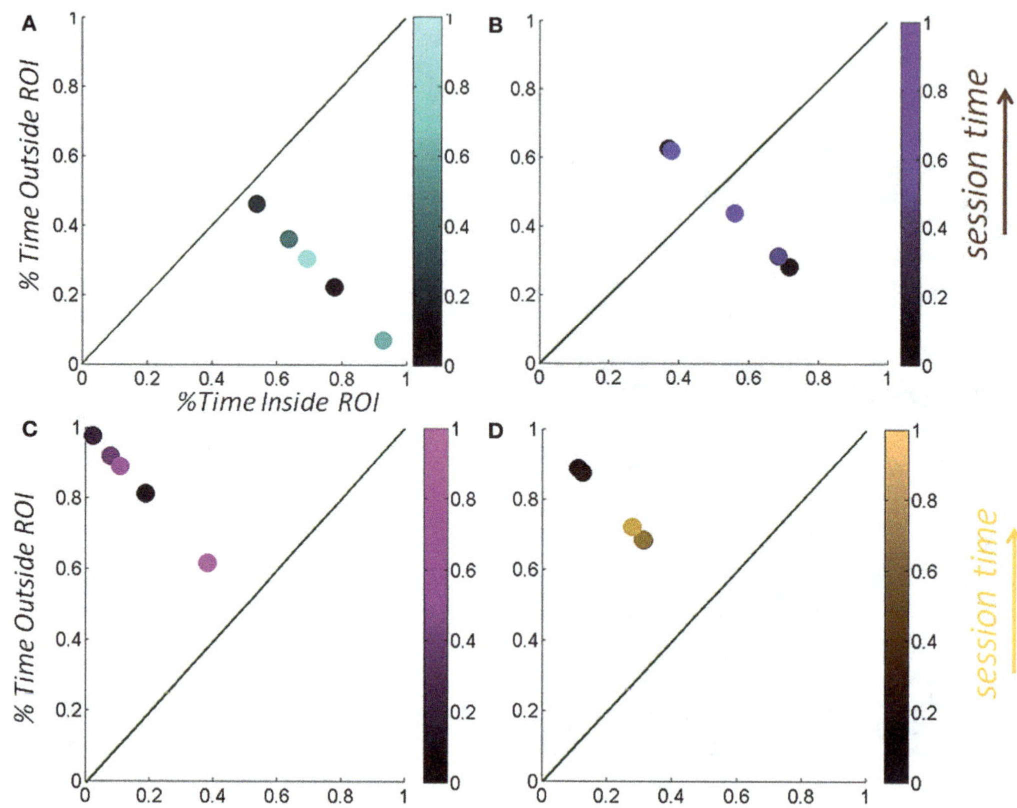

FIGURE 10 | Temporal progression of the validation metric as a function of session time-length. (A,B) Quantification of the percentage of session time that the hand spent inside the vRoI (goal-contacting) vs. outside the vRoI (goal-seeking) **(C,D)** as a function of session length. Notice the progression of the bright colors toward the lower right as the recording goes on in **(C)** and **(D)**.

between the patterns of spontaneous variations and those from intended motions. **Figure 11** shows for a subset of the participants (each represented by a point) the changes in their performance across different sessions (we focus only on the participants that returned a month later) to compare their performance in terms of reliability and predictability of the estimated probability distributions.

Across all participants we obtained the worst (most unreliable and most random) and the best (most reliable and most predictable) performances. **Figures 11A,B** show the ASD and TD participants. These are the most random patterns (minimum values of the shape parameter) and the most unreliable distributions (the highest Fano factor denoting the largest dispersion given by the variance to the mean ratio). Notice that in both cases the distinction between the stochastic signatures of the random motions exploring outside the vRoI and those from the ones homing into the vRoI is larger in TD than ASD, but in both cases the slopes do tilt. In the best performance cases (**Figures 11C,D**) the slopes of the IN and OUT vRoI scatters begin to separate. This separation is more evident in TD participants. The difference in slope tilt shows a faster rate of change in the overall progression of the group towards the discrimination between variability patterns that come from spontaneous random and goal-seeking movements OUT vRoI, as well as patterns from the intentional goal-contacting movements IN vRoI. The former include random motions whereas the latter include very deliberate motions (as in the example of the child in **Figure 9** lower panel, actually holding the hand IN vRoI to continuously play the media).

SBV SERVES AS A PROXY TO INDUCE AND SHARPEN IBV

Across all subjects the changes in the patterns of SBV associated with random motions in peripersonal space searching outside the vRoI supported the gains in predictability outside the vRoI. They were associated as well with changes in the patterns of intended behavioral variability (IBV) that the children acquired as they repeatedly aimed to the IN vRoI; and as they eventually made repeated contact with the goal, until they continuously sustained the hand at the goal. The motor variability associated with the spontaneous search movements (both random and goal-seeking) also accelerated implicit learning of secondary goals and their shifts in goal priority. These included: (1) shifting from crossing the vRoI in order to trigger the media ON; (2) shifting to actually holding the hand inside the vRoI so as to play the media continuously. As the patterns of SBV became more predictive so did the patterns of IBV. The latter variability was more directly associated with the achievement of the self-discovered goals. **Table A4** lists for all subjects the Fano Factor and the change in predictability for both the SBV and the IBV linked respectively to the initially random and the acquired goal-directed motions.

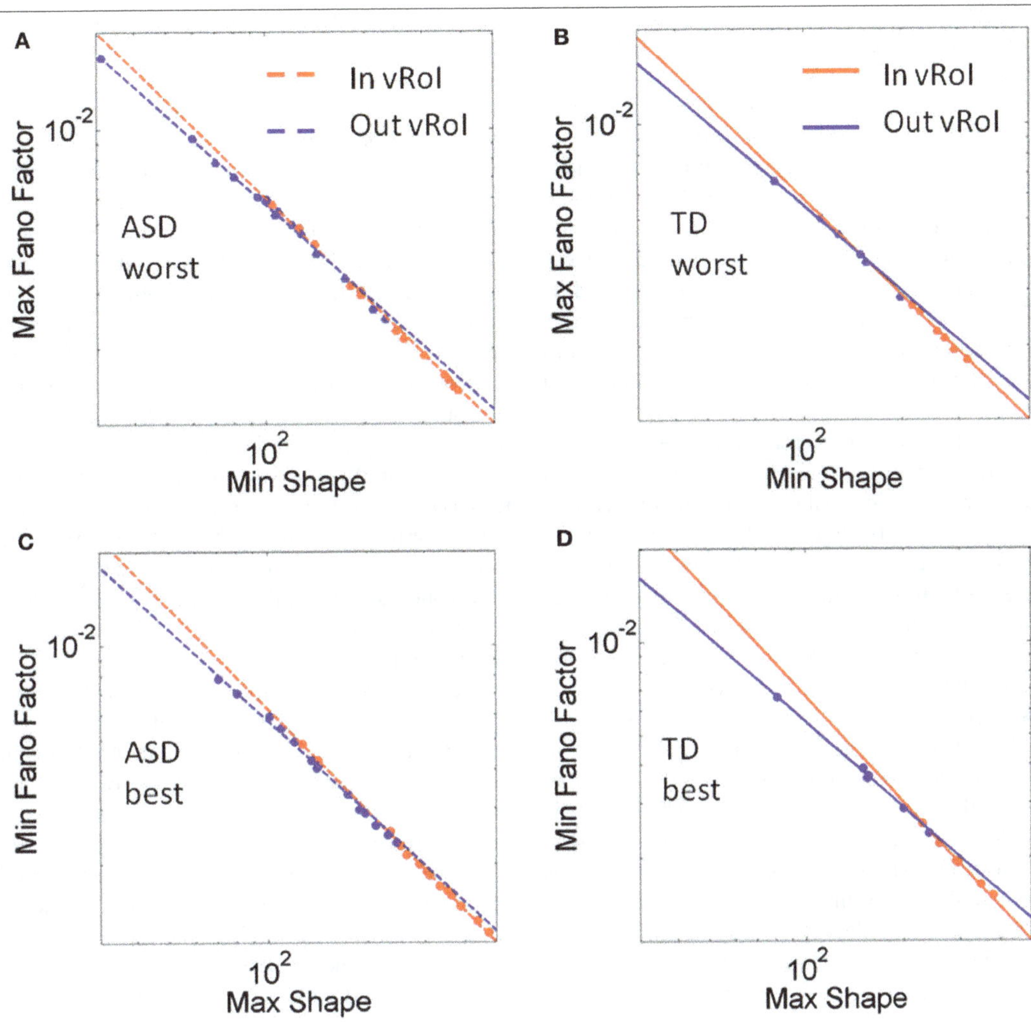

FIGURE 11 | Lack of differentiation between randomly searching motions and goal-directed motions in ASD. (A,B) Worst performance of ASD and TD participants given by their highest Fano Factor values; lowest shape parameter values and poorest distinction between IN and OUT vRoI patterns (i.e., poor separation of the slopes). **(C,D)** Best performance in ASD and TD participants given by lower values of the Fano Factor, higher values of the shape parameter and larger separation of the slopes of the power relation (**Table A4** lists the values of the power fit.)

CONCLUSIONS AND FUTURE STEPS

This work introduces a new concept that combines the notion of co-adapting in closed feedback loops the statistics of the real-time hand motions of the child and the statistics of the states of external stimuli. From these settings, with minimal to no instructions the child self-discovered the implicit goals of a task and naturally learned how to prioritize them in order to maximize the reward of the task. We were able to quantify in real time, with precise statistical indexes, the levels of predictability and reliability of their movements as they transitioned from random, to exploratory, to goal-seeking, and goal-contacting motions until they turned into intended anticipatory behavior.

We quantified the transitions from goal-directness to intentionality when the children deliberately held their hand in the vRoI in order to continuously play the media. This progression towards connecting the child's actions and intentions occurred in a matter of seconds within one session. The transient shifts in stochastic patterns of one session were retained weeks later and even improved without practicing the task during the time period between visits. The children independently drove the flow of the experimental intervention as the real-time feedback from their movements helped them self-discover cause and effect between the statistics of their hand motions and those of the media states. The child's self-discovery of such relations unlocked the volitional control of his/her actions and helped them modulate the position and orientation of the hand in space so as to sustain the media playing to reliably maximize this rewarding outcome.

This closed loop concept is rooted in the basic Brain Machine (Computer) Interface paradigms, (BMI or BCI; Vidal, 1973). The novelty in our approach is that instead of tracking/adapting a central neural signal to control an external device; the present experimental intervention co-adapts the real time statistical signals recorded from the peripheral physical micro-movements of the body with those statistical patterns reflecting the state of the external media. The methods use both statistics (externally and internally driven) as feedback signals to modify the stochastic patterns of the child's behavior. In this regard the statistical patterns from the periphery (the limbs movements) are continuously feeding back into the central centers of the brain via afferent channels. This continuous flow of re-afferent peripheral information harnessed from the motor behavior was systematically used here as a proxy to evoke better modulation of the central control of their motor patterns. The child learned to better regulate and eventually anticipate centrally sent efferent motor signals according to the patterns of peripheral hand movement variability, which we could read out in real time. These patterns transformed from random and noisy to predictable and reliable in a matter of minutes.

Under these settings the non-verbal children with ASD became engaged in the task, improved the autonomy over their limb-hand linkage and self-discovered the implicit goals and the hidden priorities that the experimenter defined. All children resolved the very problem that they self-discovered. In tandem they shifted the stochastic signatures of their hand micro-motions from random, noisy, and restricted to predictive and reliable with higher explorative bandwidth. Moreover, these positive gains were retained over time despite no training during the intermediate weeks.

We used a new SPBA (Torres and Jose, 2012). This new platform permits the real-time objective dynamic tracking of the non-stationary statistical features of the continuous flow of natural behaviors. We can thus during a session, detect shifts in their stochastic trajectories as a function of preferred forms of sensory guidance, context, etc. The term "preferred" in this case is revealed by the maximal shift toward the formation of a motor expectation (predictive and reliable). That maximal shift tells the forms of sensory guidance, context, etc. causing maximal rates of change in the stochastic toward the desirable statistical regimes.

The combination of this new experimental paradigm concept (encouraging spontaneous self-discovery of the goals) with the SPBA enables the automatic assessment of the continuous flow of natural behaviors. It also enables the discovery and real-time tracking of exploratory patterns in the children. These patterns in the present settings evolved from random motions to deliberate trial-and-error, then to goal-directed motions and finally to intentional actions. Importantly we were able to automatically select the media type that most likely accelerated this learning process, based on this real-time automatic tracking.

All the children with ASD had goal-directed behaviors, a fact that is currently used by behavioral approaches reinforcing such behaviors through commands and explicit goal-directed instructions. Such therapeutic regimes have provided a working platform for early interventions and treatments. In some cases the child visibly changes and can be mainstreamed into public or private schools hosting TD peers. Without a doubt behavioral therapies are very important. Whether relaxed (music therapy, horse therapy, dancing therapy, etc.) or structured (speech therapy, occupational therapy, physical therapy, Applied Behavioral Analyses, rapid prompting methods, etc.), these therapies, each one in its own right, have played and are bound to continue playing a critical role in the treatments of some autism type and in general research. Nonetheless, two aspects have been lacking in all methods: objective quantification and assessment of spontaneous aspects of the behavior, occurring largely beneath awareness. Furthermore, their reliance on explicit instructions when the individual with ASD—particularly the non-verbal individual—may not be able to follow instructions on command; their reliance on stimuli that is inferred by the clinician to be the best for the child without methods for blind validation; their general reliance on observation and hand-written scores and their overall subjective tracking methods call for a dramatic change in traditional therapeutic regimes. With the advent of current computational technological advances and algorithms these therapies can do better. They already have in place the infrastructure necessary to provide the means to revolutionize the ways in which ASD is treated and tracked over time. But they need major changes for a truly optimal and effectively reproducible outcome that could potentially uncover universal principles invariably leading to success in ASD interventions. The need for objective, automatic, computerized methods has been imminent for quite some time now. Such methods would provide "the neutral outsider" to anyone's agenda and biases, and would help reconcile senseless controversies in autism exclusively based on opinion and observations.

Our results show improvements with retention over time. They call for a major transformation in the philosophy of the current therapeutic interventions in ASD and in the rigor and objectivity with which the outcome of such methods are currently assessed. The methods presented in this report provide a precise prescription to achieve positive changes toward anticipatory behaviors. The results also invite the field to shift from being exclusively command/instruction driven to allow the person with ASD to spontaneously explore and self-discover the purpose(s) of a given task whenever possible.

Every individual in our study, independent of the degree of verbal capabilities and reported IQ score, was capable of performing this implicitly defined task with minimal to no instruction. By engaging their sensory motor systems and implicitly driving the child with the external input we were able to close the corrupted feedback loops and sensory-substitute the noisy-random-restricted peripheral limb's motions (which are a form of continuous kinesthetic feedback) with the external media of their liking. In this augmented physical reality setting, as the children embodied the statistics of the external media states, they self-discovered cause and effect relations. This self-realization prompted predictive statistical regimes in the media states that helped reinforce the volitional control over their own motor actions in closed loop with the media.

The children with ASD in this study developed more reliable, anticipatory motor statistics that were retained and even improved weeks later even without practice. More importantly we could backtrack exactly which media type was the most effective in the acquisition of precise indexes of reliability and predictability and reconstruct for each child the path of least resistance during this experimental intervention: the path with the fastest rate-of-change toward anticipatory behavior. We could do so for both intentional segments of their behavior and for co-existing spontaneous segments as well. The results reinforce the notion that beneath our awareness other aspects of our behaviors are co-occurring with the deliberate aspects and revealing fundamental information about the learning process. Under the presently proposed concept we can automatically and objectively register and dynamically track such implicit changes in parallel with the changes in deliberate control (Torres, 2011, 2012, 2013; Torres et al., 2013).

We have discovered here a way to (1) engage individuals with autism in spontaneous exploration; (2) modulate the peripheral motor output as a function of external stimuli statistics; (3) extract the form of sensory guidance that most likely accelerates shifts toward predictive and reliable statistical regimes of motor behavior; (4) make the gains long-term rather than transient; (5) automatically backtrack the learning trajectories of deliberate and spontaneous aspects of the behavior as well as their precise rates of change—unique to each child. All of it could be done in real time and checked again longitudinally in a novel way where the child, rather than the therapist/researcher, was the leading party. All throughout the session, the researcher merely intervened to gently steer the child's self-discovery process. This is in stark contrast with the therapist/researcher assuming the leading role. The latter is routinely done in current approaches to ASD treatments and research. In this regard, the variability from the spontaneous segments of the behavior played a fundamental role in the self-discovery process that the children underwent.

The spontaneous motor variability patterns from the periphery, which are currently not tracked in traditional behavioral interventions, turned out to be critical in order to evoke and sustain centrally driven intentionality and autonomous control in the actions of these non-verbal children with ASD. Here we pose the question to the field of whether the sensory feedback from peripherally driven changes could systematically impact the development of central centers of the brain. We further ask whether in ASD the levels of gain-retention would be better and more effective in some children when the interventions were based on spontaneous self-discovery rather than exclusively based on explicit commands.

We propose that sub-cortically based and peripherally based anticipatory control of movement may typically develop along different time scales than anticipatory control from the neocortex. It is known that philogenetically there is an order of appearance in the development of such structures that evolution has imposed (Porges, 2003). Furthermore, recent neuromagnetic developmental studies on motor anticipation during button presses have revealed that between the 4 and 6 years of age TD children do not yet have the patterns of anticipatory motor control that they later on develop by 12 years of age (Gaetz et al., 2010). In contrast we have recently found that in TD children the statistical signatures of anticipatory motor control patterns from the peripheral limbs are already in place after 4 years of age (Torres et al., 2013). Future research to address these issues during typical development is warranted in our lab: (1) whether there is an order of appearance for statistically anticipatory motor control, for example, starting at the peripheral synapses, following at the sub-cortical structures, and later appearing in the neocortex; (2) whether peripheral feedback can be used to reshape central structures during development; (3) whether spontaneous self-discovery evokes, sustains, and modulates intentional control. Finally we plan to investigate how anticipatory motor control evolves in ASD upon an early developmental glitch that may fundamentally alter the order of systemic maturation and result in a very different form of adaptive cognition, one which we cannot at present access or even know how to begin defining.

This new conceptual paradigm and statistical platform are simple and easy to use. They go well with current computational technological advancements and complement in non-trivial ways the present approaches to autism research and treatments. These methods are inclusive of the self-discovery abilities and sensory strengths of the individual with ASD. We invite others to try them out and unleash the potential of all the children according to the sensory-motor capabilities and predispositions that they already have. As Esther Thelen taught us in her seminal work (Thelen and Smith, 1994), p. 305, "*Development does not happen because internal maturation processes tell the system how to develop. Rather, development happens through and because of the activity of the system itself.*"

ACKNOWLEDGMENTS

We thank all the children and the parents who participated in the study. We thank Dr. Robert W. Isenhower for data collection. We thank the personnel from the Douglass Developmental Disability Center at Rutgers University for clinical evaluations and help; all the personnel from the Christian Sarkine Autism Treatment Center at the Indiana University Medical School at Indianapolis for clinical records and support throughout the study. This work was supported by NSF Cyber Enabled Discovery and Innovation Type I (Idea) grant # 0941587 "A novel quantitative framework to study lack of social interactions in Autism Spectrum Disorders" to Elizabeth B. Torres and Dimitris N. Metaxas.

REFERENCES

Bernstein, N. (1967). *The Co-ordination and Regulation of Movements.* Oxford: Oxford Press.

Bhat, A. N., and Galloway, J. C. (2006). Toy-oriented changes during early arm movements: hand kinematics. *Infant Behav. Dev.* 29, 358–372. doi: 10.1016/j.infbeh.2006.01.005

Bhat, A. N., and Galloway, J. C. (2007). Toy-oriented changes in early arm movements III: constraints on joint kinematics. *Infant Behav. Dev.* 30, 515–522. doi: 10.1016/j.infbeh.2006.12.007

Bhat, A. N., Lee, H. M., and Galloway, J. C. (2007). Toy-oriented changes in early arm movements II–joint kinematics. *Infant Behav. Dev.* 30, 307–324. doi: 10.1016/j.infbeh.2006.10.007

Black, A. H., Gilbert, R. M., and Millenson, J. R. (1972). *Reinforcement; Behavioral Analyses.* New York, NY: Academic Press.

Bonnel, A., McAdams, S., Smith, B., Berthiaume, C., Bertone, A., Ciocca, V., et al. (2010). Enhanced pure-tone pitch discrimination among persons with autism but not Asperger syndrome. *Neuropsychologia* 48, 2465–2475. doi: 10.1016/j.neuropsychologia.2010.04.020

Caron, M. J., Mottron, L., Rainville, C., and Chouinard, S. (2004). Do high functioning persons with autism present superior spatial abilities? *Neuropsychologia* 42, 467–481. doi: 10.1016/j.neuropsychologia.2003.08.015

Cole, J. (1995). *Pride and a Daily Marathon.* Cambridge, MA: MIT Press.

Cooper, J. O., Heron, T. E., and Heward, W. L. (1987). *Applied Behavior Analysis.* Columbus: Merrill Publishing Company.

De Volder, A. G., Catalan-Ahumada, M., Robert, A., Bol, A., Labar, D., Coppens, A., et al. (1999). Changes in occipital cortex activity in early blind humans using a sensory substitution device. *Brain Res.* 826, 128–134.

Dusing, S. C., and Harbourne, R. T. (2010). Variability in postural control during infancy: implications for development, assessment, and intervention. *Phys. Ther.* 90, 1838–1849. doi: 10.2522/ptj.2010033

Fano, U. (1947). Ionization yield of radiations. II. The fluctuations of the number of ions. *Phys. Rev.* 72:26. doi: 10.1103/PhysRev.72.26

Fetters, L. (2010). Perspective on variability in the development of human action. *Phys. Ther.* 90, 1860–1867. doi: 10.2522/ptj.2010090

Fournier, K. A., Hass, C. J., Naik, S. K., Lodha, N., and Cauraugh, J. H. (2010a). Motor coordination in autism spectrum disorders: a synthesis and meta-analysis. *J. Autism Dev. Disord.* 40, 1227–1240. doi: 10.1007/s10803-010-0981-3

Fournier, K. A., Kimberg, C. I., Radonovich, K. J., Tillman, M. D., Chow, J. W., Lewis, M. H., et al. (2010b). Decreased static and dynamic postural control in children with autism spectrum disorders. *Gait Posture* 32, 6–9. doi: 10.1016/j.gaitpost.2010.02.007

Gaetz, W., MacDonald, M., Cheyne, D., and Snead, O. C. (2010). Neuromagnetic imaging of movement-related cortical oscillations in children and adults: age predicts post-movement beta rebound. *Neuroimage* 51, 792–807. doi: 10.1016/j.neuroimage.2010.01.077

Gidley Larson, J. C., Bastian, A. J., Donchin, O., Shadmehr, R., and Mostofsky, S. H. (2008). Acquisition of internal models of motor tasks in children with autism. *Brain* 131, 2894–2903. doi: 10.1093/brain/awn226

Goddard, P., Goddard, D., and Cujec, C. (2012). *I Am Intelligent: From Heartbreak to Healing–A Mother and Daughter's Journey through Autism.* Guilford, CT: Globe Pequot Press.

Gowen, E., Stanley, J., and Miall, R. C. (2008). Movement interference in autism-spectrum disorder. *Neuropsychologia* 46, 1060–1068. doi: 10.1016/j.neuropsychologia.2007.11.004

Hadders-Algra, M. (2010). Variation and variability: key words in human motor development. *Phys. Ther.* 90, 1823–1837. doi: 10.2522/ptj.20100006

Haswell, C. C., Izawa, J., Dowell, L. R., Mostofsky, S. H., and Shadmehr, R. (2009). Representation of internal models of action in the autistic brain. *Nat. Neurosci.* 12, 970–972. doi 10.1038/nn.2356

Hausdorff, J. M., Zemany, L., Peng, C., and Goldberger, A. L. (1999). Maturation of gait dynamics: stride-to-stride variability and its temporal organization in children. *J. Appl. Physiol.* 86, 1040–1047.

Heathcock, J. C., Bhat, A. N., Lobo, M. A., and Galloway, J. C. (2005). The relative kicking frequency of infants born full-term and preterm during learning and short-term and long-term memory periods of the mobile paradigm. *Phys. Ther.* 85, 8–18.

Helders, P. (2010). Variability in childhood development. *Phys. Ther.* 90, 1708–1709. doi: 10.2522/ptj.2010.90.12.1708

Izawa, J., Pekny, S. E., Marko, M. K., Haswell, C. C., Shadmehr, R., and Mostofsky, S. H. (2012). Motor learning relies on integrated sensory inputs in ADHD, but over-selectively on proprioception in autism spectrum conditions. *Autism Res.* 5, 124–136. doi: 10.1002/aur.1222

Jansiewicz, E. M., Goldberg, M. C., Newschaffer, C. J., Denckla, M. B., Landa, R., and Mostofsky, S. H. (2006). Motor signs distinguish children with high functioning autism and Asperger's syndrome from controls. *J. Autism Dev. Disord.* 36, 613–621. doi: 10.1007/s10803-006-0109-y

Jones, V., and Prior, M. (1985). Motor imitation abilities and neurological signs in autistic children. *J. Autism Dev. Disord.* 15, 37–46. doi: 10.1007/BF01837897

Kuipers, J. B. (1999). *Quaternions and Rotation Sequences: A Primer with Applications to Orbits, Aerospace, and Virtual Reality.* Princeton, NJ: Princeton University Press.

Lee, H. M., Bhat, A., Scholz, J. P., and Galloway, J. C. (2008). Toy-oriented changes during early arm movements IV: shoulder-elbow coordination. *Infant Behav. Dev.* 31, 447–469. doi: 10.1016/j.infbeh.2007.12.018

Levy-Tzedek, S., Novick, I., Arbel, R., Abboud, S., Maidenbaum, S., Vaadia, E., et al. (2012). Cross-sensory transfer of sensory-motor information: visuomotor learning affects performance on an audiomotor task, using sensory-substitution. *Sci. Rep.* 2:949. doi: 10.1038/srep00949

Limpert, E., and Stahel, W. A. (2011). Problems with using the normal distribution–and ways to improve quality and efficiency of data analysis. *PLoS ONE* 6:e21403. doi: 10.1371/journal.pone.0021403

Limpert, E., Stahel, W. A., and Abbt, M. (2001). Log-normal distributions across the sciences: keys and clues. *Bioscience* 51, 341–352.

Lleonart, J., Salat, J., and Torres, G. J. (2000). Removing allometric effects of body size in morphological analysis. *J. Theor. Biol.* 205, 85–93. doi: 10.1006/jtbi.2000.2043

Minshew, N. J., Sung, K., Jones, B. L., and Furman, J. M. (2004). Underdevelopment of the postural control system in autism. *Neurology* 63, 2056–2061. doi: 10.1212/01.WNL.0000145771.98657.62

Mosimann, J. E. (1970). Size allometry: size and shape variables with characterizations of the lognormal and generalized gamma distributions. *J. Am. Stat. Assoc.* 65, 930–945. doi: 10.1080/01621459.1970.10481136

Mostofsky, S. H., Dubey, P., Jerath, V. K., Jansiewicz, E. M., Goldberg, M. C., and Denckla, M. B. (2006). Developmental dyspraxia is not limited to imitation in children with autism spectrum disorders. *J. Int. Neuropsychol. Soc.* 12, 314–326. doi: 10.1017/S1355617706060437

Mottron, L., and Belleville, S. (1993). A study of perceptual analysis in a high-level autistic subject with exceptional graphic abilities. *Brain Cogn.* 23, 279–309. doi: 10.1006/brcg.1993.1060

Mottron, L., and Belleville, S. (1995). Perspective production in a savant autistic draughtsman. *Psychol. Med.* 25, 639–648. doi: 10.1017/S0033291700033547

Mottron, L., Belleville, S., Stip, E., and Morasse, K. (1998). Atypical memory performance in an autistic savant. *Memory* 6, 593–607. doi: 10.1080/741943372

Mottron, L., Burack, J. A., Stauder, J. E., and Robaey, P. (1999). Perceptual processing among high-functioning persons with autism. *J. Child Psychol. Psychiatry* 40, 203–211. doi: 10.1111/1469-7610.00433

Mottron, L., Peretz, I., and Menard, E. (2000). Local and global processing of music in high-functioning persons with autism: beyond central coherence? *J. Child Psychol. Psychiatry* 41, 1057–1065. doi: 10.1111/1469-7610.00693

Noterdaeme, M., Mildenberger, K., Minow, F., and Amorosa, H. (2002). Evaluation of neuromotor deficits in children with autism and children with a specific speech and language disorder. *Eur. Child Adolesc. Psychiatry* 11, 219–225. doi: 10.1007/s00787-002-0285-z

Porges, S. W. (2003). The polyvagal theory: phylogenetic contributions to social behavior. *Physiol. Behav.* 79, 503–513. doi: 10.1016/S0031-9384(03)00156-2

Rinehart, N. J., Bradshaw, J. L., Brereton, A. V., and Tonge, B. J. (2001). Movement preparation in high-functioning autism and Asperger disorder: a serial choice reaction time task involving motor reprogramming. *J. Autism Dev. Disord.* 31, 79–88. doi: 10.1023/A:1005617831035

Riso, R. R. (1999). Strategies for providing upper extremity amputees with tactile and hand position feedback–moving closer to the bionic arm. *Technol. Health Care* 7, 401–409.

Rogers, S. J., Bennetto, L., McEvoy, R., and Pennington, B. F. (1996). Imitation and pantomime in high-functioning adolescents with autism spectrum disorders. *Child Dev.* 67, 2060–2073. doi: 10.2307/1131609

Rovee-Collier, C. (1989). "The 'memory system' of prelinguistic infants," in *The Development and Neural Bases of Higher Cognitive Functions*, ed A. Diamond (New York, NY: Annals of the New York Academy of Sciences), 517–536.

Samson, F., Hyde, K. L., Bertone, A., Soulieres, I., Mendrek, A., Ahad, P., et al. (2011). Atypical processing of auditory temporal complexity in autistics. *Neuropsychologia* 49, 546–555. doi: 10.1016/j.neuropsychologia.2010.12.033

Samson, F., Mottron, L., Soulieres, I., and Zeffiro, T. A. (2012). Enhanced visual functioning in autism: an ALE meta-analysis. *Hum. Brain Mapp.* 33, 1553–1581. doi: 10.1002/hbm.21307

Smith, L. (2006). Movement matters: the contributions of esther thelen. *Biol. Theor.* 1, 87–89.

Soulieres, I., Dawson, M., Samson, F., Barbeau, E. B., Sahyoun, C. P., Strangman, G. E., et al. (2009). Enhanced visual processing contributes to matrix reasoning in autism. *Hum. Brain Mapp.* 30, 4082–4107. doi: 10.1002/hbm.20831

Stergiou, N., Buzzi, U., Kurz, M., and Heidel, J. (2004). *Non-Linear Tools in Human Movement.* Champaign, IL: Human Kinetics Publishers.

Thelen, E. (1994). Three-month-old infants can learn task-specific patterns of interlimb coordination. *Psychol. Sci.* 5, 280–285. doi: 10.1111/j.1467-9280.1994.tb00626.x

Thelen, E., Corbetta, D., and Spencer, J. P. (1996). Development of reaching during the first year: role of movement speed. *J. Exp. Psychol. Hum. Percept. Perform.* 22, 1059–1076. doi: 10.1037/0096-1523.22.5.1059

Thelen, E., Corbetta, D., Kamm, K., Spencer, J. P., Schneider, K., and Zernicke, R. F. (1993). The transition to reaching: mapping intention and intrinsic dynamics. *Child Dev.* 64, 1058–1098. doi: 10.2307/1131327

Thelen, E., and Fisher, D. M. (1983a). From spontaneous to instrumental behavior: kinematic analysis of movement changes during very early learning. *Child Dev.* 54, 129–140. doi: 10.2307/1129869

Thelen, E., and Fisher, D. M. (1983b). The organization of spontaneous leg movements in newborn infants. *J. Mot. Behav.* 15, 353–377.

Thelen, E., and Smith, L. B. (1994). *A Dynamic Systems Approach to the Development of Cognition and Action.* Cambridge, MA: MIT Press.

Todorov, E. (2005). Stochastic optimal control and estimation methods adapted to the noise characteristics of the sensorimotor system. *Neural Comput.* 17, 1084–1108. doi: 10.1162/089976605 3491887

Todorov, E. (2009). Efficient computation of optimal actions. *Proc. Natl. Acad. Sci. U.S.A.* 106, 11478–11483. doi: 10.1073/pnas. 0710743106

Torres, E. B. (2011). Two classes of movements in motor control. *Exp. Brain Res.* 215, 269–283. doi: 10.1007/s00221-011-2892-8

Torres, E. B. (2012). Atypical signatures of motor variability found in an individual with ASD. *Neurocase* 1, 1–16. doi: 10.1080/13554794.2011.654224

Torres, E. B. (2013). Signatures of movement variability anticipate hand speed according to levels of intent. *Behav. Brain Funct.* 9:10. doi: 10.1186/1744-9081-9-10

Torres, E. B., and Jose, J. V. (2012). *Novel Diagnostic Tool to Quantify Signatures of Movement in Subjects with Neurobiological Disorders, Autism and Autism Spectrum Disorders.* New Brunswick, NJ: US patent application.

Torres, E. B., Brincker, M., Isenhower, R. W., Yanovich, P., Stigler, K. A., Nurnberger, J. I., et al. (2013). Autism: the micro-movement perspective. *Front. Integr. Neurosci.* 7:32. doi: 10.3389/fnint.2013.00032

Torres, E. B., Heilman, K. M., and Poizner, H. (2011). Impaired endogenously evoked automated reaching in Parkinson's disease. *J. Neurosci.* 31, 17848–17863. doi: 10.1523/JNEUROSCI.1150-11.2011

Torres, E. B., Raymer, A., Gonzalez Rothi, L. J., Heilman, K. M., and Poizner, H. (2010). Sensory-spatial transformations in the left posterior parietal cortex may contribute to reach timing. *J. Neurophysiol.* 104, 2375–2388. doi: 10.1152/jn.00089.2010

Torres, E. B., and Zipser, D. (2002). Reaching to grasp with a multi-jointed arm. I. Computational model. *J. Neurophysiol.* 88, 2355–2367. doi: 10.1152/jn. 00030.2002

Torres, E. B., and Zipser, D. (2004). Simultaneous control of hand displacements and rotations in orientation-matching experiments. *J. Appl. Physiol.* 96, 1978–1987. doi: 10.1152/japplphysiol.00872.2003

van der Meer, A. L., van der Weel, F. R., and Lee, D. N. (1995). The functional significance of arm movements in neonates. *Science* 267, 693–695. doi: 10.1126/science.7839147

van Wermeskerken, M., van der Kamp, J., Te Velde, A. F., Valero-Garcia, A. V., Hoozemans, M. J., and Savelsbergh, G. J. (2011). Anticipatory reaching of seven- to eleven-month-old infants in occlusion situations. *Infant Behav. Dev.* 34, 45–54. doi: 10.1016/j.infbeh.2010.09.005

Veraart, C., Cremieux, J., and Wanet-Defalque, M. C. (1992). Use of an ultrasonic echolocation prosthesis by early visually deprived cats. *Behav. Neurosci.*106, 203–216. doi: 10.1037/0735-7044.106.1.203

Vereijken, B. (2010). The complexity of childhood development: variability in perspective. *Phys. Ther.* 90, 1850–1859. doi: 10.2522/ptj.20100019

Vidal, J. J. (1973). Toward direct brain-computer communication. *Annu. Rev. Biophys. Bioeng.* 2, 157–180. doi: 10.1146/annurev. bb.02.060173.001105

Von Hofsten, C. (1982). Eye-hand coordination in the newborn. *Dev. Psychol.* 18, 450–461. doi: 10.1037/0012-1649.18.3.450

Von Hofsten, C. (2004). An action perspective on motor development. *Trends Cogn. Sci.* 8, 266–272. doi: 10.1016/j.tics.2004.04.002

Williams, J. H., Whiten, A., Suddendorf, T., and Perrett, D. I. (2001). Imitation, mirror neurons and autism. *Neurosci. Biobehav. Rev.* 25, 287–295. doi: 10.1016/S0149-7634(01)00014-8

Yanovich, P., Isenhower, R. W., Sage, J., and Torres, E. B. (in press). Spatial-orientation priming impedes rather than facilitates the spontaneous control of hand-retraction speeds in patients with Parkinson's disease. *PLoS ONE.*

Conflict of Interest Statement: The authors declare that the research was conducted in the absence of any commercial or financial relationships that could be construed as a potential conflict of interest.

8

Rhythm and timing in autism: learning to dance

Pat Amos*

Training and Private Consultation, Ardmore, PA, USA

Edited by:
Anne M. Donnellan, University of Wisconsin-Madison, University of San Diego, USA

Reviewed by:
Elizabeth B. Torres, Rutgers University, USA
Trevor McDonald, Education Associates Inc., USA

****Correspondence:***
Pat Amos, 635 Ardmore Avenue, Ardmore, PA 19003-1831, USA.
e-mail: pat.amos@verizon.net

In recent years, a significant body of research has focused on challenges to neural connectivity as a key to understanding autism. In contrast to attempts to identify a single static, primarily brain-based deficit, children and adults diagnosed with autism are increasingly perceived as out of sync with their internal and external environments in dynamic ways that must also involve operations of the peripheral nervous systems. The noisiness that seems to occur in both directions of neural flow may help explain challenges to movement and sensing, and ultimately to entrainment with circadian rhythms and social interactions across the autism spectrum, profound differences in the rhythm and timing of movement have been tracked to infancy. Difficulties with self-synchrony inhibit praxis, and can disrupt the "dance of relationship" through which caregiver and child build meaning. Different sensory aspects of a situation may fail to match up; ultimately, intentions and actions themselves may be uncoupled. This uncoupling may help explain the expressions of alienation from the actions of one's body which recur in the autobiographical autism literature. Multi-modal/cross-modal coordination of different types of sensory information into coherent events may be difficult to achieve because amodal properties (e.g., rhythm and tempo) that help unite perceptions are unreliable. One question posed to the connectivity research concerns the role of rhythm and timing in this operation, and whether these can be mobilized to reduce overload and enhance performance. A case is made for developmental research addressing how people with autism actively explore and make sense of their environments. The parent/author recommends investigating approaches such as scaffolding interactions via rhythm, following the person's lead, slowing the pace, discriminating between intentional communication and "stray" motor patterns, and organizing information through one sensory mode at a time.

Keywords: autism, cross-modal perception, movement, rhythm, sensory perception, synchrony, timing

"...*movement must itself be considered a perceptual system.*"
(Thelen and Smith, 1994, p. 193; emphasis in original)

Everyday descriptions of social interaction are rich in figures of speech that derive from rhythm and timing in general, and dance or music in particular. If we are in love, we may describe the feeling as "two hearts beating as one," being "swept off our feet," feeling "in the groove," or experiencing "good vibes." We joke that "it takes two to tango," and may patronize a well-known online dating site that sums up its promise as "harmony." Encountering socially maladroit individuals, we describe them as having two left feet, being out of step, being off beat, or stepping on our toes. "Timing," we declare, "is everything."

Yet we have the capacity to empathize with people who move differently, and have popularized many affirmations based on Thoreau's advice to those who hear "a different drummer." Researchers and therapists seem drawn to these images as well, characterizing developmentally vital interactions between parent and child as a dance of relationship and writing about how to support children who fall out of synch in that dance (Fogel, 1993; Maurer, 1994, 1996; Stern, 2000; Wieder and Greenspan, 2005; Trevarthen, 2011). Is it possible that the choice of these terms is far more than a literary flourish, embodying something intuitive and essential about how human beings relate? Could a closer examination of what is happening when people on the autism spectrum seem to move to a different drummer encourage breakthroughs in how we partner with them, and create better vibes all around? As a parent, that would be music to my ears.

It has been my privilege to observe the development of my own children (and others with whom I have worked) at a micro level over many years, and to have emerged with skepticism about the prevailing narrative which portrays people with autism as essentially aimless, unmotivated carriers of static deficits or traits. When my children were very young, it became clear that the typical diagnostic process did not recognize the limitations of its "snapshot viewed from afar," and that the field was neither disposed nor equipped to notice the dynamic adaptations of which parents become acutely aware. In particular, I became impressed by the ways in which autism, explained in the literature as a brain-based challenge to cognition, in fact presented as deeply embodied: my children appeared to be constantly negotiating with their bodies via strategies that looked quite complicated, were very dependent on task conditions, yielded highly variable results, disintegrated in demand situations, and sometimes looked startlingly similar to the struggles with neurodegenerative conditions experienced by older family members. It surprised me that sustaining a dance of relationship could take so much concentration. When my oldest son, around age six, started to search his body for imaginary buttons, pressing them hopefully to make it function, the metaphorical light bulb turned on: we needed an approach to autism that would recognize and join him in exploring movement and perception. We still do, but are getting closer. This review will trace some converging lines of enquiry.

NERVOUS SYSTEMS AND CONNECTIVITY

The flow of information in our bodies involves two basic sets of systems: the central nervous systems or CNS (brain and spinal cord) and the peripheral nervous systems (composed of the sensory nervous system, which sends information to the CNS from the external environment and internal organs, and the motor nervous system which sends information from the CNS to muscles, glands, and organs, including the skin). As information is constantly adjusted through an ongoing stream of internal and external motion, it moves in two directional flows: from the central to the peripheral nervous systems, and from the peripheral to the central nervous systems. Challenges to bodily rhythm and timing can take a variety of forms depending on which of these flows is involved, and also on whether the "beat of a different drummer" is emerging from involuntary or automatic responses of the nervous systems (e.g., the fight or flight responses of fear, reflexes) or from a lack of voluntary control (e.g., paralysis, dyspraxia, the results of illness or disease).

Dangerous and dramatic central to peripheral disruptions of brain and body rhythm may occur when the usual periodicities of brain waves suddenly veer into chaotic states, resulting in the seizures experienced by many people with autism. Although the comorbidity rate is not well-defined, the Autism Society (2012) estimates that somewhere between 11 to 39% of people with autism develop seizures; published research cites rates as high as 40% (Gabis et al., 2005). In comparison, the prevalence rate for active epilepsy in the general population is between 0.4% and 1% (World Health Organization, 2009). A recent EEG study of children with autism indicated that over 85% had abnormal brain-wave patterns, even if they did not result in overt seizures (Yasuhara, 2010). Non-convulsive seizure activity may manifest as changes in affect and behavior, including dissociative experiences and altered perceptions of body and environment.

These types of central to peripheral disruptions of bodily rhythms are relatively easy to diagnose, and have received a large share of research attention. But human lives are shaped and defined by many other kinds of rhythms, often involving the peripheral to central flow of information. Among people diagnosed with autism spectrum disorders (ASDs), difficulties with sensory modulation (often visible as hyper- or hypo-reactivity) and with voluntary motor activity (Donnellan et al., 2013), as well as unusual registration and/or expression of pain—an understudied area due to difficulties in identifying pain behavior (Nader et al., 2004)—may indicate challenges to the functioning of the afferent somatic systems, while frequent reports of unusual diet and gastrointestinal problems may indicate dysregulation of the enteric systems (Horvath and Perman, 2002). These challenges affect not only the efficiency of peripheral flows of information within the body, but the functioning of those predictably-timed cyclic flows between the natural (and, ultimately, the social) environment and peripheral nervous systems which are known as circadian rhythms.

The circadian rhythms give us daily cycles of sleep and wakefulness, hunger, body temperature, and brain waves, as well as hormonal peaks and ebbs. Associated with these short-term natural rhythms may be fluctuating states of sensory arousal and alertness. People diagnosed with an ASD often appear to experience states that fluctuate more widely and more often, sending them out of sync with typical daily rhythms. Parents may report that their offspring experience unpredictable daily cycles including difficulty registering hunger and shortened, sporadic intervals of sleep (Malow, 2004; Hu et al., 2009; Glickman, 2010). One study found sleep disturbances among 52% of subjects with autism vs. 7% of their typically developing siblings (Horvath and Perman, 2002). Evidence has also been found for "clock gene" anomalies in autism, which may affect sleep, memory, and timing (Nicholas et al., 2007).

Many parents and teachers of children with autism also report significant challenges to the regulation of mood and activity that appear linked to seasonal changes, such as the daylight-related Seasonal Affective Disorder with its apt acronym of SAD. In this case we might argue that an overall pattern of behavior *does* predictably track a biological temporal rhythm; unfortunately, unless one is a hibernating mammal it represents an adaptation to the wrong situation at the wrong time-scale; as such it can interfere with reception of the shorter-term behavioral cues to which humans must attend.

Preliminary research into the effects of disruptions of circadian timing suggests that "Behavioral disturbances in ASD may arise in part from an inability of an individual's circadian oscillator to entrain to environmental and social cues" (Barnard and Nolan, 2008, para. 15). When the internal clock cannot reliably, consistently match or mirror the environmental and social rhythms of typical activity, long-term consequences may be profound. The circadian time of brain rhythms and physiological cycles is tightly entwined with developmental time, the engine of which is the time sensitive everyday experiences in which all children engage—and in which children with autism appear to engage in different ways, over different periods, using different strategies.

The "dance of relationship" by which newborn child and caregiver begin to make mutual sense of their world is understood to be based on the co-production, or entrainment, of their actions (Fogel, 1993; Stern, 2000). Clearly we need to know more about how this dance works when the different metronomes of different nervous systems do not readily fall into sync. It seems possible that all of these levels of rhythm and timing, from circadian time to developmental time, and from the real time self-synchrony of perception and movement to the real time interactional synchrony of communication and social activity, might one day be woven into a unified field theory that makes sense of the amazingly diverse ways humans move to the rhythm of time.

AUTISM RESEARCH: A MISSING PIECE?

Over the last few decades, a significant body of research has zeroed in on challenges to neural connectivity as key to understanding autism (Belmonte et al., 2004). Previous theories have been laid successively to rest, including the early suggestion that autism may be a traumatic response to cold parenting [Bettelheim, 1967; see response in Rimland (1964)]; an extreme language impairment (see Bartak et al., 1975), a single basic learning impediment such as a limited attention span, an amnesiac disorder, or an auditory processing deficit (see Minshew and Rattan, 1994); or closely correlated with intellectual disability (see Edelson, 2006). Recent interest in the supposed inability of children with autism to invoke a Theory of Mind (ToM) (Baron-Cohen et al., 1985) faltered once this multidimensional concept was deconstructed (see Rogers et al., 2007). Many researchers now argue that no such inborn mental mechanism exists, and look instead to the study of dynamic systems to understand different embodied experiences (Shanker, 2004).

The study of dynamic systems offers autism researchers a way out of the old debate between genetics and environment, the heavyweight determinisms that traditionally stood sentinel over child development studies. To the autism field they brought the dubious gifts of prognosis at the time of diagnosis, and of an aggressive form of behaviorism constructed on an engineering model. Viewed as a dynamic system, however, the development of *any* child can be seen to emerge without a top-down genetic script or one-way environmental chutes and ladders, through ongoing perceptions and actions. Knowledge itself appears as an action-based process (Thelen and Smith, 1994, p. 247). The movement perspective on autism offers evidence of an overabundance of variability in this process of assembling reliable embodiments of knowledge: the process continues, but is overloaded and precarious; the categories generated may increasingly reflect the elaboration and playing out of a different perceptual system. Instead of approaching such children as non-learners, the new research task becomes one of discovering the dynamic adaptations of their individual learning trajectories and intervening to decrease the noisiness that seems to occur in both directions of neural flow. Such research may suggest the neurological basis of a dynamic model to explain the challenges to movement and sensing, and ultimately the differences in developmental trajectories, found across the autism spectrum.

In overviews of decades of autism research, Donnellan (1999), Donnellan and Leary (1995), Donnellan et al. (2010, 2013), and Gowen and Hamilton (2012) identified the exploration of movement differences and their impact on the rhythms of daily life as crucial to a better understanding of the experiences of people on the autism spectrum. Developmental approaches to children with autism recommend "following the child's lead" sympathetically (Greenspan, 1992, 1997; Greenspan and Wieder, 1997, 2006) and emphasize the importance of the dance of relationship; occupational science, with its emphasis on fostering sensory integration and regulation, has become increasingly valued as a source of approaches for enhancing bodily synchrony and *praxis,* the ability to plan actions and engage meaningfully with the world (Williamson et al., 2000). Speech-language pathologists, providers of assistive and alternative communication supports, and various types of music therapists also emphasize the use of rhythm and timing as scaffolding to build social and communicative interactions (Schögler, 2008; Hardy and LaGasse, 2013).

The recognition of movement difficulties, however, has not necessarily led to accurate interpretations of their nature. A persistent belief is that sensory uptake at the level of the primary sensory organs must not function accurately; people with autism are sometimes described as unable to receive basic sensory information from their environment. To the contrary, a significant body of research confirms that the sensory systems function properly at their initial tasks of registering input (Minshew and Rattan, 1994), including the proprioceptive sense of limb position (Fuentes et al., 2011). It is the ability to make reliable, intentional use of this input that appears to malfunction, a finding consistent with the descriptions of self-advocates such as Nick Pentzell:

> *To have autism is like having a short in a computer. I know what I want to do, but my body gets confused and it does not correctly carry out the order my brain sends it. I take in information, but my body scrambles the output* (Young, 2011, p. 164).

For such individuals, unusual challenges and exceptional skills can exist side by side, in the same brain domains (Williams et al., 2006). Self-advocate Sue Rubin reflects:

> *It is funny how we are considered strange or different, even though our recollection of complex patterns, memory for precise detail, and overall capabilities many times exceed those of the people who are pointing or staring* (Young, 2011, p. 107).

This research does not implicate certain types of information, such as language or social interaction, as inherently too complex; rather, it suggests that something about the ways information is structured or becomes available may overwhelm a highly sensitive processing system (Williams et al., 2006). The whole then becomes less than the sum of its parts.

One question we can put to the connectivity research concerns the role of rhythm and timing in this delicate operation and, in particular, whether they can be mobilized to reduce overload and enhance performance. To respond, researchers will need to move beyond the well-documented connectivity challenges in the cortical regions that dominate current autism research, and recognize that this brain-based model remains partial because it is disembodied. The missing piece may be a consideration of connectivity challenges in the peripheral nervous systems. Replicable, testable theories about what occurs in these systems for children with ASDs have been scarce to non-existent, which may help explain the widespread bias toward envisioning autism as fully rooted in the neural processing of key cortical regions, and the disinclination to attach much significance to sensorimotor phenomena, which tend to be reflected in diagnostic protocols as secondary or optional criteria. In contrast to studying people with autism as if only central cortical structures and connections contribute to development, researchers need to look at movement itself: as sensed and organized, conscious and unconscious, volitional and non-volitional, as it plays out at different levels in the peripheral nervous systems, and as these systems interface with the CNS to develop a dynamic, self-organizing map of the body in space and time.

RHYTHM AND TIMING IN EARLY DEVELOPMENT

It may be helpful to consider how sensory input is organized in typical child development, and then bring to bear some observations of infants who were later diagnosed with autism. Newborn infants capture our attention precisely because they do not respond as "blank slates"; instead, infants quickly begin to organize responses to sensory input, charming caregivers with tightly-timed reflections of their own actions. The development of proprioception and vestibular processing involve them in learning not only how their bodies move in space, but how they move in time. The trajectory of any action involving coordinated movement, from walking through a moving crowd to jumping into a conversation, can only be projected if time is accurately weighed in the equation. Time can also be seen as *emerging* from the equation because time perception is bound up with movement; we talk about approaching "points in time," "moving through time," and events being "distant in time" because we sense that movements of the body, both external and internal, are involved in assembling a perception of time's "placement" relative to our trajectory. Like our movements, time is perceived consciously and unconsciously, deliberately and unintentionally; it both flows from bodily motion and flows back to guide its course.

We call the dual-natured, split-second calculation that guides our coordinated movements "timing" and, when it is part of a broader ability to plan and strategize, we refer to a person as having a "sense of time." Yet a sense of time is not associated with any specific sensory system; it is registered through the peripheral nervous systems as they carry motor and sensory information to and from the CNS. In the CNS, time perception is associated with a highly distributed brain system including the cerebral cortex, cerebellum, and basal ganglia—areas of the brain generally associated with autism (Bauman and Kemper, 2005). As was the case with the connectivity challenges discussed earlier, however, researchers have paid more attention to the function of the cortical regions in time perception than to the peripheral nervous systems. In assuming that the neocortex is the only source of the intelligent forces—timing, decision making, planning—driving development, much of the autism field continues to ignore the ways that intelligence is embodied and may be engaged through a dance of relationship.

Timing seems to operate as the common link that binds sensory experiences into a coherent whole. Infants move in carefully-timed synchrony with caregivers in a dance-like exchange that creates the framework for a child's first experiences of actors, actions, and things acted upon. The importance of the shared information that emerges through this engagement is profound, as child development and autism researcher Colwyn Trevarthen makes clear:

> Most impressively, an alert newborn can draw a sympathetic adult into synchronized negotiations of arbitrary action, which can develop in coming weeks and months into a mastery of the rituals and symbols of a germinal culture, long before any words are learned (Trevarthen, 2011, p. 121).

When the timing of these early experiences is "off" it can trigger a cascade of consequences for development (Trevarthen et al., 1998; Greenspan and Shanker, 2007). Many parents of infants who were later diagnosed with autism report that their baby was difficult to engage, following either a pattern of muscle tension and hyperarousal which left them difficult to sooth, or being "floppy" and difficult to arouse; babies may also oscillate between these states (Williamson et al., 2000). However, some parents recall what they felt was a typical infancy, and in most cases the early motor milestones of these babies reportedly are met on time (Centers for Disease Control and Prevention, 2010).

Even families who do not recall particular concerns in the first few months tend to start reporting them around the 12–15 month mark, when the child's preverbal communication appears to lag. As developmental experts point out, this is the time period when social development—manifested through rapid leaps in language, reciprocal interactions, and joint attention—begins to heat up. The beat gets faster, the steps more complex, and the perception of difficulty keeping up with peers is heightened (Greenspan and Shanker, 2007). Somewhere in the second or third year, it becomes obvious that the child needs support in the dance of relationship (Greenspan, 1992). But the question remains: what has been happening in the child's development before social and communication differences became pronounced, and before autism was suspected? Answering that question might lead to an understanding of the dynamics of autism, and help us discover the *kinds* of support needed. We would not need to untangle the complex etiologies of the ASDs or the origins of a particular child's autism; instead, we would need to discover how the child operates in and makes sense of the world, and how the child's experiences are creating—or not creating—a stable and reliable basis from which to extrapolate into new situations and timeframes.

Several lines of investigation may be converging on an intriguing answer to this question of child development, and may deeply implicate the rhythm and timing of sensorimotor experience. They include demonstrations that, even in the first months of life, when those first motor milestones are being met, babies on their way to an autism spectrum diagnosis are meeting them differently (Teitelbaum et al., 1998, 2004). These findings are supported by recent data from a variety of studies using different measures, which suggest that "80–90% of children with ASD show some degree of motor abnormality" (Hilton et al., 2011, p. 4), "with 95% of one sample demonstrating" some degree of sensory processing dysfunction (Tomchek and Dunn, 2007, p. 198). They are underscored by the observations and that "over 90% of children with autism had sensory abnormalities and had sensory symptoms in multiple sensory domains" (Leekam et al., 2007, p. 894), and are underscored by the observations of numerous self-advocates with ASDs.

Unfortunately, the existence of separate studies confirming motor differences and sensory differences also suggests that the lines of investigation are not converging seamlessly: in the autism literature motor differences remain isolated from sensory challenges, a situation which obscures their nature and neurological dynamics. Movement is, as Thelen and Smith insisted in their groundbreaking work on cognition and action, a perceptual system (1994, p. 193); to move is to perceive, and to perceive is to move. Yet the current generation of parents and therapists, drawing on and popularizing the bifurcated research literature, is now glossing children's motor difficulties as "clumsiness" and making a clumsy distinction between "sensory" challenges and "behavior" challenges. The exploration and dissemination of a neurologically-grounded, fully embodied and dynamic developmental model for thinking about movement needs to become a priority.

Starting in the mid-1990's, a team of researchers at the University of Florida began gathering home videos made by the parents of infants and toddlers who were later diagnosed with autism (Teitelbaum et al., 1998) and Asperger syndrome (Teitelbaum et al., 2004). In each case, researchers found differences in the ways these babies used their bodies to interact with their environments. Within the first collection of videos there appeared a number of challenges that continuing research confirmed as characteristic, among them: difficulties in self-synchronizing the body to roll over and to crawl; a lack of superimposed movements; a lack of protective reflexes; failure to exploit allied reflexes to enhance movement; the preservation of motor patterns from an earlier stage of development, as if physical development itself were occurring out of sync; and difficulty coordinating arms and head to explore objects. The researchers suggested that these differences had gone unremarked because the action *does* get performed. The story, they emphasized, is in *how* it gets performed.

Watching the subtle struggles embodied in these videos, viewers are reminded of the ways typically developing children proceed to capture their bodies' spontaneous movements in increasingly intentional and goal-directed ways (Thelen and Smith, 1994), and of the profound ways that a lack of predictable movements and reflexes would alter that dynamic, creating a developmental cascade that flows with increasing velocity toward an autism diagnosis (Maurer and Damasio, 1982). A related observation made by viewers of the video clips is that they are witnessing the unfolding of adaptive developmental *differences* rather than a display of static deficits. These children are co-adapting with their environment, determinedly brokering complex and probably exhausting deals with their bodies in order to keep moving and exploring. The video vignettes tell a very different story from the presumption of autistic indifference, and refute the conflation of movement challenges with lesser intelligence, "task avoidance," or the desire to self-injure or aggress. Witnessed at an early age, without judgmental interpretations, it is easier to confirm the words of self-advocates such as Tom Page, who states: "*My senses and body parts did not work as a unit*" (Young, 2011, p. 166).

DYSSYNCHRONY AND SUBROUTINES

These observations of early development fit well with data from a variety of fields, including neuropsychology, neurophysiology, and neuroimaging, which suggest that autism is fundamentally a "Temporo-Spatial Processing Disorder (TSPD) of multi-sensory flows":

> TSPDs include various degrees of disability in i) processing multi-sensory stimuli online, ii) associating them into meaningful and coherent patterns and iii) producing real-time sensory-motor adjustments and motor outputs (Gepner and Féron, 2009, abstract).

TSPDs, defined to include a range of conditions from attention deficit disorder and dyslexia to Parkinson's disease, reflect "disconnectivity" or "dyssynchrony" across multiple neurofunctional systems and would be expected to play out in the realm of "perceiving, imitating, understanding and producing emotional and verbal events on time, and therefore in interacting here and now with (the) human and social environment" (2009, p 1238).

These predictable expressions of connectivity challenges parallel, and may help explain, the diagnostic "autism triad" centering on impairments in communication, impairments in social interaction, and restrictive interests and repetitive behavior (American Psychiatric Association, 2000). Communication and social interaction are highly sensitive to mis-timing; an appearance of impairment may arise from processing demands the system cannot meet. Repetition or restriction of experiences may represent an actual adaptation to dyssynchrony: if you cannot slow the pace of demands, at least limit their number. Significantly, the proposed effects of TSPDs are reflected in the self-reports of people diagnosed with autism. As Tom Page recalls:

> *In the beginning of my life, I was a frightened little boy. I remember being confused most of the time. People were doing things for no reason that I could make out. I seemed to be doing things for no reason they could make out. Neither could understand each other's actions. Their mouths moved and made sounds that made little sense to me* (Young, 2011, p. 76).

Page and many others relate experiences of profound dyssynchrony, in which the different sensory aspects of a situation fail to match up coherently; ultimately, intentions and actions may themselves be uncoupled. This may occur temporarily and without warning as automatic movement "subroutines" cease to function as team players and emerge into prominence on their own. Subroutines are fixed action patterns that we all rely on, and don't notice as long as they are working in sync under the auspices of our general intentions (MacLean, 1990). We stand up "automatically" when called upon; appropriately produce a social smile; or effortlessly turn a corner as we continue to walk onward, uniting two action patterns in a superimposed movement (which children in the Teitelbaum et al. (1998) and Teitelbaum et al. (2004) videos were unable to effect). We don't have to plan these subroutines consciously because they are triggered by and subservient to the larger scheme of action in which we are involved, and that scheme in turn is coupled or entrained to social and environmental cues.

But for people with autism (and other familiar conditions, such as traumatic brain injury and Parkinson's) these fixed action patterns can take on a life of their own that may look—and feel to the person—confusing and even alien, as if they were coming from somewhere else. My own daughter, taken to task for her wandering ways when she repeatedly left her elementary school classroom, put her case succinctly: "*My brain doesn't tell my legs what to do; my legs tell my brain what to do.*" Several of my adult acquaintances with autism will unexpectedly reach out to touch objects while disavowing any interest in doing so. Nor is this phenomenon limited to the gross motor domain; for example, Sue Rubin warns others to attend to her typed communication and not necessarily to her speech, which may be unrelated (Biklen et al., 2005, pp. 92–93). Barb Rentenbach cautions, "*My facial expressions don't always match my emotions* (Young, 2011, p. 163), and indeed many people with autism are faulted for displaying the "wrong" affect, which may be interpreted by others as signifying insensitivity. Nick Pentzell, a gifted college scholar, writes candidly of disagreeing with his body's activities:

> *I tell (my body) to go to sleep, but it leaps on my bed. I tell it to want good and it goes for bad. I open the door to maturity and it slams it in my face* (Young, 2011, p.163).

Similar reflections account for a large portion of the autobiographical autism literature. A person whose body is running competing subroutines is easily misperceived as failing to employ willpower. Yet as Barbara Moran memorably put it:

> *If only people knew the reason why autistic people get upset so easily. Self-control is much harder because there is so much "self" to control* (Autism Support and Advocacy in Pennsylvania, n.d.).

Overstimulation of a delicately-balanced sensorimotor system appears to be a frequent factor in this uncoupling of intention and action (Markram et al., 2007). The peripheral nervous systems are involved: stress is placed on the autonomic systems that control visceral responses, and in particular on the sympathetic and parasympathetic systems, which must function in a complementary manner to regulate physiological responses and ultimately social behavior (Porges, 2003). As the balance between arousal and inhibition goes awry, the results are unintentional and unanticipated. This unpredictability of how and when one's body will lose balance is another frequent theme in the autobiographical literature of autism. As Sue Rubin observes:

> *Autism plays on a person's five senses. It can vary from day to day and is not something one can control or see coming* (Biklen et al., 2005, p. 103).

For "neurotypical" individuals who take their neurosynchrony for granted, it can be difficult to envision what transient connectivity challenges would feel like. One useful image might be the croquet game in Lewis Carroll's *Alice's Adventures in Wonderland*: (Carroll, 2002, orig. 1866) when the components of the game (i.e., flamingo for the mallet, hedgehog for the ball, the Queen's guards for hoops) are pursuing their own subroutines, the game is impossible to play. Despite her knowledge of the rules, at those times Alice will be mocked as incompetent. But we also know that there will be fortunate moments when all systems are in sync and a structured, non-chaotic game will emerge. Similarly, parents and teachers report incidents when people with autism surpass their typical level of performance with a virtuoso display, such as the "non-speaking" individual who suddenly makes a highly articulate statement, only to lapse back into silence, or the person who executes a perfectly coordinated gymnastic move once every few years. These may be occasions when a delicately balanced sensorimotor system momentarily achieves full harmony.

The existence of this non-volitional performance variability may encourage us to wonder about the ways in which typical education and treatment goals for people with autism are structured, with success defined and knowledge measured in predictable repetitions of a task (e.g., 9 times out of 10, with 90% accuracy), and with connectivity further destabilized by mounting pressure, time constraints, and increased demands to repeat a successful act. If these speculations about neural connectivity are correct, we inadvertently may be creating the very types of expectations and circumstances most likely to frustrate performance and to lead to underestimations of knowledge.

People with Parkinson's and related conditions may devise ways to trigger missing subroutines (such as those that help initiate walking), or to re-integrate and utilize intentionally movement patterns that have gone astray, by means of movement and rhythm accommodations (Sacks, 1990). The triggering of allied reflexes—using intact movement patterns to indirectly initiate the desired but inaccessible movement—is a potentially useful strategy. Some approaches to autism support attempts to restart or reintegrate movement through similar accommodations, including modeling the action to be performed; moving with the person; using indirection to trigger a recalcitrant movement; enhancing proprioception via touch, deep pressure, or rhythm; and incorporating subroutines via the Rapid Prompting Method (Chen et al., 2012).

TIMING AND THE BINDING WINDOW

In autism, the typical rhythms of sensory and social connectivity may be disrupted in a number of ways, only a few of which have begun to be investigated in any depth. Starting in the 1960's, William Condon looked at the importance of self-synchrony (the effective coordination of one's own body) and interactional synchrony (coordination of one's own movements with those of others) for communication and social interaction. He suggested that these core processes were challenging for people with autism because sound processing was both delayed and triggered multiple responses, as if a sound were echoing. Condon found that children with autism would "entrain" or respond to the sound first on their left side, followed by a delayed response on the right (the opposite pattern occurred with children who had dyslexia) (Condon, 1974, 1975, 1985).

Condon theorized that these disruptions would compromise the crucial sharing of experiences from an early stage of development, causing the closely-timed, rhythmic interactions between child and caregiver—and the unified audiovisual experiences they create—to falter (Condon, 1979). Such babies would appear highly distracted; due to mistiming, they would perceive their sensory world to lack pattern and focus.

Condon became interested in the use of carefully attuned rhythm-based interventions in helping to support both self-synchrony and interactional synchrony; the film "Looking for Me," (1970) in which dance teacher Janet Adler works to communicate at the body level with two young children with autism, grew out of one of his projects of that era. These same concerns about how to conduct a dance of relationship with children on the autism spectrum reemerged in the Developmental, Individual-difference, Relationship-based (DIR) approach which took shape during the 1980's and came to prominence in the 1990's (Greenspan, 1992, 1997; Greenspan and Wieder, 1997, 2006).

While this early work suggested that registering and responding to sounds is not a tight, efficient process for people with autism, recent research on audiovisual processing has found that the "binding window"—the window of time in which the input from different sensory modes occurs closely enough to ascribe it to the same event—was twice as long for subjects with autism as for the control group (Foss-Feig et al., 2010). The times involved may seem vanishingly small—600 ms vs. 300 ms, respectively—but at the neurological level that can be enough to inhibit or prevent multisensory experiences from binding into a single well-integrated perception. Sights, sounds, and perhaps other sensory information, would not match up smoothly; unrelated events might be perceived as connected, while aspects of the same event might be experienced without the precise timing (e.g., of speech sound and facial movement) that creates meaning. This would leave the person straining for coherence and, perhaps, adapting by trying to limit input coming through the "window" to one perceptual mode at a time. Foss-Feig and colleagues suggest possible outcomes of a wide binding window, including interferences in responding to input, difficulty identifying the source modality of input, and changes in information content sufficient to "endow social interaction with confusing and irrelevant associations" (2010, pp. 387–388).

The biographical autism literature may offer instances of "confusing and irrelevant associations" that have become locked in, to the detriment of social interaction. For example, Sean Barron, who with his mother wrote *There's a Boy in Here*, vividly recalls his anger when bus 24 at his elementary school arrived late, depriving him of the pleasure of seeing the entire fleet lined up (Barron and Barron, 1992, p. 108). So strong was this initial association of the number 24 with disappointment that over time it attached to other things designated with that number (e.g., marbles and playing cards that he felt compelled to purge), eventually including a teacher whose friendly overtures he repeatedly rejected upon learning that she was 24 years old (Barron and Barron, 1992, pp. 151–152).

Linking his unhappy experience with bus 24 with his teacher's age was unfortunate for Sean, since it removed the possibility of getting to know her as more than a number. But seeing such activities not as examples of irrational or asocial behavior, but as emerging from an active process of trying to associate perceptions—perhaps in the presence of an extended binding window that opens upon an overly generous array of possibilities—profoundly changes the usual autism narrative. There is also no reason why unusual perceptual associations need be detrimental; some may reveal interesting perspectives and creative possibilities, as suggested in the anecdotal literature about the prevalence of synesthesia on the autism spectrum and the pleasurable, imaginative uses to which such associations may be put (Tammet, 2006).

MULTI-MODAL/CROSS-MODAL COORDINATION

Research on typical infant development offers important clues to what may be happening when people with autism try to assemble or bind coherent multi-sensory experiences. Called multi-modal, cross-modal, inter-sensory, or multi-channel coordination, it involves the crucial ability to create a unified whole out of perceptions from different sensory channels, as when a baby registers visual recognition of an object she previously has only explored by touch, or recognizes that a certain sound is associated with his cup hitting the floor rather than with other nearby events. Infants are born ready to start building stable multi-modal perceptions out of sensory stimuli; it is this emergent capacity that keeps their experiences from being, in the oft-quoted words of William James, "one great blooming, buzzing confusion" (1890, p. 462).

The question is how infants, or any of us, take the multi-modal stimuli arriving through different senses and construct a unitary event. The answer appears to be that infants make use of *amodal* stimulation that cuts across the boundaries of different sensory modes:

> Amodal information is information, such as synchrony, rhythm, tempo, and intensity, that can be detected in more than one sense modality. Detecting this information promotes the processing of unitary multimodal events in young infants (Bahrick and Lickliter, 2004, p. 137).

Amodal properties may act as universal attractors that pull diverse sensory input into recognizable patterns. When the amodal information perceived though one sensory channel is also perceived through another channel, a match is made, supporting the unification of both streams of information into a seamless whole. Bahrick and Lickliter cite extensive research demonstrating the use of amodal information by infants to link the experience of faces and voices, and specifically of lip movements with speech; to detect visual and auditory indicators of emotion; and to "match objects and sounds on the basis of temporal synchrony, tempo, rhythm, and temporal microstructure specifying the substance and composition of objects" (2004, p. 137).

This research on how typically-developing infants bind sensory perceptions references the very types of experiences with which infants and children with autism are known to struggle. It seems possible that, if the detection of amodal properties that should unite such basic sensory experiences were perturbed by mis-timing, the experience of synchrony that allows even arbitrary, socially-mediated relations, such as that between an object and a speech sound, to be detected by an infant (Gogate and Bahrick, 1998) would be inhibited (Guiraud et al., 2012). The difficulty experienced by children with autism in constructing coherent perceptions of basic but multimodal social and emotional cues could be a predictable outcome of a wide binding window that leaves the different sensory aspects of an event confusingly out of sync. The frequent preference many of these children demonstrate for unimodal stimuli—for exploring the world one sensory channel at a time (Grandin and Scariano, 1986; Grandin, 1995, 2000)—may constitute a reasonable alternative strategy, and tend to result over time in increasingly different ways of organizing attention and perceptual categories (Marco et al., 2011).

Our ability to synchronize stimulation from different sensory modes into a coherent experience is not just a curiosity of brain science; it reveals a process vital to cognition. In their groundbreaking work on infant development as a dynamic and emergent, rather than pre-scripted, process, Thelen and Smith review the research on cross-modal or intersensory performance and suggest:

> ...the developmental significance may be far more than that intersensory coordination exists. Indeed, we believe that what we are observing in experiments is the very mechanism of development—not a product, but the process through which intelligent commerce with the world is selected and maintained. In our view, what experimental tests of cross-model performance do is reveal how perception-action categories—the fundamental stuff of cognitive development—are selected in real time (Thelen and Smith, 1994, p. 192).

Thelen, Smith, and colleagues used the principles of dynamic systems theory to explore how sensorimotor systems, thought processes, and the self develop through ongoing entrainment with the physical and social environments. If development is an ongoing process of coordination through which body and environment are mutually shaped and explored, then the not-yet-diagnosed babies in the home videos studied by Teitelbaum et al. (1998) and Teitelbaum et al. (2004) are caught in the act of developing and creating their worlds, not of demonstrating deficits. People with autism are, of course, continually perceiving and moving, just as they are undertaking "intelligent commerce with the world" as they continue to evaluate and revise their perceptual categories. But, to quote the memorable title of Sue Rubin's 2004 documentary about her life, "*Autism is a World*"; intelligent commerce with that world may need to recognize a different currency and the existence of a different economy.

That economy may turn out to be based less on the real time coordination of the different currencies represented by our different sensory modes, than on the opportunity to pay them out one at a time, at different rates and over different time periods. Williams (1992, 1994, 1996, 1998) and other self-advocates have recounted their challenges in processing multimodal stimuli, especially for long periods or when trying to assimilate new information. Alberto Frugone writes of his difficulty processing auditory and visual information simultaneously:

> *For example, I'm sitting in front of the TV set, I hear the words and I can decipher their meaning, but I don't use my visual perception simultaneously, otherwise my attention would go* (Biklen et al., 2005, p. 196).

My second son found his own solution to this problem in the close captioning feature of the TV, which he used to reduce stimulation to one (visual) mode. My daughter took the opposite approach, "watching" her favorite cartoon show by retreating to the upstairs hallway so that only the distant sound was available. To prevent processing overload, my oldest son's conversational rhythm involves frequent pacing in and out of the room. Given a computer, he immediately developed a preference for emailing—even with people under the same roof. The ability to organize communication according to his own rhythms pays great dividends: his typed conversations are long and eloquent, in contrast to the more cursory messages of his "live" conversation.

A preference for uni-modal and highly systematized patterns of exploration is common on the autism spectrum, and may represent an accommodation to sensory differences. *There's a Boy in Here* chronicles episodes that may suggest how the young Sean worked to piece together the developmental experiences he needed, in the face of frustrating connectivity challenges. For example, Sean recollects how, as a preschooler, he was engrossed in certain types of activities:

> *I got enormous pleasure from throwing things into a big tree in our backyard. It didn't matter to me what shape or size the object was—I took toys out of the sandbox or things from the kitchen ... I wanted to see how high they would go and where they would get caught. I loved the pattern: throwing the object as high as I could, seeing where it hit the tree, following its downward movement with my eyes, and watching where it got stuck* (Barron and Barron, 1992, p. 44).

Years later Sean's investigations expanded beyond his backyard:

> *I had an intense interest in dead-end streets. The things I liked to do, in general, were those that offered some variation but were still repetitious. So dead-end streets were perfect. I knew the different ways that such streets could look. Two neighboring streets could both be dead-ends but look and feel totally unlike each other. Yet they both ended, and in that way they were the same* (Barron and Barron, 1992, p. 89).

It would be easy to label this behavior as "perseverative" or to classify it as a sign of intellectual disability, but that would not respond to Sean's obvious intelligence or to his memory of actively experimenting with patterns and categories. Other self-advocates have reported similar motivations for similar activities:

> *The inability to get consistent meaning through any of my senses in an environment that demanded that I did, meant that I developed another side; a side with an acute ability to respond, not to meaning but to patterns* (Williams, 1996, p. 242).

Such observations might encourage us to ask: Was Sean trying to establish satisfying patterns among various perceptions in the face of difficulties (such as an enlarged binding window) that made each experience potentially novel and challenging to align and compare? Did the controlled variations in dead-end streets attract exploration for similar reasons?

It seems possible that some of the play strategies of children with autism, many of which involve the exploration of small differences introduced into repeated enactments of an established pattern, may represent adaptations to sensory processing challenges and attempts to overcome them by self-imposing a rhythm, pace, and finely-detailed scale acceptable to the demands of their sensorimotor systems. Seeking and systematizing fundamental patterns may be an intelligent and sensible strategy if experience is often overwhelming and refractory at the perceptual level. In the absence of a reliable sense of embodied movement through space and time, these repeated patterns may provide a frame of reference—a sort of prosthesis for the nervous systems. So far, however, exploratory play on the autism spectrum remains understudied and is discounted by some as a negligible domain. These possibilities are raised in a spirit of humility, because we have known so little (and have been content to assume there was so little to know) about how children and adults with autism explore their environments, and about the timeframes and rhythms through which their movement and perceptual systems operate.

A SENSE OF TIME

It is often observed that the sense of time appears to work differently for many people with autism. That would not be surprising, given the increasing evidence that autism involves challenges to neural connectivity and different ways of assembling experiences. What has to be connected in order to accurately sense time is something even more complicated than, for example, connecting speech sounds with facial movements. Time is not a mode or channel of sensory experience, but an amodal property that unites the perceptions of different senses. We sense time through comparisons of our experiences, bootstrapping from events of known duration to establish expectations about other events; repeated events in the world and familiar rhythms of the body come to stand for intervals of time, with which new events can be compared (Lakoff and Johnson, 1999, pp. 128–139).

If these embodied experiences are unreliable for people on the autism spectrum, it might make sense that the comparison process also would prove challenging, resulting in a panicked feeling of being adrift in a sea of time. Preliminary research has suggested that development of an accurate perception of temporal duration may be delayed among people with autism, and that this delay may help explain certain key diagnostic features (Allman, 2011; Allman et al., 2011). It seems possible that the deep satisfaction many people with autism find in repetitious activities—such as my oldest son's strong inclination, in early childhood, to repeatedly turn lights on and off—may have something to do with a need to ingrain the experience of these temporal units by participating in a pattern as replicable and predictable as a pendulum or metronome. Oliver Sacks has noted that patients with Parkinson's disease (a movement disorder with certain similarities to autism, including slowed gait and speech, and difficulty initiating actions) can be "activated and regulated, ordered and organized" by measures such as

> . . .stairs, steps painted on the ground, clocks, metronomes, and devices that count in a simple, regular, and orderly manner; or by co-action and co-ordination with a concrete, living activity or agent (1990, p. 347).

It remains to be seen whether and how people with autism might be inventing similar mechanisms to self-regulate and, if so, how the possibility of co-action with other persons—skilled partners in the dance of relationship—might be more deftly exploited to enhance temporal awareness and praxis.

Sensing time with reasonable accuracy has enormous consequences for anticipating, planning, inhibiting unwanted responses, and mitigating anxiety, which flourishes when expectations are violated or not established. Caregivers often note the rising panic of a child with autism who faces a non-preferred task and seems unable to call upon any guiding sense of when or whether it will end. Similarly, a person with autism may be unable to be guided by a sense of time in anticipating desirable events. In the book *Strange Son*, many of Tito Mukhopadhyay's challenges are described in terms of his difficult relationship with time:

> He did not experience time the way most people did... He was anxious all the time because he could not anticipate what was next. When (his mother) told him anything having to do with future events, his anxiety redoubled because he could not tolerate the thought of getting from the present moment to a designated time in the future. If he wanted something, he had to have it right now (Iversen, 2006, p. 143).

Time-based challenges to perception and action may turn out to be highly varied, involving not only time future but time present. Leary and Hill (1996) compiled descriptions of many movement differences in autism that may present as difficulties in timing, including instances of individuals becoming stuck in an activity (time never stops), or frozen in catatonic states (time never starts). Damasio and Maurer (1978), Vilensky et al. (1981) identified Parkinsonian symptoms in the gait of people with autism that involved moving to a slower internal clock, and more recent studies have confirmed related challenges manifested in arm movements (Mari et al., 2003). Respecting, and not disrupting, that internal clock can be a powerful accommodation. During my oldest son's adolescence, when his self-regulation seemed especially challenged, I was frequently baffled by his tendency to "freeze" in place for extended periods just as we were running late. I queried Ralph Maurer, a psychiatrist and director of a university-based autism center, who suggested that these abrupt stops, usually followed by a period of rapidly shaking a string or fingers near his eyes, may be my son's way of resetting his internal clock when my fast pace had jammed the gears. (Many people with autism describe the latter activity as a way to slow the demands of perception by segmenting it into still frames, like viewing a "flip book" animation). Considered from this angle, the situation improved enormously when I slowed down or waited silently, so that my rhythms would not overwhelm his own.

TIMING AND EMOTION

Timing our actions to accord with the actions of others is vital to our experience of emotion, and the success or failure of mutual timing can profoundly influence our relationships with and feelings about others. An out of sync phone conversation, with both parties repeatedly talking at once, will probably end in negative feelings; movies in which the sound is out of sync with the actors' lips prevent us from engaging emotionally. Research into the Social Engagement System of people with autism and related conditions suggests that dyssynchronies of the autonomic nervous system are deeply implicated in the kinds of timing breakdowns that can subvert the dance of relationship and emotional development (Porges, 2003). Facial expression, head gesture, the ability to rapidly extract speech sounds from ambient noise, the prosody or rhythm and timing of spoken language, and social interaction in general can be compromised; as the phylogenetically more recent and more directly socially-mediated mechanisms falter, the nervous system reorganizes around "the adaptive defensive strategies of mobilization (i.e., fight or flight behaviors) or immobilization (i.e., shutdown)" (Porges, 2003, p. 508). These non-volitional responses are frequently observed among people diagnosed with autism. Since the peripheral and central nervous systems are bidirectional and intertwined, they may both exacerbate and reflect the dysregulated cardiopulmonary and digestive activities found on the autism spectrum, inhibiting entrainment with the circadian rhythms around which key aspects of social life are organized.

Successful social engagement therefore may need to be approached as an alert, intentional process that is deeply embodied and meets the person with autism on their own terms, avoiding the triggering of defenses. If emotional and social communication is to occur, it cannot be a disembodied one-way process like feeding data into a computer; participants must rise to the challenge of co-creating a synchronous experience (De Jaegher, 2006, p. 186). Sean Barron offers a rare inside view of what a successfully coordinated interaction could feel like to a person who has seldom been able to sustain one. He recounts how, after his family relocated to California, he entered a new high school. His school experiences had previously been confusing and lonely, and his expectations were low as his sister Megan introduced him to her new friend Dianne:

> *Megan and Dianne went to sit down under a large tree, and I stood where I was. Meg looked back at me. "Sean, come and join us!" I did. Several other kids came over and sat down, and I was introduced to all of them. Everyone chatted about school, but I couldn't really hear them—there was a kind of hum inside me that I later realized was happiness. I was very aware that as they talked, they looked at me, too, that they were including me in their group. I believe I'll never forget that day.... Sitting under that tree, I had the first relaxed moments of my life. I began to feel safe enough to listen to the other kids, and the amazing thing was that I understood what they were saying! It all made sense to me* (Barron and Barron, 1992, p. 218).

It seems significant that Sean's surprise over feeling safe and relaxed, followed by his sudden realization that he can access the emotion and understand the communication taking place, matches the prediction that "the perception of safety is the primary requirement" in successful intervention, since it prevents "degrading of the function of the Social Engagement System" (Porges, 2003, p. 511). Given a safe and respectful setting in which to organize his perceptions, Sean displays intelligent and highly motivated efforts to piece together experiences that did not immediately present in a unified way: the hum inside and the outer event, leading to the dawning realization that this is what is meant by happiness. We note the time required (in both minutes of real time and years of developmental time) for him to make sense of the unfolding situation. Above all, we note the dance of relationship that takes place, and the "meaningfulness" that it supports (De Jaegher, 2013).

The ability and determination to connect experiences and probe unexpected similarities also drives creativity, art, imagination, and insight; it makes humans unpredictable and sometimes mistaken, but more than just automata. By now the phenomenon of people with autism, including the most severe challenges, excelling in various creative endeavors has become almost a commonplace; from Tito Mukhopadhyay's heartfelt poetry to Larry Bissonnette's (Biklen et al., 2005) witty and allusive paintings, we recognize that people with autism are interested in, and able to create, new and unexpected conceptual linkages out of the raw stuff of experience.

The formation of, and often intense emotional investment in, unusual categories of things by people on the spectrum might also be explicable as a tendency of this developmental difference to support a wide variety of unusual, creative associations (including complex algorithms for calculating and recalling them). Referred to as "preferred interests" or "passions," and sometimes rising to the level of "savant skills," they can be a motivating force that powers development if approached respectfully. Even an enthusiasm which at first glance seems narrow can ultimately be linked to a potentially limitless array of other topics. From the time he was a toddler, my oldest son was fascinated with big industrial storage tanks. While this was not a category of object that appealed to most children, he experienced them as awe-inspiring. We took trips to admire storage tanks the way others travel to view the Pyramids. Examining them visually may have served an exploratory function similar to the play with buckets and boxes through which his age peers developed the concept of containment (Lakoff and Johnson, 1980, pp. 30–32), but on a more heroic scale. We engaged with him around this interest, eventually introducing him to laboratory beakers, which were "like objects" that also stored chemicals in rounded containers. When, in adolescence, he made the leap from beakers to an interest in test tubes, we began to glimpse a career; as an adult, he is now employed as a phlebotomy technician, enthusiastically filling test tubes at a local hospital.

Engaging in these intense interests with a person with autism can be the first step in a dance of relationship that introduces us to the world they perceive, and allows us to become more in sync with their rhythms of exploration and development (Stillman, 2009, pp. 139–147). Objects and activities to which a person with autism gravitates may turn out to be no stranger than the typical objects and "rituals" that most people use to reassure themselves that the world is orderly, knowable, and meaningful. The impetus to find it so seems universal. That person who looks disconnected and out of step may, for all we know, be engaged in a deeply felt activity that evokes an experience of transcendent connectivity and harmony. As Sue Rubin explains:

> *As someone would carry around a lucky coin or rabbit's foot, I tend to walk about with a plastic item such as a spoon or plastic button in hand.... Water, in which I also find great comfort and joy, is something that falls with an unexplainable grace. For that split second that the water falls, I can almost see into another world* (Biklen et al., 2005, pp. 83–84).

SUGGESTIONS FOR RESEARCH AND PRACTICE

These observations about rhythm and timing are not intended to suggest yet another thing that is "wrong with" people diagnosed with autism. Nor are they intended to provide a new set of instant explanations for why a particular person does certain particular things. As Douglas Biklen reminds us,

> The traverse from neurology to behavior is a remarkably elusive one, yet the tendency to treat it as direct, obvious, and specific can occur without hesitation (Biklen et al., 2005, p. 35).

Perhaps bringing rhythm and timing into our field of vision *will* cause us to hesitate, and orient us in a better direction: away from static depictions of behavior as discrete items with firm boundaries, and away from the kind of indiscriminate reductionism that requires the sacrifice of more dynamic questions and observations. Colwyn Trevarthen speaks for and with a growing cohort of researchers in lamenting that in much of current psychology

> Neither the purposes of the individual human being, nor the meaning built by sharing of purposes, experiences and feelings between consciously active and mutually aware subjects, are explained (Gallese and Lakoff, 2005) (Trevarthen, 2011, p. 122).

When we consider rhythm and timing, the significance of evolving relationships, of personal history, and of the process of striving for meaning, come back into focus. We start to recognize the ways people respond to sensorimotor obstacles by negotiating hard-won and fragile internal treaties that allow them to keep operating. We give ourselves permission to think about how people develop, moment by moment, as the sum of their entire, irreducible history of embodied perceptual experiences. We listen seriously to self-advocates like Barbara Moran, who assures us, "*My mind gets there in the end; but it takes the scenic route*" (Donnellan and Leary, 1995, p. 45).

Clearly there is a huge impact on development when a child's perceptual experiences are out of sync and he or she struggles with challenges to bodily and social connectivity. Attending to rhythm and timing may offer new, more insightful ways to respond. With such a goal in mind, here are some possible directions we could explore more thoroughly, both as everyday practitioners and as researchers:

(1) Bring relationships and their development to the forefront of our work; emphasize reciprocal relationships in which both partners give and take. Reciprocity is not the same as teaching, training, modifying behavior, overseeing a child's play, or general caretaking. It should be understood as an intentional, active process of sharing the child's world, one in which we "need to become something of a detective to discern the ways that the child is expressing joint attention and social and emotional reciprocity" (Gernsbacher, 2006, p. 145). Ralph Maurer suggests that if we commit ourselves to learn how relationship works we might discover "a missing behavior technology ....that uses concurrent stimuli to exploit oscillators"—in other words, one with the power to "compensate for the children's deficiencies in that dance of relationship, like Arthur Murray [dance] instructors, and then work from within the dance to expand the child's world, like mothers do with infants" (Maurer, 1995, p. 2).

(2) Work with, not on, people with autism (Lovett, 1996); support them to explore their preferred interests and to expand them in directions that others can share, rather than controlling access to these interests and exploiting them contingently. Remember that the things that motivate and make sense to people with autism can become the foundation for their explorations of the larger environment. Researchers might consider the complex connections between sensory and motor challenges and the emergence of particular kinds of experiential categories as key features of a child's motivational landscape, and seek ways to engage more substantially around a child's interests and support their elaboration and connection with categories that are meaningful to caregivers, peers, and the child's culture.

(3) Avoid the tendency to concentrate on abstractions at the expense of real life experiences (e.g., memorizing rote "facts" without seeking ways to apply them; learning to identify pictures of activities rather than engaging in them) or to create simulated, out-of-context experiences (e.g., token economies, "pretend" shopping, "job-like settings" with pointless tasks). Self-advocate Alberto Frugone puts it this way:

> *It's necessary for me to gain real experience. While trying to perform an action, even if my gestures are difficult, I obtain valid practice. But it has to be a practical, contextual action not an artificial situation* (Biklen et al., 2005, p. 187).

Lack of access to meaningful, typical experiences may result in knowledge gaps that lead to low appraisals of a person's intelligence and to stigmatization. Now that decades of research and practice have assured us that discrete skills rehearsed in isolation do not tend to generalize well (Koegel and Koegel, 1996, 2006), researchers might seek new ways to support "valid practice" while avoiding the perils of prompt dependence and unnecessarily intrusive physical support.

(4) Value exploration over replication as new activities are learned and transitions are negotiated. It is possible to place too high a priority on having a person with autism do things the same way and follow the same routine every time. Our growing understanding of dynamic systems suggests that encouraging flexibility and supporting a person to experiment with different solutions to a task may be crucial for successful adaptation. Researchers may wish to reconsider their data collection to incorporate variability itself (Thelen and Smith, 1994, pp. 86–88), not as randomness or noise in the system (or, in the diagnostic terms of autism, self-stimulation or off-task behavior) but as developmental data worthy of closer attention.

(5) Slow down; work and communicate at a longer, slower rhythm. Give longer wait times to allow the person to process meaning and formulate a response. Create safety; reduce anxiety through techniques that relax body and mind, such as deep breathing, yoga, and "mindfulness" (Kabat-Zinn, 1991). Many parents and therapists successfully utilize music, rhythm, and dance to support and explore emotions and scaffold communication. Researchers have found useful therapeutic models in the coordination of body rhythms between typically developing infants and caregivers, and could explore new ways to adapt them to infants and children whose sensorimotor systems may not be disposed to find that early social dance coherent or compelling. as well as to older individuals for whom the dance faltered at an early stage.

(6) Try communicating via a single sensory channel or mode at a time; minimize multisensory stimulation, especially when teaching something new, or when a person is tired or

stressed. Consider whether multimodal goals, such as making eye contact while conversing, are furthering or frustrating comprehension and performance. Given that proprioceptive feedback for many people with autism may be inadequate, researchers might consider whether it is possible to devise more salient ways to present and guide proprioceptive experiences, such as by re-routing them through a preferred perceptual channel (e.g., so that body location and position could be experienced through sounds, lights, or haptic feedback triggered by movement).

(7) Create accommodations for sensory and movement differences. Since these differences are generally not under a person's direct control and don't respond well to demand situations, we can respond instead by supporting the person to "work around" these challenges via personalized solutions (Donnellan et al., 2010; Leary and Donnellan, 2012), and by exploring environmental, interactional, and self-regulatory adjustments that enhance praxis. It may be useful to examine the supports and accommodations that are known to work for people with neurologically similar experiences, such as the challenges to gait and timing in Parkinson's, to determine whether they can be successfully adapted to support timely initiation and enhanced coordination for people with autism.

(8) Assume that the person on the autism spectrum is intelligent, has the capacity to learn, and is motivated to make sense of his or her experiences. Make decisions based on the criterion of the least dangerous assumption, which states that:

> ...in the absence of conclusive data, educational decisions ought to be based on assumptions which, if incorrect, will have the least dangerous effect on the likelihood that students will be able to function independently as adults (Donnellan, 1984, p. 141)

and that

> ...there is less danger to students if teachers assume that poor performance is due to instructional inadequacy rather than to student deficits (Donnellan, 1984, p. 147).

The implications of this principle for research may prove to be profound: with the connectivity research suggesting that performance among people with autism is highly sensitive to internal and external conditions, and easily disrupted, research design deserves increased scrutiny. Factors that were once considered to have no impact, or to be cleanly separable from the experimental situation, may have to be reconsidered. The results of some past experiments may become open to reinterpretation—possibly in very exciting and productive ways—based on new questions about task design and presentation.

(9) Explore schedules, checklists, images and pictures, flow charts, and timelines; clocks and timers with visual representations and sound cues; the use of songs, melodies, or simple beats to establish a predictable rhythm and timeframe; and similar customized strategies and devices that appeal to different senses to make the passage of time easier to experience and to track. The importance of structuring tasks and information clearly, assuring that essential features are salient and minimizing sensory and conceptual clutter, is widely appreciated. These features of task design appear to compensate for difficulties with rhythm and timing, but are under-researched and in need of experimental refinement.

(10) Consider that some people may be more talented than others at finding and matching the rhythms of people with autism. Training can help, but not always. The presence or absence of this ability may be a non-trivial factor in providing successful support. The support of a sensitive "dance" partner may also turn out to be the active ingredient that explains the efficacy of certain methods and approaches "for autism" which otherwise defy explanation. It would be helpful to reevaluate puzzling or inconclusive data on treatment efficacy, particularly from studies that posited a significant placebo effect, with an eye toward analyzing the movement, rhythm, timing, and overall impact of the person(s) partnering or interacting with the subject(s) with autism; they may be, or be supplying, the active ingredient that is driving the change.

ON RESEARCH FOCUS AND DESIGN

In summary, this parent proposes that it is time to take a break from the enumeration of what people with autism appear to be "not doing" and construct a research agenda based on the assumption that they *are* exploring and developing, and that investigating *how* that is occurring will open new vistas. If any area of study can force us to leave teleology at the door, as the price of admission, it is autism. Measured as progress toward predefined and self-obvious goals, development in autism becomes a dry account of missed marks; when activity and adaptation are given primacy in research and practice, we begin to see differently.

What we are seeing is a developmental difference that appears to be marked by profound challenges to neurological connectivity, resulting in a cascade of confusing perceptual experiences that disrupts the finely-tuned choreography of social interaction. A promising question researchers might ask concerns the role of rhythm and timing in the rapid, yet highly sensitive, operations involved in piecing together coherent sensory and motor experience, and whether temporal accommodations and supports can be mobilized to reduce an overloaded processing system and enhance performance. Is there plasticity in the perceptual and motor systems of children diagnosed with autism, and does it differ in speed and degree according to type of sensory input, task structure, and the type of accommodations and supports utilized to guide them?

Evidence is mounting that this may be so: for example, research on Musical Interaction Therapy suggests interventions that can be used to overcome social timing challenges and build a scaffold for the emergence of communication and language (Wimpory and Nash, 1999; Wimpory et al., 2007); similar work is being done through Neurologic Music Therapy by practitioners such as Hardy (Hardy and LaGasse, 2013). An ongoing study by neuroscientist Elizabeth Torres is developing computer-based supports that may assist children with autism to cope with the randomness and noisiness of their actions, which seem to involve a reduced distinction between intentional and unintentional movement

(DeWeerdt, 2012). Documenting such plasticity, and identifying the types of supports and accommodations to which it responds, would be a significant step toward improving praxis so that people with autism can more effectively realize their potential.

In researching performances that are highly sensitive to many variables, we must face an issue that many autism researchers have so far been content to set aside: accountability for the impact of researchers themselves on the test situation, including their place in a complex history of beliefs and assumptions about autism, and how these might impact their ability to design and engage subjects in meaningful test protocols. A lab coat is not a Harry Potter-style cloak of invisibility, and it is only the now-fading presumption that people with autism operate independently of and indifferently to the environment and social world that has allowed much research to go forth without addressing such issues. A dedicated research focus on what individuals with autism actually experience, what they intend and attempt to do (and how this happens in the context of movements their bodies inadvertently produce), how they play and explore, and the accommodations and supports they require to make sense of daily life, may prove enlightening (Robledo et al., 2012), and encourage us to include people with autism (and their families) in designing future research. There is much to be said for self-advocates' concept of autism not as a pathology but as a culture or way of perceiving—as Sue Rubin says, "*a world*"—and the way to approach a culture or world is to engage with it open-mindedly, in the spirit of harmonizing with the rhythms of a different drummer and "learning to dance."

REFERENCES

Adler, J. (Writer/Producer), (1970). *Looking for Me.* (Documentary, black and white: VHS and DVD). Berkeley, CA: Berkeley Media, L. L. C.

Allman, M. J. (2011). Deficits in temporal processing associated with autistic disorder. *Front. Integr. Neurosci.* 5:2. doi: 10.3389/fnint.2011.00002

Allman, M. J., DeLeon, I. G., and Wearden, J. H. (2011). A psychophysical assessment of timing in individuals with autism. *Am. J. Intellect. Dev. Disabil.* 116, 165–178.

American Psychiatric Association. (2000). *Diagnostic and Statistical Manual of Mental Disorders, 4th Edn.* Text revision. Washington, DC: American Psychiatric Association.

Autism Society. (2012). *About Autism–Related Conditions.* Retrieved from http://www.autism-society.org/about-autism/diagnosis/related-conditions.htmlan

Autism Support and Advocacy in Pennsylvania. (n.d.). *Look Again: An Inside View of Autism/PDD.* Retrieved from http://www.aspergersyndrome.org/Articles/Look-Again-An-Inside-View-of-Autism-PDD-There%E2%80%99.aspx

Bahrick, L. E., and Lickliter, R. (2004). Infants' perception of rhythm and tempo in unimodal and multimodal stimulation: a developmental test of the intersensory redundancy hypothesis. *Cogn. Affect. Behav. Neurosci.* 4, 137–147.

Barnard, A. R., and Nolan, P. M. (2008). When clocks go bad: neurobehavioural consequences of disrupted circadian timing. *PLoS Genet.* 4:e1000040. doi: 10.1371/journal.pgen.1000040

Baron-Cohen, S., Leslie, L., and Frith, U. (1985). 'Does the autistic child have a "theory of mind"?' *Cognition* 21, 37–46.

Barron, J., and Barron, S. (1992). *There's a Boy in Here.* New York, NY: Simon and Schuster.

Bartak, L., Rutter, M., and Cox, A. (1975). A comparative study of infantile autism and specific developmental language disorders. I. The children. *J. Autism Child. Schizophr.* 7, 383–396.

Bauman, M. L., and Kemper, T. L. (2005). Neuroanatomic observations of the brain in autism: a review and future directions. *Int. J. Dev. Neurosci.* 23, 183–187.

Belmonte, M. K., Allen, G., Beckel-Mitchener, A., Boulanger, L. M., Carper, R. A., and Webb, S. J. (2004). Autism and abnormal development of brain connectivity. *J. Neurosci.* 24, 9228–9231.

Bettelheim, B. (1967). *The Empty Fortress.* New York, NY: Free Press.

Biklen, D., Attfield, R., Bissonette, L., Blackman, L., Burke, J., Frugone, A., et al. (2005). *Autism and the Myth of the Person Alone.* New York, NY: New York University.

Carroll, L. (2002, original 1866). *Alice's Adventures in Wonderland.* New York, NY: Sea Star Books.

Centers for Disease Control and Prevention. (2010). *Autism Spectrum Disorders (ASDs): Signs and Symptoms.* Retrieved from http://www.cdc.gov/ncbddd/autism/signs.html

Chen, G. M., Yoder, K. J., Ganzel, B. L., Goodwin, M. S., and Belmonte, M. K. (2012). Harnessing repetitive behaviours to engage attention and learning in a novel therapy for autism: an exploratory analysis. *Front. Psychol.* 3:12. doi: 10.3389/fpsyg.2012.00012

Condon, W. S. (1974). "Multiple response to sound in autistic-like children," in *Proceedings of the National Society for Autistic Children Conference* (Washington, DC).

Condon, W. S. (1975). Multiple response to sound in dysfunctional children. *J. Autism Child. Schizophr.* 5, 37–56.

Condon, W. S. (1979). "Neonatal entrainment and enculturation," in *Before Speech: The Beginnings of Interpersonal Communication,* ed M. Bullowa (New York, NY: Cambridge University Press), 131–148.

Condon, W. S. (1985). "Sound-film microanalysis: a means of correlating brain and behavior," in *Dyslexia, A Neuro-Scientific Approach,* eds F. Duffy and N. Geschwind (Boston, MA: Little, Brown, and Company), 123–156.

Damasio, A. R., and Maurer, R. G. (1978). A neurological model for childhood autism. *Arch. Neurol.* 35, 777–786.

De Jaegher, H. (2006). *Social Interaction Rhythm and Participatory Sense-Making: An Embodied, Interactional Approach to Social Understanding, With Some Implications for Autism.* (Doctoral dissertation, University of Sussex, Brighton, UK). Retrieved from http://hannedejaegher.files.wordpress.com/2011/09/cv_hannedejaeghersept2011.pdf

De Jaegher, H. (2013). Embodiment and sense-making in autism. *Front. Integr. Neurosci.* 7:15. doi: 10.3389/fnint.2013.00015

DeWeerdt, S. (2012). "Movement patterns may distinguish autism subgroups," *Simons Foundation Autism Research Initiative Report on the 2012 Society for Neuroscience Annual Meeting.* Retrieved from http://sfari.org/news-and-opinion/conference-news/2012/society-for-neuroscience-2012/movement-patterns-may-distinguish-autism-subgroups

Donnellan, A. (1984). The criterion of the least dangerous assumption. *Behav. Disord.* 9, 141–150.

Donnellan, A. (1999). Invented knowledge and autism: highlighting our strengths and expanding the conversation. *JASH* 24, 230–236.

Donnellan, A., Hill, D., and Leary, M. (2010). Rethinking autism: implications of sensory and movement differences. *Disabil. Stud. Q.* 30, [Online].

Donnellan, A., Hill, D., and Leary, M. (2013). Rethinking autism: implications of sensory and movement differences for understanding and support. *Front. Integr. Neurosci.* 6:124. doi: 10.3389/fnint.2012.00124

Donnellan, A., and Leary, M. (1995). *Movement Differences and Diversity in Autism/Mental Retardation: Appreciating and Accommodating People with Communication and Behavior Challenges.* Madison, WI: DRI Press.

Edelson, M. G. (2006). Are the majority of children with autism mentally retarded? A systematic evaluation of the data. *Focus Autism Other Dev. Disabil.* 21, 66–83.

Fogel, A. (1993). *Developing Through Relationships.* Chicago, IL: The University of Chicago Press.

Foss-Feig, J., Kwakye, L. D., Cascio, C. J., Burnette, C. P., Kadivar, H., Stone, W. L., et al. (2010). An extended multisensory temporal binding window in autism spectrum disorders. *Exp. Brain Res.* 203, 381–389.

Fuentes, C. T., Mostofsky, S. H., and Bastian, A. J. (2011). No proprioceptive deficits in autism despite movement-related sensory and execution impairments. *J. Autism Dev. Disord.* 41, 1352–1361.

Gabis, L., Pomeroy, J., and Andriola, M. R. (2005). Autism and epilepsy: cause, consequence, comorbidity, or coincidence? *Epilepsy Behav.* 7, 652–656.

Gallese, V., and Lakoff, G. (2005). The brain's concepts: the role of the sensory-motor system in conceptual knowledge. *Cogn. Neuropsychol.* 22, 455–479.

Gepner, B., and Féron, F. (2009). Autism: a world changing too fast for a mis-wired brain? *Neurosci. Biobehav. Rev.* 33, 1227–1242.

Gernsbacher, M. A. (2006). Toward a behavior of reciprocity. *J. Dev. Process.* 1, 139–152.

Glickman, G. (2010). Circadian rhythms and sleep in children with autism. *Neurosci. Biobehav. Rev.* 34, 755–768.

Gogate, L., and Bahrick, L. (1998). Intersensory redundancy facilitates earning of arbitrary relations between vowel sounds and objects in seven-month-old infants. *J. Exp. Child Psychol.* 69, 1–17.

Gowen, E., and Hamilton, A. (2012). Motor abilities in autism: a review using a computational context. *J. Autism Dev. Disord.* 1–22.

Grandin, T. (1995). *Thinking in Pictures: Other Reports from My Life with Autism.* New York, NY: Doubleday.

Grandin, T. (2000). Visual thinking, sensory problems, and communication difficulties. *Autism Spectrum Disorders Fact Sheet.* Retrieved from http://www.autism-help.org/story-sensory-communication.htm

Grandin, T., and Scariano, M. (1986). *Emergence: Labeled Autistic.* Novato, CA: Arena Press. (Republished by Warner Books, 1996).

Greenspan, S. (1992). Reconsidering the diagnosis and treatment of very young children with autistic spectrum or pervasive developmental disorder. Zero to Three. *Bull. Natl. Center Clin. Infants Prog.* 13, 1–9.

Greenspan, S. (1997). *The Growth of the Mind.* New York, NY: Addison-Wesley Publishing.

Greenspan, S., and Shanker, S. (2007). The developmental pathways leading to pattern recognition, joint attention, language and cognition. *New Ideas Psychol.* 25, 128–142.

Greenspan, S., and Wieder, S. (1997). Developmental patterns and outcomes in infants and children with disorders in relating and communicating: a chart review of 200 cases of children with autistic spectrum diagnoses. *J. Dev. Learn. Disord.* 1, 1–38.

Greenspan, S., and Wieder, S. (2006). *Engaging Autism: Using the Floortime Approach to Help Children Relate, Communicate, and Think.* Cambridge, MA: Da Capo Press.

Guiraud, J. A., Tomalski, P., Kushnerenko, E., Ribeiro, H., Davies, K., Charman, T., et al. (2012). Atypical audiovisual speech integration in infants at risk for autism. *PLoS ONE* 7:e36428. doi: 10.1371/journal.pone.0036428

Hardy, M., and LaGasse, A. (2013). Rhythm, movement, and autism: using rhythmic rehabilitation research as a model for autism. *Front. Integr. Neurosci.* 7:19. doi: 10.3389/fnint.2013.00019

Hilton, C. L., Zhang, Y., Whilte, M. R., Klohr, K. L., and Constantino, J. (2011). Motor impairment in sibling pairs concordant and discordant for autism spectrum disorders. *Autism* 16, 430–441.

Horvath, K., and Perman, J. (2002). Autistic disorder and gastrointestinal disease. *Curr. Opin. Pediatr.* 14, 583–587.

Hu, V. W., Sarachana, T., Kim, K. S., Nguyen, A. T., Kulkarni, S., Steinberg, M. E., et al. (2009). Gene expression profiling differentiates autism case–controls and phenotypic variants of autism spectrum disorders: evidence for circadian rhythm dysfunction in severe autism. *Autism Res.* 2, 78–97.

Iversen, P. (2006). *Strange Son: Two Mothers, Two Sons, and the Quest to Unlock the Hidden World of Autism.* New York, NY: Riverhead Books.

James, W. (1981, original 1890). *The Principles of Psychology.* Cambridge, MA: Harvard University Press.

Kabat-Zinn, J. (1991). *Full Catastrophe Living: Using the Wisdom of Your Body and Mind to Face Stress, Pain, and Illness.* New York, NY: Delta Trade Paperbacks.

Koegel, R. L., and Koegel, L. K. (1996). *Teaching Children with Autism: Strategies for Initiating Positive Interactions and Improving Learning Opportunities.* Baltimore, MD: Paul, H. Brookes Publishing.

Koegel, R. L., and Koegel, L. K. (2006). *Pivotal Response Treatments for Autism: Communication, Social, and Academic Development.* Baltimore, MD: Paul, H. Brookes Publishing.

Lakoff, G., and Johnson, M. (1980). *Metaphors We Live By.* Chicago, IL: The University of Chicago Press.

Lakoff, G., and Johnson, M. (1999). *Philosophy in the Flesh: The Embodied Mind and its Challenge to Western Thought.* New York, NY: Basic Books.

Leary, M., and Donnellan, A. (2012). *Autism: Sensory-Movement Differences and Diversity.* Cambridge, WI: Cambridge Book Review Press.

Leary, M., and Hill, D. (1996). Moving on: autism and movement disturbance. *Mental Retard.* 34, 39–53.

Leekam, S. R., Nieto, C., Libby, S. J., Wing, L., and Gould, J. (2007). Describing the sensory abnormalities of children and adults with autism. *J. Autism Dev. Disord.* 37, 894–910.

Lovett, H. (1996). *Learning to Listen: Positive Approaches and People with Difficult Behavior.* Baltimore, MD: Paul, H. Brookes Publishing.

MacLean, P. D. (1990). *The Triune Brain in Evolution: Role in Paleocerebral Functions.* New York, NY: Plenum.

Malow, B. (2004). Sleep disorders, epilepsy, and autism. *Mental Retard. Dev. Disabil. Res. Rev.* 10, 122–125.

Marco, E. J., Hinckley, L. B., Hill, S. S., and Nagarajan, S. S. (2011). Sensory processing in autism: a review of neurophysiologic findings. *Pediatr. Res.* 69(5 Pt 2), 48R–54R.

Mari, M., Castiello, U., Marks, D., Marraffa, C., and Prior, M. (2003). The reach-to-grasp movement in children with autism spectrum disorder. *Philos. Trans. R. Soc. B Biol. Sci.* 358, 393–403.

Markram, H., Rinaldi, T., and Markram, K. (2007). The intense world syndrome–An alternative hypothesis for autism. *Front. Neurosci.* 1, 77–96. doi: 10.3389/neuro.01/1.1.006.2007

Maurer, R. (1994). "Autism, the brain, and the dance of relationships," in *Rethinking Autism/PDD, the Annual Conference of the Autism National Committee* (King of Prussia, PA).

Maurer, R. (1995). "Why study movement in autism? Statement of the autism national committee," in *Statement of the Autism National Committee. NIH State-of-the Science in Autism Conference* (Bethesda, MD).

Maurer, R. (1996). "Autism and the cerebellum: a neurophysiological basis for intervention," in *The Communicator, Newsletter of the Autism National Committee,* 7. Retrieved from http://www.autcom.org/articles/Cerebellum.html

Maurer, R., and Damasio, A. (1982). Childhood autism from the point of view of behavioral neurology. *J. Autism Dev. Disord.* 12, 195–205.

Minshew, N. J., and Rattan, A. (1994). "The clinical syndrome of autism," in *Handbook of Neuropsychology, Vol. 7: Child Neuropsychology,* eds S. J. Segalowitz and I. Rapin (Amsterdam: Elsevier Science Ltd.).

Nader, R., Oberlander, T., Chambers, C., and Craig, C. (2004). Expression of pain in children with autism. *Clin. J. Pain* 20, 88–97.

Nicholas, B., Rudrasingham, V., Nash, S., Kirov, G., Owen, M. J., and Wimpory, D. C. (2007). Association of Per1 and Npas2 with autistic disorder: support for the clock genes/social timing hypothesis. *Mol. Psychiatry* 12, 581–592.

Porges, S. W. (2003). The Polyvagal Theory: phylogenetic contributions to social behavior. *Physiol. Behav.* 79, 503–513.

Rimland, B. (1964). *Infantile Autism.* East Norwalk, CT: Appleton-Century-Crofts.

Robledo, J., Donnellan, A. M., and Strandt-Conroy, K. A. (2012). An exploration of sensory and movement differences from the perspective of individuals with autism. *Front. Integr. Neurosci.* 6:107. doi: 10.3389/fnint.2012.00107

Rogers, K., Dziobek, I., Hassenstab, J., Wolf, O. T., and Convit, A. (2007). Who cares? Revisiting empathy in Asperger syndrome. *J. Autism Dev. Disord.* 37, 709–715.

Rubin, S. (Writer), and Wurtzburg, G., (Producer/Director), (2004). *Autism is a World.* Atlanta GA: CNN Productions.

Sacks, O. (1990). *Awakenings.* New York, NY: Harper Perennial.

Schögler, B. (2008). "Rhythm in communication: the fundamental basis of music therapy," in *Handicap, Education and Participation–Encyclopaedia of Special Education,* eds O. Braun and U. Lüdke (Stuttgart; Germany: Kohlhammer) [Online].

Shanker, S. G. (2004). Autism and the dynamic developmental model of emotions. *Philos. Psychiatry Psychol.* 11, 219–233.

Stern, D. N. (2000). *The Interpersonal World of the Infant.* New York, NY: Basic Books.

Stillman, W. (2009). *Empowered Autism Parenting: Celebrating (and defending) your Child's Place in the World.* San Francisco, CA: Jossey-Bass.

Tammet, D. (2006). *Born on a Blue Day: A Memoir of Aspergers and an Extraordinary Mind.* New York, NY: Hodder and Stoughton Ltd.

Teitelbaum, O., Benton, T., Shah, P. K., Prince, A., Kelly, J. L., and Teitelbaum, P. (2004). Eshkol-Wachman movement notation in diagnosis: the early detection of Asperger's syndrome. *Proc. Natl. Acad. Sci. U.S.A.* 101, 11909–11914.

Teitelbaum, P., Teitelbaum, O., Nye, J., Fryman, J., and Maurer, R. G. (1998). Movement analysis in infancy may be useful for early diagnosis of autism. *Proc. Natl. Acad. Sci. U.S.A.* 95, 13982–13987.

Thelen, E., and Smith, L. B. (1994). *A Dynamic Systems Approach to the Development of Cognition and Action.* Cambridge, MA: MIT Press/Bradford Books.

Tomchek, S. D., and Dunn, W. (2007). Sensory processing in children with and without autism: a comparative study using the Short Sensory Profile. *Am. J. Occup. Ther.* 61, 190–200.

Trevarthen, C. (2011). What is it like to be a person who knows nothing? Defining the active intersubjective mind of a newborn human being. *Infant Child Dev.* 20, 119–135.

Trevarthen, C., Aitken, K., Papoudi, D., and Robarts, J. (1998). *Children with Autism: Diagnosis and Intervention to Meet their Needs, 2nd Edn.* London: Jessica Kingsley Publishers.

Vilensky, J. A., Damasio, A., and Maurer, R. G. (1981). Gait disturbances in patients with autistic behaviour. *Arch. Neurol.* 38, 646–649.

Wieder, S., and Greenspan, S. (2005). Can children with autism master the core deficits and become empathetic, creative, and reflective? *J. Dev. Learn. Disord.* 9, 39–61.

Williams, D. (1992). *Nobody Nowhere.* London: Doubleday.

Williams, D. (1994). *Somebody Somewhere.* New York, NY: Times Books.

Williams, D. (1996). *Autism–An Inside-Out Approach.* London: Jessica Kingsley Publishers.

Williams, D. (1998). *Like Color to the Blind.* New York, NY: Random House.

Williams, D. L., Goldstein, G., and Minshew, N. J. (2006). Neuropsychologic functioning in children with autism: further evidence for disordered complex information processing. *Child Neuropsychol.* 12, 279–298.

Williamson, G. G., Anzalone, M. E., and Hanft, B. E. (2000). "Assessment of sensory processing, praxis, and motor performance," in *The Interdisciplinary Council on Developmental and Learning Disorders (ICDL) Clinical Practice Guidelines,* ed ICDL (Bethesda, MD: ICDL Press), 155–184.

Wimpory, D. C., Hobson, R. P., and Nash, S. (2007). What facilitates social engagement in preschool children with autism? *J. Autism Dev. Disord.* 37, 564–573.

Wimpory, D. C., and Nash, S. (1999). Music interaction therapy–therapeutic play for children with autism. *Child Lang. Teach. Ther.* 15, 17–28.

World Health Organization. (2009). *Epilepsy Fact Sheet #999.* Retrieved from http://www.who.int/mediacentre/factsheets/fs999/en/index.html

Yasuhara, A. (2010). Correlation between EEG abnormalities and symptoms of autism spectrum disorder (ASD). *Brain Dev.* 32, 791–798.

Young, S. (2011). *Real People, Regular Lives: Autism, Communication, and Quality of Life.* Madison, WI: Lifeline Typing, L.L.C.

Conflict of Interest Statement: The author declares that the research was conducted in the absence of any commercial or financial relationships that could be construed as a potential conflict of interest.

9

Embodiment and sense-making in autism

Hanne De Jaegher[1,2]*

[1] Department of Logic and Philosophy of Science, IAS-Research Centre for Life, Mind, and Society, University of the Basque Country, San Sebastián, Spain
[2] Department of Informatics, Centre for Computational Neuroscience and Robotics, Centre for Research in Cognitive Science, School of Life Sciences, University of Sussex, Brighton, UK

Edited by:
Anne Donnellan, University of San Diego, USA

Reviewed by:
Antonio Pereira, Federal University of Rio Grande do Norte, Brazil
Elizabeth B. Torres, Rutgers University, USA
Martha R. Leary, Private Practice, Canada

***Correspondence:**
Hanne De Jaegher, Department of Logic and Philosophy of Science, IAS-Research Centre for Life, Mind, and Society, University of the Basque Country, Avenida de Tolosa 70, 20018 San Sebastián, Spain.
e-mail: h.de.jaegher@gmail.com

In this article, I sketch an enactive account of autism. For the enactive approach to cognition, embodiment, experience, and social interaction are fundamental to understanding mind and subjectivity. Enaction defines cognition as sense-making: the way cognitive agents meaningfully connect with their world, based on their needs and goals as self-organizing, self-maintaining, embodied agents. In the social realm, the interactive coordination of embodied sense-making activities with others lets us participate in each other's sense-making (social understanding = participatory sense-making). The enactive approach provides new concepts to overcome the problems of traditional functionalist accounts of autism, which can only give a piecemeal and disintegrated view because they consider cognition, communication, and perception separately, do not take embodied into account, and are methodologically individualistic. Applying the concepts of enaction to autism, I show:

(1) How embodiment and sense-making connect, i.e., how autistic particularities of moving, perceiving, and emoting relate to how people with autism make sense of their world. For instance, restricted interests or preference for detail will have certain sensorimotor correlates, as well as specific meaning for autistic people.
(2) That reduced flexibility in interactional coordination correlates with difficulties in participatory sense-making. At the same time, seemingly irrelevant "autistic behaviors" can be quite attuned to the interactive context. I illustrate this complexity in the case of echolalia.

An enactive account of autism starts from the embodiment, experience, and social interactions of autistic people. Enaction brings together the sensorimotor, cognitive, social, experiential, and affective aspects of autism in a coherent framework based on a complex non-linear multi-causality. This foundation allows to build new bridges between autistic people and their often non-autistic context, and to improve quality of life prospects.

Keywords: autism, enaction, sense-making, participatory sense-making, embodiment, social interaction, coordination dynamics

INTRODUCTION

Autism is primarily seen as a combination of social, communicative, and cognitive deficits. However, there is growing awareness that autism is also characterized by different ways of perceiving and moving, as well as particular emotional-affective aspects. Evidence ranges from hypo- and hyper-sensitivities, over difficulties with the timing, coordination, and integration of movement and perception, painfulness of certain stimuli, muscle tone differences, rigid posture, movement, attention, and saliency problems, to differences in bodily coordination during social interactions.

If the social, communicative, and cognitive deficits were difficult to pull together under one explanation, now, as the many and divergent aspects of what we may call autistic embodiment are gaining interest, an integrative explanation seems still further off.

In this paper, I explain why three of the main autism theories [theory of mind (ToM), weak central coherence (WCC), and executive function (EF)] are inherently piecemeal, and why this is a problem.

Then, I sketch a proposal to bring the many aspects of autism together, by doing justice to the experience of autism. The proposal is based on the enactive approach to cognition, which uses the notion of *sense-making* to define cognition as the meaningful way in which an agent connects with her world. It brings a dimension of personal significance right to the core of cognition. Sense-making is based in the inherent needs and goals that come with being a bodily, self-organizing, self-maintaining, precarious being with a singular perspective on the world. Sense-making plays out and happens through the embodiment and situatedness of the cognitive agent: her ways of moving and perceiving, her affect and emotions, and the context in which she finds herself, all determine the significance she gives to the world, and this significance in turn influences how she moves, perceives, emotes, and is situated.

The social side of this—important in cognition in general, and also for understanding autism—is captured by the notion of *participatory sense-making*, which describes how individual sense-making is affected by inter-individual coordination. If sense-making is a thoroughly embodied activity, and we can coordinate our movements, perceptions, and emotions in interactions with each other, then, in social situations, we can literally *participate in each other's sense-making*. This notion brings the dynamics of interactive encounters into the foreground and provides novel elements for the study of autism, such as the idea of the rhythmic capacity (discussed below). The notion connects ways of measuring coordination (using dynamical systems tools) with the investigation of the 1st and 2nd person experience of autism.

These are the central items that I apply to autism research in order to uncover the relation between what I call "autistic embodiment" and "autistic psychology." On the basis of empirical research, I show that autism is characterized by a different embodiment, and propose hypotheses based on the dimensions of significance that are inherent in sense-making. I suggest that their great attention to detail, preference for repetition and sameness, and restricted interests may be inherently meaningful for people with autism, and not just, as they have often been conceived, inappropriate behaviors to be treated away. In the social and communication realm, I suggest that social interaction difficulties are not to be considered exclusively as individually based, but that the patterns in the interaction processes that autistic people engage in play an important role in them. Evidence shows that people on the spectrum have difficulties with temporal coordination in social interactions, but also unexpected capacities in this area. I propose that people with autism are less flexible in dealing with the wide range of interactional styles that characterize social life, but that how they can deal with this depends not just on individual capacities, but also on the interactions they engage in. Different measurable aspects of the dynamics of interactions involving people with autism illustrate this. Finally, I discuss some implications for diagnosis, remediation, integration, and quality of life.

CURRENT UNDERSTANDING OF AUTISM

THREE THEORIES

Autism is most often seen as a combination of social, communicative, and cognitive deficits. The three explanatory theories addressing these aspects are ToM, WCC, and EF (Baron-Cohen, 2003; Frith, 2003).

ToM theory aims to explain non-autistic social cognition in functional/computational terms. Underlying it is the assumption that what other people think and feel is internal and hidden from us, and the only clue we have to go on is their perceptible behavior. From this, we supposedly infer their intentions, using dedicated neural and/or cognitive mechanisms. People with autism are thought to have more trouble than usual doing this, and to find it difficult to "read other people's minds," or to imagine what they are thinking or feeling. The suggestion is that autistic people lack or have a broken "ToM"—the purported neural or cognitive device that computes others' underlying intentions from their perceived behaviors—or to have difficulties with "mindreading" or "mentalizing" (Baron-Cohen et al., 1985, 1986; Baron-Cohen, 1995; Goldman, 2012). This proposal underlies much of the traditional understanding of autism, and has been very fruitful in terms of research output. It has been around since the 1970s, and many studies today, not just of autism but of social cognition generally, are still built on its basis (see e.g., Sterck and Begeer, 2010), although more recent findings also suggest that people with autism tend to be better at mindreading than thought before (see e.g., Begeer et al., 2010; Lombardo et al., 2010; Roeyers and Demurie, 2010; see also Happé, 1994).

WCC theory (Frith, 1989; Shah and Frith, 1993; Frith and Happé, 1994; Happé, 1994) suggests that people with autism focus on piecemeal information and have difficulty integrating what they perceive as well as perceiving things in context. This difficulty is manifested at different levels, from perceiving whole objects to grasping the gist of a story. For example, research shows that it is difficult to read homographs in context (Frith and Snowling, 1983; Happé, 1997; López and Leekam, 2003). Francesca Happé, Uta Frith and others also call WCC a cognitive *style* (Happé, 1999; Frith, 2003). Neurotypicals[1] tend to prefer processing the overall meaning of a scene, while autistics focus on details. WCC research has generated interest in remarkable aspects of autistic perception, and has given attention to what can be seen not just as deficits, but as cognitive capacities and advantages (Happé, 1999; Frith, 2003; Happé and Frith, 2009; Mottron, 2011). Some of the more striking such capacities are making jigsaw puzzles upside down or without a picture on it (Frith and Hermelin, 1969; Frith, 1989, 2003), or finding hidden figures, e.g., triangles, in a drawing of an object like a house or baby cot (Shah and Frith, 1983).

The EF theory proposes that people with autism lack control over their actions and attention, associated with activity in the frontal lobes. This would explain, for instance, problems with the inhibition of behavior, the strong need for routines and structure, narrow interests, repetitive and stereotypic movements and thought processes, and a need for sameness (Ozonoff et al., 1991; Russell et al., 1991; Russell, 1998). It predicts that people with autism have difficulties with, for instance, the Stroop test, which assesses inhibition, and the Tower of London test, which evaluates planning capacities (Robinson et al., 2009).

PROBLEMS WITH THE THEORIES

These theories are not without problems. For instance, Boucher (2012) argues that ToM is too focused on high-level capacities, while it is not clear what could be underlying them. Also, while some people with autism do pass ToM tests, some with other disabilities (and not autism) do not pass high-level ToM tests, leading to the question of whether ToM deficits reliably pick out autism in particular (see e.g., Happé, 1994; Boucher, 2012). If language abilities and higher order reasoning are closely intertwined with ToM (Sigman et al., 1995; for a discussion, see Malle, 2002),

[1]"Neurotypicals" is a term used by autistic people to denote non-autistics, see http://isnt.autistics.org/ (a satirical website by people with autism), http://www.autistics.org/ (a site by people with autism for people with autism) and http://en.wikipedia.org/wiki/Neurotypical. I use this term interchangeably with "non-autistics."

maybe autism is rather a problem with language and reasoning? Or could it even be that people on the spectrum, good as they seem to be at literal reasoning, and strict application of structures and rules, are in fact the ones who do use an explicit ToM? As Sigman et al. (1995) found, there may be a connection between high reasoning capacities and good scores on ToM tests in people with autism, because they can "calculate" ToM-like inferences and explanations of behavior. Despite this, such calculations seem to have a limited effect since teaching people with autism about the "rules" of social interaction and perception does not necessarily lead to greater social fluency (Ozonoff and Miller, 1995).

WCC has been criticized for being overly focused on a deficit at the level of contextual, global processing, while there is also research showing a preference for local processing, with global processing sometimes intact (see e.g., Plaisted et al., 1999; Mottron et al., 2000). The theory is also questioned on the basis of how central the drive for central coherence really is, i.e., whether a deficit in integrated information processing spans all levels of cognitive processing (López et al., 2008).

Regarding EF (like for ToM), it is not clear that it is specific to autism and not other disorders, whether all people with autism have executive function deficits, and also precisely how such deficits develop (Hill, 2004a,b).

Perhaps more important than the specific criticisms is the fact that none of the theories suffices on its own to explain autism as a whole. While ToM explains the so-called triad symptoms: social, communicative, and cognitive deficits (Wing and Gould, 1979; American Psychiatric Association, 2000), WCC addresses the non-triad symptoms (narrow attention to detail, islets of ability, and context-insensitivity), and EF deals with the repetitive behaviors (Baron-Cohen, 2003; Frith, 2003). Frith argues that autism is such a complex phenomenon that it needs all these theories (Frith, 2003). She proposes to unify them by searching for the common denominator in the key symptoms of autism, which she suggests is an "absent self" or a lack of top-down control. Frith invokes the age-old idea of the homunculus to explain this. The homunculus—Latin for "little man"—is a kind of controller in the brain, who views what comes in from the sense organs, interprets the situation using these signals, and then sends commands to the muscles and executive organs, so that the human can react appropriately. The idea has a troubled history in philosophy and psychology, and many reject it altogether (Bennett and Hacker, 2003). One of the reasons is that another "little man" inside the first one would be needed to control *his* brain states, and then another one inside the latter one, and so on, *ad infinitum* (see, for instance, Dreyfus, 1992). While recognizing this problem, but also that the idea of a homunculus is, indeed, nevertheless taken for granted in much of neuroscience and psychology, Frith suggests that maybe there is an ultimate homunculus, one behind or inside of which there is not a further one anymore. She proposes that this final homunculus is self-awareness or the ultimate controller, and that this is what people with autism lack (Frith, 2003). How this might be possible is not explained. Major theoretical difficulties aside, evidence supporting such an idea is anything but conclusive. And even then, it is not clear how this lack would explain all the aspects of autism (Frith, 2008).

DISEMBODIED AND ISOLATED

When taking a step back and looking at these theories with some distance, we notice in all of them two important under-considered elements. Firstly, they show little concern for the embodiment and situatedness of the autistic person, and secondly, even in the investigation of social deficits, interactive factors do not play an explanatory role. The theories are disembodied and methodologically individualistic.

The domination of functionalist explanations of autism—at least in the Anglo-Saxon research world—has left other significant aspects of autism all but ignored (or at best informally recognized but never making an impact on research, which amounts to the same). Lately, however, there is increasing interest in the different ways of moving, perceiving, and emoting of autistic people. There is more and more research on autistic perception, hypo- and hyper-sensitivities, movement, and emotional specificities (Gepner et al., 1995, 2001; Baranek, 2002; Gepner and Mestre, 2002a; Rogers and Ozonoff, 2005; Fournier et al., 2010; Whyatt and Craig, 2012; Donnellan et al., 2013; Smith and Sharp, in press).

The embodied turn in cognitive science urges us to take the role of the body in subjectivity and cognition seriously (see Brooks, 1991; Varela et al., 1991; Dreyfus, 1992; Lakoff and Johnson, 1999; O'Regan and Noë, 2001; Gallagher, 2005; Thompson, 2007; Gallagher and Zahavi, 2008, etc.). Embodied approaches agree that the body plays a crucial role in cognition and emotion. They vary, however, as to the role for and notions of the body they propose. For extended functionalism, the body primarily simplifies cognitive information processing, "offloading" it from brain to muscles (Clark and Chalmers, 1998; Wheeler, 2010). For the sensorimotor approach, perceptual experience and cognition are grounded in the mastering of regularities in sensorimotor activity that depends on bodily structures and habits (O'Regan and Noë, 2001). For enaction, the body may play the above roles but it is in addition an organic precarious self-sustaining system with needs, and this is why embodied creatures care about their world in the first place, they have their own perspective of significance which is rooted in the body (Varela et al., 1991; Thompson, 2007; Di Paolo et al., 2010). It is this approach that forms the basis for the view on autism that I take here.

Furthermore, the trio of theories, while they are centrally concerned with autism's most striking difficulty—its social and communicative aspects—do not do justice to the possible roles played by social interaction processes (Gallagher, 2001, 2004a; McGeer, 2001). The study of social interaction processes has recently become prominent in social neuroscience, psychology, and developmental psychology (Reddy et al., 1997; Reddy and Morris, 2004; Sebanz et al., 2006; De Jaegher et al., 2010; Dumas et al., 2010; Schilbach, 2010; Di Paolo and De Jaegher, 2012; Pfeiffer et al., 2013; Schilbach et al., in press). Proponents of ToM will say that social interaction is *of course* central to their theory (Michael, 2011). But this is not so obvious. ToM is certainly concerned with social interaction, but only as an input to or an end-product of individual, brain-based, high-level cognitive processes, not as complex processes in their own right or in any of their relevant dynamic features. None of the mainstream theories provides an account of the role that interaction processes *as such* play in how autism manifests, develops, and affects the people on the spectrum as well as those around them.

What is an "interaction as such"? Let me illustrate it with some examples from everyday life. There is a way in which the interactions we engage in can take on a life of their own. This happens, for example, when we feel "in sync" with someone, or when two people speaking on the phone cannot seem to hang up, even if they both feel this is the end of the conversation (Torrance and Froese, 2011), or in cases of interactions that time and again manifest a certain atmosphere, e.g., of animosity, or of flirting—even if each participant clearly wants and even tries to avoid this dynamic (see also Granic, 2000). In these examples, the interaction process, in its extra-individual dimension, influences, modifies, and in part creates the intentions of those engaged in it (De Jaegher and Di Paolo, 2007; De Jaegher, 2009; Fuchs and De Jaegher, 2009; Gallagher, 2009; De Jaegher et al., 2010). Although this plays a great role in everyday life, and also in autism, none of it is accounted for or even considered by ToM, WCC, EF, or any combination of them.

I claim that an integrated theory of autism cannot ignore embodiment and social interaction processes. They are key elements of the enactive account I propose here.

LIMITS OF PIECEMEAL FUNCTIONALISM

There is another common ill that the three theories suffer. Given their cognitivist and functionalist background, it is no surprise that the accounts consider perception, action, and cognition as relatively separate domains that can be investigated practically in isolation (Frith, 2003; Happé et al., 2006). The overall approach is piecemeal, and the hope is that the insights and explanations will eventually be put together. *How* is another matter. In a way, this is a kind of "weak coherence" view of mind. Or, in the words of Baron-Cohen (though he does not apply this term to autism *theories*), it is a *systemizing* way of thinking, which he associates with male thinking and with autism (Baron-Cohen, 2002), and which is also associated with standard reductionist views of science (see e.g., Polanyi, 1958). Piecemeal approaches can generate partial knowledge, but they have a number of problems at the time of putting the pieces together, especially when the various elements bear intricate relations to each other, as is the case in autism.

First we can ask, what precisely is the link between the different aspects of the "autistic mind"? In general, the aim is for a unified account based on a single causal mechanism or underlying deficit (Volkmar et al., 2004, 2005; though see also Happé et al., 2006, who argue against a single underlying deficit or theory). Functionalism's answers to the question of integration are limited to a linear strategy, in which either everything is reduced to a common root, often a neural function (e.g., Frith's ultimate homunculus), or to a common higher cognitive capacity (e.g., Frith's metaphor of the absent self). But seeking an integrative view of autism does not necessarily imply adopting a monocausal approach. It can also mean adopting a framework where as many factors as possible cohere, even in the presence of multiple causal elements that relate non-linearly. The analytic, systemizing approach in much of cognitive science and autism research has delivered worthwhile insights, but there is something that remains unclear, something that can only be grasped when we look at all the issues through a synthetic lens too. This something, I suggest, is central to what makes autistic people, and others, relate in meaningful ways with the world. We come back to it below.

We can also ask the question of how the elements of autism are related in specifically developmental terms. The deficits proposed by ToM, WCC, and EF are relatively high-level, and several researchers have pointed out that something is likely to go wrong earlier in development, in so-called precursors to, for instance, a full-blown ToM mechanism (Hobson, 1991, 1993; Klin et al., 1992; Hendriks-Jansen, 1997; Gallagher, 2001, 2004a,b; McGeer, 2001; Hutto, 2003; Zahavi and Parnas, 2003). Often, within these theories, development is thought as the straight temporal sequence between a set of precursors and their concomitant trait. But, as dynamical systems researchers argue, a genuinely developmental approach is one that accounts for change *over time*, i.e., one that "sees capacities and deficits as not just following each other, but following *from* each other" (Hendriks-Jansen, 1997, p. 383, emphasis in original; see also Fogel, 1993; Thelen and Smith, 1994; Lewis and Granic, 2000; Shanker and King, 2002; Shanker, 2004). On Frith's account of autism, all the problems are tethered to a common anchor, the ultimate self-awareness, which, however, "only gradually emerges in older children and adolescents" (Frith, 2003, p. 209). The fact that the proposed central traits or deficits of autism are relatively high-level makes it difficult to see the developmental trajectory from one symptom to another, let alone how they are meaningfully connected. One keeps wondering: *why* are the symptoms connected in this way? Another way to put this is that, even though research overwhelmingly focuses on *children* with autism[2], its main explanations are adultist (Sheets-Johnstone, 1999a). That is, they posit adult capacities—or rather, deficits in adult capacities—and then work their way down from there. In this way, it has been hard to imagine that sensory and motor difficulties could be basic to autism, because traditionally it has been hard to imagine the embodied aspects of social reasoning, integrative information processing, planning, or inhibition. The same point can be made about the developmental neglect of social interaction.

If, as I suggest, autism is characterized by differences in embodiment, the question is not just: how do we connect the higher-level psychological functions and traits, but: how do we connect all of this with the differences in perceiving, moving, and emoting? What are the binding factors between autistic embodiment and autistic psychology?

TOWARD AN ENACTIVE ACCOUNT OF AUTISM: EMBODIMENT, INTERACTION, AND EXPERIENCE

Certainly, the criticisms laid out here are all directed at the "dry" theories. This does not preclude scientists, researchers,

[2]Which in itself is a problem. The research focus on children can affect the actual lives of people with autism throughout life. In many countries, care facilities are directed at children, and there are no services for those over 18. This is the case in the two countries where I have had experience with autism facilities, Belgium and the UK, and it is possibly similar in other countries.

practitioners, clinicians, teachers, people with autism and their nearest from recognizing, dealing with, and using in their daily practices the elements that I suggest these theories lack. In fact, these people often have a sophisticated intuitive practical understanding of autistic embodiment, behavior, sociality, affect, and experience. However, as long as scientific theories do not describe or explain this know-how, these issues remain poorly understood, poorly connected amongst each other, and difficult to systematically link with practice. Most people who deal with autism in some way or another, whether as a researcher, a practitioner, or personally affected, mean the best, and do their utmost to make life as good as possible with the current knowledge available. But a lot of improvement is still possible and needed, as shown by the fact that even for some of the most integrative and dynamic intervention programs, it is still difficult to bring them to those who need them, or to say why they work (see e.g., Gutstein and Sheely, 2002; Greenspan and Wieder, 2006). Such integrative, holistic programs can use the help of a comprehensive, coherent theory to back them up and provide insight into why certain practices work[3] and, in turn, the practical know-how of these programs can illuminate and inform theoretical and empirical work.

In sum, I suggest that to understand autism we should avoid piecemeal functionalist pitfalls and their reductionistic demands, while taking stock of the insights that established theories have brought us. An approach that integrates the cognitive, social, communicative, embodied, interactive, experiential, and affective aspects of autism is possible. I propose that this account, based on a coherent and comprehensive view of embodiment, subjectivity, and mind, is *enaction*. In this paper, I can only sketch its potential for understanding autism, and I hope I can at least establish that an integrative understanding of autism—one in which its various elements cohere—requires an account of the embodiment, social interaction processes, and experience of autism.

ENACTIVE COGNITIVE SCIENCE

This section provides a necessary and quick introduction to the central concepts of enactive theory. These concepts are applied to autism below, and I introduce them here with a view to this task. I build up the enactive story around two of its main concepts: *sense-making*—the enactive notion of cognition in general; and *participatory sense-making*—enactive social cognition. Along the way, important concepts to pick up are *autonomy* (both as applied to individuals and to social interaction processes), *embodiment*, *experience*, *coordination*, and *rhythm capacity*.

SENSE-MAKING

Enactive cognitive science attempts to answer fundamental questions such as: what is an agent, what is autonomy, why do cognizers care about their world, why does anything mean something to someone? Enaction is a non-reductive naturalistic approach that proposes a deep continuity between the processes of living and those of cognition. It is a scientific program that explores several phases along this life-mind continuum, based on the mutually supporting concepts of *autonomy*, *sense-making*, *embodiment*, *emergence*, *experience*, and *participatory sense-making* (Varela et al., 1991; Thompson, 2005, 2007; De Jaegher and Di Paolo, 2007; Di Paolo et al., 2010).

The organizational properties of living organisms make them paradigmatic cases of cognizers (Varela, 1997; Thompson, 2007). One of these properties is the constitutive and interactive *autonomy* of living systems. This autonomy lies in the fact that they self-generate, self-organize, and self-distinguish. That is, living systems are networks of dynamical processes (metabolic, immune, neural, sensorimotor, etc.) that generate their own identity by self-sustaining and distinguishing themselves from their environment, while at the same time constantly exchanging matter and energy with the environment. An autonomous system is composed of several processes that actively generate and sustain an identity under precarious conditions. In short, living systems are constantly producing themselves physically and regulating their interactions with the world to satisfy the needs created by their precarious condition. Constitutive and interactive properties like these have been proposed to emerge at different levels of identity-generation apart from the metabolic level, including sensorimotor and neuro-dynamical forms of autonomy (Varela, 1979, 1997; Moreno and Etxeberria, 2005; De Jaegher and Di Paolo, 2007; Thompson, 2007; Di Paolo et al., 2010).

Enactive researchers propose that autonomy is also what makes living systems cognizers (Varela, 1997; Weber and Varela, 2002; Di Paolo, 2005; Thompson, 2007). This view rejects the traditional idea that cognizers passively respond to environmental stimuli or satisfy internal demands. Instead, the organism is a center of activity in the world, spontaneously generating its own goals as well as responding to the environment (McGann, 2007). Novel identities emerge, and the coupling between the emergent processes and their context constrains and modulates the operation at underlying levels (Thompson and Varela, 2001; Thompson, 2007; Di Paolo et al., 2010). Actions and their consequences constantly shape the underlying processes and modulate autonomy such that intentions, goals, norms, and significance in general change as a result. The significant world of the cognizer is therefore not pre-given but largely *enacted*, shaped as part of its autonomous activity.

Taking seriously a principle of emergence and mutual constraining between various levels (e.g., personal and subpersonal) makes the enactive approach very skeptical about the localization of function at one level in specific components at a lower level (exemplified in the idea of the homunculus that Frith would like to revive). It rejects "boxology" as a valid method to address the "how does it work" question (De Jaegher and Di Paolo, 2007; Di Paolo, 2009).

For the enactive approach, the body is more than just anatomical or physiological structures and sensorimotor strategies. It is a precarious network of various interrelated self-sustaining identities (organic, cognitive, social), each interacting with the world in terms of the consequences for its own viability. This makes cognition inherently embodied (Sheets-Johnstone, 1999b).

The same applies to experience, which is both methodologically and thematically central for enaction. Experience is not—as it is for cognitivism—an epiphenomenon or a puzzle. It is

[3]And even physical therapists call for the development of more embodied interventions (Bhat et al., 2011).

essentially intertwined with being alive and enacting a meaningful world. Therefore, experience also forms part of the enactive method. It is not just data to be explained, but becomes a guiding force in a dialogue between phenomenology and science, resulting in an ongoing pragmatic circulation and mutual illumination between the two (Varela, 1996, 1999; Gallagher, 1997; van Gelder, 1999).

All these ideas together help us to understand the enactive characterization of cognition as sense-making: a cognizer's adaptive regulation of its states and interactions with the world, with respect to the implications for the continuation of its own autonomous identity. In other words, sense-making is concerned acting and interacting, and the concern comes directly from the sense-maker's self-organization under precarious circumstances. Unlike functionalist approaches, enactivism provides an operational definition of cognition. An organism casts a web of significance on its world. It regulates its coupling with the environment because it maintains a self-sustaining identity or identities that initiate that very same regulation. This establishes a non-neutral perspective on the world. This perspective comes with its own normativity, which is the counterpart of the agent being a center of activity in the world (Varela, 1997; Weber and Varela, 2002; Di Paolo, 2005; Di Paolo et al., 2010; Thompson, 2007). Exchanges with the world are inherently significant for the cognizer. Thus, cognition or sense-making is the creation and appreciation of meaning in interaction with the world. Sense-making is a relational and affect-laden process grounded in biological organization (Jonas, 1966; Varela, 1991, 1997; Weber and Varela, 2002; Di Paolo, 2005; Thompson, 2007). This is why and how things matter to embodied cognizers.

PARTICIPATORY SENSE-MAKING

"Social cognition" understood in enactive terms is better captured by the notion of "intersubjectivity," which is the meaningful engagement between subjects (Reddy, 2008). Three aspects here are crucial: engagement, meaning, and subject. In the section above, I explained what enactive subjects are, in their inherently meaningful, cognitive-affective interactions with the world. Here, we focus on the encounters between such sense-making subjects.

In order to explain *participatory sense-making* for understanding autism, we need the concepts of (the autonomy of) the social interaction process, engagement, coordination dynamics, and social skills (De Jaegher and Di Paolo, 2007; Fuchs and De Jaegher, 2009; McGann and De Jaegher, 2009; Di Paolo and De Jaegher, 2012), all of which are operational, as I will explain now.

Social interactions are complex phenomena involving verbal and nonverbal behavior, varying contexts, numbers of participants and technological mediation. Interactions impose timing demands, involve reciprocal and joint activity, exhibit a mixture of discrete and continuous events at different timescales, and are often robust against external disruptions. Essential to interaction is that it involves engagement between agents. Engagement (Reddy and Morris, 2004; Reddy, 2008) captures the qualitative aspect of social interactions once they start to "take over" and acquire a momentum of their own. Experientially, engagement is the fluctuating feelings of connectedness with an other, including that of being in the flow of an interaction, and tensions.

We define social interaction on the basis of the autonomy of the interaction process and that of the individuals involved. Thus, a social interaction process is "a co-regulated coupling between at least two autonomous agents, where: (1) the co-regulation and the coupling mutually affect each other, constituting an autonomous self-sustaining organization in the domain of relational dynamics and (2) the autonomy of the agents involved is not destroyed (although its scope can be augmented or reduced)" (De Jaegher et al., 2010, pp. 442–443; also De Jaegher and Di Paolo, 2007, p. 493).

Each agent involved in such a coupling contributes to its co-regulation, but the interaction process also self-organizes and self-maintains. This means that it sometimes continues in a way that none of its participants intends. To illustrate this, think of encountering someone in a narrow corridor. Sometimes, as you meet, in order to avoid bumping into each other, you both step in front of each other a few times, each moving to the same side at the same time—when all you both wanted was to continue on your way. This is a very simple example of the interaction process becoming, for a brief while, autonomous. We defined autonomy above as a self-distinguishing network of processes that sustain themselves under precarious conditions (Varela, 1997; Di Paolo, 2005, 2009; Thompson, 2007). The individual participants as interactors are also autonomous (point 2). If one of them loses their autonomy, for the other it would be like interacting with an object or a tool (De Jaegher and Di Paolo, 2007).

This has a resonance for those with experience of autism. Sometimes a person with autism will take another person by the hand and direct her to something that is out of reach for him. This can feel strange and alienating. The feeling makes sense because, following the definition, this situation would not count as a social interaction, and there would only be a shallow kind of engagement or none at all. One person in the interaction determines the situation (or at least attempts to do so). To neurotypicals, this can be both uneasy and uncanny, because they generally expect even rather instrumental interactions to have some element of mutuality. When this is absent, it is experienced as somehow wrong.

While they last, interactions self-organize and self-maintain through processes of coordination, including its breakdowns and repairs (De Jaegher and Di Paolo, 2007; Di Paolo and De Jaegher, 2012). Coordination is "the non-accidental correlation between the behaviors of two or more systems that are in sustained coupling, or have been coupled in the past, or have been coupled to another, common, system" (De Jaegher and Di Paolo, 2007, p. 490). Coordination is typically easily achieved by simple mechanical means and, when cognitive systems are involved, it does not necessarily require cognitively complicated skill. Coordination can happen at multiple timescales (Winfree, 2001). Temporal coordination is not the only kind; appropriately patterned behaviors, such as mirroring, anticipation, imitation, etcetera are all forms of coordination according to the definition given here. Coordination does not have to be absolute or permanent. There are degrees of coordination and coupled systems may undergo changes in the level of coordination over time (Tronick and Cohn, 1989; Kelso, 1995; Oullier et al., 2008).

Analyses of social interactions and conversations show that participants unconsciously coordinate their movements and utterances (Condon, 1979; Scollon, 1981; Davis, 1982; Kendon, 1990; Grammer et al., 1998; Issartel et al., 2007; Richardson et al., 2007). For instance, listeners coordinate their movements, however small, with the changes in speed, direction and intonation of the movements and utterances of the speaker (Bavelas et al., 2002). Studies of the way musicians play together also show this (see for instance Maduell and Wing, 2007; Moran, 2007). These findings suggest that interactors' perception-action loops are coupled and interlaced with each other (Marsh et al., 2006; Fuchs and De Jaegher, 2009). This includes processes of synchronization and resonance, in-phase or phase-delayed behavior, rhythmic co-variation of gestures, facial or vocal expression, etc. This complexity of interpersonal coordination is already present in early development (Condon and Sander, 1974; Tronick and Cohn, 1989; Malloch, 1999; Jaffe et al., 2001; Stern, 2002/1977; Trevarthen and Malloch, 2002; Malloch and Trevarthen, 2009).

We coordinate in different modalities (movement of different parts of our bodies, gestures, language, thoughts, etc.). We can distinguish a range of different kinds of coordination, such as pre-coordination, one-sided and bi-directional coordination (Fuchs and De Jaegher, 2009). Patterns of interpersonal coordination can directly influence the continuing disposition of the individuals involved to sustain or modify their encounter (De Jaegher and Di Paolo, 2007; Oullier et al., 2008). This is due to the fact that the interactors, generally, are highly plastic, and susceptible to being affected by the history of coordination. When this double influence is in place (from the coordination onto the unfolding of the encounter and from the dynamics of the encounter onto the likelihood to coordinate), we are dealing with a social interaction. This emerging level is sustained and identifiable as long as the processes described (or some external factor) do not terminate it.

With the concept of coordination and other dynamical systems tools, interaction dynamics can be measured (see e.g. Kelso, 2009a,b). Moreover, they can be related to neural activity. The field of second-person neuroscience is growing (Schilbach et al., in press) and the investigation of people interacting live has produced interesting results (e.g. Lindenberger et al., 2009; Dumas et al., 2010, 2012; Cui et al., 2012; Konvalinka and Roepstorff, 2012). This is a welcome development and we have formulated enactive proposals of what taking the interaction process seriously means for understanding brain mechanisms involved in social interactions (Di Paolo and De Jaegher, 2012).

The consequence of these developments for social understanding—and here we come to the concept of *participatory sense-making*—is that, when we engage in interaction, not only the participants, *but also* the interaction process as such modulates the sense-making that takes place. This means that intentions can be truly understood as generated and transformed interactionally. Sometimes, it is impossible to say who is the "author" of the intention, whether it be an emotion, a thought, a belief, or something else. Interacting with each other thus opens up new domains of sense-making that we would not have on our own. There are, moreover, degrees of participation; we sometimes participate a lot (joint meaning-making) and sometimes minimally (one-sided coordination, where, for instance, we point out an object or an idea to someone).

With this view comes a particular approach to social skill (McGann and De Jaegher, 2009). Social skill is evidenced in interactive performance that cannot be conceived purely as an individual feat. Social skill is the flexibility to deal with the regularities (and irregularities) of the social domain provided by the actions of others. This flexibility, though partly determined individually, is also determined by the process of interaction. Moreover, social skills involve "acting through socially constructed norms and practices" (ibid. p. 430). These societal norms and practices are coordinated and negotiated in interaction with others, "rather than simply acted out without sensitivity to the actions of the other" (ibid. p. 431).

Specifically, as regards timing and coordination, one aspect of social skill is what we call the *rhythm capacity* (De Jaegher, 2006). This is the skill to flexibly switch between different interaction rhythms, or "a mastery of mutual coordination" (McGann and De Jaegher, 2009, p. 431). The notion of social skill can be applied to an individual interactor by considering his performance along a certain scale of interest across different interactions, and can be tested, for example, by investigating range of flexibility.

The rhythm capacity is only manifested in interaction processes. It is always also dependent on other interactors' behaviors and the dynamics of the interaction processes. In contrast to an individual skill like typewriting, the rhythmic capacity is also dependent on a relation of mutuality and coherence with the social skill of other interactors involved. It is impossible to test this in the absence of another person who also brings their own rhythmic capacity, and the interaction between them. The performance of rhythmic capacity is partly determined by the interaction process. It can be empirically measured in terms of frequencies and timescales of recoveries from coordination breakdowns (e.g., infrequent breakdowns and/or fast recoveries would be indicative of a high rhythm capacity).

In short, the argument for participatory sense-making is this: If, as indicated above, we make sense of the world by moving around in it and with it (sense-making is thoroughly embodied), and we coordinate our movements with others when interacting with them, this means that we can coordinate our sense-making activities, affecting not only how we make sense of the world but also of others and of ourselves. That is, we literally *participate in each other's sense-making*. We generate and transform meaning together, in and through interacting.

SENSE-MAKING AND PARTICIPATORY SENSE-MAKING IN AUTISM

The enactive approach to autism considers the particular difficulties of sense-making and participatory sense-making in autism. Underlying sense-making in general are a person's organismic self-organization, embodiment, needs, skills, and situation. In section "Evidence for a Different Sense-Making in Autism," we delve into aspects of sense-making in autism, on the basis of evidence from studies of autistic perception, movement, and affect. Differences in these domains, I propose, correspond with a different enactment and understanding of the world. In section "Participatory Sense-Making in Autism," we discuss how this works in the social realm, where a further important factor is the interaction process, and take a look at participatory sense-making in autism. In each area, I propose novel hypotheses for further research.

EVIDENCE FOR A DIFFERENT SENSE-MAKING IN AUTISM

Here, I review evidence for what I call autistic embodiment, i.e., the particular ways in which the biology, neurophysiology, affective, and sensorimotor structures and skills of people with autism differ from those of non-autistics.

Current research investigates "autistic embodiment" as if it consisted of distinct parts. Perception is mostly studied separately from movement and affect, and different pre-supposed sub-aspects of each (e.g., feature detection, categorization, pattern recognition; movement planning and execution; expression and recognition of emotion) are investigated in isolation from each other (see e.g., Rinehart et al., 2001, 2006; Gowen and Hamilton, 2013). Questions that dominate research on sensorimotor aspects of autism are: which kind of processing is primary (e.g. "low-level" vs. "high-level"); what are the differences between autistic and non-autistic perception, movement, and sensation; are we dealing with underperformance or with superior performance; is the connection between motoric/perception particularities and the social/emotional aspects of autism one of correlation, precedence, causation, or amplification (e.g. Happé, 1999; Mottron et al., 2006; Papadopoulos et al., 2012). There is no agreement on whether people with autism are indeed "differently embodied" and if so, precisely how, but research on these matters is on the rise (Leary and Donnellan, 2012; Donnellan et al., 2013).

Often, the particularities of the ways in which people with autism behave are seen as disturbed or disruptive and consequently as "to be treated away." Two questions *not* generally asked in current research are: *why do people with autism move and perceive in the way that they do*, and *what does this have to do with how they engage with and understand the world, others, and themselves*? If we consider embodiment and sense-making as fundamentally interwoven, these questions are basic. When a person with autism moves, perceives, or emotes differently, this relates inextricably to how he understands the world. This fact is under-recognized in research that considers perceptual, motor, and affective behaviors in view of their role in the functional whole of cognition, instead of in relation to what matters to the person. We need to find out the precise link between sensorimotor-affective characteristics of autism and the way in which autistic people make sense of their world (Savarese, 2010; Robledo et al., 2012; Torres, 2012; Donnellan et al., 2013).

I propose that the notion of sense-making—integrative as it is of perceptual meaning and affective value—is particularly well-placed to interpret the wide-ranging evidence on the sensorimotor-affective aspects of autism. The concept of sense-making may also help integrate the evidence into a comprehensive, coherent framework that can generate further refined research hypotheses[4].

Perception, movement, and affect in autism

Autistic perception was a legitimate area of study in the 1960s (see e.g., Rimland, 1964; Hermelin and O'Connor, 1965, 1970; Frith and Hermelin, 1969). In 1987, Frith and Baron-Cohen asserted that there were no low-level perceptual problems in autism, and that perceptual differences were due to cognitive processing deficits (Frith and Baron-Cohen, 1987). This is also a basic assumption of the WCC theory, which Frith proposed a few years later in recognition of those aspects of autism that could not be easily explained by ToM, like the islets of ability or the attention to detail (Frith, 1989). While WCC inspired a shift in research focus toward autistic perception, including investigations of so-called low-level perception (Happé, 1996), it considers perception as regulated, top-down, by cognitive processes and thus these cognitive processes as central (Happé and Frith, 2006). Therefore, even if WCC put autistic perception on the research map, its focus is on cognitive processing.

While sensory and perceptual differences are not considered centrally in the main explanatory theories of autism introduced above, they feature prominently in many autobiographical accounts (Williams, 1992; Grandin, 1995; Sacks, 1995; Gerland, 1996; Chamak et al., 2008; Robledo et al., 2012). Everyday sensations that non-autistics generally are not aware of, like the touch of the fabric of a pair of new trousers on the skin, can hurt people with autism. Some loud noises, especially sudden ones, may be unpleasant, while others are pleasurable. Autistic people may not notice other people talking to or touching them, thus being hypo-sensitive to particular events. There are no general patterns of hyper- or hypo-sensitivity, and sensory responses vary greatly across the spectrum, and manifest both toward social and non-social stimuli (Baranek, 2002; Rogers and Ozonoff, 2005; Kern et al., 2006).

Sensory sensitivity has been linked to problems with attention and attention-shifting (Liss et al., 2006). Attention-shifting has been found to be slower in autism than in the non-autistic population (Casey et al., 1993; Courchesne et al., 1994; Townsend et al., 1996), and Liss et al. (2006) hypothesize that hyper- and hypo-sensitivity are due to a decreased ability to modulate attention (see also Landry and Bryson, 2004). It would therefore seem to be a kind of strategy to deal with overstimulation (Markram et al., 2007; Markram and Markram, 2010).

Research suggests that children with autism perceive visual motion differently. Gepner et al. (1995), for instance, found

[4]Note that my use of the term sense-making differs from that of Noens and van Berckelaer-Onnes (2005). They use the notion in the context of the WCC theory, without defining it. Sense-making, in their usage, is to do with "meaning perception," for instance in organizing elements of perception into a functional whole (e.g., seeing a gestalt), and sometimes, with communication, as in "the exchange of meanings" (Noens and van Berckelaer-Onnes, 2004, p. 202). Their use of the term has none of the enactive background in terms of embodiment, experience, self-organization, and autonomy, and is not connected with a wider sense of subjectivity, even if, again, their ultimate concern is with providing a better fit between the person with autism and his world.

that children with autism have a weaker postural response to the perception of movement compared to non-autistic children, especially when the movement is very fast (Gepner and Mestre, 2002a). Gepner and Mestre (2002b) also propose that there is a "rapid visual motion integration deficit" in autism, manifesting, for instance, in rapid blinking or looking at things while moving the fingers rapidly in front of the eyes (see also Williams, 1992). Gepner and Mestre propose that the "world moves too fast" for children with autism, and that this is why they need to "slow it down" by exploring it in ways like those just mentioned. One of their experiments suggests that the effect of the rapid, rhythmic, involuntary eye-movements when perceiving fast-moving objects (optokinetic nystagmus, this happens for instance when looking outside while you are in a fast train) is weaker in autistic than in non-autistic children (Gepner and Massion, 2002; Gepner and Mestre, 2002b). Furthermore, people with autism find it easier to perceive emotion in moving displays of faces when the images are shown slowed down[5] (Gepner et al., 2001). Research suggests that autistic people have a higher threshold for perceiving motion coherence (Milne et al., 2002), direction of motion (Bertone et al., 2003), and biological motion (Blake et al., 2003 and Klin et al., 2009). Gepner and Mestre (2002b) also propose possible underlying neurological mechanisms, mainly involving the cerebellum[6]. The research by Gepner and colleagues combines insights into autistic movement (e.g., postural reactions) with the perception of movement, and thus integrates some aspects of autistic embodiment that fit together also on an enactive logic.

Mari et al. (2003) suggest that movement problems should be considered basic to autism. They investigated "reach-to-grasp movement" and found that children with autism had more difficulties in planning and execution than the non-autistic control group. Leary and Hill (1996), in their review article on movement disturbances in autism, also argue that movement difficulties should be seen as core to the condition and that they are at the basis of the social difficulties of people affected. According to them, movement difficulties in autism include problems of movement function such as posture, muscle tone, non-goal directed movements such as nervous tics and action-accompanying movements, and difficulties with voluntary movements, which implicate language and movement planning. Papadopoulos et al. (2011, 2012) and Bhat et al. (2011) provide recent supporting evidence.

There is no real agreement on the extent and kinds of sensorimotor disturbances in autism. Several kinds of impairments have been found, and a variety of causes indicated (Vilensky et al., 1981; Jones and Prior, 1985; Bauman, 1992; Hallet et al., 1993; Gepner et al., 1995; Haas et al., 1996; Rapin, 1997; Ghaziuddin and Butler, 1998; Teitelbaum et al., 1998, 2004; Turner, 1999; Brasic, 2000; Müller et al., 2001; Rinehart et al., 2001, 2006; Gepner and Mestre, 2002b; Schmitz et al., 2003; Martineau et al., 2004; Bhat et al., 2011; Dowd et al., 2012). In contrast to this, Minshew and her colleagues did not find low-level sensorimotor deficits in autism (Minshew et al., 1997, 1999). Fournier et al. (2010) recently reviewed the literature on motor coordination deficits, and conclude that they are "a cardinal feature of ASD" (p. 1227). Other research suggests that people with autism have difficulty combining tasks that require perceiving and moving in different modalities at the same time (Bonneh et al., 2008; Hill et al., 2012). Mottron et al. (2006; Mottron and Burack, 2001) propose that there is an enhanced perceptual functioning in autism.

From embodiment to sense-making

Since embodiment and sense-making are intrinsically connected, the body partly determines how we interact with the world. "The world" is moreover that of a specific agent—not that of an external observer. That is, in the way you relate to the world, you construct and pick up as relevant that which is meaningful to you, but not necessarily to someone else. Sensory hyper- and hypo-sensitivities and particular patterns of moving, emoting, and perceiving influence autistic sense-making, and vice versa. In general, the sensorimotor and affective aspects of autism can be seen as alternative ways of perceiving the world or also as strategies to cope with it, for instance in order to slow down the world, or to avoid or modulate stimuli that switch quickly in rhythm and pattern.

Sense-making is a narrowing down of the complexity of the world. Non-autistic sense-making often ignores certain details and jumps to a particular significance (I'm thirsty, I want water, I get it but hardly care about whether the glass is tall or short, transparent, opaque, etc.). People with autism often perceive more detail, but to the detriment of not perceiving quickly enough that which is more salient in a non-autistic context (for instance, when a person with autism grabs someone else's glass of water and drinks from it, not noticing whether this is appropriate or not in the social context, Vermeulen, 2001).

If autistic embodiment is intrinsically linked with autistic sense-making, we can hypothesize that many autistic people will find joy or significance in behaviors and embodied styles of sense-making that are considered "autistic." An often-ignored factor in perception is the aesthetic element. There may be a value to some autistic sense-making which is simply that of enjoying or remarking on patterns—patterns in space, in ideas, in numbers, in size, in time. Rich patterns exist everywhere in the world, and many autistic people value them, care about them, even enjoy them. This makes ignoring the pattern or the detail doubly difficult. People with autism not only do not initially or without prompt or necessity perceive holistic meaning, but they may feel that they will lose something salient if they (are made to) try to capture the gist of something.

The enactive approach conceives of the way people with autism perceive, make sense, move, and emote, as intrinsically meaningful to them. In this, autistic people are no different from other

[5]This, on a cognitivist account, could be said to be because they have an explicit ToM approach to emotions, i.e., because they have to think about and infer what the emotions are. The argument would be that this is a slower process than emotion recognition in neurotypicals, and that this is the reason why it is easier like this for them. An enactive account would conjecture that they do not have the interactive experience, and that this is why, indeed, they may have to "figure out" the emotions, rather than relate to them via connection, interaction processes, "direct perception" (Gallagher, 2008), and participatory sense-making.

[6]The role of the cerebellum is very relevant, and a possibly fruitful topic for future research, as it is implicated in movement and timing.

people. An easy way to test this idea is to see whether persons with autism enjoy or suffer from that which they do and which seems strange to non-autistics.

For instance, in relation to their compulsion for detail, we can ask whether people with autism are, in general, at ease with their disposition for piecemeal processing. Do they regret missing the holistic sense or pity non-autistics for not enjoying detailed patterns? If the hypothesis is true, people with autism can be properly described as having a different conception of wholeness, one that has to do with order, patterns, exceptions, and perceptual richness. Anecdotal evidence for this idea comes from aesthetic appreciation, savant skills, and creativity in autistic people (see e.g., Sacks, 1985; Happé and Frith, 2009). Stronger evidence for WCC having a potential value or significance for people with autism is harder to find. WCC has been described positively as a cognitive style (Happé, 1999), and Happé and Frith (2009, p. 1348) suggest that there is a "rage to learn" and an intrinsic motivation in special talents, indicating that the special skills, as well as their learning and the learning of certain information can be interesting in their own right.

However, savant skills and high creativity are not representative of the whole autistic population (Hacking, 2009). Also, most of this research is concerned with how the processing style relates to other isolated aspects of the functioning of the person with autism, not with their personal significance or more general value. What enaction predicts goes beyond the cognitivist conception in which functioning and adaptation are considered as adequate fit to the non-autistic context. Enaction is concerned with functioning as valued and significant from the perspective of the person herself, in her context. Cognitive, perceptual, sensorimotor, and affective styles should in the first instance be approached from the point of view of the situated self-organizing sense-maker, not just that of an "objective" observer. What is such an observer objective about if he studies cognition but misses the *meaning for the subject* whose cognition he is studying?

An area in which there is evidence that people with autism derive pleasure from their specialized activities or thinking styles is restricted interests and repetitive behaviors. Circumscribed interests are highly frequent in autism, with between 75–88% of the autistic population engaging in them (Klin et al., 2007; Spiker et al., 2012). In direct support of the enactive hypothesis, repetitive activities in autism—unlike obsessions and compulsions in obsessive compulsive disorder—have been found to be "beloved activities apparently associated with great positive valence" (Klin et al., 2007, p. 97; see also Baron-Cohen, 1989; Klin et al., 1997). It has been found that circumscribed interests are highly motivating for children with autism, and that allowing them to engage in these behaviors can help them produce appropriate behaviors (Hung, 1978), and increase social interactions with non-autistic peers and with siblings (Baker et al., 1998; Baker, 2000). Lovaas also considers repetitive interests as intrinsically motivating for the perceptual reinforcement and self-stimulation that they provide, even connecting this to the sensory joys of gourmet food, art, recreational drugs, and smoking (Lovaas et al., 1987).

In a qualitative interview assessing how people with autism and their siblings and parents experience the restricted interests, Mercier et al. (2000) found that they "provide a sense of well-being, a positive way of occupying one's time, a source of personal validation, and an incentive for personal growth" (p. 406). The interviewees also recognized negative aspects of repetitive and circumscribed activities, such as their invasiveness, the amount of time they occupy, and (fear of) potentially socially unacceptable behaviors they may provoke. One of the participants sums up the tension between the positive and negative aspects as follows: "Basically, what others will tell me is that I monopolize time that could have been used for better things. But sometimes I can't think of better things to do when I have my free time" (p. 414).

In contrast to Mercier et al.'s subject-oriented approach, a recent study attempted to show a link between anxiety and restricted interests based on the assumption that restricted interests are a (maladaptive) way of coping with distress (Spiker et al., 2012). The study found that particular kinds of restricted interests were associated with anxiety, while others were not. However, the kind that was associated with anxiety, viz. "symbolically enacted restricted interests," is not defined or even described in the paper. Moreover, the authors themselves say that it might be that "symbolically enacted RI [restricted interests] only appear coupled to anxiety in children with high functioning ASD because these problems have overlapping behavioral manifestations, such that RI-related behaviors may be misinterpreted as anxiety-related behaviors" (ibid. p. 316). Furthermore, unlike in Mercier et al.'s (2000) study, the nature and incidence of restricted interests was gathered from interviews with the parents, not with the children themselves, and all the children involved in the study were diagnosed as having an anxiety comorbidity (thus biasing the answer to the question of a relation between anxiety and restricted interests in the cases studied).

Restricted interests, focus on detail, and other autistic sensorimotor and affective particularities often interfere with everyday life, and this can make them difficult to deal with, both for the person with autism and for their social and familial environment. However, this does not imply that they could not in themselves be relevant, salient, or significant for the person with autism. It might be that these behaviors are disruptive as a consequence of their manifesting in a context that can or will not accommodate them. This is not to suggest that such behaviors should simply be accepted. Rather it is to suggest that dealing with them should also start from the meaning they have for the person with autism, not just from the question of whether they are appropriate. The interviews conducted by Mercier and colleagues show that doing this can help find suitable ways to deal with the restricted, repetitive behaviors, even to the point of converting them into acceptable activities or extinguishing them (Mercier et al., 2000).

PARTICIPATORY SENSE-MAKING IN AUTISM

Participatory sense-making relies on the capacity to flexibly engage with your social partner from moment to moment, where this engagement involves emotion, knowledge, mood, physiology, background, concepts, language, norms, and, crucially, the dynamics of the interaction process and its coordinations and breakdowns. I have conjectured that a sensorimotor interactional coordination ability is at the basis of this connection.

We have seen that sensorimotor differences imply a different sense-making in autism. Sensorimotor differences, especially those involving temporal aspects of perception and movement, will affect interaction and coordination in social encounters, and therefore introduce systematic differences in participatory sense-making. This is true the other way around as well. If social connection is basic to individual cognitive/emotional development (Hobson, 2002), embodiment and sense-making will be influenced by a history of interactive engagements. In the following, I paint an increasingly inter-individual picture of (social) sense-making in autism and its problems.

A differently salient social world

Different aspects of the social environment are relevant to people with autism than to non-autistics. Ami Klin suggests that autistic people experience the world, including and especially the social world, as differently salient (Klin et al., 2003). Using an eye-tracker, they analyzed the way persons with autism scan film scenes in comparison with neurotypicals. Autistic people looked significantly less at socially salient aspects like the eyes and mouths of protagonists, or the object of a pointing gesture than non-autistic controls (Klin et al., 2002). It also seems that children with autism do not spontaneously pay attention to social stimuli that are salient to typically developing children, such as human sounds and faces (Klin et al., 2003; Shic et al., 2011). Furthermore, they seem to prefer to attend to inanimate objects over other humans (Klin et al., 2003; Jones et al., 2008). Not only is the preference different, autistic people also seem less sensitive to biological motion, an aspect of the recognition of the motion of other humans (Blake et al., 2003).

Even though Klin and his colleagues emphasize the anchoring of cognition in embodiment and the developmental process of acquiring social cognition, their work still has an individualistic flavor. They hit the nail on the head when they say that "the (non-autistic) child "enacts the social world," perceiving it selectively in terms of what is immediately essential for social action," but when they consider the work for this to be done by "perceptually guided actions" (Klin et al., 2003, p. 349), they fall short of the logical next step. They are rightly convinced that social interaction is the basis of social cognition, and they study social capacities from an embodied perspective. The next thing to put up for investigation is the interaction process.

Interpersonal engagement in autism

On the enactive account, crucial for social understanding is the capacity to connect. This capacity is relevant both during actual interactions and during non-interactive social situations where social understanding is more observational (Di Paolo and De Jaegher, 2012). If people on the autism spectrum have difficulty connecting, we need to study the social interaction processes they engage in (or fail to engage in).

Peter Hobson argues that, generally, "a conceptual grasp of the nature of 'minds'... is acquired through an individual's experience of affectively patterned, intersubjectively co-ordinated relations *with* other people" (Hobson, 1993, pp. 4–5, emphasis in original). In other words, social cognition is based in "interpersonal engagement" (Hobson, 2002). With regard to autism, he makes the conjoined claims that what underlies the deficits of autism is a hampered "intersubjective engagement" with social partners from very early in life, and that these engagements are the foundation of flexible and creative thought. Therefore, a deficit in this area would at once explain the problems with social interaction and communication of individuals with autism and the particularities of their ways of thinking (especially literal and decontextualized thinking, well-known to anyone who regularly interacts with people with autism, see also Vermeulen, 2001).

Hobson probes autistic social interactions as they are experienced, to find out how they differ from neurotypical interactions. In this way, he investigates the qualities of relatedness and connectedness. In several imitation studies, he shows that even though children on the spectrum are able to copy actions, they generally do not copy the *way* an action is performed, for instance, whether it was performed harshly or gently (Hobson and Lee, 1999), or directed at the experimenter himself or the child (self- or other-directedness, Meyer and Hobson, 2005). For Hobson and his colleagues, these findings indicate that children with autism identify with others less than typically developing children do: "the autistic individuals were not so much abnormal in their attempts to imitate *the actions* modeled, but instead were abnormal in their attempts to imitate *the person* who modeled" (Hobson and Lee, 1999, p. 657, emphasis in original). What is missing is an imitation of the "expressive quality of another person's behavior" (ibid.).

Interestingly, Hobson also investigated the other side of this: what it is like to interact with someone with autism, in a study called "Hello and Goodbye" (Hobson and Lee, 1998). As the title says, this study analyzes the greetings and farewells of children with autism, compared with a control group of children with learning difficulties. The children were brought into a room to perform a task at a table with an experimenter (Hobson himself), who sat opposite them. The task was no more than a pretext for creating the opportunities for greetings and farewells. Upon entering the room, the children were introduced to Hobson by his colleague. The videotaped episodes of introduction, greeting and farewell were rated by independent judges naïve to the aim of the study, who counted the amount of smiling, nodding, waving and vocalizing of each participant. The hypothesis was supported: children with autism showed fewer greeting and farewell behaviors than the control group, and also combined them less. This is not so surprising given that this result bears out the diagnostic criteria for autism. However, the judges were also given a more subjective item to rate, namely how much interpersonal engagement there was between the participant and the experimenter. They judged that, in the interactions with the participants with autism, there was much less intersubjective engagement at the different stages of the interaction than in those with the non-autistic group.

In a description of this same study in his book *The Cradle of Thought*, Hobson relates something that is not reported in the paper: that, from the videotapes, one could have the impression that, regarding Hobson's own behavior as the interactor, "there was a deliberateness to my own gestures and actions [and that] I was less outgoing and more hesitant in my efforts to make contact, and my 'Goodbye' seemed forced. It was clear that I was doing my best to be relaxed and engaging, but I did a poor job when I did not have an engaging partner." He adds: "The lesson is: interpersonal engagement is just that—interpersonal" (Hobson, 2002, pp. 50–51). For a similar point, made through a study of sharing humor and laughter in autism, see Reddy et al. (2002).

The central issue here—which remains insufficiently investigated—is the interaction process as such. If there are sensorimotor and coordination differences in autism, and we take the embodied interaction process as defined in section "Participatory Sense-Making" as central to social understanding, then we can suspect that the interaction process will be hampered in autism. Is this the case?

Interaction rhythm and rhythmic capacity in autism

People with autism often seem awkward in the way they coordinate with others in interactions. Some studies suggest, however, that children with autism have more mastery of the basics of interactional capacity than previously thought. Dickerson et al. (2007), for instance, argue that persons with autism can temporally appropriately place their interventions in social encounters. They investigated interactions between two autistic children and their tutors during question-and-answer sessions involving answer cards, in which both children tapped the answer cards—a seemingly meaningless action. However, Dickerson and colleagues found that the tapping was placed temporally just after the tutor asked the question and before the child started answering, continuing sometimes into the answer of the child. This suggests, first, that the tapping displayed engagement, an engagement that could also have been shown through eye contact, something known to be difficult for people with autism (American Psychiatric Association, 2000). And second, it suggests that the tapping indicated that the child was about to answer the question, i.e., the tapping was "projecting a relevant forthcoming response on the part of the child" (Dickerson et al., 2007, p. 297). Similar findings were made in relation to gaze (Dickerson et al., 2005). Interesting in this research is that the actions of all interaction partners are being investigated, also that of non-autistic participants. This allows to query the experience (cf. Hobson above), as well as the perceived appropriateness of the behavior. The tutors in the tapping study, for instance, took the behavior as interactionally relevant and appropriate (Dickerson et al., 2007).

Other research suggests that people with autism have timing differences. In a study in which participants were asked to tap in synchrony with an auditory stimulus, Sheridan and McAuley (1997) found that the autistic participants' tapping was more variable than that of the non-autistic group (see also Isenhower et al., 2012, for a similar result in an intra-individual bi-manual drumming task). Trevarthen and Daniel (2005) report on interactional timing and rhythmic difficulties in autism in a study of the interactions between a father and his twin daughters, one of whom was later diagnosed with autism (see also St. Clair et al., 2007). With this twin, the father was unable to engage in rhythmic interaction. This is reminiscent of Hobson's Hello and Goodbye study, which also showed that an interaction partner is less able to engage with a partner who is less rhythmically able. Again, it becomes apparent that social capacity is interactional and not just individual.

Another set of investigations centers around the contingency detection hypothesis (Watson, 1979; Gergely and Watson, 1999; Nadel et al., 1999). Gergely (2001) hypothesized that, in normal development, there is a transition from an expectancy of perfect contingency to one of less than perfect contingency. Before they are 3 months old, Gergely conjectures, infants expect to perceive effects of their actions that immediately follow those actions. These are found mostly in their own actions (what Piaget calls "circular reactions," 1936). Around 3 months, infants start to search for "high-but-imperfect" contingency, which is found in games with other people and in effects of the infant's actions on the environment. With this shift the infant supposedly starts to engage in interactions with the social world. With regard to autism, Gergely reckons that this shift does not take place, or not fully. As a result, the child with autism would continue to seek perfect contingency throughout life. There is no direct evidence for this theory yet, even though it is an interesting hypothesis. Jacqueline Nadel, who has also worked on contingency detection in children both with and without autism, found that children with autism do not spontaneously detect and expect social contingency, although they can learn to do it after an experimental phase in which the adult experimenter has imitated them (see Nadel et al., 2000; Field et al., 2001).

While there is a general and rather vague idea that people with autism are "awkward" in their interactions, until we investigate those interactions, we do not know what this means or entails. If interactional timing is awkward, and one or both partners do not have the flexibility to adapt to the other's timing, the *rhythmic capacities* (see above) will be of a low quality, and this will result in interactional problems. Although further research is needed, the evidence points to various problems with interaction timing in autism, but also unexpected capabilities. On an enactive perspective, both of these will impact on the dynamics of social interaction, specifically on the quality of coordination, the frequency of coordination breakdowns, the ability to repair them, and the experience of the interactors with and without autism, supporting Hobson's observations. Interactions involving people with autism do not fully lack flexibility, but its scope is reduced due to motor and timing differences. This can be both the cause and the symptom of difficulties with connecting. Findings like the ones reported allow to keep searching for and refine hypotheses about what precisely characterizes "autistic interactions."

One way in which to test rhythmic capacity and other interactional capacities of and with people with autism, is to study how often breakdowns occur, as well as how easily they are recovered from. Dynamical measures of coordination can be used to construct an index of how quickly the pair achieves coordination again after breakdown (see e.g., Kelso, 1995, 2009a,b; van Orden et al., 2003, 2005; Riley et al., 2011). Immediate or fast recovery would indicate a high rhythmic capacity, and slow, absent, "jumpy," or unclear recoveries would indicate a lower or narrower rhythmic capacity, i.e., little interactional flexibility overall. The prediction is that interactions of people with autism show a marked reduction in rhythm capacity compared to those of non-autistics. Recently, Marsh and colleagues tested this in a study of unconscious rocking (in rocking chairs) between children with and without autism and their parents, finding that children with autism had a lower tendency to rock in symmetrical timing with their parents (Marsh et al., 2013; see also Schmidt and O'Brien, 1997). A similar difference is expected between interactions of people with autism who do or do not have an interaction history with each other (i.e., whether they have interacted before, and how much). The case of interactions between people with autism who have an interaction history is especially interesting, because it brings several predictions together. We predict both that people who have interacted before will have a smoother rhythm capacity, and that people with autism will have a more reduced rhythm capacity. If these two elements come together, i.e., in an interaction between two autistic people with a long interaction history between them, this will have its own specific rhythmic characteristics.

So far, we have discussed interactional capacities, but what about participatory sense-making?

What is participatory sense-making like in autism?

Penny Stribling and her colleagues have studied the behavior and speech of autistic children in an interactional context, using conversation analysis. One of their studies evaluates instances of echolalia, produced by a boy with autism in a single session of play with a robot (Stribling et al., 2005/2006). Echolalia is the repetition of utterances (one's own or an other's), and is often considered meaningless and uncommunicative, and the general advice is to ignore it. However, Stribling demonstrates that the repeated utterances of the boy had an interactional function. He repeated a phrase that seemed communicationally irrelevant because of its literal content, yelling 'spelling assertions' such as "please has got an A in it!" By taking a panoramic view of the situation, i.e., by studying the utterance in its interactive context, as well as its prosodic characteristics, Stribling et al. found that the boy's supposedly irrelevant utterances were in fact a protest at losing control over the robot, and an attempt to regain it. They suggest this because, first, all the instances of the echoed utterance that they recorded happened when another person was starting to play with the robot, and second, the way the utterances were made had strong prosodic similarities to how a protest generally sounds (rising loudness and emphasis). Further to their explanation, we can add that the utterance could also have an intrinsic meaning. From the enactive point of view, in which a cognizer self-maintains and self-organizes, it can be proposed that the boy is self-affirming his place in an interaction in which he feels that something is taken away from him, by uttering knowledge that he has. These utterances could be a way of maintaining individual autonomy in an interactional situation. This possibility can be further researched using the notions of self-organization and individual and interactional autonomy as conceptual tools for deepening the understanding of phenomena like echolalia.

Difficulties with coordinating and interacting in autism will lead to hampered participatory sense-making because, as we have seen, participatory sense-making is the inter-individual coordination of embodied and situated sense-making. As regards the new domains of sense-making that are generated in interaction it is clear to see that, if there are such difficulties in autistic interaction as I have just described, the range of orientations, from one-sided (or instructive) coordination of a person in their individual cognitive domain to closely coupled mutual orientation of sense-making, will be difficult to achieve. Additionally, because of the experience of negative affect that results from more frequent coordination breakdowns, social interaction may be less often sought by people with autism, resulting in fewer opportunities to engage in participatory sense-making.

One of Hobson's proposals is that flexible thinking develops from affective interpersonal engagement, and that, in autism, hampered interpersonal relating throughout development leads to the cognitive problems of autism, which are characterized by inflexibility of thinking, lack of creativity, and literal and decontextualized understanding (Vermeulen, 2001; Hobson, 2002). Similarly, if, as proposed by Reddy (2003), complex self-conscious emotions develop out of infants' early interactive experiences (in particular the awareness of being the object of another's attention), then a history of non-fluid interactions must impact on the development and understanding of social emotions, such as embarrassment, pride, and shame.

On the present proposal, if the developmental trajectory of participatory sense-making is hindered in specific ways, among others in the area of interactional coordination, this will reinforce a lack of flexibility in thinking and in dealing with self-conscious emotions. In order to specify in detail why this is the case, the present work needs to be extended with a developmental strand. For now, we can conclude that, if there is less flexibility in social interactional timing and coordination, the creation of new domains of sense-making that rely on participation by others is impeded. It is likely that flexibility in both of these areas is strongly related, especially if there is such a strong developmental interaction between them. Further research is needed to find out the precise relationship between interactional flexibility and flexibility in thinking and emoting.

Some implications for intervention and diagnosis

Underlying the interactional difficulties of people with autism we could find neurological and/or sensorimotor differences, but such individual differences do not suffice to explain where specific autistic ways of making sense of the world come from. Social understanding is a constitutive aspect of cognition in general, and it is at its basis truly inter-individual (even the personal skills that permit remote observational social understanding, I propose, are dependent on interactive skills and experiences, see Di Paolo and De Jaegher, 2012). Therefore, interventions for autism—w.r.t. social difficulties, cognition, affect, and sensorimotor capacities—need to pay special attention to interactional coordination, rhythmic capacity and participatory sense-making (this is the basis of, for instance, music therapy, and dance and body movement interventions, Wigram and Gold, 2006; Samaritter and Payne, 2013). This is the context that affords the best interpretation of neurological and other individual factors.

Putting things in the appropriate rhythmic and interactive context is not a novelty for many parents, caregivers, teachers, and friends who successfully motivate, adapt to, and engage autistic partners. Such is the case with approaches like Relationship Development Intervention (Gutstein and Sheely, 2002), or intensive interaction (Caldwell, 2006) and similar ones. The gist of these approaches is to gently introduce the child to flexible interactions with both the social and the "non-social" world in playful settings. At the heart of Relationship Development Intervention sits the idea that people with autism have problems with dynamic, but not with static intelligence. The suggestion has been made before that people with autism are good at scientific-style cognition, but have less adaptive, engaged, know-how intelligence (Kanner, 1973; Baron-Cohen, 2002, 2003). The development of flexibility in interaction can aid the development of flexibility and creativity in behavior and thinking in general, as the present work also predicts, in line with Hobson's ideas (Hobson, 2002), and enhance daily support, friendships, and love relationships.

CONCLUSION

In this paper, I have looked at autism through an enactive lens in order to help integrate the diverse aspects of autism that have up to now been examined in isolation. Unlike the search for a common root or key causal factors, enaction strives for a coherent picture of autism, while embracing a complex, non-linear multi-causality. In this effort, two elements that I aimed to do justice to are the experience of autism—both that of people with autism and that of those interacting with them—and the differences in embodiment that seem present in autism.

I suggest that people with autism make sense of the world differently, and that, in the social realm, they are differently able to participate in sense-making with others.

This leads to the following methodological considerations. If we base autism research on the question of why something means something for someone, we can connect autistic styles of sense-making with particular ways of moving, perceiving, and emoting. Hypotheses based in a subject-oriented approach to cognition and mind in autism will be better able to connect the elements that up to now have remained disconnected. For instance, I proposed that restricted interests and repetitive behaviors, if given a place in the actions and interactions of people with autism, can help them, among other things, to improve their social flexibility. I suggested that a focused treatment is needed of a surprising blind spot in autism research: the social interaction process itself. Once we do that, we will be better able to understand both the difficulties and the capacities that people with autism have in this domain. Behaviors that seem irrelevant can acquire significance from the context of the social interaction. To understand this, we must abandon disembodied individualism.

I have hinted at the possible developmental questions that may arise from considering both subjective and interactive factors. This is one of the directions where further work is needed. Another such open direction is to draw further implications for diagnosis, therapy, and interventions.

Ethically, the approach put forward here is not one of *laissez faire*. On the contrary, it is one that starts from *also* taking seriously the perspective and subjectivity of people with autism themselves, in a principled, coherent, and comprehensive way. It is then that we can expect to be able to build bridges that are well-informed by both autistic and non-autistic experience.

ACKNOWLEDGMENTS

I would like to thank Ezequiel Di Paolo, Miriam Kyselo, Thomas Fuchs, Shaun Gallagher, Steve Torrance, Sanneke de Haan, Mieke Koppers, Luc De Jaegher, the reviewers, and the editor for their invaluable suggestions and shared experience. This work is supported the Marie-Curie Initial Training Network "TESIS: toward an Embodied Science of InterSubjectivity" (FP7-PEOPLE-2010-ITN, 264828); Marie-Curie Fellowship "INDYNAUTS, Interaction dynamics and autonomy in social cognition" (FP7-PEOPLE-2009-IEF, 253883), and by the Spanish Government project: El concepto de autonomía en bioética e investigación biomédica, MICINN (FFI2008-06348-C02-02/FISO).

REFERENCES

American Psychiatric Association. (2000). *Diagnostic and Statistical Manual of Mental Disorders, 4th Edn. DSM-IV-TR (text revision)*. Washington, DC: American Psychiatric Association.

Baker, M. J. (2000). Incorporating the thematic ritualistic behaviors of children with autism into games: increasing social play interactions with siblings. *J. Posit. Behav. Intervent.* 2, 66–84.

Baker, M. J., Koegel, R. L., and Koegel, L. K. (1998). Increasing the social behavior of young children with autism using their obsessions. *J. Assoc. Pers. Sev. Handicaps* 23, 300–309.

Baranek, G. T. (2002). Efficacy of sensory and motor interventions for children with autism. *J. Autism Dev. Disord.* 32, 397–422.

Baron-Cohen, S. (1989). Do autistic children have obsessions and compulsions? *Br. J. Clin. Psychol.* 28, 193–200.

Baron-Cohen, S. (1995). *Mindblindness: An Essay on Autism and Theory of Mind*. Cambridge, MA: MIT Press.

Baron-Cohen, S. (2002). The extreme male brain theory of autism. *Trends Cogn. Sci.* 6, 248–254.

Baron-Cohen, S. (2003). A mature view of autism. *Trends Cogn. Sci.* 7, 380–383.

Baron-Cohen, S., Leslie, A. M., and Frith, U. (1985). Does the autistic child have a theory of mind? *Cognition* 21, 37–46.

Baron-Cohen, S., Leslie, A. M., and Frith, U. (1986). Mechanical, behavioural and intentional understanding of picture stories in autistic children. *Br. J. Dev. Psychol.* 4, 113–125.

Bauman, M. L. (1992). "Motor dysfunction in autism," in *Movement Disorders in Neurology and Psychiatry*, eds A. B. Joseph and R. R. Young (Boston, MA: Blackwell), 660–663.

Bavelas, J. B., Coates, L., and Johnson, T. (2002). Listener responses as a collaborative process: the role of gaze. *J. Commun.* 52, 566–580.

Begeer, S., Malle, B. F., Nieuwland, M. S., and Keysar, B. (2010). Using theory of mind to represent and take part in social interactions: comparing individuals with high-functioning autism and typically developing controls. *Eur. J. Dev. Psychol.* 7, 104–122.

Bennett, M. R., and Hacker, P. M. S. (2003). *Philosophical Foundations of Neuroscience*. Oxford: Blackwell.

Bertone, A., Mottron, L., Jelenic, P., and Faubert, J. (2003). Motion perception in autism: a 'complex' issue. *J. Cogn. Neurosci.* 15, 218–225.

Bhat, A. N., Landa, R. J., and Galloway, J. C. (2011). Current perspectives on motor functioning in infants, children, and adults with autism spectrum disorders. *Phys. Ther.* 91, 1116–1129.

Blake, R., Turner, L. M., Smoski, M. J., Pozdol, S. L., and Stone, W. L. (2003). Visual recognition of biological motion is impaired in children with autism. *Psychol. Sci.* 14, 151–157.

Bonneh, Y. S., Belmonte, M. K., Pei, F., Iversen, P. E., Kenet, T., Akshoomoff, N., et al. (2008). Cross-modal extinction in a boy with severely autistic behaviour and high verbal intelligence. *Cogn. Neuropsychol.* 25, 635–652.

Boucher, J. (2012). Putting theory of mind in its place: psychological explanations of the socio-emotional-communicative impairments in autistic spectrum disorder. *Autism* 16, 226–246.

Brasic, J. R. (2000). Neuromotor assessment and autistic disorder. *Autism* 4, 287–298.

Brooks, R. (1991). Intelligence without representation. *Artif. Intell.* 47, 139–159.

Caldwell, P. (2006). *Finding You Finding Me.* London: Jessica Kingsley.

Casey, B. J., Gordon, C. T., Mannheim, G. B., and Rumsey, J. (1993). Dysfunctional attention in autistic savants. *J. Clin. Exp. Neuropsychol.* 15, 933–946.

Chamak, B., Bonniau, B., Jaunay, E., and Cohen, D. (2008). What can we learn about autism from autistic persons? *Psychother. Psychosom.* 77, 271–279.

Clark, A., and Chalmers, D. J. (1998). The extended mind. *Analysis* 58, 7–19.

Condon, W. S. (1979). "Neonatal entrainment and enculturation," in *Before Speech*, ed M. Bullowa (Cambridge, MA: Cambridge University Press), 131–148.

Condon, W. S., and Sander, L. W. (1974). Neonate movement is synchronized with adult speech: Interactional participation and language acquisition. *Science* 183, 99–101.

Courchesne, E., Townsend, J., Akshoomoff, N. A., Saitoh, O., Yeung-Courchesne, R., Lincoln, et al. (1994). Impairment in shifting attention in autistic and cerebellar patients. *Behav. Neurosci.* 108, 848–865.

Cui, X., Bryant, D. M., and Reiss, A. L. (2012). NIRS-based hyperscanning reveals increased interpersonal coherence in superior frontal cortex during cooperation. *Neuroimage* 59, 2430–2437.

Davis, M. (ed.). (1982). *Interaction Rhythms. Periodicity in Communicative Behavior.* New York, NY: Human Sciences Press.

De Jaegher, H. (2006). *Social Interaction Rhythm and Participatory Sense-Making: An Embodied, Interactional Approach to Social Understanding, with Implications for Autism.* Unpublished, D. Phil. Thesis, University of Sussex, Brighton.

De Jaegher, H. (2009). Social understanding through direct perception? Yes, by interacting. *Conscious. Cogn.* 18, 535–542.

De Jaegher, H. (2010). "Enaction versus representation: an opinion piece," in *The Embodied Self: Dimensions, Coherence and Disorders*, eds T. Fuchs, H. Sattel, and P. Henningsen (Stuttgart: Schattauer), 218–224.

De Jaegher, H., and Di Paolo, E. (2007). Participatory Sense-Making: an enactive approach to social cognition. *Phenomenol. Cogn. Sci.* 6, 485–507.

De Jaegher, H., Di Paolo, E. A., and Gallagher, S. (2010). Can social interaction constitute social cognition? *Trends Cogn. Sci.* 14, 441–447.

Dickerson, P., Rae, J., Stribling, P., Dautenhahn, K., and Werry, I. (2005). "Autistic children's co-ordination of gaze and talk: re-examining the 'asocial' autist," in *Applying Conversation Analysis*, eds K. Richards and P. Seedhouse (London: Palgrave Macmillan), 19–37.

Dickerson, P., Stribling, P., and Rae, J. (2007). Tapping into interaction: how children with autistic spectrum disorders design and place tapping in relation to activities in progress. *Gesture* 7, 271–303.

Di Paolo, E. A. (2005). Autopoiesis, adaptivity, teleology, agency. *Phenomenol. Cogn. Sci.* 4, 97–125.

Di Paolo, E. A. (2009). Extended life. *Topoi* 28, 9–21.

Di Paolo, E. A., and De Jaegher, H. (2012). The interactive brain hypothesis. *Front. Hum. Neurosci.* 6:163. doi: 10.3389/fnhum.2012.00163

Di Paolo, E. A., Rohde, M., and De Jaegher, H. (2010). "Horizons for the enactive mind: values, social interaction, and play," in *Enaction: Towards a New Paradigm for Cognitive Science*, eds J. Stewart, O. Gapenne, and E. Di Paolo (Cambridge, MA: MIT Press), 33–87.

Dreyfus, H. L. (1992). *What Computers Still Can't Do.* Cambridge, MA: MIT Press.

Donnellan, A., Hill, D. A., and Leary, M. R. (2013). Rethinking autism: implications of sensory and movement differences for understanding and support. *Front. Integr. Neurosci.* 6:124. doi: 10.3389/fnint.2012.00124

Dowd, A., McGinley, J., Taffe, J., and Rinehart, N. (2012). Do Planning and visual integration difficulties underpin motor dysfunction in autism? A kinematic study of young children with autism. *J. Autism Dev. Disord.* 42, 1539–1548.

Dumas, G., Martinerie, J., Soussignan, R., and Nadel, J. (2012). Does brain know who is at the origin of what in an imitative interaction? [Original Research]. *Front. Hum. Neurosci.* 6:128. doi: 10.3389/fnhum.2012.00128

Dumas, G., Nadel, J., Soussignan, R., Martinerie, J., and Garnero, L. (2010). Inter-brain synchronization during social interaction. *PLoS ONE* 5:e12166. doi: 10.1371/journal.pone.0012166

Field, T., Field, T., Sanders, C., and Nadel, J. (2001). Children with autism display more social behaviours after repeated imitation sessions. *Autism* 5, 317–323.

Fogel, A. (1993). *Developing Through Relationships: Origins of Communication, Self and Culture.* London: Harvester Wheatsheaf.

Fournier, K., Hass, C., Naik, S., Lodha, N., and Cauraugh, J. (2010). Motor coordination in autism spectrum disorders: a synthesis and meta-analysis. *J. Autism Dev. Disord.* 40, 1227–1240.

Frith, U. (1989). *Autism. Explaining the Enigma.* Oxford: Blackwell.

Frith, U. (2003). *Autism. Explaining the Enigma, 2nd Edn.* London: Blackwell.

Frith, U. (2008). *Autism: A Very Short Introduction.* Oxford: Oxford University Press.

Frith, U., and Baron-Cohen, S. (1987). "Perception in autistic children," in *Handbook of Autism and Pervasive Developmental Disorders*, eds D. J. Cohen, A. M. Donnellan, and P. Rhea (Winston, MD: Silver Spring), 85–102.

Frith, U., and Happé, F. (1994). Autism: beyond "theory of mind". *Cognition* 50, 115–132.

Frith, U., and Hermelin, B. (1969). The role of visual and motor cues for normal, subnormal and autistic children. *J. Child Psychol. Psychiatry* 10, 153–163.

Frith, U., and Snowling, M. (1983). Reading for meaning and reading for sound in autistic and dyslexic children. *J. Dev. Psychol.* 1, 329–342.

Fuchs, T., and De Jaegher, H. (2009). Enactive intersubjectivity: participatory sense-making and mutual incorporation. *Phenomenol. Cogn. Sci.* 8, 465–486.

Gallagher, S. (1997). Mutual enlightenment: recent phenomenology and cognitive science. *J. Conscious. Stud.* 4, 195–214.

Gallagher, S. (2001). The practice of mind: theory, simulation or primary interaction? *J. Conscious. Stud.* 8, 83–108.

Gallagher, S. (2004a). Understanding interpersonal problems in autism: interaction theory as an alternative to theory of mind. *Philos. Psychiatry Psychol.* 11, 199–217.

Gallagher, S. (2004b). The interpersonal and emotional beginnings of understanding: a review of Peter Hobson's the cradle of thought: exploring the origins of thinking. *Philos. Psychiatry Psychol.* 11, 253–257.

Gallagher, S. (2005). *How the Body Shapes the Mind.* Oxford: Oxford University Press.

Gallagher, S. (2008). Direct perception in the intersubjective context. *Conscious. Cogn.* 17, 535–543.

Gallagher, S. (2009). Two problems of intersubjectivity. *J. Conscious. Stud.* 16, 298–308.

Gallagher, S., and Zahavi, D. (2008). *The Phenomenological Mind: An Introduction to Philosophy of Mind and Cognitive Science.* London: Routledge.

Gepner, B., Deruelle, C., and Grynfeltt, S. (2001). Motion and emotion: a novel approach to the study of face processing by young autistic children. *J. Autism Dev. Disord.* 31, 37–45.

Gepner, B., and Massion, J. (2002). L'autisme: une pathologie du codage temporel? *TIPA* 21, 177–218.

Gepner, B., and Mestre, D. (2002a). Postural reactivity to fast visual motion differentiates autistic from children with Asperger syndrome. *J. Autism Dev. Disord.* 32, 231–238.

Gepner, B., and Mestre, D. (2002b). Rapid visual-motion integration deficit in autism. *Trends Cogn. Sci.* 6, 455.

Gepner, B., Mestre, D., Masson, G., and de Schonen, S. (1995). Postural effects of motion vision in young autistic children. *Neuroreport* 6, 1211–1214.

Gergely, G. (2001). The obscure object of desire: "Nearly, but clearly not, like me": contingency preference in normal children versus children with autism. *Bull. Menninger Clin.* 65, 411–426.

Gergely, G., and Watson, J. S. (1999). "Early socio-emotional development: contingency perception and the social-biofeedback model," in *Early Social Cognition*, ed P. Rochat (Hillsdale, NJ: Erlbaum), 101–137.

Gerland, G. (1996). *A Real Person. Life on the Outside.* London, Souvenir Press.

Ghaziuddin, M., and Butler, E. (1998). Clumsiness in autism and Asperger syndrome: a further report. *J. Intellect. Disabil. Res.* 42, 43–48.

Goldman, A. I. (2012). "Theory of mind," in *The Oxford Handbook of Philosophy of Cognitive Science*, eds E. Margolis, R. Samuels, and S. Stich (Oxford: Oxford University Press), 402–424.

Gowen, E., and Hamilton, A. (2013). Motor abilities in autism: a review using a computational context. *J. Autism Dev. Disord.* 43, 323–344.

Grammer, K., Kruck, K. B., and Magnusson, M. S. (1998). The

courtship dance: patterns of nonverbal synchronization in opposite-sex encounters. *J. Nonverbal Behav.* 22, 3–29.

Grandin, T. (1995). *Thinking in Pictures: and Other Reports from My Life with Autism.* New York, NY: Vintage.

Granic, I. (2000). "The self-organization of parent-child relations: beyond bidirectional models," in *Emotion, Development, and Self-Organization. Dynamic Systems Approaches to Emotional Development*, eds M. D. Lewis and I. Granic (Cambridge: Cambridge University Press), 267–297.

Greenspan, S. I., and Wieder, S. (2006). *Engaging Autism: Using the Floortime Approach to Help Children Relate, Communicate, and Think.* Cambridge, MA: Da Capo Press.

Gutstein, S. E., and Sheely, R. K. (2002). *Relationship Development Intervention with young children. Social and Emotional Development Activities for Asperger Syndrome, Autism, PDD and NLD.* London: Jessica Kingsley.

Haas, R. H., Townsend, J., Courchesne, E., Lincoln, A. J., Schreibman, L., and Yeung_Courchesne, R. (1996). Neurologic abnormalities in infantile autism. *J. Child Neurol.* 11, 84–92.

Hacking, I. (2009). Autistic autobiography. *Philos. Trans. R. Soc. Lond. B Biol. Sci.* 364, 1467–1473.

Hallet, M., Lebiedowska, M. K., Thomas, S. L., Stanhope, S. J., Denckla, M. B., and Rumsey, J. (1993). Locomotion of autistic adults. *Arch. Neurol.* 50, 1304–1308.

Happé, F. (1994). *Autism: An Introduction To Psychological Theory.* Hove: Psychology Press.

Happé, F. (1996). Studying weak central coherence at low levels: children with autism do not succumb to visual illusion. A research note. *J. Child Psychol. Psychiatry* 37, 873–877.

Happé, F. (1997). Central coherence and theory of mind in autism: reading homographs in context. *Br. J. Dev. Psychol.* 15, 1–12.

Happé, F. (1999). Autism: cognitive deficit or cognitive style? *Trends Cogn. Sci.* 3, 216–222.

Happé, F., and Frith, U. (2006). The weak coherence account: detail-focused cognitive style in autism spectrum disorders. *J. Autism Dev. Disord.* 36, 5–25.

Happé, F., and Frith, U. (2009). The beautiful otherness of the autistic mind. *Philos. Trans. R. Soc. Lond. B Biol. Sci.* 364, 1345–1350.

Happé, F., Ronald, A., and Plomin, R. (2006). Time to give up on a single explanation for autism. *Nat. Neurosci.* 9, 1218–1220.

Hendriks-Jansen, H. (1997). The epistemology of autism: making a case for an embodied, dynamic and historical explanation. *Cybern. Syst.* 28, 359–415.

Hermelin, B., and O'Connor, N. (1965). Visual imperception in psychotic children. *Br. J. Psychiatry* 56, 455–460.

Hermelin, B., and O'Connor, N. (1970). *Psychological Experiments with Autistic Children.* Oxford: Pergamon Press.

Hill, E. L. (2004a). Executive dysfunction in autism. *Trends Cogn. Sci.* 8, 26–32.

Hill, E. L. (2004b). Evaluating the theory of executive dysfunction in autism. *Dev. Rev.* 24, 189–233.

Hill, E. L., Crane, L., and Bremner, A. J. (2012). "Developmental disorders and multisensory perception," in *Multisensory Development*, eds A. L. Bremner, D. J. Lewkowicz, and C. Spence (Oxford: Oxford University Press), 273–300.

Hobson, R. P. (1991). Against the theory of 'Theory of Mind'. *Br. J. Dev. Psychol.* 9, 33–51.

Hobson, R. P. (1993). The emotional origins of social understanding. *Philos. Psychol.* 6, 227–249.

Hobson, R. P. (2002). *The Cradle of Thought.* London: Macmillan.

Hobson, R. P., and Lee, A. (1998). Hello and goodbye: a study of social engagement in autism. *J. Autism Dev. Disord.* 28, 117–127.

Hobson, R. P., and Lee, A. (1999). Imitation and identification in autism. *J. Child Psychol. Psychiatry* 40, 649–659.

Hung, D. (1978). Using self-stimulation as reinforcement for autistic children. *J. Autism Child. Schizophr.* 8, 355–366.

Hutto, D. D. (2003). Folk psychological narratives and the case of autism. *Philos. Pap.* 32, 345–361.

Isenhower, R. W., Marsh, K. L., Richardson, M. J., Helt, M., Schmidt, R. C., and Fein, D. (2012). Rhythmic bimanual coordination is impaired in young children with autism spectrum disorder. *Res. Autism Spectr. Disord.* 6, 25–31.

Issartel, J., Marin, L., and Cadopi, M. (2007). Unintended interpersonal coordination: "can we march to the beat of our own drum?" *Neurosci. Lett.* 411, 174–179.

Jaffe, J., Beebe, B., Feldstein, S., Crown, C. L., and Jasnow, M. D. (2001). *Rhythms of Dialogue in Infancy: Coordinated Timing in Development (Vol. 66).* Oxford: Blackwell.

Jonas, H. (1966). *The Phenomenon of Life. Toward a Philosophical Biology.* Evanston, IL: Northwestern University Press.

Jones, V., and Prior, M. (1985). Motor imitation abilities and neurological signs in autistic children. *J. Autism Dev. Disord.* 15, 37–45.

Jones, W., Carr, K., and Klin, A. (2008). Absence of preferential looking to the eyes of approaching adults predicts level of social disability in 2-year-old toddlers with autism spectrum disorder. *Arch. Gen. Psychiatry* 65, 946–954.

Kanner, L. (1973). *Childhood Psychoses: Initial Studies and New Insights.* Washington, DC: V. H. Winston.

Kelso, J. A. S. (1995). *Dynamic Patterns: The Self-Organization of Brain and Behaviour.* Cambridge, MA: MIT Press.

Kelso, J. A. S. (2009a). "Synergies: atoms of brain and behavior," in *Progress in Motor Control: A Multidisciplinary Perspective*, ed D. Sternad (New York, NY: Springer), 83–92.

Kelso, J. A. S. (2009b). "Coordination dynamics," in *Encyclopedia of Complexity and System Science*, ed R. A. Meyers (Heidelberg: Springer), 1537–1564.

Kendon, A. (1990). *Conducting Interaction: Patterns of Behavior in Focused Encounters.* Cambridge, Cambridge University Press.

Kern, J. K., Trivedi, M. H., Garver, C. R., Grannemann, B. D., Andrews, A. A., Savla, J. S., et al. (2006). The pattern of sensory processing abnormalities in autism. *Autism* 10, 480–494.

Klin, A., Danovitch, J. H., Merz, A. B., and Volkmar, F. R. (2007). Circumscribed interests in higher functioning individuals with autism spectrum disorders: an exploratory study. *Res. Pract. Pers. Sev. Disabil.* 32, 89–100.

Klin, A., Jones, W., Schultz, R., and Volkmar, F. (2003). The enactive mind, or from actions to cognition: lessons from autism. *Philos. Trans. R. Soc. Lond. B Biol. Sci.* 358, 345–360.

Klin, A., Jones, W., Schultz, R., Volkmar, F., and Cohen, D. (2002). Visual fixation patterns during viewing of naturalistic social situations as predictors of social competence in individuals with autism. *Arch. Gen. Psychiatry* 59, 809–816.

Klin, A., Lin, D. J., Gorrindo, P., Ramsay, G., and Jones, W. (2009). Two-year-olds with autism orient to non-social contingencies rather than biological motion. *Nature* 459, 257–261.

Klin, A., McPartland, J. C., and Volkmar, F. R. (1997). "Asperger's syndrome," in *Handbook of Autism and Pervasive Developmental Disorders*, eds D. J. Cohen, and F. R. Volkmar (New York, NY: Wiley), 88–125.

Klin, A., Volkmar, F., and Sparrow, S. S. (1992). Autistic social dysfunction: some limitations of the theory of mind hypothesis. *J. Child Psychol. Psychiatry* 33, 861–876.

Konvalinka, I., and Roepstorff, A. (2012). The two-brain approach: how can mutually interacting brains teach us something about social interaction? [Review]. *Front. Hum. Neurosci.* 6:215. doi: 10.3389/fnhum.2012.00215

Lakoff, G., and Johnson, M. H. (1999). *Philosophy in the Flesh: The Embodied Mind and Its Challenge to Western Thought.* New York, NY: Basic Books.

Landry, R., and Bryson, S. E. (2004). Impaired disengagement of attention in young children with autism. *J. Child Psychol. Psychiatry* 45, 1115–1122.

Leary, M. R., and Donnellan, A. (2012). *Autism: Sensory-Movement Differences and Diversity.* Cambridge: Cambridge Book Review Press.

Leary, M. R., and Hill, D. A. (1996). Moving on: autism and movement disturbance. *Ment. Retard.* 34, 39–53.

Lewis, M. D., and Granic, I. (eds.). (2000). *Emotion, Development, and Self-Organization Dynamical Systems Approaches to Emotional Development, 1st Edn.* Cambridge, MA: Cambridge University Press.

Lindenberger, U., Li, S., Gruber, W., and Müller, V. (2009). Brains swinging in concert: cortical phase synchronization while playing guitar. *BMC Neurosci.* 10:22. doi: 10.1186/1471-2202-10-22

Liss, M., Saulnier, C., Fein, D., and Kinsbourne, M. (2006). Sensory and attention abnormalities in autistic spectrum disorders. *Autism* 10, 155–172.

Lombardo, M., Chakrabarti, B., Bullmore, E., and Baron-Cohen, S. (2010). Shared neural circuits for mentalizing about the self and others. *J. Cogn. Neurosci.* 277, 1623–1635.

López, B., and Leekam, S. R. (2003). Do children with autism fail to process information in context? *J. Child Psychol. Psychiatry* 44, 285–300.

López, B., Leekam, S. R., and Arts, G. R. J. (2008). How central is central coherence? *Autism* 12, 159–171.

Lovaas, I., Newsom, C., and Hickman, C. (1987). Self-stimulatory behavior and perceptual reinforcement. *J. Appl. Behav. Anal.* 20, 45–68.

Maduell, M., and Wing, A. M. (2007). The dynamics of ensemble: the case for flamenco. *Psychol. Music* 35, 591–627.

Malle, B. F. (2002). "The relation between language and theory of mind in development and evolution," in *The Evolution of Language out of Pre-Language*, eds T. Givón and B. F. Malle (Amsterdam: Benjamins), 265–284.

Malloch, S., and Trevarthen, C. (eds.). (2009). *Communicative Musicality: Exploring the Basis of Human Companionship*. Oxford: Oxford University Press.

Malloch, S. N. (1999). Mothers and infants and communicative musicality. *Musicae Sci.* 1999–2000, 29–57. (Special issue).

Mari, M., Castiello, U., Marks, D., Marraffa, C., and Prior, M. (2003). The reach-to-grasp movement in children with autism spectrum disorder. *Philos. Trans. R. Soc. Lond. B Biol. Sci.* 358, 393–403.

Markram, K., and Markram, H. (2010). The intense world theory - a unifying theory of the neurobiology of autism. *Front. Hum. Neurosci.* 4:224. doi: 10.3389/fnhum.2010.00224

Markram, H., Rinaldi, T., and Markram, K. (2007). The intense world syndrome – an alternative hypothesis for autism. *Front. Neurosci.* 1, 77–96. doi: 10.3389/neuro.01.1.1.006.2007

Marsh, K. L., Isenhower, R. W., Richardson, M. J., Helt, M., Verbalis, A. D., Schmidt, R. C., et al. (2013). Autism and social disconnection in interpersonal rocking. *Front. Integr. Neurosci.* 7:4. doi: 10.3389/fnint.2013.00004

Marsh, K. L., Richardson, M. J., Baron, R. M., and Schmidt, R. C. (2006). Contrasting approaches to perceiving and acting with others. *Ecol. Psychol.* 18, 1–38.

Martineau, J., Schmitz, C., Assaiante, C., Blanc, R., and Barthélémy, C. (2004). Impairment of a cortical event-related desynchronisation during a bimanual load-lifting task in children with autistic disorder. *Neurosci. Lett.* 367, 298–303.

McGann, M. (2007). Enactive theorists do it on purpose. *Phenomenol. Cogn. Sci.* 6, 463–483.

McGann, M., and De Jaegher, H. (2009). Self-other contingencies: enacting social perception. *Phenomenol. Cogn. Sci.* 8, 417–437.

McGeer, V. (2001). Psycho-practice, psycho-theory and the contrastive case of autism. How practices of mind become second-nature. *J. Conscious. Stud.* 8, 109–132.

Mercier, C., Mottron, L., and Belleville, S. (2000). A psychosocial study on restricted interests in high functioning persons with pervasive developmental disorders. *Autism* 4, 406–425.

Meyer, J. A., and Hobson, R. P. (2005). Orientation to self and other: the case of autism. *Interact. Stud.* 5, 221–244.

Michael, J. (2011). Interactionism and mindreading. *Rev. Philos. Psychol.* 2, 559–578.

Milne, E., Swettenham, J., Hansen, P., Campbell, R., Jeffries, H., and Plaisted, K. (2002). High motion-coherence thresholds in children with autism. *J. Child Psychol. Psychiatry* 43, 255–263.

Minshew, N., Goldstein, G., and Siegel, D. J. (1997). Neuropsychologic functioning in autism: profile of a complex information processing disorder. *J. Int. Neuropsychol. Soc.* 3, 303–316.

Minshew, N. J., Luna, B., and Sweeny, J. A. (1999). Oculomotor evidence for neocortical systems but not cerebellar dysfunction in autism. *Neurology* 52, 917–922.

Moran, N. (2007). *Measuring Musical Interaction: Analysing Communication in Embodied Musical Behaviour*, Unpublished, D. Phil Thesis, Open University, Milton Keynes.

Moreno, A., and Etxeberria, A. (2005). Agency in natural and artificial systems. *Artif. Life* 11, 161–176.

Mottron, L. (2011). Changing perceptions: the power of autism. *Nature* 479, 33–35.

Mottron, L., and Burack, J. (2001). "Enhanced perceptual functioning in the development of autism," in *The Development of Autism: Perspectives from Theory and Research*, eds J. Burack, T. Charman, N. Yirmiya, and P. Zelazo (Mahwah, NJ: Erlbaum), 131–148.

Mottron, L., Dawson, M., Soulières, I., Hubert, B., and Burack, J. (2006). Enhanced perceptual functioning in autism: an update, and eight principles of autistic perception. *J. Autism Dev. Disord.* 36, 27–43.

Mottron, L., Peretz, I., and Ménard, E. (2000). Local and global processing of music in high-functioning persons with autism: beyond central coherence? *J. Child Psychol. Psychiatry 41*, 1057–1065.

Müller, R. A., Pierce, K., Ambrose, J. B., Allen, G., and Courchesne, E. (2001). Atypical patterns of cerebral motor activation in autism: a functional magnetic resonance study. *Biol. Psychiatry* 49, 665–676.

Nadel, J., Carchon, I., Kervella, C., Marcelli, D., and Réserbat-Plantey, D. (1999). Expectancies for social contingency in 2-month-olds. *Dev. Sci.* 2, 164–173.

Nadel, J., Croué, S., Mattlinger, M.-J., Canet, P., Hudelot, C., Lécuyer, C., et al. (2000). Do children with autism have expectancies about the social behaviour of unfamiliar people? A pilot study using the still face paradigm. *Autism* 4, 133–145.

Noens, I., and van Berckelaer-Onnes, I. (2004). Making sense in a fragmentary world: communication in people with autism and learning disability. *Autism* 8, 197–218.

Noens, I., and van Berckelaer-Onnes, I. (2005). Captured by details: sense-making, language and communication in autism. *J. Commun. Disord.* 38, 123–141.

O'Regan, J. K., and Noë, A. (2001). A sensorimotor account of vision and visual consciousness. *Behav. Brain Sci.* 24, 883–917.

Oullier, O., de Guzman, G. C., Jantzen, K. J., Lagarde, J., and Kelso, J. A. S. (2008). Social coordination dynamics: measuring human bonding. *Soc. Neurosci.* 3, 178–192.

Ozonoff, S., and Miller, J. N. (1995). Teaching theory of mind: a new approach to social skills training for individuals with autism. *J. Autism Dev. Disord.* 25, 415–433.

Ozonoff, S., Pennington, B. F., and Rogers, S. J. (1991). Executive function deficits in high-functioning autistic individuals: relationship to theory of mind. *J. Child Psychol. Psychiatry* 32, 1081–1105.

Papadopoulos, N., McGinley, J., Tonge, B., Bradshaw, J., Saunders, K., Murphy, A., et al. (2011). Motor proficiency and emotional/behavioural disturbance in autism and Asperger's disorder: another piece of the neurological puzzle? *Autism* 16, 627–640.

Papadopoulos, N., McGinley, J., Tonge, B. J., Bradshaw, J. L., Saunders, K., and Rinehart, N. J. (2012). An investigation of upper limb motor function in high functioning autism and Asperger's disorder using a repetitive Fitts' aiming task. *Res. Autism Spectr. Disord.* 6, 286–292.

Pfeiffer, U. J., Timmermans, B., Vogeley, K., Frith, C. D., and Schilbach, L. (2013). Towards a neuroscience of social interaction. *Front. Hum. Neurosci.* 7:22. doi: 10.3389/fnhum.2013.00022

Piaget, J. (1936). *La Naissance de l'Intelligence chez l'Enfant*. Neuchâtel: Delachaux.

Plaisted, K., Swettenham, J., and Rees, L. (1999). Children with autism show local precedence in a divided attention task and global precedence in a selective attention task. *J. Child Psychol. Psychiatry* 40, 733–742.

Polanyi, M. (1958). *Personal Knowledge. Towards a Post Critical Epistemology*. London: Routledge and Kegan Paul.

Rapin, I. (1997). Autism. *New Engl. J. Med.* 337, 97–104.

Reddy, V. (2003). On being the object of attention: implications for self-other consciousness. *Trends Cogn. Sci.* 7, 397–402.

Reddy, V. (2008). *How Infants Know Minds*. Cambridge, MA: Harvard University Press.

Reddy, V., Hay, D., Murray, L., and Trevarthen, C. (1997). "Communication in infancy: mutual regulation of affect and attention," in *Infant Development: Recent Advances*, eds G. Bremner, A. Slater, and G. Butterworth (Hove: Psychology Press), 247–273.

Reddy, V., and Morris, P. (2004). Participants don't need theories: knowing minds in engagement. *Theory Psychol.* 14, 647–665.

Reddy, V., Williams, E., and Vaughan, A. (2002). Sharing humour and laughter in autism and Down's syndrome. *Br. J. Psychol.* 93, 219–242.

Richardson, M. J., Marsh, K. L., Isenhower, R. W., Goodman, J. R. L., and Schmidt, R. C. (2007). Rocking together: dynamics of intentional and unintentional interpersonal coordination. *Hum. Mov. Sci.* 26, 867–891.

Riley, M. A., Richardson, M., Shockley, K., and Ramenzoni, V. C. (2011). Interpersonal synergies. *Front. Psychol.* 2:38. doi: 10.3389/fpsyg.2011.00038

Rimland, B. (1964). *Infantile Autism. The Syndrome and Its Implications for a Neural Theory of Behavior*. New York, NY: Appleton-Century-Crofts.

Rinehart, N. J., Bellgrave, M. A., Tonge, B. J., Brereton, A. V., Howells-Rankin, D., and Bradshaw, J. L. (2006). An examination of movement kinematics in young people with high-functioning autism and Asperger's Disorder: further evidence for a motor planning deficit. *J. Autism Dev. Disord.* 36, 757–767.

Rinehart, N. J., Bradshaw, J. L., Brereton, A. V., and Tonge, B. J. (2001). Movement preparation in high-functioning autism and Asperger disorder: a serial choice reaction time task involving motor reprogramming. *J. Autism Dev. Disord.* 31, 79–88.

Robinson, S., Goddard, L., Dritschel, B., Wisley, M., and Howlin, P. (2009). Executive functions in children with autism spectrum disorders. *Brain Cogn.* 71, 362–368.

Robledo, J., Donnellan, A. M., and Strandt-Conroy, K. (2012). An exploration of sensory and movement differences from the perspective of individuals with autism. [Original Research]. *Front. Integr. Neurosci.* 6:107. doi: 10.3389/fnint.2012.00107

Roeyers, H., and Demurie, E. (2010). How impaired is mind-reading in high-functioning adolescents and adults with autism? *Eur. J. Dev. Psychol.* 7, 123–134.

Rogers, S. J., and Ozonoff, S. (2005). Annotation: what do we know about sensory dysfunction in autism? A critical review of the empirical evidence. *J. Child Psychol. Psychiatry* 46, 1255–1268.

Russell, J. (ed.). (1998). *Autism as an Executive Disorder.* Oxford: Oxford University Press.

Russell, J., Mauthner, N., Sharpe, S., and Tidswell, T. (1991). The 'windows' task as a measure of strategic deception in preschoolers and autistic subjections. *Br. J. Dev. Psychol.* 9, 331–349.

Sacks, O. (1985). *The Man Who Mistook His Wife for a Hat, and Other Clinical Tales.* London: Picador.

Sacks, O. (1995). *An Anthropologist on Mars.* New York, NY: Vintage.

Samaritter, R., and Payne, H. (2013). Kinaesthetic intersubjectivity: a dance informed contribution to self-other relatedness and shared experience in non-verbal psychotherapy with an example from autism. *Arts Psychother.* 40, 143–150.

Savarese, R. J. (2010). Toward a postcolonial neurology: autism, Tito Mukhopadhyay, and a new geopoetics of the body. *J. Lit. Cult. Disabil. Stud.* 4, 273–290.

Schilbach, L. (2010). A second-person approach to other minds. *Nat. Rev. Neurosci.* 11, 449.

Schilbach, L., Timmermans, B., Reddy, V., Costall, A., Bente, G., Schlicht, T., et al. (in press). Towards a second-person neuroscience. *Behav. Brain Sci.*

Schmidt, R. C., and O'Brien, B. (1997). Evaluating the dynamics of unintended interpersonal coordination. *Ecol. Psychol.* 9, 189–206.

Schmitz, C., Martineau, J., Barthélémy, C., and Assaiante, C. (2003). Motor control and children with autism: deficit of anticipatory function? *Neurosci. Lett.* 348, 17–20.

Scollon, R. (1981). "The rhythmic integration of ordinary talk," in *Georgetown University Round Table on Languages and Linguistics*, ed D. Tannen (Washington, DC: Georgetown University Press), 335–349.

Sebanz, N., Bekkering, H., and Knoblich, G. (2006). Joint action: bodies and minds moving together. *Trends Cogn. Sci.* 10, 70–76.

Shah, A., and Frith, U. (1983). An islet of ability in autistic children: a research note. *J. Child Psychol. Psychiatry* 24, 613–620.

Shah, A., and Frith, U. (1993). Why do autistic individuals show superior performance on the block design task? *J. Child Psychol. Psychiatry* 34, 1351–1364.

Shanker, S. (2004). Autism and the dynamic developmental model of emotions. *Philos. Psychiatry Psychol.* 11, 219–233.

Shanker, S., and King, B. J. (2002). The emergence of a new paradigm in ape language research. *Behav. Brain Sci.* 25, 605–656.

Sheets-Johnstone, M. (1999a). *The Primacy of Movement.* Amsterdam: John Benjamins.

Sheets-Johnstone, M. (1999b). Emotion and movement: a beginning empirical-phenomenological analysis of their relationship. *J. Conscious. Stud.* 6, 259–277.

Sheridan, J., and McAuley, J. D. (1997). "Rhythm as a cognitive skill: temporal processing deficits in autism," in *Proceedings of the Fourth Australiasian Cognitive Science Conference* (Newcastle, NSW).

Shic, F., Bradshaw, J., Klin, A., Scassellati, B., and Chawarska, K. (2011). Limited activity monitoring in toddlers with autism spectrum disorder. *Brain Res.* 1380, 246–254.

Sigman, M., Yirmiya, N., and Capps, L. (1995). "Social and cognitive understanding in high-functioning children with autism," in *Learning and Cognition in Autism*, eds E. Schopler and G. B. Mesibov (New York, NY: Plenum).

Smith, R., and Sharp, J. (in press). Fascination and isolation: a grounded theory exploration of unusual sensory experiences in adults with Asperger syndrome. *J. Autism Dev. Disord.* 1–20. doi: 10.1007/s10803-012-1633-6

Spiker, M. A., Lin, C. E., Van Dyke, M., and Wood, J. J. (2012). Restricted interests and anxiety in children with autism. *Autism* 16, 306–320.

St. Clair, C., Danon-Boileau, L., and Trevarthen, C. (2007). "Signs of autism in infancy: Sensitivity for rhythms of expression in communication," in *Signs of autism in infants: Recognition and Early Intervention*, ed S. Acquarone (London: Karnac), 21–45.

Sterck, E. H. M., and Begeer, S. (2010). Theory of mind: specialized capacity or emergent property? *Eur. J. Dev. Psychol.* 7, 1–16.

Stern, D. N. (2002/1977). *The First Relationship: Infant and Mother, 2nd Edn.* London: Harvard University Press.

Stribling, P., Rae, J., and Dickerson, P. (2005/2006). "Spelling it out": the design, delivery and placement of 'echolalic' utterances by a child with an autism spectrum disorder. *Issu. Appl. Linguist.* 15, 3–32.

Teitelbaum, O., Benton, T., Shah, P. K., Prince, A., Kelly, J. L., and Teitelbaum, P. (2004). Eshkol-Wachman movement notation in diagnosis: the early detection of Asperger's syndrome. *Proc. Natl. Acad. Sci. U.S.A.* 101, 11909–11914.

Teitelbaum, P., Teitelbaum, O., Nye, J., Fryman, J., and Maurer, R. (1998). Movement analysis in infancy may be useful for early diagnosis of autism. *Proc. Natl. Acad. Sci. U.S.A.* 95, 13982–13987.

Thelen, E., and Smith, L. B. (1994). *A Dynamic Systems Approach to the Development of Cognition and Action*. London: Bradford.

Thompson, E. (2005). Sensorimotor subjectivity and the enactive approach to experience. *Phenomenol. Cogn. Sci.* 4, 407–427.

Thompson, E. (2007). *Mind in Life: Biology, Phenomenology, and the Sciences of Mind.* Cambridge, MA: Harvard University Press.

Thompson, E., and Varela, F. J. (2001). Radical embodiment: neural dynamics and consciousness. *Trends Cogn. Sci.* 5, 418–425.

Torrance, S., and Froese, T. (2011). An inter-enactive approach to agency: participatory sense-making, dynamics, and sociality. *Humana Mente* 15, 21–53.

Torres, E. B. (2012). Atypical signatures of motor variability found in an individual with ASD. *Neurocase.* doi: 10.1080/13554794.2011.654224. [Epub ahead of print].

Townsend, J., Harris, N. S., and Courchesne, E. (1996). Visual attention abnormalities in autism: delayed orienting to location. *J. Int. Neuropsychol. Soc.* 2, 541–550.

Trevarthen, C., and Daniel, S. (2005). Disorganized rhythm and synchrony: early signs of autism and Rett syndrome. *Brain Dev.* 27(Suppl. 1), S25–S34.

Trevarthen, C., and Malloch, S. N. (2002). Musicality and music before three: human vitality and invention shared with pride. *Zero Three* 23, 10–18.

Tronick, E. Z., and Cohn, J. F. (1989). Infant-mother face-to-face interaction: age and gender differences in coordination and the occurrences of miscoordination. *Child Dev.* 60, 85–92.

Turner, M. (1999). Annotation: repetitive behaviour in autism: a review of psychological research. *J. Child Psychol. Psychiatry* 40, 839–849.

van Gelder, T. (1999). "Wooden iron? Husserlian phenomenology meets cognitive science," in *Naturalizing Phenomenology,* eds J. Petitot, F. J. Varela, B. Pachoud, and J.-M. Roy (Stanford, CA: Stanford University Press), 245–265.

van Orden, G. C., Holden, J. G., and Turvey, M. T. (2003). Self-organization of cognitive performance. *J. Exp. Psychol.* 132, 331–350.

van Orden, G. C., Holden, J. G., and Turvey, M. T. (2005). Human cognition and 1/f scaling. *J. Exp. Psychol.* 134, 117–123.

Varela, F. J. (1979). *Principles of Biological Autonomy.* New York, NY: Elsevier (North Holland).

Varela, F. J. (1991). "Organism: a meshwork of selfless selves," in *Organism and the Origin of Self,* ed A. Tauber (Dordrecht: Kluwer), 79–107.

Varela, F. J. (1996). Neurophenomenology: a methodological remedy for the hard problem. *J. Conscious. Stud.* 3, 330–349.

Varela, F. J. (1997). Patterns of life: intertwining identity and cognition. *Brain Cogn.* 34, 72–87.

Varela, F. J. (1999). "The specious present: a neurophenomenology of time consciousness," in *Naturalizing Phenomenology: Issues in Contemporary Phenomenology and Cognitive Science*, eds J. Petitot, F. J. Varela, B. Pachoud, and J.-M. Roy (Stanford, CA: Stanford University Press), 266–314.

Varela, F. J., Thompson, E., and Rosch, E. (1991). *The Embodied Mind: Cognitive Science and Human Experience, 6th Edn.* Cambridge, MA: MIT Press.

Vermeulen, P. (2001). *Autistic Thinking. This is The Title.* London: Jessica Kingsley.

Vilensky, J. A., Damasio, A. R., and Maurer, R. G. (1981). Gait disturbances in patients with autistic behavior: a preliminary study. *Arch. Neurol.* 38, 646–649.

Volkmar, F., Chawarska, K., and Klin, A. (2005). Autism in infancy and early childhood. *Annu. Rev. Psychol.* 56, 315–336.

Volkmar, F. R., Lord, C., Bailey, A., Schultz, R. T., and Klin, A. (2004). Autism and pervasive developmental disorders. *J. Child Psychol. Psychiatry* 45, 135–170.

Watson, J. (1979). "Perception of contingency as a determinant of social responsiveness," in *The Origin of the Infant's Responsiveness,* ed E. Thoman (New York, NY: Erlbaum), 33–64.

Weber, A., and Varela, F. J. (2002). Life after Kant: natural purposes and the autopoietic foundations of biological individuality. *Phenomenol. Cogn. Sci.* 1, 97–125.

Wheeler, M. (2010). "In defence of extended functionalism," in *The Extended Mind,* ed R. Menary (Harvard, MA: MIT Press), 245–270.

Whyatt, C., and Craig, C. (2012). Motor skills in children aged 7–10 years, diagnosed with autism spectrum disorder. *J. Autism Dev. Disord.* 42, 1799–1809.

Wigram, T., and Gold, C. (2006). Music therapy in the assessment and treatment of autistic spectrum disorder: clinical application and research evidence. *Child Care Health Dev.* 32, 535–542.

Williams, D. (1992). *Nobody Nowhere.* London: Jessica Kingsley.

Winfree, A. T. (2001). *The Geometry of Biological Time.* London: Springer.

Wing, L., and Gould, J. (1979). Severe impairments of social interaction and associated abnormalities in children: epidemiology and classification. *J. Autism Dev. Disord.* 9, 11–29.

Zahavi, D., and Parnas, J. (2003). Conceptual problems in infantile autism research. Why cognitive science needs phenomenology. *J. Conscious. Stud.* 10, 53–71.

Conflict of Interest Statement: The author declares that the research was conducted in the absence of any commercial or financial relationships that could be construed as a potential conflict of interest.

10

Autism as a developmental disorder in intentional movement and affective engagement

***Colwyn Trevarthen* [1]* *and Jonathan T. Delafield-Butt* [2]**

[1] *Department of Psychology, College of Humanities and Social Sciences, University of Edinburgh, Edinburgh, UK*
[2] *Early Years, School of Education, Faculty of Humanities and Social Sciences, University of Strathclyde, Glasgow, UK*

Edited by:
Elizabeth B. Torres, Rutgers University, USA

Reviewed by:
Antonio Pereira, Federal University of Rio Grande do Norte, Brazil
Nandakumar Narayanan, Yale, USA

****Correspondence:***
Colwyn Trevarthen, Department of Psychology, College of Humanities and Social Sciences, University of Edinburgh, 7 George Square, Edinburgh EH8 9JZ, UK
e-mail: c.trevarthen@ed.ac.uk

We review evidence that autistic spectrum disorders have their origin in early prenatal failure of development in systems that program timing, serial coordination and prospective control of movements, and that regulate affective evaluations of experiences. There are effects in early infancy, before medical diagnosis, especially in motor sequencing, selective or exploratory attention, affective expression and intersubjective engagement with parents. These are followed by retardation of cognitive development and language learning in the second or third year, which lead to a diagnosis of ASD. The early signs relate to abnormalities that have been found in brain stem systems and cerebellum in the embryo or early fetal stage, before the cerebral neocortex is functional, and they have clear consequences in infancy when neocortical systems are intensively elaborated. We propose, with evidence of the disturbances of posture, locomotion and prospective motor control in children with autism, as well as of their facial expression of interest and affect, and attention to other persons' expressions, that examination of the psychobiology of motor affective disorders, rather than later developing cognitive or linguistic ones, may facilitate early diagnosis. Research in this area may also explain how intense interaction, imitation or "expressive art" therapies, which respond intimately with motor activities, are effective at later stages. Exceptional talents of some autistic people may be acquired compensations for basic problems with expectant self-regulations of movement, attention and emotion.

Keywords: autism, motor development, emotional expression, communication, education, therapy

INTRODUCTION TO A DIFFERENT, PSYCHOBIOLOGICAL APPROACH

> "**Generality of the problem of Syntax**: Not only speech, but all skilled acts seem to involve the same problems of serial ordering . . . Analysis of the nervous mechanisms underlying order in the more primitive acts, may contribute ultimately to the resolution even of the physiology of logic."
>
> (Lashley, 1951, pp. 121–122)
>
> "**A Different Approach to the Problem:** In so far as an organism perceives a given object, it is prepared to respond with reference to it. This preparation-to-respond is absent in an organism that has failed to perceive."
>
> (Sperry, 1952, p. 296)

Lashley (1951) and Sperry (1952) observed that perception, intelligent action and thinking depend upon impulses that move the body purposefully. The animal brain contributes systematic and serial organization, in time and space, to muscle activity under expectant perceptual and emotional control. It is always active, not passively reactive to stimuli. Nor is the human brain ever animated by thoughts of external events alone. All mental and behavioral skills depend on preparation to respond with serial ordering of acts. "The sole product of brain function is motor coordination" (Sperry, 1952, p. 297). This is a psychobiological theory of motives and affects in the mind, clearly articulated before the advent of the "cognitive revolution" that divorced mind from vital body in the 1960's (Miller, 2003).

The motor theory of consciousness was inspired by the research of Charles Sherrington (1906) on "the integrative action of the nervous system." It has support from developmental neurobiology and neuroembryology (Trevarthen, 1986a; Prechtl, 2001), from ethology of the adaptive action patterns of animals and how they communicate emotional evaluations for social cooperation (Gallistel, 1980; Marler, 1984; Fentress and Gadbois, 2001; Panksepp, 2005), and from infant psychology and communication (Trevarthen, 1986b, 2001a, 2009a; Stern, 2000, 2010).

Research focused on cognitive disorders of perceptual information processing, selective awareness, and representational thinking articulated in language, all of which skills develop after infancy—disregards the developmental foundations of experience in motor coordination, and in the expression of vital states as emotions for regulation of social life. In an animal's perceived world, its "Umwelt" (von Uexküll, 1957), conceptions of objects are created by the intentional subject's attempts to locate and perceive "sign stimuli" detected in the environment by dedicated receptors (Buchanan, 2008; Berthoz and Christen, 2009). Self-regulation of knowing, with emotional assessments of risks and benefits, becomes in humans the source of cultural sign systems of social cooperation—for sustaining health, for reproduction and for learning how to use environmental resources collaboratively (Sebeok, 1990; Trevarthen, 1990; Stern, 2010; Porges and Furman, 2011).

We relate autistic disturbance of cognitive functions to growth errors in creative agency attributable to events in brain development of embryo, fetus and infant (Trevarthen et al., 1998, 2006; Trevarthen, 2000; Trevarthen and Daniel, 2005; St. Clair et al., 2007). We address development of the autopoetic subcortical neurobiology that makes possible manifestations of intentions and emotions before birth (Delafield-Butt and Trevarthen, 2013), and the cooperation of movements after birth within an intimate infant-parent intentional system (Sander, 2008), which sustains itself by the primary emotional processes of consciousness (Solms and Panksepp, 2012). The motivation of the developing human organism is environment expectant, ready for sharing agency and emotions in movement, but this sharing is "anoetic"; that is, not dependent on acquired categorical knowledge of the structure and uses of the environment (Vandekerckhove and Panksepp, 2011). The infant is adapted physically and motivated psychologically to receive not only vital care in attachment to the mother, but also "companionship" for the young mind's growing purposes in imaginative movement and the uptake of new experience (Trevarthen, 2005, 2013). Shared health and meaning are created in human awareness by primary processes of joint agency and emotional sympathy between the movements of human bodies (Trevarthen, 1986b, 2012; Reddy, 2008; Stuart, 2010).

We need to have a clear conception of the nature of animal movement and its affective sociability if we wish to understand how children with autism fail to organize and time their movements effectively, hesitate to become affectively engaged with their parents as infants (Muratori and Maestro, 2007), and fall behind their peers in learning how to share and use knowledge of the human world playfully (Reddy et al., 2002).

Based on evidence of early neural growth errors in core brainstem systems during fetal ontogenesis, and on new evidence of disturbance of primary *prospective motor control* of expressive action, we present the following hypothesis on the etiology of autism for testing and argument:

(1) A primary cause of autism spectrum disorders is an error in early growth of intrinsic motive and motor systems of the brainstem during prenatal ontogenesis.
(2) This interferes with efficient integration of sensory information with motor timing, and is accompanied by disturbance of autonomic functions, disrupting timing and control of prospective sensory perception in movement as well as vital regulation of functions within the body. All these disorders become most obvious in early childhood, when a toddler normally gains many new powers of movement in engagement with the environment, including speech.
(3) Social isolation, socio-emotional and cognitive delay, and language disorder in children and adults with autism are *secondary consequences* developed within socio-emotional systems as experience-dependent compensations for primary sensori-motor and affective integration errors and poorly regulated motor intentions. These compensations are elaborated mainly by cortical systems that grow after birth.

AUTISM IS A DISORDER OF SELF-RELATED MOTOR-AFFECTIVE PROCESSES, WHICH CONTROL DEVELOPMENT OF SHARED COGNITIVE REPRESENTATIONS

People diagnosed as autistic exhibit disabilities in regulation of the order and timing of moving, in the feelings of their bodies and emotional control, in selective expectation of objects for experience, in attention to other persons expressions, in the playfulness and humor of their social engagements, and in collaborative learning (Baron-Cohen et al., 2000; Reddy et al., 2002, 2010; Rogers and Williams, 2006; Mundy et al., 2009; Hobson and Hobson, 2011; Torres, 2013). cognitive disabilities attributed to failure in special modular mental functions of perceptual selection, of conceptual grouping, or of a capacity to conceive and think about the emotions behind other persons" face expressions, orientations and practical actions, or to imagine the representational contents of their minds (Baron-Cohen et al., 1985; Frith, 1989/2003; Morton, 2004), may only be identified after infancy. Similarly, definition of autistic disturbance by reference to neuropsychological tests that identify faults in praxis, gnosis, reasoning and language in adults after local brain injury ignores the large transformations in brain function and behavior that take place during psychological development (Karmiloff-Smith, 2009; Thomas and Karmiloff-Smith, 2002; Karmiloff-Smith, 2009).

We propose that faults in higher mind functions of persons with autism arise out of disorder in the early development of primary, non-reflective sensori-motor factors that regulate moving-with-awareness of an integrated Self. These affect vitality dynamics, the qualities of motor control that express essential expectancies of action and enable communication of emotion in purposes (Stern, 2010; Gowen, 2012; Gowen and Hamilton, 2013; Rochat et al., 2013). The primary processes of mental agency do not require conceptual representation or explicit reference to external events; they are primary conscious experience (Vandekerckhove and Panksepp, 2011). Growth errors found in formation of brain stem motor control and emotional systems of the embryo and fetus (Prechtl, 2001; Rodier and Arndt, 2005), interfere with the maturation of sensory-motor skills at significant periods in a child's early life, impairing cultural learning mediated in postnatal elaborations of the neocortex and dependent on creative emotional engagement with human company (Trevarthen et al., 2006). Interpreting autism in these terms requires attention to the environment–expectant processes of morphogenesis by which human bodies and brains are formed *in utero*, with special adaptations for intersubjective communication (Trevarthen, 2001a,b), and information on how additional brain networks grow and learn after birth (Thomas and Karmiloff-Smith, 2002). This is a "developmental psychobiology," not a "developmental cognitive neuroscience" based on the neuropsychological definition of disorders inferred retrospectively from effects of damage to parts of the adult brain (Baron-Cohen et al., 2000). Psychological theory must also explain how individuals with high-functioning autism and Asperger's disorder perform certain feats of perception or action with remarkable precision, but with inadequate awareness of the context, or "weak central coherence," in their self-related conceptions and plans for action (Frith, 1989/2003; Rinehart et al., 2001).

No single genetic, neurobiological or environmental factor has been identified as the cause of autism, which is also not attributable to the loss of a single cerebral function or capacity (Bauman and Kemper, 2005; Aitken, 2010). The complex and varied cognitive problems of people with autism, and the abnormalities in habits of action and of social response or use of language, are consequences of core disabilities, manifestations of which might be recognized, and compensated for, in infancy, before the development at the end of the first year of "joint attention" (Trevarthen, 2000).

A new scientific recognition of these core disabilities in autism, and their relationship to imagination for action and to qualities of movement, is emerging from attention to the emotions that evaluate other persons actions (Hobson, 1993, 2002/04; Reddy et al., 2002, 2010; Reddy, 2008; Hobson and Hobson, 2011), and from a brain science of intentions in movement and the intersubjective sharing of their dynamics of expression (Gallese, 2006; Stern, 2010; Gowen, 2012; Gallese and Rochat, 2013; Rochat et al., 2013).

AUTISM COMPROMISES AFFECTIVE SHARING, AND REQUIRES CREATIVE RESPONSE TO THIS

When Leo Kanner (Kanner, 1943) distinguished "autistic disturbances of affective contact" in 1943, he accentuated that the disorder is emotional. Hobson and Hobson (2011) quote examples from Kanner's sensitive case studies that identify a difficulty in engagement with other person's intentions, experiences and feelings. Kanner also recorded that parents of these children were often concerned from the first year about their child's detachment or aloneness. Reddy (2008, 2011) cites a large number of studies that prove normally developing infants "know minds" and learn complex cooperative activities by deliberately engaging playfully and inquisitively with the way other persons display their interests, experiences and feelings. This eagerness for enjoyment of shared experience, a sympathetic activity, which goes beyond "joint attention to objects," is weakened in autism.

The cognitive deficiencies of autism measured by tests of perceptual recognition, rational choice, and language are skills that must be gained by learned *accommodation* to objective experience, and normally depend on deliberate adult instruction. But all can be attributed to deep subjective causes that impair imaginative moving, the pleasures of the body in explorative action, and a motivation to deliberately share this "seeking" in inventive and playful, *assimilatory*, communication, going "beyond the information given" (Bruner, 1974). It appears likely that autism results from disorders of imaginative and sociable playfulness itself, for which the motives and emotions are apparent from birth. Such disorders can be traced back to creative developments of movement and awareness in body and mind before birth (Trevarthen and Delafield-Butt, 2013), to disorders of sensory-motor circular reactions that become the tools for mastery of engagement with the world (Piaget, 1951, 1954) and for the development of shared cultural understanding (Baldwin, 1902).

Though some medical treatments lead to improvements in associated conditions, there is no drug or surgical intervention for autism. A prescribed course of training or instruction in behaviors, cognitive abilities or communication by learned symbolic language may help, but can have adverse consequences, increasing the subject's anxiety, isolation and dependency (Trevarthen et al., 1998). Moreover, the activity, cognitive capacities, relationships and emotional well-being of a child or older person with autism can be improved by a variety of non-verbal, non-cognitive activities in which a therapist, who engages sensitively with the individuality of their impulses and felt experiences, accompanies the autistic person in the emotions of intimate engagement to more productive and less defensive states of activity and awareness. This type of relational and creative "art" therapy, which responds to and guides the primary actions, interests and feelings of individuals with autism, much as mother engages her affections with her animated infant from birth, can benefit language learning and both social and practical education (Malloch and Trevarthen, 2009; Stern, 2010).

Evidence that autistic behaviors express abnormalities of prenatal development of the brain stem (Rodier and Arndt, 2005) relate to evidence that early postnatal communication, if it is to support social and cognitive development, must be ready to protect the infant against autonomic reactions of protective withdrawal and depression, as well as to support positive initiatives promoting advances in social communication (Panksepp and Sahley, 1987; Panksepp and Watt, 2011; Porges, 2011; Porges and Furman, 2011). Infant psychology and paediatric practice have been transformed by abundant confirmation that precise coordination of well-formed intentions, interests and feeling may occur within the child and between the child and an attentive and affectionate adult from the neonate stage (Brazelton and Nugent, 1995; Trevarthen, 1977, 1998, 2009a; Stern, 2000; Sander, 2008; Nagy, 2011). This is the arena in which we must be alert for weaknesses in developing human sense and for special support it may need from the parental and social environment (Narvaez et al., 2013).

PSYCHOBIOLOGY OF HUMAN MENTAL FUNCTIONS

DEVELOPMENTAL NEUROBIOLOGY OF SELF-CONSCIOUS INTENTIONS WITH EMBODIED FEELINGS, AND SOCIAL AWARENESS

Evidence concerning the generation of animate intentions, awareness and emotion in deep processes of the brain (Panksepp and Biven, 2012) questions the "thalamo-cortico-centric" theory of conscious awareness, thought and memory, which focuses on abilities that depend on learned definition of objects from information picked up *outside* the body, on the routines of fine articulate skills for using the environment, and on educated conventions of representation and reflective thought about objective information. Functional brain research shows that the primate neocortex is excited to regulate motor activities prospectively in reference to their goals, seeking perceptual confirmation by imaginatively simulating the completion of the action within an established context of multimodal information (Fogassi et al., 2005; Pezzulo et al., 2008; Pezzulo and Castelfranchi, 2009; Hesslow, 2012; Gallese and Rochat, 2013). The process of intending to act in a particular way is not a consequence of backward coupling of frontal cortex "executive functioning" to recollections of the past objects and events mediated impersonally in the temporal lobe. It is the product of a forward-looking creative imagination that builds an episodic memory of past events related to an intentional personal self (Tulving, 2002), with an autopoetic imagination equipped from the start with "implicit experiential and procedural memory processes that generate non-reflective qualia" (Vandekerckhove and Panksepp, 2011, p. 7).

These animating functions of the primate brain mediate intersubjective coordination of self-related experiences in intimate direct communication of purposes and feelings with others. The anticipations of experience are charged with emotional values linked in the brain stem with autonomic regulation of vitality within the body (Damasio, 2010; Solms and Panksepp, 2012), and these affections are communicated between subjects by a reciprocal *sympathetic* cooperation of purposes and experiences (not a one way imitation or shadowing of emotional processes now commonly called "empathy"). Human relationships and mutual awareness depend on relational emotions that promote social cooperation in performance of creative actions and thinking, to increase collective well-being (Stern, 1993; Hobson, 1993, 2002/04; Trevarthen, 2009a).

The well-coordinated performances and expressions of affect of newborn infants in expectant orientation to real or imagined objects, and to persons (Trevarthen, 1984, 1986b; Nagy, 2011), the development of intentional movements and rhythmic emotional expressions of fetuses (Trevarthen and Delafield-Butt, 2013), and the behaviors of anencephalic children (Merker, 2007) support phylogenetic evidence that primary conscious states and emotional evaluations, which are essential regulations in all goal directed consciousness, are indeed first generated and regulated sub-cortically (Solms and Panksepp, 2012), without neocortical involvement. These motor-emotional systems are elaborated in the orbito-frontal cortex and the temporal lobe of human beings, which continue to develop to adult stages (Schore, 1994, 2005). Before these developments they play a central role in maternal care, and in the repair of emotional disorders (Schore, 2003).

Affective self-regulation and emotional communication to regulate engagement with other individuals have evolved in vertebrates by elaboration of intrinsic neurochemical systems in the brain stem linked to the hypothalamus (Trevarthen et al., 2006). Regulation by the vagal nerve of essential self-related vital processes of heart activity, respiration and feeding is adapted for intersubjective coordination in the primate social brain by means of communication employing expressive movements of eyes, face, and vocalization. Throughout development of a child, from the time of maternal support of the infant through birth and nursing, there is a dynamic process that balances changes in self-regulation against the need for collaborative regulations of relationships with other persons in various degrees of intimacy (Porges and Furman, 2011; Carter and Porges, 2013). These have particular significance for identifying and explaining autism (Patriquin et al., 2013).

The importance of rhythmic emotionally expressive hand gestures in human communication from infancy (Trevarthen, 1986b; Trevarthen et al., 2011), indicates that forebrain systems for guiding action of the hands in complex manipulations have been recruited into the brain stem and limbic systems for assisting autonomic regulations by self-touching or holding and further adapted to the service of social coordination. Hands are part of the human emotional motor system (Holstege et al., 1996). Indeed, movements of "mimesis" for social celebration in dance and song, appears likely to have preceded evolution of speech and contributed to its power to communicate thoughts as *Homo sapiens sapiens* evolved (Donald, 2001; McNeill, 2005; Mithen, 2009; Gillespie-Lynch et al., 2013). The roots of this human talent for expressive gestural mimicry is apparent in infancy and an essential contributor to the intimacy of parental care (Trevarthen, 1999, 2013; Dissanayake, 2000).

Both gestural and linguistic languages develop in intense interpersonal communication mediated by vitality dynamics and expressions of emotional investment that provide a basis for the transmission of more differentiated semantic references by symbols (Stern, 2010; Lüdtke, 2012). Dynamic communications carried by consistent innate measures of moving in time (Pöppel and Wittmann, 1999), over intervals from fractions of a second to minutes and longer, are cultivated in all human societies in the arts of music, dance and theatre. They begin as a universal human regulation of rhythms of the mind or "biochronology," active before birth and elaborated in the communicative musicality and rhythmic action games parents play with infants in the middle of the first year (Trevarthen, 1999, 2009b; Malloch and Trevarthen, 2009).

Autistic children show abnormalities in production and reception of communication by both speech and gesture, and in writing (Rapin and Allen, 1983).

THE NEUROLOGY OF COMMUNICATION BY TRANSFER OF THE DYNAMICS AND FORM OF INTENTIONS AND FEELINGS IN MOVEMENT

New data from social neuroscience confirm the "common sense" that we are aware of other person's states of mind by immediate or direct engagement with the Other's *motor* intentions, by whatever modality or movement these intentions are expressed, matching them by instantaneous "affect attunement" (Stern, 1993, 2010) to the animation by which we generate intentions of our own Self (Gallese, 2006; Bråten, 2009). Sensitivity for the intentions, interests and feelings of other individuals, for the social affordances of their behaviors, must depend upon matching regulatory processes that govern the rhythm or pulse and expressive tonality or quality of movements of the human body as well as by "mirroring" their body-related form (Trevarthen, 1986b, 1999; Stern, 2010).

Regions in the adult cerebral hemispheres of a monkey or human being that are sensitive to organism-object relations, and that respond selectively to perceived *capacities for action* of the self, also respond to the possible actions available to, and enacted by others (Gallese, 2007). The same neural system is responsible for perceiving one's own possibilities for action *and* the possibilities for action of another. Direct *intra-personal* neural resonance within the "mirror neuron system," reflecting the Self, gives one individual direct *inter-personal* access in "felt immediacy" (Bråten, 2009) with intentions in the mind of an Other made manifest in their body movement, in "intersubjectivity" (Trevarthen, 1979, 1998; Trevarthen and Aitken, 2001). Further, data from imaging of brain activities show there exists substantial overlap in activity of this system for awareness of actions with activity excited by merely *thinking about* an intentional act (Decety and Grezes, 2006).

Direct resonance between preparation, execution, observation and thought in action depends on "motor images" (Bernstein, 1967), which underpin perception, observation, and planning of goal-directed action, and also integrate Self-related experience (Llinàs, 2001; Northoff and Panksepp, 2008). An amodal perception-action system is also the means by which complex embodied human intentions may be communicated between agents across many channels of expression, in a "consensuality," which, when further elaborated and mediated by language, becomes a tool for sharing abstract concepts and plans (Maturana et al., 1995).

Disruption of the neural systems of motor planning in time and space, by epigenetic dysregulation of early development in the brain stem, or by environmental insult to the growing brain, will have pervasive effects in maturation of consciousness, behavior and social engagement, such as occurs in autism (Aitken and Trevarthen, 1997; Trevarthen et al., 1998; Trevarthen, 2000).

PRENATAL GENESIS OF AUTISM

We have described the coordinative mechanisms in the brain as an "intrinsic motive formation" (IMF), "ready at birth to share emotion with caregivers for regulation of the child's cortical development, upon which cultural cognition and learning depend. ... many psychological disorders of childhood can be traced to faults in early stages of brain development when core motive systems form." (Trevarthen and Aitken, 1994, p. 597). The IMF, laid out in development of the fetus, is a core component of all of the sensory-motor mechanism of human communication—by gesture and dance, speech and song, or by writing, playing musical instruments and other manual or digital media (Trevarthen, 2001a,b). Rodier and Arndt (2005) relate autistic behaviors that limit expressive movements of the eyes, face and vocal productions, and anticipatory attention to expressive movements of other persons, to malformation in the embryo of core regulatory systems in the midbrain, the brain stem visceral efferent and afferent nuclei, and the olivary nuclei and cerebellum. They conclude, "there is no region but the brain stem for which so many lines of evidence indicate a role in autism" (Rodier and Arndt, 2005, p. 146).

IMAGINATIVE INTENTIONS AND EMOTIONS OF THE PRIMARY SELF

There has been, in the last two decades, a highly significant re-evaluation of the relationship between emotion and cognition, and their functional inseparability in human experience and in communication at all stages of development (Damasio, 2010; Panksepp and Biven, 2012). Comparative studies of the mammalian emotional system demonstrates that an *affective* core sense of the Self (Northoff and Panksepp, 2008; Solms and Panksepp, 2012) does not depend on learned conceptual knowing. This "anoetic" consciousness of a live body (Vandekerckhove and Panksepp, 2011) develops before a child becomes familiar with the external world through practice of intention and testing of actions which explore the affordances of situations and objects. At all stages of the development of human conscious intelligence this mobile self-with-feelings remains active, generating an innate spatio-temporal context for the arousal of movements to engage with the environment, and affective values for sustaining core vitality (Stern, 2010). From mid gestation through infancy the developing self is sensitive to other persons' responses to its activities and vitality, first showing signs of vital state to achieve shared "amphoteronomic" regulation of its own autonomics with those of the mother. After birth the infant signals its own rhythmically intended and affectively measured acts in responsive ways that lead to the "synrhythmic" communication for cooperative learning and cultural development (Maturana et al., 1995; Donald, 2001; Trevarthen et al., 2006; Malloch and Trevarthen, 2009; Porges and Furman, 2011).

DEVELOPMENT OF HUMAN AGENCY IN INFANCY, AND BEFORE BIRTH

MEASURES OF INFANT SENSORY-MOTOR INTELLIGENCE, SELF-REGULATION AND SOCIABILITY

Movements of a baby under 2 months old are coordinated and integrated within a rhythmic awareness of a single intentional subjectivity (Trevarthen, 1979, 1984). These movements were described by Prechtl (2001) and Einspieler and Prechtl (2005) as "general movements" (GM), which, "involve the whole body in a variable sequence of arm, leg, neck, and trunk movements. They wax and wane in intensity, force and speed, and they have a gradual beginning and end. Rotations along the axis of the limbs and slight changes in the direction of movements make them fluent and elegant and create the impression of complexity and variability. If the nervous system is impaired, GMs loose their complex and variable character and become monotonous and poor." (Einspieler and Prechtl, 2005, p. 61). General movements are not precisely focused, intentional and directed by discrimination of discrete objects, but they can orient head, eyes and limbs to external events in coordinated sequences within a body-related space (Trevarthen, 1984). Visually directed reaching in newborns compensates for changes in the "load" of a limb, which proves the responsiveness of this non-reflex imaginative coordination to proprioceptive reafference, or "body self awareness" (Van der Meer et al., 1996).

A newborn infant's movements are especially sensitive to sight, hearing and touch of an attentive the mother in face-to-face engagement, and they can take a creative part in a shared narrative of expressive action (Trevarthen and Delafield-Butt, 2013). Her voice was learned *in utero* (DeCasper and Fifer, 1980) and its sound motivates rapid visual learning of her face. Imitation tests, made with care to allow the infant to focus attention and regulate a state of responsive arousal, prove that a newborn can initiate eye-movements, face expressions, vocal sound patterns and hand gestures of another person (Meltzoff and Moore, 1977; Maratos, 1982; Field et al., 1983; Heimann et al., 1989; Kugiumutzakis, 1999; Nagy and Molnar, 2004; Nagy, 2011). These behaviors signaling a "second person other-awareness" are adapted for sharing curiosity for others' mental states of interest and affective appraisal (Reddy, 2011).

At 2 months, after a period of rapid maturation of sub-cortical and cortical visual-motor regulations of foveal sight (Trevarthen, 1986a), the infant's precisely timed responses of looking, smiling, and vocalization give evidence of preparation for sharing ritual practices and language (Bateson, 1979). Electroencephalic data on the activity of a 9-week-old infant's brain when looking at the photograph of a woman's face (Tzourio-Mazoyer et al., 2002) confirmed that complementary neocortical areas in left and right brain, which 2 years later will become involved in a child's learning of expression and reception of spoken language, are already components in cerebral regulation of interpersonal contact by a "social brain," long before the training of a "social intelligence" by life with other persons (Frith and Frith, 1999). The subcortical visual and auditory systems that mature from the early fetal period show an asymmetry related to differences in left and right parts of the brain stem that mediate in complementary autonomic regulations (Trevarthen, 1996). Schore (1994, 2005) proposes that the early developing right brain motivates shared learning of perception and articulation of meaning in language when the left cerebral hemisphere shows an acceleration of growth in the second and third year, the period when diagnosis of autism becomes possible.

Developments around 3–5 months correlate with more differentiated movements of the baby's extremities when new neocortical sensory-motor functions are developing. Einspieler and Prechtl, label these subtle gestures "fidgety," and describe them as, "small movements of moderate speed with variable acceleration of neck, trunk, and limbs in all directions" (Einspieler and Prechtl, 2005, p. 61). They lead the infant to make more discriminating orientations of head, eyes and hands intending to reach for and touch or take hold of objects at a distance from the body, and are accompanied by a fall in attention to the mother. This incites the mother to be more animated and playful, and to incorporate the baby's selective interest in objects into "person-person-object" games (Hubley and Trevarthen, 1979; Reddy, 2011).

PROGRAMMED DEVELOPMENT OF THE INFANT-PARENT SYSTEM

Longitudinal studies of developments in actions, perception and communication in the first two years, with information on internally regulated brain growth changes, confirm that there are transformations in the motives and emotions of the child for collaboration with parental care (Trevarthen and Aitken, 2003). Sander's studies of infants with their mothers from birth over the first 36 months showed that growth of a human life is sustained by a series of stages of adjustment within a system of human-to-human engagement (Sander, 2008). Both mother and child are significant actors, but in the creative process of development the child must normally set the pace and the times of important advance. Brazelton extended Sander's system approach to an interpersonal paediatrics accepting the conscious and personal powers of the newborn, and defining "touch points" in the developing life with parents and in the community (Brazelton and Nugent, 1995; Brazelton and Sparrow, 2006). Periods of change in developing powers that are both sensitive and significant, are symptoms of advances in motivation for learning and for communication (Johnson, 2005). Their consequences depend on collaboration with parents who are "attuned" to the infant (Stern, 2000), and both intimate and playful in their accommodation to the child's impulses.

Data from a review of the literature on changes in the child's psychology and brain over the first 18 months (Trevarthen and Aitken, 2003) point to natural emergence in the child of new levels of mastery of action and awareness at around 6 weeks, 4 months, 7 months, 9 months, and between 15 and 18 months. These agree with longitudinal studies of infant's capacity to take initiative in joint activities (Trevarthen, 1977; Hubley and Trevarthen, 1979; Reddy, 2011). These five advances in adaptive processes correlate with temperamental changes commonly referred to as "regressions." They adapt to cultural differences in the frequency of parental initiatives or directives (Reddy et al., 2012). They are products of the active system of "intent participation" in the environment with companions that drive cultural learning (Trevarthen, 2013).

SENSORI-MOTOR INTENTIONALITY BEFORE BIRTH: GENESIS OF PRIMARY SELF-CONSCIOUSNESS AND THE FIRST INTERSUBJECTIVITY

Spontaneous movements develop in the late embryo and fetus, showing increased sensory awareness of their purposes (Delafield-Butt and Trevarthen, 2013). The first integrative actions of the nervous system are to move the body, and the first nerve tracts in the central nervous system are those that will activate movements to express different orientations and emotional states (Trevarthen, 1986a). After 8 weeks the core neurochemical systems of the subcortical brain that will link motor centers and select and evaluate experiences throughout life make their appearance. At this stage the fetus makes the general movements of Prechtl (2001). These become increasingly differentiated and controlled with the benefit of re-afference from sensory systems that grow in the following weeks. Detailed studies of by real-time ultrasonography demonstrate a fetus's exploratory sensation-testing to touch their own body, their face, the placenta, umbilicus, and the uterine wall with their hands at 11 weeks. They make jaw movements and swallow amniotic fluid, expressing pleasure or disapproval at tastes, sucking and smiling or grimacing with disgust. Complex movements of trunk, arms, and legs position the body, and may react to movements of the mother's body and to the contractions of the muscles of her uterus (Lecanuet et al., 1995; Trevarthen et al., 2006; Piontelli, 2010). In weeks 10–14 fetal movements become differentiated into individual, isolate actions with increasing goal-direction to particular parts of the body (Prechtl, 2001; Piontelli, 2010). The arms and hands "test" sensitive zones of the body, especially to the face and head, exploring the border of sensory innervation on the top of the head (Piontelli, 2010, p. 61–67).

In singleton pregnancies motor planning of action patterns adapted for different goals is evident before 22 weeks gestational age (Zoia et al., 2007). In twin pregnancies, movements directed by one twin to the other are "carefully" slowed, even by 18 weeks, which the researchers interpret as evidence of a primary "social awareness" (Castiello et al., 2010). At this time the motor centers of the brain stem and spinal cord are directing the coordinated behavior of the fetus (Okado, 1980). Neocotical cells do not develop dendrites until after 26 weeks of gestation (Hevner, 2000).

This natural history of human movement at a stage of development when the sensori-motor environment can only be the properties of an organized body itself appears to support Lashley's conclusion that propositional thought may depend on, and indeed be derived from, the spontaneous syntactic ordering of movement sequences (Lashley, 1951, p. 122). The fetus has an imaginative "motor intelligence" and can formulate orderly projects without neocortical skills.

Expressions in fetuses, in addition to twisting movements of distress and tentative exploration by touch, give evidence of emotions—of discomfort, curiosity or pleasure, adapted for communication of interests and feelings. In the third trimester, movements of the face visualized by 4D ultrasound develop into complexes that define a "cry face gestalt" or a "laughter gestalt," expressing emotions that will communicate powerfully immediately after birth in the regulation of parental care (Reissland et al., 2011). Maternal hunger with depletion of energy supply to the fetus drives "anxious" patterns of fetal movement. The mother and the fetus are already affectively connected. These discoveries prompt a revolution in psychological theory and medical ethics. There is a consensus in modern paediatrics that by 24 weeks the fetus should be considered a conscious agent deserving the same standard of sympathetic medical care as adults (Royal College of Obstetricians and Gynaecologists, 2010).

READINESS FOR SUPPORT OF THE BODY IN RHYTHMS OF MOVEMENT, AWARE OF SURROUNDINGS, AND ATTENTIVE TO HUMAN COMPANY IN MOVEMENT

Infants demonstrate the regulations of an innate time for life in movement. Research on their dynamics and coordination with a parent's movements have led to a natural science of human "musicality" (Trehub, 1990; Papoušek, 1996; Malloch, 1999; Malloch and Trevarthen, 2009). Inspired by discoveries of precise analysis of films, revealing self-synchrony of movements of individual actors and inter-synchrony between actors in conversations (Birdwhistell, 1970; Jaffe and Felstein, 1970; Condon and Ogston, 1971) researchers found that infants and adults share matching rhythms (Condon and Sander, 1974; Beebe et al., 1985; Jaffe et al., 2001). One remarkable video recording made by Saskia van Rees of a 2 month premature infant in precisely timed coordination of dialogue of simple "coo" sounds vividly demonstrates how this shared sense of time for combining syllables in phrases may lead to a narrative in wordless dialogue (Trevarthen, 1999).

Two bands of time are shown to be fundamental in dialogues, games and songs between young infants and their parents (Trevarthen, 1999, 2009b). Faster rhythms of syllables and phrases in speech and song, or dancing steps and gestures, correspond with arm and hand grasping for object manipulation, or of the head and eye rotations that perform visual inspection. These range from the median syllable frequency of 1.5–3 per second—the same as a running or fast stepping, a glance or eyebrow rise, a laugh or a hand wave—to every 3–5 s for a visual scan, a manipulative sequence, a phrase of speaking or song, and a cycle of deep breathing. These are somato-motor coordinations that achieve use of the environment and pickup of information for perception, or of a communicative message, in the "psychological present," the "here and now" of consciousness in action.

Slower periods of sensed vitality, as expressed in the "extended present" of an episode in a story, a verse of singing or a stanza of poetry, occupy 10–25 s. Longer times of imagined activity and narrations form natural elements of 25–50 s in the rhythmic verses, playful or calming, of baby songs in all languages. These slower events are identified with autonomic events that regulate arousal, hunger and wakefulness throughout life, and regulation of the rate of heartbeat and breathing by the vagal nerve (Delamont et al., 1999). They are accompanied by bursts of electrical activity in the cerebral cortex that have a role in the fluctuating experiences of dreaming. They link the imagination with the economy of life energy in the body, and with the expressive arts.

Stern (1993, 2000, 2010) called the cycles of arousal or variations in vitality dynamics in mother infant play "emotional narratives" expressing "implicit relational knowing." Malloch analysed the controlled patterns of change in voice qualities and pitch of the voices of mothers and infants in dialogues and baby songs as "narratives" that, "allow two persons to share a sense of passing time, and to create and share the emotional envelopes that evolve through this shared time. They express innate motives for sharing emotion and experience with other persons and for creating meaning in joint activity." (Malloch, 1999, p. 45). These shared "routines" are identified by Bruner (1999) as the medium for reference in language. We have recently been finding evidence of the same "narrative" cycles of arousal in the "general movements" of newborn infants, which may be shared with a sensitive mother who coordinates with her baby by modulated vocal sounds, touches or rocking. They participate in tides of consciousness of being together that later will regulate the changes of meaning in a story or the recollections of episodic memory (Delafield-Butt and Trevarthen, 2013; Trevarthen and Delafield-Butt, 2013).

SENSORI-MOTOR DIS-COORDINATION IN AUTISM, FROM INFANCY

DEFICIT IN PROSPECTIVE MOTOR CONTROL IN AUTISM AND ITS CONSEQUENCES FOR DEVELOPING INTENTIONALITY AND LEARNING

The complex disorder of childhood autism, and how it has serious effects on a young child's life, may be described as follows:

> "By about one to two years after birth . . . at a time when infants usually become acutely aware of other people and what they are doing, full of playful imagination and eager for new experiences, these babies became strangely self-contained or isolated in their own world and increasingly unresponsive or irritable, and difficult to understand; their vocalizations movements often seemed repetitious and pointless, and their gestures and postures were also odd. Throughout their childhood they continued to express themselves in ways that made parents, teachers and other children feel unable to make contact.
>
> As pre-schoolers, the children are not insensitive to others or unaffectionate, and they can show strong likes and dislikes for particular people. Sometimes they imitate or seek to interact, but never in a free and easy way, and sometimes with a peculiar ritualistic insistence, and remarkable inattention to their effects on other people. Strange postures and movements and a need for sameness, combined with obsessive interest in certain objects and experiences, cut them off from others. At times they seem to be in a trance, "floating off," "looking" or "listening" when nothing is there, often with strange flapping of the hands, or an enigmatic smile, and they only make unintelligible baby-like vocalizations. They may get into inexplicable panics and seem very distressed, anxious or terrified, especially when forced to have close contact with people or in strange environments. In general they do

> not like, or fear, unfamiliar places or routines. They protest at irregularities in their world and repeat seemingly trivial actions for their own interest. Some, in panicky states or anger, may injure themselves. Most of the time, however, they seem content to amuse themselves, often performing favorite actions over and over. Their behaviors can be frightening and distressing to parents who need help to understand what is wrong and how to cope with a child who looks healthy enough, but who won't respond."
>
> (Trevarthen et al., 1998, p. 1–2).

Odd behaviors like these are seen in children who do not have autism, but they are momentary and easily regulated by the child's playful resourcefulness or by affectionate attentions of parents, and in shared enjoyment with other children. The autistic child has persistent problems in both self-regulated actions and emotions, and in awareness of other person's intentions, interests and feelings. There are conflicting ideas on the causes of these problems and how to respond, especially for the early stages.

Disorders of movement in children with autism particularly affect expressive movements in communication (Ricks and Wing, 1975; Damasio and Maurer, 1978; Gillberg and Coleman, 1992; Frith and Frith, 1999; Oller et al., 2010). These have lead to an interpretation in terms of a deficit in "executive functioning" (Rumsey, 1985) attributed to a developmental fault in the frontal lobes that manifests itself in the second year. Recent data point to a more basic and probably earlier developing deficit in prospective control of movements (Mari et al., 2003; Rinehart et al., 2006a; Dowd et al., 2012; Gowen and Hamilton, 2013). For example, in an automated vocal analysis of a large body of data recorded from natural expressive behavior of infants 10–50 months of age, Oller et al. (2010) identified massive delay in development of movements of vocal articulation in children developing autism or language delay. Such disorders affecting communication behavior can be explained as originating as faults in the timing and integration capacities of the brainstem sensorimotor system, which develops prenatally and affords prospective control for later developments in psychological functions. Failure in cognitive strategies of "action planning" and "action execution" (e.g., Rinehart et al., 2001; Nazarali et al., 2009) attributable to change in mirror neuron systems (e.g., Cattaneo et al., 2007; Fabbri-Destro et al., 2009), require higher-order cortical processing, which develops after birth.

Children with ASD differ from typically developing children in the efficiency of three types of prospective motor control:

(i) Generation of *single actions*, such as when extending the hand to touch, or indicate, an object of interest;
(ii) Organization of a *series of actions* to perform more complex tasks or projects, including speaking, and
(iii) Simultaneous *coordination of multiple action units* to achieve coherent purpose, as in postural accommodations when standing or walking.

Simple "action units" and serially organized "action chains" both require precise coordination of muscle actions that are conceived or imagined "ahead-in-time" so that they achieve a desired future effect efficiently (Bernstein, 1967; von Hofsten, 1993; Lee, 2009). And an integrative control of movement is a necessary foundation for learning more advanced and complex tasks, such as speaking and reading (von Hofsten, 2004, 2007). Awareness of others' intentions requires detecting prospective control in their movements, and this is apparent in how infants participate in dialog and games (Trevarthen, 1986b). Failure to time movements prospectively and meet expectation in movement will thwart efficient goal acquisition, confuse awareness and frustrate a sense of success, causing negative emotions of self-protection and avoidance (Bower et al., 1970; Rovee-Collier et al., 1978).

(i) Evidence for disturbance in prospective control of single action units.

Autistic persons exhibit significant differences in the timing and patterning of single movements (Rinehart et al., 2001, 2006a; Mari et al., 2003; Nazarali et al., 2009; Dowd et al., 2012). The type of disturbance varies with the task and the sub-group examined. For example, in a reach-to-grasp task individuals with ASD grouped by low or average to high intellectual ability, with full-scale I.Q. scores below and above 80, exhibited different kinematics, and both groups acted significantly less efficiently than typically developing children (Mari et al., 2003). Differences between ASD groups were thought to reflect different compensatory coping strategies for a primary deficit in motor planning. The autistic individuals also failed to coordinate the two subactions in the reach-to-grasp task, i.e., reaching of the arm and the opening of the fingers. They performed one act and then the other separately. Typical children coordinate the sequence of arm and hand actions in "pre-reaching" and gesturing fluently from early infancy (Trevarthen, 1984; Rönnqvist and von Hofsten, 1994; Prechtl, 2001).

(ii) Evidence for disturbance in serial organization of multiple action units.

The progressive planning of "action chains" communicate intentions. When we see someone grasping a bottle, for example, the initial reaching movement of the arm differs depending on whether the goal is to shelve it or to serve some wine (Jeannerod, 1999). The postural preparation of the body and extension of the arm, with shifts of gaze, are adjusted from the start in different ways depending on the final goal. Children with ASD have deficits in this preparatory coordination for motor sequencing or action chaining (Cattaneo et al., 2007; Fabbri-Destro et al., 2009). Typically developing children, when asked to perform an object manipulation task, such as turning an upside-down drinking glass right-side up, adjust their body posture at the start of the action so that their final posture is comfortable (Rosenbaum et al., 1990). Children with autism begin with a comfortable posture and conclude it in an uncomfortable one, suggesting a deficit of motor "knowledge" of how the action will proceed.

Cattaneo and colleagues (2007) used electromyographic recordings of the mylohyoid muscle movements that lower the jaw and raise the tongue for reaching-to-grasp-to-eat, and they compared this sequence with the muscle activity during a movement of reaching-to-grasp-to-place. They found that typically-developing children anticipated eating the food with mylohyoid activation beginning well before their hand had grasped the piece of food. In contrast, this activation did not start in children with ASD until the food was already grasped in the hand and traveling toward their mouth, demonstrating a failure to couple the action chains efficiently. This lack of anticipation was also evident when the children were asked to watch another person perform the reach-to-grasp-to-eat action. The mylohyoid activation occurred in typically-developing children at the onset of the other's movement toward the food, but in autistic individuals there was no mylohyoid activation at all.

(iii) Evidence for failure in simultaneous integration of multiple action units.

Measurements of children's postural adjustments and muscle tensions during load shifting shows that prospective control of whole-body posture and perception of body-space goals, which require synchronizing and co-ordinating action units throughout the body in shifts of the legs, chest, back, and arms, are also disrupted in autism (Schmitz et al., 2003). Disturbances of prospective control for the whole body are confirmed by data on gait differences in individuals with autism, showing an increase stride length and variability of the width of stride, but also significant differences in postural adjustments of the upper-body to maintain balance (Hallett et al., 1993; Vernazza-Martin et al., 2005; Rinehart et al., 2006b; Calhoun et al., 2011; Nayate et al., 2011). They also have difficulties in perceiving the environmental context for their movements (Gowen and Hamilton, 2013).

DIFFERENCES IN PROSPECTIVE MOTOR TIMING AFFECT SOCIAL EXPECTATION AND UNDERSTANDING

The subtle deficits in prospective motor control of children with ASD must be involved in the symptoms of social isolation and emotional distress that they show. They have difficulties in communicating their intention in gestural acts, and in sensing the dynamics of another's intentions from their movements (Cattaneo et al., 2007; Zalla et al., 2010; Gowen, 2012). Imitation-based or interaction therapies for ASD employing sensitive response to signs of intended movement are able to assist because they facilitate both anticipation of actions and psychological and emotional connection (Escalona et al., 2002; Nadel, 2006; Zeedyk, 2008; Field et al., 2011; Solomon et al., 2012). The therapist acts to excite anticipation, which simplifies and supports the performance of desired actions. It also explains why insistence on evidence from repeated measures of performance in tasks to test perceptual preferences or cognitive mastery can fail to detect or explain the cause of failure (Wigram and Gold, 2012). Such external measures, focusing on achievement of goals or response to facts, neglect the temporo-spatial phenomena of prospective motor control within the subject.

Problems of intentionality and its perceptual guidance in autism, and pathological defense against sensory overload (Rosenhall et al., 1999; Foxton et al., 2003), may be due to faults in motor regulations of sense organs; of the inner ear to adjust the sensitivity of hearing, and of head and eye movements to control selection of detail by foveal fixation which is guided by pick-up of global information from the ambient field. Hearing and production of speech sounds, which autism impairs in differing degrees, is particularly demanding, requiring detection and control of affective expression transmitted by small modulations in the timbre, pitch and loudness of vowel sounds, and their constraint by consonants produced in rapid sequences to articulate intelligible words in information-rich phrases. Autism, however, interferes not only with the motor controls of selective hearing and seeing, but with attention to all the expressive movements of other persons.

In high functioning persons with autism, exceptional abilities in detecting, separating and combining visual details or pitches of sounds (O'Riordan et al., 2001; Bonnel et al., 2003; Mottron et al., 2006) may be a consequence of compensatory hypertrophy in higher cortical sensory systems driven by a bias to detect affective self-related feedback or support. Ockleford's experience with supporting exceptional performative talents in autistic children who cannot speak suggest that pleasure from control of pitch in sounds from musical instruments activates a primary reward system different from that which discriminates speech components (Ockleford, 2012, 2013). In confrontation with another, a person with autism avoids looking at the eyes, directing attention to the mouth (Senju and Johnson, 2009). Given that rapid movements of the eyes transmit important information about the direction and intensity of *interest*, in preparation for shifts in locomotion, posture or reaching by hand, as well as selective attention to individuals in a group, they implicate tracking of sequences of intended action to engage with others' prospective control in thought and action (Bal et al., 2010). Lower face expressions and mouth movements express *affect* and are essential for emotional sympathy. They attract attention of an observer for judging another person's feelings.

Failure to appreciate playful teasing and humor and avoidant or defensive reaction to strangers, as well as preference for familiar surroundings and consistency in placement of objects or execution of routines, characteristics of ASD, all point to a disturbance of imaginative curiosity for prospects of action. They are as much disorders of self-regulation of pleasurable movement-with-awareness as of affective other-awareness, and they impair intentional and emotional engagement (Hobson and Hobson, 2011; Reddy, 2011)

DISORDERS OF AUTISM IN THE FIRST YEAR

Teitelbaum and colleagues (1998, 2002), studying home movies of infants later diagnosed as autistic, made a comparative analysis of the developmental stages of turning over, crawling, sitting, standing and walking, which infants typically master in the first year. Using the Eshkol-Wachman Movement Notation for temporal and spatial parameters of human body movement they showed deficits in whole body control and sequencing of the movements of trunk, head and limbs to control balance and posture changes, which were interpreted as disordered sensory-motor reflexes. These detailed observations have been helpful for parents who suspect their infant may be developing autism, assisting them to engage the attention of medical specialists and therapists (Teitelbaum and Teitelbaum, 2008)

Similar disturbance of anticipatory regulations of whole body postures were found by Danon-Boileau (2007) in films made of two sisters while they were being bathed by their mother; one, at five months, who later developed autism, and the other who developed normally, at 3 months. The films show the anxiety and awkwardness of the first girl who scarcely looked at her mother, and an analysis of the mother's speech shows she was not "in contact" and was using her voice with a detached tone, to draw response. With the normally developing sister the mother's speech is lively and addressed to the child as person seeking to share the experience. This infant keeps eye contact with the mother and reacts expressively. Similar observations were made in an analysis of home movies of identical twin girls at 10 months, when their father was helping them to walk or playing a game with them in the family living room (Trevarthen and Daniel, 2005; St. Clair et al., 2007). One girl later diagnosed as autistic, and who did not speak until the age of 3, showed clear delay in motor coordination for stepping and for regulation of her sitting posture. She lacked attention to other persons' eyes and made fleeting smiles and she could not participate in a teasing game with her father that required anticipation of his rhythmically phrased behaviors and speech. The rhythms and expressions in response to teasing and tickling with the father were different from those of the typically developing twin, and the father was unable to reciprocate, creating confusion in games and interactions. Her sister who had a mild retardation at school age, developed normally through the first years showing no evidence of autism.

The lack of responsive attention by the infant developing autism to her father's attempts to play caused him to become irregular and insistent in his solicitations, which afterwards he could see only confused the child. The same transformation of parents' responses to avoidant or disengaged behavior of an infant developing autism have been noted in other studies of home movies and in prospective studies of siblings of autistic children, i.e., a change to a more insistent and monotonous mode that tries to excite a response (Baranek, 1999; Saint-Georges et al., 2010, 2011). For example, there is a lack of the affective modulation of the parent's voice in speech to an infant who later develops autism (Mahdhaoui et al., 2011). Disorder in development of the child's vocal control on the way to mastery of speech, such as that demonstrated by Oller et al. (2010) for the crucial period from 1–4 years, will affect the parents ability to share talking, and prompt them to use stimulating or coercive ways of engaging with the child.

Two research strategies have been used to search for evidence of abnormal development before medical diagnosis is possible: prospective study of the infant siblings of older children with autism. The two procedures confirm important conclusions about manifestations of autistic disorder that are developing in the first 18 months after birth (Zwaigenbaum et al., 2005; Saint-Georges et al., 2010). They highlight effects of the "flatness" and lack of seeking for engagement and also changes associated with the phases of motor development which were recorded by Teitelbaum (Teitelbaum et al., 1998, 2002), and the development of interest in objects. Attention to objects was normal in the first six months in infants developing autism when their attention to social engagement was significantly low (Maestro et al., 2002). There is a specific loss of interest in other persons" expressions early in infancy (Muratori and Maestro, 2007).

Expression of intentions and affects is achieved with cross-modal fluency between voice and gesture that promotes sympathetic action and shared experience with "affect attunement" (Trevarthen, 1986b, 2009a; Tronick, 1989; Stern, 2000; Reddy, 2008). Expressive acts, like all goal-directed voluntary movement, require prospective control, and by assimilation of the form and flow of the movements of the body and voice of one subject states of intention, affect, arousal and interest are conveyed to the awareness of the other in "felt immediacy" (Bråten, 2009; Stern, 2010; Trevarthen et al., 2011). If predictive control of the timing and harmonization of these expressive body movements are disrupted, then psycho-motor attunement with the perceptual and motor experiences of others will be confused.

Magnetic resonance imaging of the brains of autistic children indicate reduction in size of the brainstem and midbrain at birth, a loss of tissue more than compensated for by excessive growth of the brain as a whole postnatally (Hashimoto et al., 1995). Detailed neuroanatomical investigation of brains from children with ASD also indicate limbic midbrain structures and brainstem regions are affected (Rodier and Arndt, 2005). Of particular note is an abnormality in the inferior olivary nucleus, a prominent lower brainstem nucleus known to be involved in perceiving and controlling of the timing of movement (Welsh et al., 1995), indicating a likely primary site of disruption underpinning ASD motor deficit (Welsh et al., 2005).

The data on motor impairments in ASD and their early manifestation in infancy confirm a primary deficit in the capacity to perceive and move the body in a planned way, which limits the capacity to control the timing of actions of the body and their perceptual consequences, and thence impairs the communication of intentions and ideas.

AN INTERACTIVE RELATIONAL APPROACH TO THERAPY AND TEACHING, NURTURING INTIMACY AND CREATIVEY OF MOVEMENT

> "Musical structure in improvisation can provide a framework for creative development, and . . . more creative skills may well-emerge given a structure than one might see from a purely free form of improvisation—where a lack of direction and model may leave the "non-musician" client struggling to find out how they can "create" music.... Creativity is a key process in improvisational music therapy, and demands substantial skill and flexibility in the therapists to nurture in clients for therapeutic benefit."
>
> (Wigram, 2006).

Interactive music therapy for both diagnosis and treatment of autism indicates that the aim of a therapist or teacher is to provide support for creativity, and that this requires both a "direction and model" and "skill and flexibility." It requires a guide that protects the learner from "struggling to find out how they can create." And it requires descriptive evidence from single case studies (Wigram and Gold, 2012). In the controversial field of therapy for children with autism there is a bewildering range of theories and advice for procedures, which range from strict teaching of skills to control disordered actions and feelings and to coax communication, to permissive environments where possible distractions are eliminated and attempts are made to give comfort (Trevarthen et al., 1998; Teitelbaum and Teitelbaum, 2008). Given the evidence that the core deficit in autism concerns prospective sensori-motor control and affective self-regulation, especially for activities of communication, we focus our final comments on evidence that intimate or intensive engagement with the impulses of affected children in ways that bring pleasure from control of actions and mutual recognition may bring benefit for creative learning of practical skills and artificial rituals of shared experience, including language.

Finely measured pulse, form and flow of the enactments of the sensuous body and voice convey psychological states of intention, affect, arousal, and interest (Trevarthen, 1986a,b; Stern, 2010; Trevarthen et al., 2011; Hardy and Blythe LaGasse, 2013). Gestures made in communication are controlled and directed in body-space and by selecting transitory goals with precise timing of muscular energies that display affective content in "narrative" sequences (Schögler et al., 2008; Trevarthen and Delafield-Butt, 2013). It follows that, if the common control of body movements is disrupted, then the individual will have difficulty finding psycho-motor attunement with the perceptual and motor experiences of typical others.

Understanding of the fundamental and deeply felt disorder in autism as failure of integrative brain activity for carrying out sensori-motor intentions with ease and creativity, that it is a disorder that also affects communicative expression and perceiving the motor intentions of others, may help explain how intensive, imitation-based therapies attentive to emotions may be effective and may foster enjoyable response and interest (Nind, 1999; Field et al., 2002, 2011; Nadel, 2006; Nordoff and Robbins, 2007; Zeedyk, 2008; Caldwell, 2010; Frank and Trevarthen, 2012; Lüdtke, 2012; Solomon et al., 2012). By consciously "attuning" to the motor acts of the autistic patient and feeling their affective and intentional content in "intense interaction," before re-enacting creative collaborations with adaptation to responses, the therapist provides an exterior pattern of actions that are timed and directed sensitively to compensate for repetition of uncertain, anxious attempts (Hardy and Blythe LaGasse, 2013). A responsive, "listening" makes communication possible, as well as progress to new self-confident and joyful experience, which may free an exceptional talent (Ockleford, 2013).

Sensorimotor attunement in therapy embodies mental/affective components as much as it does the motor expression, and in so doing is able to open up a co-regulation of arousals, interests, and intentions in a person otherwise unavailable and isolated. All movements are considered valid expressions of purposeful states, and even stereotypies are regarded as affective sensori-motor acts capable of initiating communication, not disregarded an unintentional, non-mental motor acts. As the therapist attends to the movements of the person, attuning to them with her own body movements, so they begin to generate an implicit, affective, and inter-subjective psycho-motor connection. Such therapy can aid not only the autistic child to achieve communication, but can be of great help to a parent. It may bring an autistic person of any age and to more self-confident and articulate participation in an intimate community of knowledge (Frank and Trevarthen, 2012; Lüdtke, 2012).

It is the experience of any therapist who works with persons suffering from autism that a conscious care must be taken to "stand back" and allow any impulse the child or adult may show to take its course, indeed shadowing or mirroring it to aid its motivation. This is the principle put into the practice of interactive music therapy (Robarts, 1998; Wigram and Gold, 2006; Nordoff and Robbins, 2007; Wigram and Elefant, 2009; Ockleford, 2013). A more explicit standing back, called "asocial," is practiced by the method developed by the paediatric neurologist Waldon to assist persons with a wide range of disabilities in acting and thinking. The therapist places him or herself behind the client, holding the arms to guide the hands in performance of tasks to move objects in such a way that a goal or project is completed bringing a sense of satisfaction. This method has proved effective in helping young children overcome the confusion and isolation of autism in a way that makes productive and progressive motor learning possible (Solomon et al., 2012).

REFERENCES

Aitken, K. J. (2010). *An A-Z of Genetic Factors in Autism: A Handbook for Professionals.* London: Jessica Kingsley.

Aitken, K. J., and Trevarthen, C. (1997). Self-other organization in human psychological development. *Dev. Psychopathol.* 9, 651–675. doi: 10.1017/S0954579497001387

Bal, E., Harden, E., Lamb, D., Vaughan-Van Hecke, A., Denver, J. W., and Porges, S. W. (2010). Emotion recognition in children with autism spectrum disorders: relations to eye gaze and autonomic state. *J. Autism Dev. Disabil.* 40, 358–370. doi: 10.1007/s10803-009-0884-3

Baldwin, J. M. (1902). *Social and Ethical Interpretations in Mental Development, 3rd Edn.* New York, NY: Macmillan.

Baranek, G. T. (1999). Autism during infancy: a retrospective video analysis of sensory-motor and social behaviors at 9–12 months of age. *J. Autism Dev. Disord.* 29, 213–224. doi: 10.1023/A:1023080005650

Baron-Cohen, S., Leslie, A., and Frith, U. (1985). Does the autistic child have a theory of mind. *Cognition* 21, 37–46. doi: 10.1016/0010-0277(85)90022-8

Baron-Cohen, S., Tager-Flusberg, H., and Cohen, D. (Eds.) (2000). *Understanding Other Minds: Perspectives From Developmental Cognitive Neuroscience.* Oxford: Oxford University Press.

Bateson, M. C. (1979). "The epigenesis of conversational interaction: a personal account of research development," in *Before Speech: The Beginning of Human Communication,* ed M. Bullowa (London: Cambridge University Press), 63–77.

Bauman, M. L., and Kemper, T. L. (2005). *The Neurobiology of Autism, 2nd Edn.* Baltimore, MD: Johns Hopkins University Press.

Beebe, B., Jaffe, J., Feldstein, S., Mays, K., and Alson, D. (1985). "Interpersonal timing: the application of an adult dialogue model to mother-infant vocal and kinesic interactions," in *Social Perception in Infants,* eds F. M. Field and N. Fox (Norwood, NJ: Ablex), 217–248.

Bernstein, N. (1967). *Coordination and Regulation of Movements.* New York, NY: Pergamon.

Berthoz, A., and Christen, Y. (Eds.) (2009). *Neurobiology of "Umwelt": How Living Beings Perceive the World.* Vienna, NY: Springer.

Birdwhistell, R. (1970). *Kinesics and Context.* Philadelphia: University of Pennsylvania Press.

Bonnel, A., Mottron, L., Peretz, I., Trudel, M., Gallun, E., and Bonnel, A.-M. (2003). Enhanced pitch sensitivity in individuals with autism: a signal detection analysis. *J. Cogn. Neurosci.* 15, 226–235. doi: 10.1162/089892903321208169

Bower, T. G. R., Broughton, J. M., and Moore, M. K. (1970). Demonstration of intention in the reaching behavior of neonate humans. *Nature 228,* 679–681. doi: 10.1038/228679a0

Bråten, S. (2009). *The Intersubjective Mirror in Infant Learning and Evolution of Speech.* Amsterdam/Philadelphia: John Benjamins Publishing Company.

Brazelton, T. B., and Nugent, J. K. (1995). *The Neonatal Behavioral Assessment Scale.* Cambridge: Mac Keith Press.

Brazelton, T. B., and Sparrow, J. D. (2006). *Touchpoints 0-3: Your Child's Emotional and Behavioral Development.* Vol. I. Cambridge, MA: DaCapo Press.

Bruner, J. S. (1974). *Beyond the Information Given.* London: George Allen and Unwin Ltd.

Bruner, J. S. (1999). "The intentionality of referring," in *Developing Theories of Intention: Social Understanding and Self-Control,* eds P. D. Zelazo, J. W. Astington, and D. R. Olson (Mahwah, NJ: Erlbaum), 329–339.

Buchanan, B. (2008). *Onto-Ethologies: The Animal Environments of Uexküll, Heidegger, Merleau-Ponty, and Deleuze.* New York, NY: SUNY Press.

Caldwell, P. (2010). *Autism and Intense Interaction.* London: Jessica Kingsley.

Calhoun, M., Longworth, M., and Chester, V. L. (2011). Gait patterns in children with autism. *Clin. Biomech.* 26, 200–206. doi: 10.1016/j.clinbiomech.2010.09.013

Carter, C. S., and Porges, S. W. (2013). "Neurobiology and the evolution of mammalian social behavior," in *Evolution, Early Experience and Human Development: From Research to Practice and Policy,* eds D. Narvaez, J. Panksepp, A. Schore, and T. Gleason (New York, NY: Oxford University Press), 132–151.

Castiello, U., Becchio, C., Zoia, S., Nelini, C., Sartori, L., Blason, L., et al. (2010). Wired to be social: the ontogeny of human interaction. *PLoS ONE* 5:e13199. doi: 10.1371/journal.pone.0013199

Cattaneo, L., Fabbri-Destro, M., Boria, S., Pieraccini, C., Monti, A., Cossu, G., et al. (2007). Impairment of actions chains in autism and its possible role in intention understanding. *Proc. Natl. Acad. Sci. U.S.A.* 104, 17825–17830. doi: 10.1073/pnas.0706273104

Condon, W. S., and Ogston, W. (1971). "Speech and body motion synchrony of the speaker-hearer," in *The Perception of Language,* eds D. Horton and J. Jenkins (Columbus, OH: Charles E. Merrill), 150–184.

Condon, W. S., and Sander, L. S. (1974). Neonate movement is synchronized with adult speech: Interactional participation and language acquisition. *Science* 183, 99–101. doi: 10.1126/science.183.4120.99

Damasio, A. (2010). *The Self Comes to Mind.* New York, NY: Pantheon.

Damasio, A. R., and Maurer, M. G. (1978). A neurological model for childhood autism. *Arch. Neurol.* 35, 777–786. doi: 10.1001/archneur.1978.00500360001001

Danon-Boileau, L. (2007). "Early signs related to posture and communication: the child's attitude and the mother's reaction," in *Signs of Autism In Infants: Recognition and Early Intervention,* ed S. Acquarone (London: Karnac), 63–79.

DeCasper, A. J., and Fifer, W. P. (1980). Of human bonding: newborns prefer their mother's voice. *Science* 208, 1174–1176. doi: 10.1126/science.7375928

Decety, J., and Grezes, U. (2006). The power of simulation: imagining one's own behavior and other's behavior. *Brain Res.* 1079, 4–14. doi: 10.1016/j.brainres.2005.12.115

Delafield-Butt, J. T., and Trevarthen, C. (2013). "Theories of the development of human communication," in *Handbook of Communication Science, Vol. 1: Theories and Models of Communication,* eds P. Cobley and P. J. Schultz (Berlin: De Gruyter Mouton), 199–221.

Delamont, R. S., Julu, P. O. O., and Jamal, G. A. (1999). Periodicity of a noninvasive measure of cardiac vagal tone during non-rapid eye movement sleep in non-sleep-deprived and sleepdeprived normal subjects. *J. Clin. Neurophysiol.* 16, 146–153.

Dissanayake, E. (2000). *Art and Intimacy: How the Arts Began.* Seattle; London: University of Washington Press.

Donald, M. (2001). *A Mind So Rare: The Evolution of Human Consciousness.* New York; London: Norton.

Dowd, A. M., McGinley, J. L., Taffe, J. R., and Rinehart, N. J. (2012). Do planning and visual integration difficulties underpin motor dysfunction in autism. A kinematic study of young children with autism. *J. Autism Dev. Disord.* 42, 1539–1548. doi: 10.1007/s10803-011-1385-8

Einspieler, C., and Prechtl, H. F. (2005). Prechtl's assessment of general movements: a diagnostic tool for the functional assessment of the young nervous system. *Mental Retard. Dev. Disabil. Res. Rev.* 11, 61–67. doi: 10.1002/mrdd.20051

Escalona, A., Field, T., Nadel, J., and Lundy, B. (2002). Imitation effects on children with autism. *J. Autism Dev. Disord.* 32, 141–144. doi: 10.1023/A:1014896707002

Fabbri-Destro, M., Cattaneo, L., Boria, S., and Rizzolatti, G. (2009). Planning actions in autism. *Exp. Brain Res.* 192, 521–525. doi: 10.1007/s00221-008-1578-3

Fentress, J. C., and Gadbois, S. (2001). "The development of action sequences," in *Handbook of Behavioral Neurobiology,* ed E. Blass (New York, NY: Kluver Academic/Plenum Publishers), 393–431.

Field, N. J., and Lundy, B. (2002). Imitation effects on children with autism. *J. Autism Dev. Disord.* 32, 141–144.

Field, T., Nadel, J., and Ezell, S. (2011). "Imitation therapy for young children with autism, autism spectrum disorders," in *Autism Spectrum Disorders - From Genes to Environment,* ed T. Williams (New York, NY: InTech), 287–298.

Field, T., Woodson, R., Cohen, D., Greenberg, R., Garcia, R., and Collins, K. (1983). Discrimination and imitation of facial expressions by term and preterm neonates. *Infant Behav. Dev.* 6, 485–489. doi: 10.1016/S0163-6383(83)90316-8

Fogassi, L., Ferrari, P. F., Gesierich, B., Rozzi, S., Chersi, F., and Rizzolatti, G. (2005). Parietal lobe: from action organization to intention understanding. *Science* 308, 662–667. doi: 10.1126/science.1106138

Foxton, A. M., Stewart, M. E., Barnard, L., Rodgers, J., Young, A. H., O'Brien, G., et al. (2003). Absence of auditory 'global interference' in autism. *Brain* 126, 2703–2709.

Frank, B., and Trevarthen, C. (2012). "Intuitive meaning: supporting impulses for interpersonal life in the sociosphere of human knowledge, practice and language," in *Moving Ourselves, Moving Others: Motion and Emotion in Intersubjectivity, Consciousness and Language,* eds A. Foolen, U. M. Ludtke, T. P. Racine, and J. Zlatev (Amsterdam: Benjamins), 261–303.

Frith, C. D., and Frith, U. (1999). Interacting minds: a biological basis. *Cogn. Sci. Rev. Sci.* 286, 1695–1698. doi: 10.1126/science.286.5445.1692

Frith, U. (1989/2003). *Autism: Explaining the Enigma.* Oxford: Blackwell.

Gallese, V. (2006). Intentional attunement: a neurophysiological perspective on social cognition and its disruption in autism. *Brain Res.* 1079, 15–24. doi: 10.1016/j.brainres.2006.01.054

Gallese, V. (2007). Before and below theory of mind: embodied simulation and the neural correlates of social cognition. *Philos. Trans. R. Soc. Lond. B Biol. Sci.* 362, 659–669. doi: 10.1098/rstb.2006.2002

Gallese, V., and Rochat, M. (2013). "The evolution of motor cognition: its role in the development of social cognition and implications for autism spectrum disorder," in *The Infant Mind: Origins of the Social Brain,* eds M. Legerstee, D. Haley, and M. Bornstein (New York, NY: Guildford Press), 19–47.

Gallistel, C. R. (1980). *The Organization of Action.* Hillsdale, NJ: Erlbaum.

Gillberg, C., and Coleman, M. (1992). *The Biology of the Autistic Syndromes, 2nd Edn.* London: MacKeith Press, Clinics in Developmental Medicine, 126.

Gillespie-Lynch, K., Greenfield, P. M., Feng, Y., Savage-Rumbaugh, S., and Lyn, H. (2013). A cross-species study of gesture and its role in symbolic development: implications for the gestural theory of language evolution. *Front. Psychol.* 4:160. doi: 10.3389/fpsyg.2013.00160

Gowen, E. (2012). Imitation in autism: why action kinematics matter. *Front. Integr. Neurosci.* 6:117. doi: 10.3389/fnint.2012.00117

Gowen, E., and Hamilton, A. (2013). Motor abilities in autism: a review using a computational context. *J. Autism Dev. Disord.* 43, 323–344. doi: 10.1007/s10803-012-1574-0

Hallett, M., Lebiedowska, M. K., Thomas, S. L., Stanhope, S. J., Denckla, M. B., and Rumsey, J. (1993). Locomotion of autistic adults. *Arch. Neurol.* 50, 1304–1308. doi: 10.1001/archneur.1993.00540120019007

Hardy, M. W., and Blythe LaGasse, A. (2013). Rhythm, movement, and autism: using rhythmic rehabilitation research as a model for autism. *Front. Integr. Neurosci.* 7:19. doi: 10.3389/fnint.2013.00019

Hashimoto, T., Tayama, M., Murakawa, K., Yoshimoto, T., Muyazaki, M., Harada, M., et al. (1995). Development of the brainstem and cerebellum in autistic patients. *J. Autism Dev. Disord.* 25, 1–18. doi: 10.1007/BF02178163

Heimann, M., Nelson, K. E., and Schaller, J. (1989). Neonatal imitation of tongue protrusion and mouth opening: methodological aspects and evidence of early individual differences. *Scand. J. Psychol.* 30, 90–101. doi: 10.1111/j.1467-9450.1989.tb01072.x

Hesslow, G. (2012). The current status of the simulation theory of cognition. *Brain Res.* 1428, 71–79. doi: 10.1016/j.brainres.2011.06.026

Hevner, R. F. (2000). Development of connections in the human visual system during fetal midgestation: a DiI-tracing study. *J. Neuropathol. Exp. Neurol.* 59, 385–392.

Hobson, R. P. (1993). *Autism and the Development of Mind.* Hove: Lawrence Erlbaum.

Hobson, R. P. (2002/04). *The Cradle of Thought: Exploring the Origins of Thinking.* London: Macmillan/New York: Oxford University Press.

Hobson, R. P., and Hobson, J. A. (2011). "Joint attention or joint engagement? Insights from autism," in *Joint Attention: New Developments in Philosophy,*

Psychology, and Neuroscience, ed A. Seemann (Cambridge, MA: MIT Press), 115–135.

Holstege, G., Bandler, R., and Saper, C. B. (eds.). (1996). *The Emotional Motor System.* Vol. 107. Amsterdam: Elsevier.

Hubley, P., and Trevarthen, C. (1979). "Sharing a task in infancy," in *Social Interaction During Infancy: New Directions for Child Development 4,* ed I. Uzgiris (San Francisco, CA: Jossey-Bass), 57–80.

Jaffe, J., Beebe, B., Felstein, S., Crown, C., and Jasnow, M. D. (2001). Rhythms of dialogue in infancy: coordinated timing and social development. *Monogr. Soc. Res. Child. Dev.* 66, i–viii, 1–132.

Jaffe, J., and Felstein, S. (1970). *Rhythms of Dialogue.* New York, NY: Academic Press.

Jeannerod, M. (1999). To act or not to act: perspectives on the representation of actions. *Q. J. Exp. Psychol.* 52A, 1–29.

Johnson, M. H. (2005). Sensitive periods in functional brain development: problems and prospects. *Dev. Psychobiol.* 46, 287–292. doi: 10.1002/dev.20057

Kanner, L. (1943). Autistic disturbances of affective contact. *Nervous Child* 2, 217–250.

Karmiloff-Smith, A. (2009). Nativism versus neuroconstructivism: rethinking the study of developmental disorders. *Dev. Psychol.* 45, 56–63. doi: 10.1037/a0014506

Kugiumutzakis, G. (1999). "Genesis and development of early infant mimesis to facial and vocal models," in *Imitation in Infancy,* eds J. Nadel and G. Butterworth (Cambridge: Cambridge University Press), 127–185.

Lashley, K. S. (1951). "The problems of serial order in behavior," in *Cerebral Mechanisms in Behavior,* ed L. A. Jeffress (New York, NY: Wiley), 112–136.

Lecanuet, J.-P., Fifer, W. P., Krasnegor, N. A., and Smotherman, W. P. (1995). *Fetal Development: A Psychobiological Perspective.* Hillsdale; Hove: Erlbaum.

Lee, D. N. (2009). General Tau Theory: evolution to date. *Perception* 38, 837–858. doi: 10.1068/pmklee

Llinàs, R. R. (2001). *I of the Vortex: From Neurons to Self.* Cambridge, MA: MIT Press.

Lüdtke, U. (2012). "Relational emotions in semiotic and linguistic development: towards an intersubjective theory of language learning and language therapy," in *Moving Ourselves, Moving Others: Motion and Emotion in Consciousness, Intersubjectivity and Language,* eds A. Foolen, U. M. Luďtke, T. P. Racine, and J. Zlatev (Amsterdam: Benjamins), 305–346.

Maestro, S., Muratori, F., Cavallaro, M. C., Pei, F., Stern, D., Golse, B., et al. (2002). Attentional skills during the first 6 months of age in autism spectrum disorder. *J. Am. Acad. Child Adolesc. Psychiatry* 41, 1239–1245. doi: 10.1097/00004583-200210000-00014

Mahdhaoui, A., Chetouani, M., Cassel, R. S., Saint-Georges, C., Parlato, E., Laznik, M.-C., et al. (2011). Computerized home video detection for motherese may help to study impaired interaction between infants who become autistic and their parents. *Int. J. Methods Psychiatry Res.* 20, e6–e18. doi: 10.1002/mpr.332

Malloch, S. (1999). "Mothers and infants and communicative musicality," in *Rhythms, Musical Narrative, and the Origins of Human Communication. Musicae Scientiae, Special Issue, 1999-2000,* ed I. Deliège (Liège: European Society for the Cognitive Sciences of Music), 29–57.

Malloch, S., and Trevarthen, C. (eds.). (2009). *Communicative Musicality: Exploring the Basis of Human Companionship.* Oxford: Oxford University Press.

Maratos, O. (1982). "Trends in development of imitation in early infancy," in *Regressions in Mental Development: Basic Phenomena and Theories,* ed T. G. Bever (Hillsdale, NJ: Erlbaum), 81–101.

Mari, M., Castiello, U., Marks, D., Marraffa, C., and Prior, M. (2003). The reach-to-grasp movement in children with autism spectrum disorder. *Philos. Trans. R. Soc. Lond. Ser. B Biol. Sci.* 358, 393–403. doi: 10.1098/rstb.2002.1205

Marler, P. (1984). "Animal communication: affect or cognition?" in *Approaches to Emotion,* ed K. R. Scherer and P. Ekman (Hillsdale, NJ: Erlbaum), 345–365.

Maturana, H., Mpodozis, J., and Letelier, J. C. (1995). Brain, language and the origin of human mental functions. *Biol. Res.* 28, 15–26.

McNeill, D. (2005). *Gesture and Thought.* Chicago, IL: University of Chicago Press doi: 10.7208/chicago/9780226514642.001.0001

Meltzoff, A. N., and Moore, M. K. (1977). Imitation of facial and manual gestures by human neonates. *Science* 198, 75–78. doi: 10.1126/science.198.4312.75

Merker, B. (2007). Consciousness without a cerebral cortex: a challenge for neuroscience and medicine. *Behav. Brain Sci.* 30, 63–134. doi: 10.1017/S0140525X07000891

Miller, G. A. (2003). The cognitive revolution: a historical perspective. *Trends Cogn. Sci.* 7, 141–144. doi: 10.1016/S1364-6613(03)00029-9

Mithen, S. (2009). The music instinct: the evolutionary basis of musicality. *Ann. N.Y. Acad. Sci.* 1169, 3–12. doi: 10.1111/j.1749-6632.2009.04590.x

Morton, J. (2004). *Understanding Developmental Disorders: A Cognitive Modeling Approach.* Oxford: Blackwell. doi: 10.1002/9780470773307

Mottron, L., Dawson, M., Soulières, I., Hubert, B., and Burack, J. (2006). Enhanced perceptual functioning in autism: An update, and eight principles of autistic perception. *J. Autism Dev. Disord.* 36, 27–43. doi: 10.1007/s10803-005-0040-7

Mundy, P., Sullivan, L., and Mastergeorge, A. M. (2009). A parallel and distributed-processing model of joint attention, social cognition and autism. *Autism Res.* 2, 2–21. doi: 10.1002/aur.61

Muratori, F., and Maestro, S. (2007). Autism as a downstream effect of primary difficulties in intersubjectivity interacting with abnormal development of brain connectivity. *Int. J. Dial. Sci.* 2, 93–118.

Nadel, J. (2006). "Does imitation matter to children with autism?" in *Imitation and the Social Mind,* eds S. Rogers and J. Williams (NewYork, NY: The Guilford Press), 118–137.

Nagy, E. (2011). The newborn infant: a missing stage in developmental psychology. *Infant Child Dev.* 20, 3–19. doi: 10.1002/icd.683

Nagy, E., and Molnar, P. (2004). Homo imitans or homo provocans. The phenomenon of neonatal initiation. *Infant Behav. Dev.* 27, 57–63. doi: 10.1016/j.infbeh.2003.06.004

Narvaez, D., Panksepp, J., Schore, A., and Gleason, T. (Eds.). (2013). *Evolution, Early Experience and Human Development: From Research to Practice and Policy.* New York, NY: Oxford University Press.

Nayate, A., Tonge, B. J., Bradshaw, J. L., McGinley, J. L., Iansek, R., and Rihehart, N. J. (2011). Differentiation of high-functioning autism and Asperger's disorder based on neuromotor behavior. *J. Autism Dev. Disord.* 42, 707–717. doi: 10.1007/s10803-011-1299-5

Nazarali, N., Glazebrook, C. M., and Elliott, D. (2009). Movement planning and reprogramming in individuals with autism. *J. Autism Dev. Disord.* 39, 1401–1411. doi: 10.1007/s10803-009-0756-x

Nind, M. (1999). Intensive interaction and autism: a useful approach. *Br. J. Spec. Edu.* 26, 96–102. doi: 10.1111/1467-8527.t01-1-00114

Nordoff, P., and Robbins, C. (2007). *Creative Music Therapy: A Guide to Fostering Clinical Musicianship.* Revised Edn. New York, NY: John Day, Gilsum, NH: Barcelona Publishers.

Northoff, G., and Panksepp, J. (2008). The trans-species concept of self and the subcortical–cortical midline system. *Trends Cogn. Sci.* 12, 259–264. doi: 10.1016/j.tics.2008.04.007

Ockleford, A. (2012). "Songs without words: exploring how music can serve as a proxy language in social interaction with autistic children," in *Music, Health, and Wellbeing,* eds R. MacDonald, G. Kreutz, and L. Mitchell (Oxford: Oxford University Press), 289–323.

Ockleford, A. (2013). *Music, Language and Autism: Exceptional Strategies for Exceptional Minds.* London: Jessica Kingsley.

Okado, N. (1980). Development of the human cervical spinal cord with reference to synapse formation in the motor nucleus. *J. Comp. Neurol.* 191, 495–513. doi: 10.1002/cne.901910311

Oller, D. K., Niyogi, P., Gray, S., Richards, J. A., Gilkerson, J., Xu, D., et al. (2010). Automated vocal analysis of naturalistic recordings from children with autism, language delay, and typical development. *Proc. Natl. Acad. Sci. U.S.A.* 107, 13354–13359. doi: 10.1073/pnas.1003882107

O'Riordan, M. A., Plaisted, K. C., Driver, J., and Baron-Cohen, S. (2001). Superior visual search in autism. *J. Exp. Psychol. Hum. Percept. Perform.* 27, 719–730.

Panksepp, J. (2005). Affective consciousness: core emotional feelings in animals and humans. *Conscious. Cogn.* 14, 19–69. doi: 10.1016/j.concog.2004.10.004

Panksepp, J., and Biven, L. (2012). *The Archaeology of Mind: Neuroevolutionary Origins of Human Emotions.* New York, NY: Norton.

Panksepp, J., and Sahley, T. (1987). "Possible brain opioid involvement in disrupted social intent and language development of autism," in *Neurobiological Issues in Autism,* eds E. Schopler and G. Mesibov (New York, NY: Plenum Press), 357–382.

Panksepp, J., and Watt, D. (2011). Why does depression hurt. Ancestral Primary-Process Separation-Distress (PANIC/GRIEF) and Diminished Brain Reward (SEEKING) processes in the genesis of depressive affect. *Psychiatry* 74, 5–13. doi: 10.1521/psyc.2011.74.1.5

Papoušek, H. (1996). "Musicality in infancy research: biological and cultural origins of early musicality," in *Musical Beginnings: Origins and Development of Musical Competence*, eds I. Deliège and J. Sloboda (Oxford; New York; Tokyo: Oxford University Press), 37–55. doi: 10.1093/acprof:oso/9780198523321.003.0002

Patriquin, M. A., Scarpa, A., Friedman, B. H., and Porges, S. W. (2013). Respiratory sinus arrhythmia: a marker for positive social functioning and receptive language skills in children with autism spectrum disorders. *Dev. Psychobiol.* 55, 101–112. doi: 10.1002/dev.21002

Pezzulo, G., Butz, M. V., Sigaud, O., and Baldasarre, G. (eds.). (2008). *From Sensorimotor to Higher-Level Cognitive Processes: An Introduction to Anticipatory Behavior Systems.* Berlin: Springer Verlag.

Pezzulo, G., and Castelfranchi, C. (2009). Thinking as the control of imagination: a conceptual framework for goal-directed systems. *Psychol. Res.* 73, 559–577. doi: 10.1007/s00426-009-0237-z

Piaget, J. (1951). *Play, Dreams and Imitation in Childhood.* London: Heinemann.

Piaget, J. (1954). *The Construction of Reality in the Child.* New York, NY: Basic Books. doi: 10.1037/11168-000

Piontelli, A. (2010). *Development of Normal Fetal Movements: The First 25 Weeks of Gestation.* Wien; New York: Springer-Verlag. doi: 10.1007/978-88-470-1402-2

Pöppel, E., and Wittmann, M. (1999). "Time in the mind," in *The MIT Encyclopedia of the Cognitive Sciences,* eds R. Wilson and F. Keil (Cambridge, MA: The MIT Press), 836–837.

Porges, S. W. (2011). *The Polyvagal Theory: Neurophysiological Foundations of Emotions, Attachment, Communication, and Self-Regulation.* New York; London: W. W. Norton.

Porges, S. W., and Furman, S. A. (2011). The early development of the autonomic nervous system provides a neural platform for social behavior: a polyvagal perspective. *Infant Child Dev.* 20, 106–118. doi: 10.1002/icd.688

Prechtl, H. F. R. (2001). "Prenatal and early postnatal development of human motor behavior," in *Handbook on Brain and Behavior in Human Development,* eds A. F. Kalverboer and A. Gramsbergen (Dordrecht: Kluwer Academic Publishers), 415–427.

Rapin, I., and Allen, D. A. (1983). "Developmental language disorders: nosological considerations," in *Neuropsychology of Language, Reading and Spelling,* ed U. Kirk (New York, NY: Academic Press), 155–184.

Reddy, V. (2008). *How Infants Know Minds.* Cambridge, MA: Harvard University Press.

Reddy, V. (2011). "A gaze at grips with me," in *Joint Attention: New Developments in Philosophy, Psychology, and Neuroscience,* ed A. Seemann (Cambridge, MA: MIT Press), 137–158.

Reddy, V., Liebal, K., Hicks, K., Jonnalagadda, S., and Chintalapuri, B. (2012). The emergent practice of infant compliance: an exploration in two cultures. *Dev. Psychol.* doi: 10.1037/a0030979. [Epub ahead of print].

Reddy, V., Williams, E., Costantini, C., and Lang, B. (2010). Engaging with the self: mirror behavior in autism, Down syndrome and typical development. *Autism* 14, 531–546. doi: 10.1177/1362361310370397

Reddy, V., Williams, E., and Vaughan, A. (2002). Sharing humour and laughter in autism and Downs syndrome. *Br. J. Psychol.* 93, 219–242. doi: 10.1348/000712602162553

Reissland, N., Francis, B., Mason, J., and Lincoln, K. (2011). Do Facial expressions develop before birth. *PLoS ONE* 6:e24081. doi: 10.1371/journal.pone.0024081

Ricks, D. M., and Wing, L. (1975). Language, communication and the use of symbols in normal and autistic children. *J. Autism Child. Schizophr.* 5, 191–221. doi: 10.1007/BF01538152

Rinehart, N. J., Bellgrove, M. A., Tonge, B. J., Brereton, A. V., Howells-Rankin, D., and Bradshaw, J. L. (2006a). An examination of movement kinematics in young people with high-functioning autism and Asperger's disorder: further evidence for a motor planning deficit. *J. Autism Dev. Disord.* 36, 757–767. doi: 10.1007/s10803-006-0118-x

Rinehart, N. J., Tonge, B. J., Bradshaw, J. L., Iansek, R., Enticott, P. G., and McGinley, J. (2006b). Gait function in high-functioning autism and Asperger's disorder: evidence for basal-ganglia and cerebellar involvement. *Eur. Child Adoles. Psychiatry* 15, 256–264. doi: 10.1007/s00787-006-0530-y

Rinehart, N. J., Bradshaw, J. L., Brereton, A. V., and Tonge, B. J. (2001). Movement preparation in high-functioning autism and Asperger disorder: a serial choice reaction time task involving motor reprogramming. *J. Autism Dev. Disord.* 31, 79–88. doi: 10.1023/A:1005617831035

Robarts, J. Z. (1998). "Music therapy and children with autism," in *Children with Autism: Diagnosis and Interventions To Meet Their Needs,* eds C. Trevarthen, K. Aitken, D. Papoudi, and J. Robarts (London: Jessica Kingsley), 172–202.

Rochat, M. J., Veroni, V., Bruschweiler-Stern, N., Pieraccini, C., Bonnet-Brilhault, F., Barthélémy, C., et al. (2013). Impaired vitality form recognition in autism. *Neuropsychologia* doi: 10.1016/j.neuropsychologia.2013.06.002. [Epub ahead of print].

Rodier, P. M., and Arndt, T. L. (2005). "The brainstem in autism," in *The Neurobiology of Autism, 2 Edn.,* eds M. L. Bauman and T. L. Kemper (Baltimore, MD: Johns Hopkins University Press), 136–149.

Rogers, S., and Williams, J. H. (eds.). (2006). *Imitation and the Social Mind: Typical Development and Autism.* New York, NY: Guilford Press.

Rönnqvist, L., and von Hofsten, C. (1994). Neonatal finger and arm movements as determined by a social and an object context. *Early Dev. Parenting* 3, 81–94. doi: 10.1002/edp.2430030205

Rosenbaum, D. A., Marchak, F., Barnes, H. J., Vaughan, J., Slotta, J. D., and Jorgensen, M. J. (1990). "Constraints for action selection: overhand versus underhand grips," in *Attention and Performance XIII,* ed. M. Jeannerod (Hillsdale, NJ: Erlbaum), 321–342.

Rosenhall, U., Nordin, V., Sandström, M., Ahlsén, G., and Gillberg, C. (1999). Autism and hearing loss. *J. Autism Dev. Disord.* 29, 349–357. doi: 10.1023/A:1023022709710

Rovee-Collier, C. K., Morrongiello, B. A., Aron, M., and Kupersmidt, J. (1978). Topographical responses differentiation and reversal in 3-month-old infants. *Infant Behav. Dev.* 1, 323–333. doi: 10.1016/S0163-6383(78)80044-7

Royal College of Obstetricians, and Gynaecologists. (2010). *Fetal Awareness: Review of Research and Recommendations for Practice.* London: Royal College of Obstetricians and Gynaecologists.

Rumsey, J. M. (1985). Conceptual problem solving ability in highly verbal, nonretarded autistic men. *J. Autism Dev. Disord.* 15, 23–36. doi: 10.1007/BF01837896

Saint-Georges, C., Cassel, R. S., Cohen, D., Chetouani, M., Laznik, M.-C., Maestro, S., et al. (2010). What studies of family home movies can teach us about autistic infants: a literature review. *Res. Autism Spect. Disord.* 4, 355–366. doi: 10.1016/j.rasd.2009.10.017

Saint-Georges, C., Mahdhaoui, A., Chetaoani, M., Cassel, R. S., Laznik, M.-C., Apicella, F., et al. (2011). Do parents recognize autistic deviant behavior long before diagnosis. Taking into account interaction using computational methods. *PLoS ONE* 6:e22393. doi: 10.1371/journal.pone.0022393

Sander, L. W. (2008). *Living Systems, Evolving Consciousness and the Emerging Person: A Selection of Papers from the Life Work of Louis Sander,* eds G. Amadei and I. Bianchi (New York; London: The Analytic Press).

Schmitz, C., Martineau, J., Barthelemy, C., and Assaiante, C. (2003). Motor control and children with autism: deficit of anticipatory function. *Neurosci. Lett.* 348, 17–20. doi: 10.1016/S0304-3940(03)00644-X

Schögler, B., Pepping, G.-J., and Lee, D. N. (2008). TauG-guidance of transients in expressive musical performance. *Exp. Brain Res.* 198, 361–372. doi: 10.1007/s00221-008-1431-8

Schore, A. N. (1994). *Affect Regulation and the Origin of the Self: The Neurobiology of Emotional Development.* Hillsdale, NJ: Erlbaum

Schore, A. N. (2003). *Affect Regulation and the Repair of the Self.* New York, NY: Norton.

Schore, A. N. (2005). Attachment, affect regulation and the developing right brain: Linking developmental neuroscience to pediatrics. *Pediatr. Rev.* 26, 204–211. doi: 10.1542/pir.26-6-204

Sebeok, T. A. (1990). *Essays in Zoosemiotics (Monograph Series of the Toronto Semiotic Circle, Number 5).* Toronto, ON: University of Toronto.

Senju, A., and Johnson, M. H. (2009). Atypical eye contact in autism: models, mechanisms and development. *Neurosci. Biobehav. Rev.*

33, 1204–1214. doi: 10.1016/j.neubiorev.2009.06.001

Sherrington, C. S. (1906). *The Integrative Action of the Nervous System.* New York, NY: Charles Scribner's Sons.

Solms, M., and Panksepp, J. (2012). The "Id" knows more than the "Ego" admits: Neuropsychoanalytic and primal consciousness perspectives on the interface between affective and cognitive neuroscience. *Brain Sci.* 2, 147–175. doi: 10.3390/brainsci2020147

Solomon, W., Holland, C., and Middleton, M.-J. (2012). *Autism and Understanding: The Waldon Approach to child Development.* Los Angeles; London; New Delhi; Singapore; Washington: Sage

Sperry, R. W. (1952). Neurology and the mind-brain problem. *Am. Sci.* 40, 291–312.

St. Clair, C., Danon-Boileau, L., and Trevarthen, C. (2007). "Signs of autism in infancy: sensitivity for rhythms of expression in communication," in *Signs of Autism In Infants: Recognition and Early Intervention,* ed S. Acquarone (London: Karnac), 21–45.

Stern, D. N. (1993). "The role of feelings for an interpersonal self," in *The Perceived Self: Ecological and Interpersonal Sources of Self-Knowledge,* ed U. Neisser (New York, NY: Cambridge University Press), 205–215.

Stern, D. N. (2000). *The Interpersonal World of the Infant: A View from Psychoanalysis and Development Psychology, 2Edn.,* New York, NY: Basic Books.

Stern, D. N. (2010). *Forms of Vitality: Exploring Dynamic Experience in Psychology, the Arts, Psychotherapy and Development.* Oxford: Oxford University Press.

Stuart, S. (2010). "Enkinaesthetia, biosemiotics and the ethiosphere," in *Signifying Bodies: Biosemiosis, Interaction and Health,* eds S. J. Cowley, J. C. Major, S. V Steffensen, and A. Dinis (Braga: The Faculty of Philosophy, Braga Portuguese Catholic University), 305–330.

Teitelbaum, O., and Teitelbaum, P. (2008). *Does Your Baby Have Autism?: Detecting the Earliest Signs of Autism.* Garden City Park, NY: Square One Publishers.

Teitelbaum, P., Teitelbaum, O., Nye, J., Fryman, J., and Maurer, R. G. (1998). Movement analysis in infancy may be useful for early diagnosis of autism. *Proc. Natl Acad. Sci. U.S.A.* 95, 13982–13987. doi: 10.1073/pnas.95.23.13982

Teitelbaum, P., Teitelbaum, O. B., Fryman, J., and Maurer, R. (2002). Reflexes gone astray in autism in infancy. *J. Dev. Learn. Disord.* 6, 15–22.

Thomas, M. S. C., and Karmiloff-Smith, A. (2002). Are developmental disorders like cases of adult brain damage. Implications from connectionist modeling. *Behav. Brain Sci.* 25, 727–788. doi: 10.1017/S0140525X02000134

Torres, E. B. (2013). Atypical signatures of motor variability found in an individual with ASD. *Neurocase* 19, 150–165. doi: 10.1080/13554794.2011.654224

Trehub, S. E. (1990). "The perception of musical patterns by human infants: the provision of similar patterns by their parents," in *Comparative Perception,* Vol. 1, Mechanisms, eds M. A. Berkley and W. C. Stebbins (New York, NY: Wiley), 429–459.

Trevarthen, C. (1977). "Descriptive analyses of infant communication behavior," in *Studies in Mother-Infant Interaction: The Loch Lomond Symposium,* ed H. R. Schaffer (London, Academic Press), 227–270.

Trevarthen, C. (1979). "Communication and cooperation in early infancy. A description of primary intersubjectivity," in *Before Speech: The Beginning of Human Communication,* ed M. Bullowa (London, Cambridge University Press), 321–347.

Trevarthen, C. (1984). "How control of movements develops," in *Human Motor Actions: Bernstein Reassessed,* ed H. T. A. Whiting (Amsterdam: Elsevier/North Holland), 223–261.

Trevarthen, C. (1986a). "Neuroembryology and the development of perceptual mechanisms," in *Human Growth, 2 Edn.,* eds F. Falkner and J. M. Tanner (New York, NY: Plenum), 301–383.

Trevarthen, C. (1986b). "Development of intersubjective motor control in infants," in *Motor Development in Children: Aspects of Coordination and Control,* eds M. G. Wade and H. T. A. Whiting (Dordrecht, Martinus Nijhof), 209–261. doi: 10.1007/978-94-009-4460-2_14

Trevarthen, C. (1990). "Signs before speech," in *The Semiotic Web, 1989,* eds T. A. Sebeok and J. Umiker-Sebeok (Berlin; New York; Amsterdam: Mouton de Gruyter), 689–755.

Trevarthen, C. (1996). Lateral asymmetries in infancy: implications for the development of the hemispheres. *Neurosci. Biobehav. Rev.* 20, 571–586. doi: 10.1016/0149-7634(95)00070-4

Trevarthen, C. (1998). "The concept and foundations of infant intersubjectivity," in *Intersubjective Communication and Emotion in Early Ontogeny,* ed S. Bråten (Cambridge: Cambridge University Press), 15–46.

Trevarthen, C. (1999). "Musicality and the intrinsic motive pulse: evidence from human psychobiology and infant communication," in *Rhythms, Musical Narrative, and the Origins of Human Communication. Musicae Scientiae, Special Issue, 1999-2000,* ed I. Deliège (Liège: European Society for the Cognitive Sciences of Music), 157–213.

Trevarthen, C. (2000). Autism as a neurodevelopmental disorder affecting communication and learning in early childhood: prenatal origins, post-natal course and effective educational support. *Prostoglandins Leucot. Essent. Fatty Acids* 63, 41–46. doi: 10.1054/plef.2000.0190

Trevarthen, C. (2001a). "The neurobiology of early communication: intersubjective regulations in human brain development," in *Handbook on Brain and Behavior in Human Development,* eds A. F. Kalverboer and A. Gramsbergen (Dordrecht: Kluwer), 841–882.

Trevarthen, C. (2001b). Intrinsic motives for companionship in understanding: their origin, development and significance for infant mental health. *Infant Ment. Health J.* 22, 95–131.

Trevarthen, C. (2005). "Stepping away from the mirror: Pride and shame in adventures of companionship Reflections on the nature and emotional needs of infant intersubjectivity," in *Attachment and Bonding: A New Synthesis. Dahlem Workshop Report 92,* eds C. S. Carter, L. Ahnert, K. E. Grossman, S. B. Hrdy, M. E. Lamb, S. W. Porges, and N. Sachser (Cambridge, MA: The MIT Press), 55–84.

Trevarthen, C. (2009a). "The functions of emotion in infancy: the regulation and communication of rhythm, sympathy, and meaning in human development," in *The Healing Power of Emotion: Affective Neuroscience, Development, and Clinical Practice,* eds D. Fosha, D. J. Siegel, and M. F. Solomon (New York, NY: Norton), 55–85.

Trevarthen, C. (2009b). "Human biochronology: on the source and functions of 'musicality'," in *Music That Works: Contributions of Biology, Neurophysiology, Psychology, Sociology, Medicine and Musicology,* eds R. Haas and V. Brandes (Vienna; New York: Springer), 221–266.

Trevarthen, C. (2012). Embodied human intersubjectivity: Imaginative agency, to share meaning. *Cogn. Semiotics* 4, *The Intersubjectivity of Embodiment,* 6–56.

Trevarthen, C. (2013). Born for art, and the joyful companionship of fiction," in *Evolution, Early Experience and Human Development: From Research to Practice and Policy,* eds D. Narvaez, J. Panksepp, A. Schore, and T. Gleason (New York, NY: Oxford University Press), 202–218.

Trevarthen, C., and Aitken, K. J. (1994). Brain development, infant communication, and empathy disorders: Intrinsic factors in child mental health. *Dev. Psychopathol.* 6, 599–635. doi: 10.1017/S0954579400004703

Trevarthen, C., and Aitken, K. J. (2001). Infant intersubjectivity: research, theory, and clinical applications. *J. Child Psychol. Psychiatry* 42, 3–48. doi: 10.1111/1469-7610.00701

Trevarthen, C., and Aitken, K. J. (2003). "Regulation of brain development and age-related changes in infants' motives: the developmental function of 'regressive' periods," in *Regression Periods in Human Infancy,* ed M. Heimann (Mahwah, NJ: Erlbaum), 107–184.

Trevarthen, C., Aitken, K. J., Papoudi, C., and Robarts, J. Z. (1998). *Children with Autism: Diagnosis and Interventions to Meet their Needs, 2 Edn.* London: Jessica Kingsley.

Trevarthen, C., Aitken, K. J., Vandekerckhove, M., Delafield-Butt, J., and Nagy, E. (2006). "Collaborative regulations of vitality in early childhood: stress in intimate relationships and postnatal psychopathology," in *Developmental Psychopathology,* Vol. 2, Developmental Neuroscience, 2 Edn. (New York, NY: Wileys), 65–126.

Trevarthen, C., and Daniel, S. (2005). Rhythm and synchrony in early development, and signs of autism and Rett syndrome in infancy. *Brain Dev.* 27, (Suppl. 1), S25–S34. doi: 10.1016/j.braindev.2005.03.016

Trevarthen, C., and Delafield-Butt, J. (2013). "Biology of shared experience and language development: regulations for the inter-subjective life of narratives," in *The Infant Mind: Origins of the Social Brain,* eds M. Legerstee, D. Haley, and M. Bornstein (New York, NY: Guildford Press), 167–199.

Trevarthen, C., Delafield-Butt, J., and Schögler, B. (2011). "Psychobiology of musical gesture: innate rhythm, harmony and melody in movements of narration," in *New Perspectives on Music and Gesture*, eds A. Gritten and E. King (Farnham, Surrey, Burlington: Ashgate), 11–43.

Tronick, E. Z. (1989). Emotions and emotional communication in infants. *Am. Psychol.* 44, 112–126. doi: 10.1037/0003-066X.44.2.112

Tulving, E. (2002). Episodic memory: from mind to brain. *Annu. Rev. Psychol.* 253, 1–25. doi: 10.1146/annurev.psych.53.100901.135114

Tzourio-Mazoyer, N., De Schonen, S., Crivello, F., Reutter, B., Aujard, Y., and Mazoyer, B. (2002). Neural correlates of woman face processing by 2-month-old infants. *Neuroimage* 15, 454–461. doi: 10.1006/nimg.2001.0979

Vandekerckhove, M., and Panksepp, J. (2011). A neurocognitive theory of higher mental emergence: From anoetic affective experiences to noetic knowledge and autonoetic awareness. *Neurosci. Biobehav. Rev.* 35, 2017–2025. doi: 10.1016/j.neubiorev.2011.04.001

Van der Meer, A. L. H., Van der Weel, F. R., and Lee, D. N. (1996). Lifting weights in neonates: developing visual control of reaching. *Scand. J. Psychol.* 37, 424–436. doi: 10.1111/j.1467-9450.1996.tb00674.x

Vernazza-Martin, S., Martin, N., Vernazza, A., Lepellec-Muller, A., Rufo, M., Massion, J., et al. (2005). Goal directed locomotion and balance control in autistic children. *J. Autism Dev. Disord.* 35, 91–102. doi: 10.1007/s10803-004-1037-3

von Hofsten, C. (1993). Prospective control – A basic aspect of action development. *Hum. Dev.* 36, 253–270. doi: 10.1159/000278212

von Hofsten, C. (2004). An action perspective on motor development. *Trends Cogn. Sci.* 8, 266–272. doi: 10.1016/j.tics.2004.04.002

von Hofsten, C. (2007). Action in development. *Dev. Sci.* 10, 54–60. doi: 10.1111/j.1467-7687.2007.00564.x

von Uexküll, J. (1957). "A stroll through the worlds of animals and men: a picture book of invisible worlds," in *Instinctive Behavior: the Development of a Modern Concept*, ed and trans. C. H. Schiller (New York, NY: International Universities Press, Inc.), 5–80.

Welsh, J. P., Ahn, E. S., and Placantonakis, D. G. (2005). Is autism due to brain desynchronization. *Int. J. Dev. Neurosci.* 23, 253–263. doi: 10.1016/j.ijdevneu.2004.09.002

Welsh, J. P., Lang, E. J., Suglhara, I., and Llinas, R. (1995). Dynamic organization of motor control within the olivocerebellar system. *Nature* 374, 453–457. doi: 10.1038/374453a0

Wigram, T. (2006). "Musical creativity in children with cognitive and social impairment," in *Musical Creativity: Multidisciplinary Research in Theory and Practice*, eds I. Deliège and G. Wiggins (London: Psychology Press, Taylor and Francis), 221–237.

Wigram, T., and Elefant, C. (2009). "Therapeutic dialogues in music: nurturing musicality of communication in children with autistic spectrum disorder and Rett syndrome," in *Communicative Musicality: Exploring the Basis of Human Companionship*, eds S. Malloch, and C. Trevarthen (Oxford: Oxford University Press), 423–445.

Wigram, T., and Gold, C. (2006). Music therapy in the assessment and treatment of autistic spectrum disorder: clinical application and research evidence. *Child Care Health Dev.* 32, 535–542. doi: 10.1111/j.1365-2214.2006.00615.x

Wigram, T., and Gold, C. (2012). "The religion of evidence-based practice: helpful or harmful to health and well-being?" in *Music, Health, and Wellbeing*, eds R. MacDonald, G. Kreutz, and L. Mitchell (Oxford: Oxford University Press), 164–182.

Zalla, T., Daprati, E., Sav, A.-M., Chaste, P., Nico, D., and Leboyer, M. (2010). Memory for self-performed actions in individuals with Asperger syndrome. *PLoS ONE* 5:e13370. doi: 10.1371/journal.pone.0013370

Zeedyk, S. (ed.). (2008). *Promoting Social Interaction for Individuals with Communication Impairments.* London and Philadelphia: Jessica Kingsley.

Zoia, S., Blason, L., D'Ottavio, G., Bulgheroni, M., Pezzetta, E., Scabar, A., et al. (2007). Evidence of early development of action planning in the human fetus: a kinematic study. *Exp. Brain Res.* 176, 217–226.

Zwaigenbaum, L., Bryson, S., Rogers, T., Roberts, W., Brian, J., and Szatmari, P. (2005). Behavioral manifestations of autism in the first year of life. *Int. J. Dev. Neurosci.* 23, 143–152. doi: 10.1016/j.ijdevneu.2004.05.001

Conflict of Interest Statement: The authors declare that the research was conducted in the absence of any commercial or financial relationships that could be construed as a potential conflict of interest.

11

Oral motor deficits in speech-impaired children with autism

Matthew K. Belmonte[1,2,3]*, Tanushree Saxena-Chandhok[4], Ruth Cherian[4], Reema Muneer[4], Lisa George[4] and Prathibha Karanth[4]

[1] The Groden Center, Providence, RI, USA
[2] Division of Psychology, Nottingham Trent University, Nottingham, UK
[3] Center for the Study of Human Development, Brown University, Providence, RI, USA
[4] The Com DEALL Trust, Bangalore, India

Edited by:
Anne M. Donnellan, University of San Diego, USA

Reviewed by:
Gary W. LaVigna, Institute for Applied Behavior Analysis, USA
A. Blythe LaGasse, Colorado State University, USA

*Correspondence:
Matthew K. Belmonte, The Groden Center, 86 Mount Hope Avenue, Providence, RI 02906-1648, USA
e-mail: belmonte@mit.edu

Absence of communicative speech in autism has been presumed to reflect a fundamental deficit in the use of language, but at least in a subpopulation may instead stem from motor and oral motor issues. Clinical reports of disparity between receptive vs. expressive speech/language abilities reinforce this hypothesis. Our early-intervention clinic develops skills prerequisite to learning and communication, including sitting, attending, and pointing or reference, in children below 6 years of age. In a cohort of 31 children, gross and fine motor skills and activities of daily living as well as receptive and expressive speech were assessed at intake and after 6 and 10 months of intervention. Oral motor skills were evaluated separately within the first 5 months of the child's enrolment in the intervention programme and again at 10 months of intervention. Assessment used a clinician-rated structured report, normed against samples of 360 (for motor and speech skills) and 90 (for oral motor skills) typically developing children matched for age, cultural environment and socio-economic status. In the full sample, oral and other motor skills correlated with receptive and expressive language both in terms of pre-intervention measures and in terms of learning rates during the intervention. A motor-impaired group comprising a third of the sample was discriminated by an uneven profile of skills with oral motor and expressive language deficits out of proportion to the receptive language deficit. This group learnt language more slowly, and ended intervention lagging in oral motor skills. In individuals incapable of the degree of motor sequencing and timing necessary for speech movements, receptive language may outstrip expressive speech. Our data suggest that autistic motor difficulties could range from more basic skills such as pointing to more refined skills such as articulation, and need to be assessed and addressed across this entire range in each individual.

Keywords: autism, non-verbal, oral motor, speech, language, dyspraxia

INTRODUCTION

Deficits in communication have long been recognised as an essential characteristic of autism, earning a place in the triad of diagnostic signs. Autism is, however, a developmental disorder not only nosologically but also ætiologically, and therefore the deficits that are most obvious, most diagnostic, and most debilitating might not necessarily be the most ætiologically primary. Viewing autism as a developmental disorder, then, compels one to seek beyond the developmental endpoints on which diagnosis is based, to identify root causes. Evidence and interpretation as to the cause of the communication deficit have ranged from a lack of social motivation or social reward (Chevallier et al., 2012), with the social cognitive capacity to develop communication presumably being intact, to specific issues in social cognition including pragmatic applications of communicative skills (Tesink et al., 2009) or theory-of-mind and perspective-taking (Frith, 1997). Debates on autism's origins, therefore, often end up framed in terms of differences between social motivational and social cognitive theories. Of course, as autism is a behaviourally diagnosed syndrome with a great degree of heterogeneity in presentation, it's likely to admit many biological causes, with different combinations of these biological causal mechanisms converging into one and the same set of diagnostic behavioural traits, and diverging into variation within the behaviourally defined phenotype (Belmonte et al., 2004). These putative causal mechanisms of social motivation and social cognition must not, therefore, be approached as exclusive of each other—or of other, even more fundamental causal mechanisms.

In both these sets of accounts, the cognitive and the motivational, the developmental endpoint combines disruptions of social communication and social reward, the only distinction being which one of these symptoms arises first and incurs the other. Seldom has the autistic disruption of social communication been conceptualised as a consequence of difficulties in acquiring and producing speech and language. Evidence to the contrary, that is, acknowledgement that at least in a subpopulation of children with autism communicative deficits may instead stem from more basic motor and oral motor issues, is now emerging. Qualitative and quantitative assessments of gross, fine, and oral motor functions in children with autism as compared to their neurotypical peers have recorded significant differences, suggesting that motor deficits could underlie some of autism's communicative and social symptoms [see Leary and Hill (1996) for a review]. A case is therefore increasingly made for screening children with autism for neuro-motor deficits and for addressing these in intervention where appropriate (Noterdaeme et al., 2002).

Amongst the motor skills, oral motor skills in particular are closely linked with speech production, fluency and clarity. Here too recent research is documenting the association between early oral motor skills and later speech fluency. Amato and Slavin (1998) noted the link between oral motor movements involving the tongue and lips and speech fluency in children with autism. Similar measures are in fact reported to be sufficiently robust as to distinguish autistic children from typically developing children, and also to distinguish between autistic children with eventually varying degrees of fluency (Gernsbacher et al., 2007). In children whose non-verbal cognitive skills are relatively intact, vocal, and other motor imitation skills at early ages—even more so than early joint attention—predict language skills at the age of 5 years (Thurm et al., 2007).

Intensive early intervention (EI) for children with autism has been shown to make a clinically significant difference for many children in multiple areas including language. The Communication DEALL EI (Karanth, 2010; Karanth et al., 2010) programme provides intensive intervention for young children (0–6 years) with autism spectrum disorders via an interdisciplinary team comprising a speech language therapist, an occupational therapist and a developmental educator/psychologist. Developmental skills are assessed and strengthened in eight domains including gross motor (GM), fine motor (FM) and activities of daily living (ADL), receptive language (RL), expressive language (EL), cognitive (C), social (S) and emotional (E) skills. Additional skills including pre-requisite learning skills (PLS), oral motor skills (OM), sensory issues (SI), and pragmatic skills are also assessed and targeted at different stages of the programme. Assessments are conducted at three intervals for each child—immediately prior to intervention (initial assessment), 6th month of intervention (mid assessment) and the 10th month (final assessment).

Our early-intervention programme develops skills prerequisite to learning and communication, including eye contact, joint attention, sitting tolerance, and compliance along with pointing or reference. Once the child shows improvement in these prerequisite learning skills, intervention tailored to the individual student's profile is provided across all domains. Over several years of clinical experience we have observed anecdotally that toddlers and young children with motor difficulties including oral motor difficulties seem more likely to remain non-verbal or to have persistent difficulties in expressive speech and language development. The increasing disparity between receptive and expressive speech and language abilities in this subgroup of children reinforces the hypothesis that, in these cases, expressive or speech deficits may be secondary to oral motor deficits. This study was undertaken to ascertain quantitatively the existence, nature, and proportion of such a subgroup amongst children diagnosed with autism within our clinical population. From a clinical viewpoint, such knowledge is a prerequisite to developing an intervention that targets this subpopulation's underlying issues early and specifically. From a pure research viewpoint, this closer characterization may help to disentangle the heterogeneity in autism's detailed phenotypes and causes.

In selecting assessments for any such clinical study a balance must be struck between the clinical measures most germane and appropriate to the clinical population and its therapeutic needs, on the one hand, and the research measures standardised and normed against typically and atypically developing populations worldwide. We have chosen to apply two indigenously developed clinical measures germane to the Indian therapeutic setting. Although cross-validation against measures developed in other cultures remains to be conducted, these measures have been normed and validated within India, have been reported in the peer-reviewed literature and codified as clinical manuals, are sensitive to the Indian population, are culturally appropriate, and emphasise clinical utility.

MATERIALS AND METHODS

SUBJECTS

Data collection took place as part of a cross-cultural comparative study of autism spectrum conditions approved by the Institutional Review Board of the Groden Center, and informed consent was obtained from each parent for research use of their children's clinical data. Case files of all children enrolled from 2009 to 2011 were reviewed, and diagnoses of autism confirmed by reference to ICD-10 criteria (World Health Organization, 1993). Cases for whom ICD-10 diagnosis of autism was in any doubt were excluded, yielding a study population of 31 children (6 females, 25 males, 4:1 male:female ratio) of middle to high socioeconomic status. Ages at enrolment ranged from 22 to 65 months, with a mean of 41 months and a standard deviation of 11 months.

Subjects attended at least one year of daily intervention with consistent monitoring at an early intervention centre and were assessed thrice (pre/mid/post-intervention) within the year. Along with the aforementioned prerequisite learning skills, the beginning of the early intervention programme addresses issues of feeding and toileting, if present. Subsequently, intensive inputs in the domains of communication, motor and cognitive, social and emotional skills are provided daily throughout the year (Karanth, 2010). It has been our clinical experience that at this stage, 2–3 months into the programme, receptive language skills begin to improve. At the same time we see a differential effect in terms of expressive language skills: Whilst in one subgroup, gains in expressive language appear commensurate with those in receptive language, in another subgroup expressive language skills are far lower. Children in this latter, expressive-impaired group are provided with more directed oral motor intervention, comprising activities related to management of oral sensory issues, improvement of tone, massages, exercises and oral motor games [see Aluri (2005), for details]. All oral motor exercises are done by the same team 2–3 times per week, with follow-up by parents.

TOOLS

Two assessment instruments developed in India and normed for Indian populations were applied:

The Com DEALL Developmental Checklist (CDDC)

The CDDC (Karanth, 2007) is a criterion referenced checklist to assess developmental skills in 8 domains—namely, gross and fine motor skills, activities of daily living, receptive and expressive language skills, and cognitive, social and emotional skills—at 6 month intervals, from 0 to 6 years of age. Questions in each domain are further subdivided in 12 age sub-groups from 0–6 months to 66–72 months. The checklist includes 36 items in each of the 8 domains assessed, for a total of 288 items. The CDDC has been field tested on urban Indian children from middle class backgrounds, has a high inter-rater reliability, and can be used as a screening measure for identification of developmental delays in specific domains (Karanth et al., 2010). The CDDC thus carries face and content validity, and shows convergent validity with independent Childhood Autism Rating Scale diagnoses (Karanth et al., 2010).

The Com DEALL Oro Motor Assessment

Children with speech language acquisition delays and disorders often have difficulties in oral motor skills. This checklist (Archana, 2008) is a standardised tool for assessing oral motor skills of children within the range of 1–4 years. It has been designed to identify clinically children who have oral motor problems, by providing developmental norms, and to inform the development of goals for intervention. It assesses 4 domains—jaw, tongue, and lip movements and speech. The 30 items cover an observation and assessment of the articulators in terms of posture (open mouth posture/extended tongue), movement (transitions from one movement to the other/raising of the tongue), function (biting/sucking), and speech production at the level of combinations of vowels and consonants in syllables, words, and phrases of varying length and complexity. All items are rated on a three-point scale, from absent, to only present spontaneously, to consistently present (on demand). For further details see (Archana, 2008). The norms are based on field testing of 90 urban Indian children.

PROCEDURE

Data collected from each case file comprised age at enrolment and raw scores along the three time points (pre-, mid-, post-intervention) for the five domains of interest: gross motor, fine motor, receptive language, expressive language, and oral motor. All daily interventions and periodic assessments were carried out by the team assigned to the group of children. This team was composed of the same clinical staff throughout all time points of measurement. The team consists of an occupational therapist, a speech language pathologist and a developmental educator/psychologist. The oral motor assessment was conducted jointly by the occupational therapist and the speech language pathologist.

Raw scores at each time point were converted to percentages by dividing by the total number of applicable items. Non-compliance in a few subjects prevented acquisition of oral motor scores from one or another time point; the mid-intervention score was unavailable from 6 subjects, and the pre-intervention score was unavailable from 3 subjects. Although the children's specific reasons for non-compliance with the oral motor tests cannot be proven, it was the impression of the clinical team that these cases of non-compliance arose because of sensory sensitivities triggered by the assessment procedures. The mouth and lips being a zone rich in tactile input, this oral motor assessment is *a priori* the most likely of our procedures to trigger tactile aversion in sensitive individuals. In contrast, had non-compliance been a consequence of receptive language difficulties it would have been equally likely to arise in the other, non-oral-motor assessments rather than arising specifically in the oral motor context. In these cases in which one of the three observations was missing because of non-compliance, slopes of the intervention scores over time were estimated from the two other time points. Scores for all measures other than these oral motor assays were available at all time points for all subjects.

STATISTICAL ANALYSIS

On the basis of the therapeutic team's clinical impression, the 31-subject sample was classified into a motor-impaired group (11 subjects) in whom expressive language difficulty seemed to occur along with oral motor impairments out of proportion to impairments in other domains, and a motor-intact group (20 subjects) in whom no such uneven profile existed (**Figure 1**). The two groups did not differ in age [motor-impaired 37.45 ± 14.36 months at enrolment, range 22–65 months, and motor-intact 43.20 ± 8.55 months at enrolment, range 29–58 months, $t_{(29)} = 1.40$, $p = 0.1711$]. As an exploratory characterization, the motor-intact group was further subdivided into a receptive-impaired subgroup with receptive language deficit out of proportion to expressive language impairments, and a receptive-intact subgroup in whom receptive and expressive language skills were on par.

Slopes for all measures as functions of time were computed from the three (or in cases of missing oral motor data, two) time points, treating the time intervals between the first and second and the second and third observations as equal.

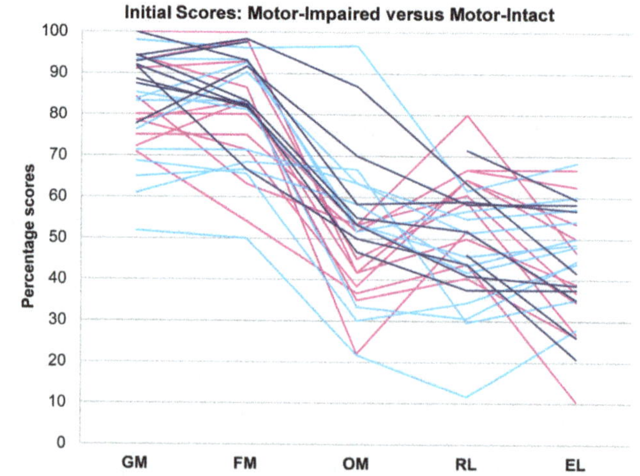

FIGURE 1 | Motor-impaired (magenta) and motor-intact (blue, with receptive-impaired subgroup in light blue and receptive-intact subgroup in dark blue) groups. The discriminant between motor-impaired and motor-intact groups −0.28·OM − 0.15·GM + 0.55·RL − 0.20·EL loaded heavily on the receptive-expressive difference and on oral motor skills, and also slightly on gross motor skills. GM, gross motor; FM, fine motor; OM, oral motor; RL, receptive language; EL, expressive language.

A linear discriminant function was constructed (SAS PROC DISCRIM, POOL=yes CROSSVALIDATE) to distinguish the motor-impaired and motor-intact groups. This procedure was attempted with three sets of inputs: once with pre-intervention values and slopes of all variables, once with slopes only, and once with pre-intervention values only. The pre-intervention values, without slopes, yielded the most accurate discrimination as assayed by leave-one-out cross-validation. Single measures then were deleted one by one from the linear discriminant input, to determine whether they were essential to discrimination. This procedure yielded a discriminant function with 100% selectivity and specificity, loading negatively on gross and oral motor skills and expressive language, and positively on receptive language. This discriminant function and its slope over time were added to the data set as derived measures. Also added as derived measures were the difference between receptive and expressive language scores, which discriminated the receptive-impaired subgroup from the receptive-intact subgroup within the motor-intact group with 100% selectivity and specificity, and the slope of this receptive-expressive difference.

Pre-intervention values and slopes of all observed and derived measures were correlated against each other. As the study was motivated by the hypothesis that expressive impairment out of proportion to receptive impairment may be secondary to oral motor impairment, correlations between oral motor and expressive skills were evaluated as planned comparisons, the other correlations as exploratory.

Outcome differences between groups were assayed via analyses of variance for each observed measure. Dependent variables were the post-intervention values of all observed measures, and the differences between pre-intervention and post-intervention values. In the three cases in which the pre-intervention oral motor score was unavailable, the mid-intervention score was used in computing this difference. Again oral motor and expressive language scores were treated as planned comparisons between motor-impaired and motor-intact groups. In addition, receptive and expressive language scores were treated as planned comparisons between the clinically classified receptive-impaired and receptive-intact subgroups of the motor-intact group. Other measures were treated as exploratory.

RESULTS

Pre-intervention score profiles for the motor-impaired and motor-intact groups are illustrated in **Figure 1**, which contains one series of line segments for each individual subject, within each of the groups, linking that individual's gross motor, fine motor, oral motor, receptive language and expressive language skills. Reading the line segments from left to right highlights scores that are out of proportion to the individual subject's overall level of functioning: Note the dips in oral motor ("OM") and expressive language ("EL") scores for members of the motor-impaired group as contrasted with members of the motor-intact group. Slopes did not contribute to the accuracy of the linear discriminant between motor-impaired and motor-intact groups, nor did fine motor scores. The final discriminant, based entirely on pre-intervention measures, reliably separated (100% sensitivity and specificity with leave-one-out cross-validation) the motor-impaired and motor-intact groups, loading negatively on oral motor skills (coefficient −0.28) and also slightly negatively on gross motor skills (−0.15), and heavily positively on the receptive-expressive language difference (+0.55 and −0.20, respectively). The gross motor score made for a slightly more accurate discriminant than the fine motor, and addition of the fine motor measure, which was highly correlated with gross motor, did not improve discrimination. The distribution of this discriminant function was bimodal (**Table 1**), with normal modes corresponding to the motor-intact and motor-impaired groups. The learning rate (slope) for receptive language was highly correlated with the motor-intact/impaired discriminant function, with the motor-impaired group learning much more slowly than the others (**Table 2**; see also **Figure 3**).

In the pre-intervention scores of the sample as a whole, gross and fine motor skills and receptive language were highly correlated with each other, and expressive language was correlated with fine (but not gross) motor skills. Oral motor skills were correlated, less strongly, with fine motor and receptive and expressive language. The learning rates (slopes) for expressive and receptive language were highly correlated with the learning rate for oral motor skills.

The motor-intact group were further characterised into two overlapping subgroups by disparity in receptive and expressive language scores. The distribution of this receptive-expressive score difference was again bimodal (**Table 3**), though the two modes were not cleanly separated, with the lesser mode comprising mostly the receptive-impaired subgroup and the greater mode including the receptive-intact subgroup along with the motor-impaired group.

In tests of group differences in outcome, the motor-impaired was distinguished from the motor-intact group by a lesser post-intervention oral motor score [motor-impaired 59.85 ± 16.62, motor-intact 75.50 ± 20.66, $F_{(1, 29)} = 10.85$, $p = 0.0026$, **Figure 2**] and also by a lesser pre-post difference in receptive language score [motor-impaired 16.72 ± 13.51, motor-intact 31.94 ± 11.63, $F_{(1, 29)} = 4.64$, $p = 0.0398$, **Figure 3**]. Within the motor-intact group, the receptive-impaired was marginally distinguished from the receptive-intact subgroup by a lesser post-intervention gross motor score [receptive-impaired 76.22 ± 14.11, receptive-intact 91.00 ± 6.13, $F_{(1, 18)} = 8.49$, $p =$

Table 1 | Histogram of values of the discriminant function −0.28·OM − 0.15·GM + 0.55·RL − 0.20·EL for members of the motor-impaired (magenta) and motor-intact (black) groups.

−22.03	1*
−19.09	1*
−16.15	5*****
−13.22	7*******
−10.28	6******
−7.34	1*
−4.40	3***
−1.46	4****
+1.48	1*
+4.42	2**

Table 2 | Correlation coefficients and associated two-tailed probabilities for slopes (s) and initial values (init) of all observed and derived measures, uncorrected for multiple comparisons.

	slope GM	slope FM	slope RL	slope EL	slope OM	slope −GM−OM+RL−EL	slope RL−EL	init GM	init FM	init RL	init EL	init OM
CORRELATIONS FOR SLOPES (s) AND INITIAL VALUES (init) OF ALL MEASURES												
slope FM	**+0.65063**											
slope RL	**+0.45181**	*+0.33220*										
slope EL	+0.22535	*+0.34574*	**+0.53471**									
slope OM	+0.25277	+0.08191	**+0.56340**	**+0.64076**								
slope −GM−OM+RL−EL		−0.01707										
slope RL−EL	+0.13596	−0.10579			−0.24157							
init GM	**−0.87684**	−0.44680	−0.16465	+0.02777	−0.03795	+0.00365	−0.17512					
init FM	**−0.65194**	**−0.66958**	+0.05686	+0.19769	+0.14333	+0.02775	−0.17640	**+0.74550**				
init RL	**−0.53856**	−0.37173	−0.39088	+0.16046	−0.07086	*-0.32631*	**−0.52376**	**+0.54302**	**+0.54727**			
init EL	−0.25380	**−0.48684**	+0.03893	+0.01430	−0.05580	+0.10532	+0.01756	+0.22412	**+0.52197**	**+0.51946**		
init OM	−0.15898	−0.04554	+0.19367	+0.26299	−0.14364	+0.29931	−0.13188	*+0.32196*	+0.41653	+0.40347	+0.38638	
init −GM−OM+RL−EL	−0.21371	−0.08900	**−0.54278**	+0.02264	+0.00398	**−0.67497**	**−0.49856**		−0.02105			
init RL−EL	−0.29170	+0.11608	−0.43897	+0.14936	−0.01556	−0.44063	**−0.55297**	*+0.32650*	+0.02747			+0.01866
	slope GM	slope FM	slope RL	slope EL	slope OM	slope −GM−OM+RL−EL	slope RL−EL	init GM	init FM	init RL	init EL	init OM
TWO-TAILED SIGNIFICANCE PROBABILITIES (UNCORRECTED FOR MULTIPLE COMPARISONS)												
slope FM	**0.00007**											
slope RL	**0.01072**	*0.06788*										
slope EL	0.22289	*0.05676*	**0.00194**									
slope OM	0.17009	0.66135	**0.00097**	**0.00010**								
slope −GM−OM+RL−EL		0.92740										
slope RL−EL	0.46584	0.57111			0.19045							
init GM	**0.00000**	0.01174	0.37610	0.88211	0.83939	0.98446	0.34605					
init FM	**0.00007**	**0.00004**	0.76127	0.28640	0.44178	0.88221	0.34250	**0.00000**				
init RL	**0.00177**	0.03949	0.02969	0.38852	0.70483	*0.07320*	**0.00249**	**0.00160**	**0.00144**			
init EL	0.16829	**0.00548**	0.83528	0.93915	0.76559	0.57285	0.92528	0.22549	**0.00260**	**0.00275**		
init OM	0.39298	0.80780	0.29653	0.15288	0.44077	0.10189	0.47946	*0.07734*	0.01976	0.02440	0.03179	
init −GM−OM+RL−EL	0.24833	0.63400	**0.00161**	0.90377	0.98307	**0.00003**	**0.00431**		0.91050			
init RL−EL	0.11134	0.53403	0.01349	0.42257	0.93378	0.01311	**0.00125**	*0.07303*	0.88337			0.92063
	slope GM	slope FM	slope RL	slope EL	slope OM	slope − GM−OM+RL−EL	slope RL−EL	init GM	init FM	init RL	init EL	init OM

*Pairs collinear by definition have been deleted. Correlations statistically significant after correction for multiple comparisons are indicated in **bold red**, exploratory correlations not significant after correction for multiple comparisons are in plain red, and suggestive trends in magenta. GM, gross motor; FM, fine motor; OM, oral motor; RL, receptive language; EL, expressive language; init, initial value; slope, slope across time points. "−GM−OM+RL−EL" denotes the discriminant function −0.28·OM − 0.15·GM + 0.55·RL − 0.20·EL.*

Table 3 | Histogram of values of the receptive-expressive language difference (RL-EL) for the motor-intact receptive-impaired (light blue) and motor-intact receptive-intact (dark blue) subgroups, and the motor-impaired (magenta) group.

−16.34	2**
−11.37	3***
−6.40	6******
−1.44	5*****
+3.53	1*
+8.50	3***
+13.47	4****
+18.44	3***
+23.40	1*
+28.37	3***

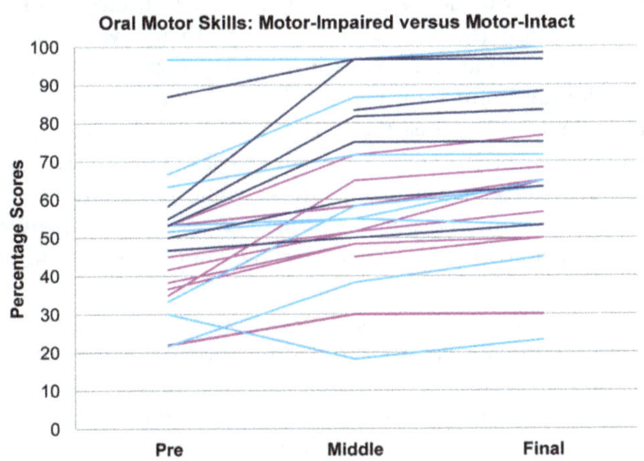

FIGURE 2 | Oral motor scores over time in motor-impaired (magenta) and motor-intact (blue) groups. Modulo a great deal of heterogeneity, the motor-impaired group on the whole began with lesser scores than the motor-intact group, by definition, but also ended with lesser scores. (For consistency with the other figures, the motor-intact group is color-coded separately as light blue for the receptive-impaired subgroup and dark blue for the receptive-intact).

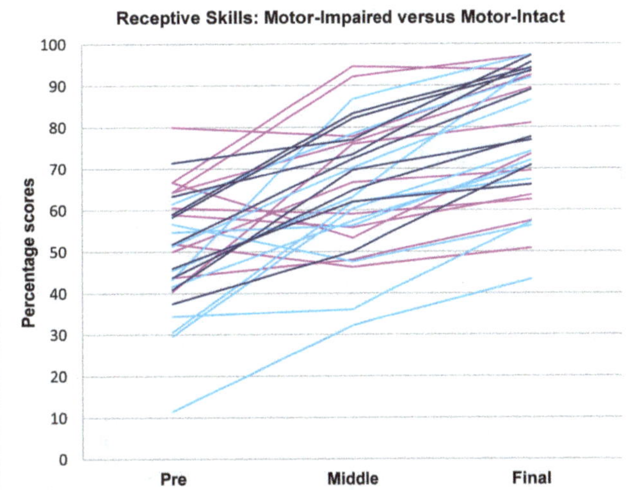

FIGURE 3 | Receptive language scores over time in motor-impaired (magenta) and motor-intact (blue) groups. The motor-impaired group improved less than the motor-intact group; note the group difference in line slopes. (For consistency with the other figures, the motor-intact group is color-coded separately as light blue for the receptive-impaired subgroup and dark blue for the receptive-intact.)

0.0093, **Figure 4**], and this difference seemed driven by many receptive-impaired individuals who began the intervention with more severe gross motor impairments and, though they progressed at rates similar to those of the receptive-intact subgroup, had not yet caught up by intervention's end. There also was a trend towards a greater pre-post difference in oral motor score [receptive-impaired 8.57 ± 7.45, receptive-intact 3.10 ± 2.96, $F_{(1, 18)} = 4.26, p = 0.0538$].

DISCUSSION

Results confirm the clinical impression that in a third of this sample, 11 of the 31 consecutively enrolled subjects with unequivocal ICD-10 diagnoses of autism, a disparity between receptive language skill and expressive speech impairment is associated with oral and other motor impairments. Motor-intact and motor-impaired groups were distinguished by a discriminant with positive loading on receptive-expressive language disparity and oral motor skills, and also somewhat on gross motor skills which were in turn highly correlated with fine motor skills. This function gives quantitative basis to the clinically observed difference between the two groups, exactly separating them into two distinct modes.

Following the period of intervention the motor-impaired group did not achieve as proficient post-intervention oral motor function, and across the entire sample the learning rates for both receptive and expressive language were highly correlated with the learning rate for oral motor skills. Even before intervention began, receptive language was correlated with gross and fine motor skills, and both receptive and expressive language were correlated with fine and oral motor skills.

Our results reinforce the notion that many people with autism experience substantial motor difficulties including deficits in gross motor, fine motor, and oral motor skills, despite the subtle presentation of these motor deficits in the context of much more obvious social cognitive symptoms, particularly at young ages. Whilst sensory issues in children on the autism spectrum have received considerable attention of late, the motor issues have not and need to be assessed in all children with autism spectrum conditions whether they appear to have motor difficulties or not. It is noteworthy that similar motor issues were neglected initially in children with a diagnosis of specific language impairment (SLI) only to be identified and documented subsequently (Hill, 2001; Marton, 2009; Rechetnikov and Maitra, 2009; Zelaznik and Goffman, 2010); in one recent study fully one third of children with SLI satisfied criteria for an additional diagnosis of Developmental Coordination Disorder (Flapper and Schoemaker, 2013). Behavioural study of twin pairs suggests a partly genetic basis for covariation of clinical communicative impairment and motor (finger-tapping) impairment (Bishop, 2002). In a large (62,944 individuals) sample

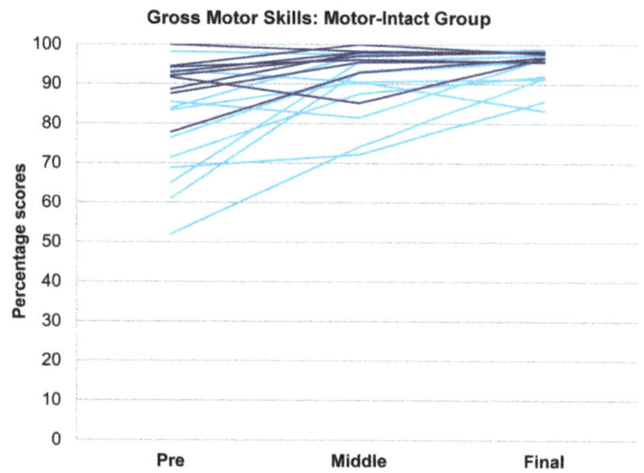

FIGURE 4 | Gross motor scores over time in the receptive-impaired (light blue) and receptive-intact (dark blue) subgroups of the motor-intact group. The receptive-impaired group ended the intervention with lesser gross motor scores, and this difference was driven by many individuals who began with more severe gross motor deficits and, though they improved at rates similar to those of the receptive-intact subgroup, did not yet approach ceiling by the end of the intervention.

of typically developing children, too, motor skills at age 1.5 years correlate with communicative skills, and predict communicative skills at age 3 (Wang et al., 2013). Speech and language acquisition in particular, seem closely linked to mastery of oral motor skills in a subgroup of children with autism. Within this subgroup, lack of expressive language skills or speech in particular, in the presence of relatively better receptive language skills, is highly correlated with poor oral motor skills.

The overall progress that children with autism make appears related to their progress in mastering and overcoming their motor issues. Our results indicate that not only do the motor deficits correlate highly with *level* of speech-language acquisition prior to intervention, but in addition the severity of the motor deficits could influence the overall rate of learning, particularly the learning of expressive language as the learning rates for expressive and receptive language were highly correlated with the learning *rate* for oral motor skills. Oral motor issues when present could pose a considerable challenge to the acquisition of speech, as the motor-impaired group was distinguished from the motor-intact group by a lesser post-intervention oral motor score. Moreover, oral motor skills in this sample vary somewhat *independently* of gross and fine motor skills, being only weakly correlated in initial level, and not at all significantly correlated in rates of development. These outcomes and characteristics highlight the need not only for individual assessment of the gross, fine, and oral motor skills in children with autism spectrum conditions but even more importantly the need for focused, individualised and child-centred intervention in all of these areas, including oral motor skills.

This small clinical study is of course not without its limitations. As this study did not involve a clinical control group, we are unable to evaluate how the therapy itself might affect the results. It was the pre-intervention motor and language scores that most effectively discriminated the motor-impaired from the motor-intact group. The question remains open, then, as to whether the same population with no intervention at all, or with an intervention not targeting oral motor skills, might spontaneously close the gap in expressive language between these motor-impaired and motor-intact groups. This study aimed not at evaluating the therapy itself—which already has been the subject of past reports—but rather at discriminating and characterizing this motor subgroup. The discriminant based on pre-intervention scores does speak to this objective.

In addition, though the measures of motor function used in this study have been evaluated and normed within India, they have not yet been cross-validated against worldwide standards such as the Mullen Scales of Early Learning or the Vineland Adaptive Behavior Scales (VABS). One of the obstacles to such cross-validation is the cost of the scales themselves which is often prohibitive for non-governmental organizations operating in developing countries (Durkin, 2013). Norming of the Mullen and/or the VABS against the CDDC and the Com DEALL Oro Motor Assessment would be a next logical step, as would a controlled study in which individuals would be randomised to distinct intervention groups so as to assay interactions between motor-impaired or motor-intact starting point, intervention, and outcome.

Correlations between speech and motor skills can arise from motor impairments *per se*, or from disconnection between motor execution and executive planning and sequencing (Hill, 2004) and/or affective motivation (Greenspan, 2001). It remains unclear from the results reported here whether the issue within the motor-impaired group might be one of oral motor execution, or of cognitive and/or affective control: that is, might autistic people with the ability to vocalise be unable to connect that ability to willed communication? This question of course relates to the debate mentioned in our introduction, between social cognitive and social motivational accounts of autism. Again we do not wish to frame cognitive, affective, and motor accounts of autism as mutually exclusive explanations; indeed, clinical, and basic science increasingly suggest that syndromes encompassing cognitive, affective, and motor coordination may be the rule rather than the exception (Gillberg, 2010).

This set of results also offers the possibility that in certain individuals with autism and oral motor impairment, expressive communication might be attained via gross and/or fine motor skills that can be somewhat more intact and may be more immediately or readily trainable relative to the level of oral motor skills. Such training of gross and fine motor skills prerequisite to communication may proceed via novel methods in traditional therapeutic settings (Chen et al., 2012) or via computer-assisted skills development as a tool for the therapist (Belmonte et al., 2013). There remains of course the potential that fine motor impairments could impede use of alternative and augmentative communication devices, because open-loop motor control which is unintegrated with sensory feedback (Haswell et al., 2009) leads to errors in pointing with a finger or hand to select amongst multiple response options. However, our current results do suggest that manual motor skills may be at least a more practical route to communication in these individuals than is spoken language. Most of all, these results highlighting autism's clinical heterogeneity in terms of motor function and ability to speak ought to prompt clinical and basic researchers and therapists to eschew a one-size-fits-all approach to autism: both therapeutic intervention and basic science must take note of such variability within the phenotype, and of the maxim that "If you've seen one person with autism, you've seen *one* person with autism."

ACKNOWLEDGMENTS

This publication was supported by an agreement with Cornell University, Department of Human Development under Faculty Early Career Development Award BCS-0846892 from the Directorate for Social, Behavioral and Economic Sciences, US National Science Foundation. Matthew K. Belmonte and Prathibha Karanth designed the study, Tanushree Saxena-Chandhok, Ruth Cherian, Reema Muneer, and Lisa George collected and curated the data, Matthew K. Belmonte designed and implemented the statistical analyses, Matthew K. Belmonte and Prathibha Karanth wrote the manuscript.

REFERENCES

Aluri, U. (2005). *Oro-Motor Kit.* Bangalore: The Com DEALL Trust.

Amato, J. J., and Slavin, D. (1998). A preliminary investigation of oromotor function in young verbal and nonverbal children with autism. *Infant-Toddler Intervent. Transdiscip. J.* 8, 175–184.

Archana, G. (2008). *A Manual from Communicaid: Assessment of Oro Motor Skills in Toddlers.* Bangalore: The Com DEALL Trust.

Belmonte, M. K., Cook, E. H. Jr., Anderson, G. M., Rubenstein, J. L. R., Greenough, W. T., Beckel-Mitchener, A., et al. (2004). Autism as a disorder of neural information processing: directions for research and targets for therapy. *Mol. Psychiatry* 9, 646–663. doi: 10.1038/sj.mp.4001499. Available online at: http://www.cureautismnow.org/conferences/summitmeetings/

Belmonte, M. K., Dhariwal, M., Saxena-Chandhok, T., and Karanth, P. (2013). Design of a touch-screen computer application to develop foundational motor communicative skills. Abstract presented at the International Meeting for Autism Research (San Sebastián).

Bishop, D. V. (2002). Motor immaturity and specific speech and language impairment: evidence for a common genetic basis. *Am. J. Med. Genet.* 114, 56–63. doi: 10.1002/ajmg.1630

Chen, G. M., Yoder, K. J., Ganzel, B. L., Goodwin, M. S., and Belmonte, M. K. (2012). Harnessing repetitive behaviours to engage attention and learning in a novel therapy for autism: an exploratory analysis. *Front. Psychol.* 3:12. doi: 10.3389/fpsyg.2012.00012

Chevallier, C., Kohls, G., Troiani, V., Brodkin, E. S., and Schultz, R. T. (2012). The social motivation theory of autism. *Trends Cogn. Sci.* 16, 231–239. doi: 10.1016/j.tics.2012.02.007

Durkin, M. (2013). The epidemiology of autism spectrum disorder: toward a more inclusive world. Keynote presented at the International Meeting for Autism Research (San Sebastián).

Flapper, B. C., and Schoemaker, M. M. (2013). Developmental Coordination Disorder in children with specific language impairment: co-morbidity and impact on quality of life. *Res. Dev. Disabil.* 34, 756–763. doi: 10.1016/j.ridd.2012.10.014

Frith, U. (1997). The neurocognitive basis of autism. *Trends Cogn. Sci.* 1, 73–77. doi: 10.1016/S1364-6613(97)01010-3

Gernsbacher, M. A., Sauer, E. A., Geye, H. M., Schweigert, E. K., and Goldsmith, H. H. (2007). Infant and toddler oral- and manual-motor skills predict later speech fluency in autism. *J. Child Psychol. Psychiatry* 49, 43–50. doi: 10.1111/j.1469-7610.2007.01820.x

Gillberg, C. (2010). The ESSENCE in child psychiatry: early symptomatic syndromes eliciting neurodevelopmental clinical examinations. *Res. Dev. Disabil.* 31, 1543–1551. doi: 10.1016/j.ridd.2010.06.002

Greenspan, S. I. (2001). The affect diathesis hypothesis: the role of emotions in the core deficit in autism and the development of intelligence and social skills. *J. Dev. Learn. Disord.* 5, 1–45.

Haswell, C. C., Izawa, J., Dowell, L. R., Mostofsky, S. H., and Shadmehr, R. (2009). Representation of internal models of action in the human brain. *Nat. Neurosci.* 12, 970–972. doi: 10.1038/nn.2356

Hill, E. L. (2001). Non-specific nature of specific language impairment: a review of the literature with regard to concomitant motor impairments. *Int. J. Lang. Commun. Disord.* 36, 149–171. doi: 10.1080/13682820010019874

Hill, E. L. (2004). Executive dysfunction in autism. *Trends Cogn. Sci.* 8, 26–32. doi: 10.1016/j.tics.2003.11.003

Karanth, P. (2007). *Communication DEALL Developmental Checklists.* Bangalore: The Com DEALL Trust.

Karanth, P. (2010). *Communication DEALL–The Program.* Bangalore: The Com DEALL Trust.

Karanth, P., Shaista, S., and Srikanth, N. (2010). Efficacy of Communication DEALL—An indigenous early intervention program for children with autism spectrum disorders. *Ind. J. Paediatr.* 77, 957–962. doi: 10.1007/S12098-010-0144-8

Leary, M. R., and Hill, D. A. (1996). Moving on: autism and movement disturbance. *Ment. Retard.* 34, 39–53.

Marton, K. (2009). Imitation of body postures and hand movements in children with specific language impairment. *J. Exp. Child Psychol.* 102, 1–13. doi: 10.1016/j.jecp.2008.07.007

Noterdaeme, M., Mildenberger, K., Minow, F., and Amorosa, H. (2002). Evaluation of neuromotor deficits in children with autism and children with a specific speech and language disorder *Eur. Child Adolesc. Psychiatry* 11, 219–225. doi: 10.1007/s00787-002-0285-z

Rechetnikov, R. P., and Maitra, K. (2009). Motor impairments in children associated with impairments of speech or language: a meta-analytic review of research literature. *Am. J. Occup. Ther.* 63, 255–263. doi: 10.5014/ajot.63.3.255

Tesink, C. M., Buitelaar, J. K., Petersson, K. M., van der Gaag, R. J., Kan, C. C., Tendolkar, I., et al. (2009). Neural correlates of pragmatic language comprehension in autism spectrum disorders. *Brain* 132, 1941–1952. doi: 10.1093/brain/awp103

Thurm, A., Lord, C., Lee, L., and Newschaffer, C. (2007). Predictors of language acquisition in preschool children with autism spectrum disorders. *J. Autism Dev. Disord.* 37, 1721–1734. doi: 10.1007/s10803-006-0300-1

Wang, M. V., Lekhal, R., Aarø, L. E., and Schjølberg, S. (2013). Co-occurring development of early childhood communication and motor skills: results from a population-based longitudinal study. *Child. Care Health Dev.* doi: 10.1111/cch.12003. [Epub ahead of print]

World Health Organization. (1993). *The ICD-10 Classification of Mental and Behavioural Disorders: Diagnostic Criteria for Research.* Geneva: World Health Organization.

Zelaznik, H. N., and Goffman, L. (2010). Generalized motor abilities and timing behavior in children with specific language impairment. *J. Speech Lang. Hear. Res.* 53, 383–393. doi: 10.1044/1092-4388(2009/08-0204)

Conflict of Interest Statement: The authors declare that the research was conducted in the absence of any commercial or financial relationships that could be construed as a potential conflict of interest.

12

Perception-action in children with ASD

Claes von Hofsten* **and Kerstin Rosander**

Department of Psychology, Uppsala University, Uppsala, Sweden

Edited by:
Elizabeth B. Torres, Rutgers University, USA

Reviewed by:
Michael Leon, University of California, USA
Patrizia Fattori, University of Bologna, Italy

Correspondence:
Claes von Hofsten, Department of Psychology, Uppsala University, Box 1225, SE-75142 Uppsala, Sweden.
e-mail: claes.von_hofsten@psyk.uu.se

How do disturbances to perception and action relate to the deficiencies expressed by children with autism? The ability to predict what is going to happen next is crucial for the construction of all actions and children develop these predictive abilities early in development. Children with autism, however, are deficient in the ability to foresee future events and to plan movements and movement sequences. They are also deficient in the understanding of other people's actions. This includes communicative actions as they are ultimately based on movements. Today there are two promising neurobiological interpretation of Autism Spectrum Disorder (ASD). First, there is strong evidence that the Mirror Neuron System (MNS) is impaired. As stated by this hypothesis, action production and action understanding are intimately related. Both these functions rely on predictive models of the sensory consequences of actions and depend on connectivity between the parietal and premotor areas. Secondly, action prediction is accomplished through a system that includes a loop from the posterior parietal cortex (PPC) through the cerebellum and back to the premotor and motor areas of the brain. Impairment of this loop is probably also part of the explanation of the prediction problems in children with ASD. Both the cortico-cerebellar loop and the MNS rely on distant neural connections. There are multiple evidence that such connections are weak in children with autism.

Keywords: autism, perception, action, anticipation, planning, mirror-neurons, diffuse tensor imaging

Perception, action and cognition are mutually dependent. Together they form functional systems, driven by motives, around which adaptive behavior develops (von Hofsten, 1993, 2004, 2007). Actions reflect all aspects of cognitive development including the motives of the child, the problems to be solved, and the constraints and possibilities of the child's body and sensory-motor system. Actions are directed into the future and their control is based on knowledge of what is going to happen next. Dysfunctions of the brain will affect the way subjects perceive the surroundings and how they organize their actions. Autism is a disorder in which the subject fails to attend to important varieties of social information and instead focuses on less informative physical aspects of the environment. In addition, actions are often compulsatory and stereotyped (see e.g., Bodfish et al., 2000; Goldman et al., 2008). Bodfish et al. (2000) found repetitive behaviors in both children with Autism Spectrum Disorder (ASD) and mentally retarded children but significantly more of them in children with autism. Furthermore, the prevalence of repetitive behavior, such as compulsion, was significantly correlated with the severity of ASD.

Deficiencies in the control of actions have not usually been considered to be core deficits of ASD or Asperger Syndrome (AS). Thus, the number of studies of action control in children with these syndromes is low compared to the studies focusing on the social aspects of the disorders. Recently, however, this picture is beginning to change. A number of studies focusing on action control in children with ASD have appeared. It is of great importance to identify the nature of the action problems associated with ASD, because this might provide crucial information for the understanding of what is failing in these children. Analyzing the physical movements has the potential of being helpful for objectively diagnose, treat and quantify performance gains starting at birth.

One widely used motor test is the Movement ABC (MABC-2) that includes a set of everyday action tasks such as walking on a line, putting beads on a string, standing on one leg, and throwing and catching objects. Green et al. (2002) used MABC-2 in a large, population-derived group of children. Definitive motor impairments were found in 79% of the children with ASD and a further 10% had borderline motor problems. Difficulty with the balance task in children with ASD stood out. In addition, the results show that children with ASD have greater difficulties in movement tasks that are both dependent on accuracy and timing, as seen in the timed peg-board tasks. Siaperas et al. (2012) tested 50 boys with AS and an equal number of typically developed boys between 7 and 14 years of age on MABC-2 and found that children with AS were especially deficient on the throwing and catching tasks, and the tasks on dexterity and balance. They also tested balance on one or both feet with open and closed eyes and found the children with AS and ASD to be deficient on all these tasks.

Although the general motor tests give clear indications of motor dysfunctions in children with ASD, they give less clear indications of what the specific problems are. From a perception-action perspective, the most important aspect of motor control is predictive control. Adaptive behavior has to deal with the fact that events precede the feedback signals about them. The only way to overcome this problem is to anticipate what is going to happen next and use that information to control one's behavior. There are many indications that children with autism are generally deficient in this kind of control.

POSTURAL CONTROL

Gravity is a potent force and when body equilibrium is disturbed, posture becomes quickly uncontrollable. Therefore, any reaction to a balance threat has to be very fast and automatic. Although several reflexes have been identified that help to control balance, postural reflexes are emergency reactions that tend to maintain balance at the cost of interrupting ongoing behavior. Disturbances to balance need to be handled by anticipating the upcoming problems and dealing with them in a predictive way.

Retrospective videos of children with autism indicate that postural control may be deficient already at an early age. For instance, Teitelbaum et al. (1998) showed a case of an 8.5-months-old boy who, when trying to maintain balance in a sitting position fell over "like a log" without using any allied reflexes to protect himself. In other cases they studied, the infant managed to sit for a few minutes at a time, but when the posture was asymmetrical as when reaching for objects or moving the arms and upper body, they fell over (Teitelbaum et al., 1998). Another less dramatic instance of poor postural control is the control of neck muscles when being pulled from a lying position. At 4 months of age an infant should be able to control his or her head position in this situation by maintaining it in line with the torso and not let it flop back. Flanagan et al. (2012) studied two groups of infants. In one group of 40 infants, all had older brothers or sisters with ASD. Ninety percent of those who went on to be diagnosed with ASD at 30–36 months had exhibited head lag at 6, 14, or 24 months. In another group of high-risk infants, Flanagan et al. (2012) tested for head lag at 6 months. They found that 15 out of 20 siblings of children who had been diagnosed with ASD exhibited head lag compared to 7 out of 21 of the low-risk siblings. Bhat et al. (2012) found that siblings of children with ASD also showed significantly more motor problems at 3 and 6 months of age compared to typically developing (TD) infants. In fact, the majority of the siblings showed both early motor delays and later communication delays.

ANTICIPATION

There is evidence that children with ASD do not anticipate upcoming actions like TD children do. In a study of feeding, Cattaneo et al. (2007) measured activation of the mouth-opening mylohyoid (MH) muscle in 6–9-years-old TD children and children with ASD. The participants were asked to watch the experimenter performing two different actions: grasping with the right hand a piece of food placed on a touch-sensitive plate, bringing it into the mouth and eating it, or grasping a piece of paper placed on the same plate and putting it into a container, located on the experimenter's right shoulder. They found that children with autism did not show any activation in the MH when observing other people who brought food to their mouth, while TD children showed proactive activity in MH in this situation. This activity demonstrates that the TD children perceive other people's actions by activating their own action system in the way suggested by the Mirror Neuron System (MNS) hypothesis but that children with ASD don't. The result is shown in **Figure 1**.

A more remarkable result was that when, in a similar experiment, subjects brought food to their own mouth or a piece of paper to a container, strong pre-activation of the MH was obtained in the typically developed children about 1 s before the food arrived at the mouth, but in the children with autism the activation of the MH only started after the food was grasped (see **Figure 1**). Thus, the children with ASD did not chain the two actions together in a predictive way, i.e., they did not prepare the opening of the mouth before they brought food to it. To test whether this lack of chaining two actions is a more general phenomenon and not just confined to bringing food to the mouth, an experiment was also performed in which two other actions were performed sequentially. The tasks were bringing food or a piece of paper to two different containers. The container for the food was to be opened by the pressing a pedal by the foot while the container for the paper was already opened. Thus, the pressing of the pedal in the food case should be performed slightly before the hand arrived with the food. Predictive pressing of the pedal was performed by the TD children but not by the children with ASD. Anticipating the effects of one's own actions is an important aspect of motor control. In children with autism this ability seems to be impaired.

Further evidence for this hypothesis comes from a lifting task by Schmitz et al. (2003). They tested how children with autism and typically developed children (mean age 8 years) could maintain the left forearm stabilized in space despite imposed or voluntary unloading of a weight attached to it. In one condition a weight was attached to the left forearm arm with an electromagnet. The magnet was inactivated at a random moment and the weight then fell to the support. In the other condition the subjects unloaded the left forearm themselves by lifting the load with the right hand from a platform resting on the left forearm. EMG was recorded from the biceps and triceps brachii. It was found that the forearm stabilization in the loading condition was as equally good in children with autism and in typically developed children. The two groups differed, however, in the unloading condition. The latency of the biceps brachii inhibition for both groups was around 60 ms in the involuntary unloading situation. In the voluntary unloading condition, the latency for the ASD group was also 60 ms while there was a proactive activation by 15 ms for the typically developed children. This shows that the TD children anticipated the voluntary unloading while the children with autism did not.

Does this deficiency in motor control appear in development together with other signs of autism or does it precede them. A recent report on feeding indicates that deficient anticipation of actions is a precursor of autism (Brisson et al., 2011). Their study is based on retrospective analysis of family home movies. The results show that 4-months-old children who later become diagnosed with ASD anticipate less often the arrival of the spoon to their mouth in a feeding situation than do children who are not at risk. Anticipation was measured by counting the number of times the mouth failed to open before the spoon arrived.

PLANNING MOVEMENT SEQUENCES

Complex goal-directed movements are usually made up of several subunits that are chained together. When a movement is

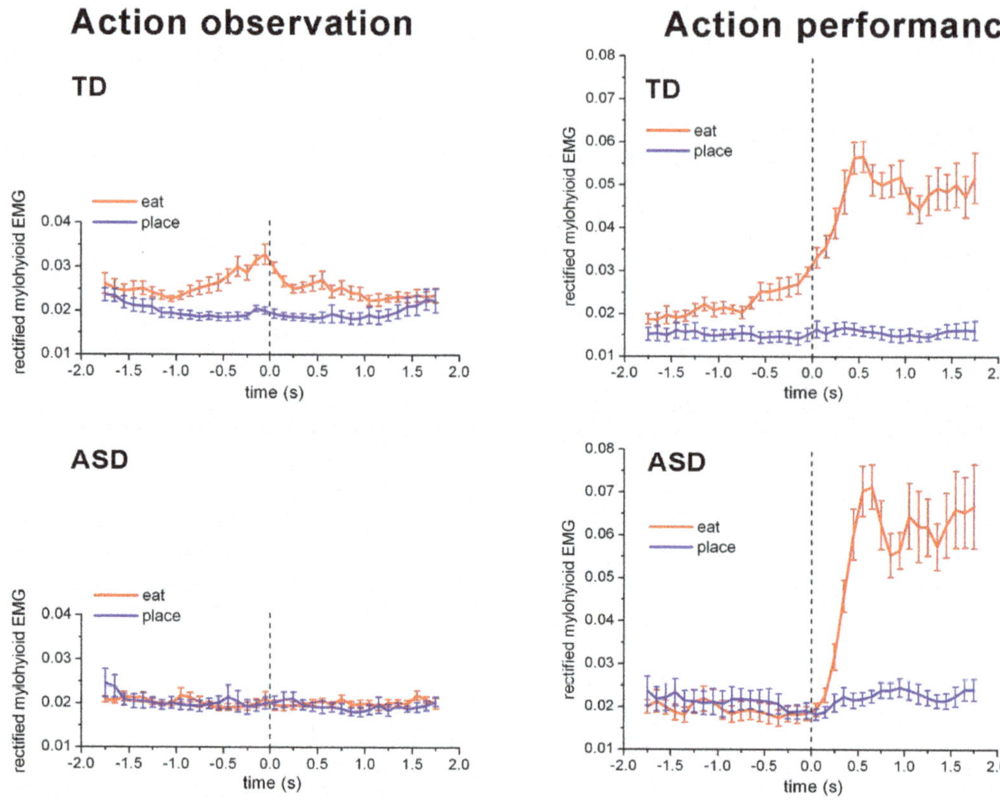

FIGURE 1 | The activation of the mylohyioid muscle during the event of bringing the food to the mouth (red) and the paper to the container (blue) in the TD children and the children with ASD. Zero is the time of grasping.

performed these subunits are linked in a predictive manner to create a continuous global action. Children with autism tend to split up such chained motor acts into unrelated movements. The result by Cattaneo et al. (2007) showing that these children do not link the approach of their hand to the mouth and the opening of the mouth is an example of such fragmentation.

To further test the hypothesis that children with ASD have a fragmented motor organization, Fabbri-Destro et al. (2009) asked children with ASD and TD children to execute two actions consisting each of three motor acts: to move the hand to and object, pick it up, and move to a container. The first two steps were identical but the last varied in difficulty. This was accomplished by varying the size of the opening of the container. The result showed that, unlike in TD children, the kinematics of the first motor act was not modulated by the task difficulty in children with autism. Similar results were obtained by Forti et al. (2011). They asked 12 high functioning preschool children with ASD and 12 TD children to grasp a ball, move it over the edge of a container, and drop it into a hole there. They found that while TD children did this in one continuous move, the children with ASD did it in a more discontinuous manner. First, they moved the ball to the container with no adjustment to what they were going to do next, then, in a discontinuous manner, turned the hand and dropped the ball. This resulted in more movement units and longer movement durations.

PROSPECTIVE LOOKING

Visual scanning the surrounding requires a plan for what to look at next. Children with ASD seem to be deficient in this ability. They do not look at the aspects of a social scene that are most informative (Klin et al., 2003) but instead fixate on insignificant details. It is not a question of being attracted by low-level visual saliency (Fletcher-Watson et al., 2009) or finding faces aversive to look at (Falck-Ytter and von Hofsten, 2011), but rather the lack of a plan of where to look next. von Hofsten et al. (2009) studied how TD preschool children and children with ASD look at when viewing a conversation between two models. They found that the TD children focused very much on the mouths of the talking models (around 70% of the time) while the children with ASD were much more scattered in their fixations and fixated the faces only 20% of the time. For instance, in contrast to the TD children they looked much at the shadow of the models. This is in line with Becchio et al. (2010) who found that instead of contributing to the perception of objects, shadows rather interfered with it. The fixation of shadows in children with autism is illustrated in **Figure 2**. An analysis was also performed on whether the subjects looked proactively at the next speaker of the conversation. It was found that this was the case in over 60% for the TD children while the children with ASD did it in less than 30% of the turns.

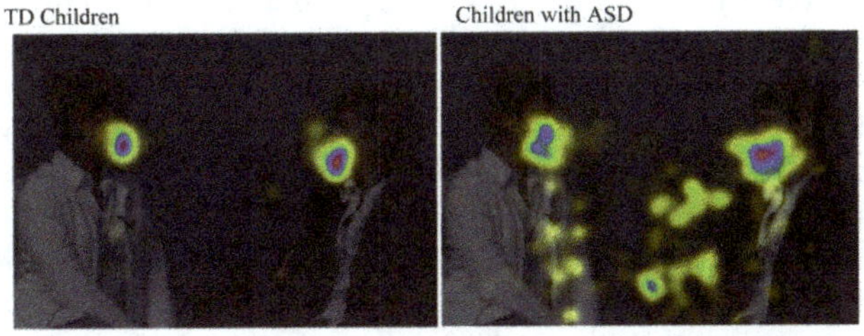

FIGURE 2 | The mean relative duration of fixations on the different parts of the display during the conversation. The durations of fixation are calculated from a group of TD 3-years-old children ($n = 12$) and a group of 3–6-years-old children with ASD ($n = 9$). The increasing amount of fixations on a specific part of the display is depicted in yellow-green-blue-red color where red corresponds to the most fixations. It can be seen that the fixations of the children with ASD are more scattered than the fixations of the TD children. In addition, the fixation highlights show that the children with ASD have a strong tendency to fixate the shadow casted by the right model. When she spoke, she tended to move her head a little and the shadow of her head attracted the gaze of the children with autism but not the TD children (From von Hofsten et al., 2009, RASD, by permission).

UNDERSTANDING ONE'S OWN ACTIONS

Children with ASD have problems with representing their own actions. Several studies have used a specific test of this ability, (the Florida Apraxia Battery modified for children, Mostofsky et al., 2006). It consists of gestures to command, gestures to imitate, and gestures with tool use. The gestures to command and gestures to imitate include both transitive gestures (those that act on or with an object, e.g., hammering a nail) and intransitive gestures (those that do not act on or with an object, e.g., waving goodbye); the gesture for tool use section contains only transitive gestures. Dowell et al. (2009) found that children with ASD had worse basic motor skill and postural knowledge than did controls. The ASD group showed significantly poorer praxis than did controls after accounting for age, IQ, basic motor skill, and postural knowledge. Dyspraxia in autism therefore appears to be associated with impaired formation of spatial representations that are primarily visual in origin. MacNeil and Mostofsky (2012) investigated a group of children with ASD and a group with ADHD and found that whereas the children from both groups show impairments in basic motor control, impairments in performance and recognition of skilled motor gestures appear to be specific to autism. The specific impairment to represent one's own movements may also be related to deficiencies in imitation.

THE RELATIONSHIP TO NEUROSCIENCE

The children with ASD express problems that raises questions as to how they relate to brain processes. The fact that prediction of upcoming events is a major problem suggests that the cerebellum is involved. Haas et al. (1996) concluded from a review of 16 quantitative magnetic resonance imaging (MRI) and autopsy studies involving more than 240 autistic cases that cerebellar abnormalities are present in ASD from at least 5 years of age and throughout development. Cerebellar deficits could also explain why balance control is impaired (Dziuk et al., 2007). The posterior parietal cortex (PPC) has strong projections to the cerebellum via pons which then connects to the premotor and motor cortex. It has been suggested that this pathway is central for the prospective control of action (Altman and Bayer, 1997). It may also be one of the major routes for visuo-motor information to reach the premotor cortex and contribute to the evolving motor command (Miall, 2003). When this network is compromised, as it is in ASD, a number of prospective control problems emerge.

Another neural network associated with this ASD is the MNS (Oberman et al., 2008). It is primarily anchored in the Superior Temporal Sulcus (STS), the Inferior Parietal Lobule (IPL) and the Premotor Area (PA) (Rizzolatti and Craighero, 2004; Rizzolatti and Sinigaglia, 2010). Hence, the mirror cells in premotor cortex may code a motoric representation of visuo-motor actions, both during action execution and during action observation, driven by the cerebellar inverse model. It has been shown that MNS is compromised in children with ASD (Iacoboni and Dapretto, 2006) and that there is a significant negative relationship between degree of activation in Pars Opercularis (premotor area) as measured by fMRI and the severity of autism as measured by the social scale of the Autism Diagnostic Interview-Revised (ADI-R) (Dapretto et al., 2006). The activation of MNS is commonly studied by measuring activation in a specific frequency band in the EEG (the mu-rhythm corresponding to 9–13 Hz in adults). During rest the amplitude is high but during motor activity it decreases due to desynchronization of the activity. It also desynchronizes when subjects observe actions and that makes it reasonable to assume that the mu-rhythm reflect MNS activation. Oberman et al. (2005) found that the mu-rhythm in a group of ASD subjects desynchronized during their own activity but not during observation of other people's actions. This indicates that these subjects do not respond to other people's actions in the way they respond to their own. These findings were replicated by Martineau et al. (2008) giving support to the suggestion that the MNS system is deficient in children with ASD.

It has been suggested that the measured deficiency in the MNS in ASD subjects could be related to weak neural connections between IPL and PA (Mostofsky and Ewen, 2011). One thing that the trans-cerebellar loop and the MNS have in common is that both rely on long connections. It has therefore been suggested that long neural connections are weak in children with ASD and that shorter connections dominate, for instance those between the somatosensory cortex and the motor cortex (Haswell et al., 2009). To test this idea, Haswell et al. (2009) measured patterns of generalization in children who learned to control a novel tool and found that the children with autism formed representations that relied more than normally on association between motor commands and proprioception, that is between the neighboring areas of somatosensory cortex and M1. They also found that the greater the reliance on proprioception, the greater was the child's impairments in social function and imitation (Haswell et al., 2009). In TD children, action representations rely more on visual and auditory information that are defined in external coordinates.

Thus, the core problem in ASD may be more fundamental than the just an impairment of MNS. Both MNS and the trans-cerebellar pathway rely on long connections. Another set of long connections that are found to be weak in children with ASD, are the ones going through Corpus Callosum. The fact that they are weak in children with autism was discovered by diffusion tensor imaging (Alexander et al., 2007). The assumption of weak long-range connections in children with ASD is also supported by Wolff et al. (2012). They conducted diffusion tensor imaging on infants from 6 to 24 months of age and found that many of the long connections in the brain started off being overdeveloped in children who were later diagnosed with ASD but were clearly underdeveloped by 2.5 years.

CONCLUSIONS

Although the most salient feature of Autism is a deficiency in communication and social ability, it is of great importance not to ignore the motor problems associated with ADS, because they might provide crucial information for the understanding of the dysfunction. It is clear that all communication consists of movements and that movement impairments give rise to disturbed communication, but it could not be the sole factor because many children with movement impairments are often good communicators. One important line of evidence suggests that children with autism are poor at predicting future events, at planning future actions and chaining action together. Prediction deficiencies are especially harmful when it comes to planning one's own actions and monitor other people's actions.

A recently discovered network in the brain, the MNS may be the mechanism that connects the motor problems and the social ones. According to the MNS hypothesis, observed actions are projected onto one's own action system together with the intentions and emotions associated with them. This facilitates the understanding of other people's actions. Impairments of the MNS will therefore have consequences both for social understanding as well as for the control of perception and action. If action planning is compromised, then the understanding of other people's actions will be compromised as well.

A number of conditions in the brain may be related to the evolution of autism but the most promising clue is the development of long connections between distant brain areas. Well-functioning long connections is crucial for the coordination of different brain areas and for the guidance of action by visual and auditory information. Impaired connections of this kind might be the ultimate reason why social function as well as prospective control are compromised in children with ASD.

ACKNOWLEDGMENTS

The research was supported by the Tercentennial Fund of the Bank of Sweden (P09-0933:1). We like to thank Terje Falck-Ytter for useful discussions.

REFERENCES

Alexander, A. L., Lee, J. E., Lazar, M., Boudo, R., DuBray, M. B., Oakes, T. R., et al. (2007). Diffusion tensor imaging of the corpus callosum in Autism. *Neuroimage* 34, 61–73.

Altman, J., and Bayer, S. A. (1997). *Development of the Cerebellar System in Relation to Its Evolution, Structure, and Functions.* Boca Raton, FL: CRC Press.

Becchio, C., Mari, M., and Castiello, U. (2010). Perception of shadows in children with autism spectrum disorder. *PLoS ONE* 5:e10582. doi: 10.1371/journal.pone.0010582

Bhat, A. N., Galloway, J. C., and Landa, R. C. (2012). Relationship between early motor delay and later communication delay in infants at risk for autism. *Infant Behav. Dev.* 35, 838–846.

Bodfish, J. W., Symons, F. J., Parker, D. E., and Lewis, M. H. (2000). Varieties of repetitive behavior in autism: comparisons to mental retardation. *J. Autism Dev. Disord.* 30,237–243.

Brisson, J., Varreyn, P., Serres, J., Foussier, S., and Adrien, L. (2011). Motor anticipation failure in infants with autism: a retrospective analysis of feeding situations. *Autism* 16, 420–429.

Cattaneo, L., Fabbri-Destro, M., Boria, S., Pieraccini, C., Monti, A., Cossu, G., et al. (2007). Impairment of actions chains in autism and its possible role in intention understanding. *Proc. Natl. Acad. Sci. U.S.A.* 104, 17825–17830.

Dapretto, M., Davies, M. S., Pfeifer, J. H., Scott, A. A., Sigman, M., Bookheimer, S. Y., et al. (2006). Understanding emotions in others: mirror neuron dysfunctions in children with autism spectrum disorders. *Nat. Neurosci.* 9, 28–30.

Dowell, L. H., Mahone, E. M., and Mostofsky, S. H. (2009). Associations of postural knowledge and basic motor skill with dyspraxia in autism: implication for abnormalities in distributed connectivity and motor learning. *Neuropsychology* 23, 563–570.

Dziuk, M. A., Gidley Larson, J. C., Apostu, A., Mahone, E. M., Denckla, M. B., and Mostofsky, S. H. (2007). Dyspraxia in autism: association with motor, social, and communicative deficits. *Dev. Med. Child Neur.* 49, 734–739.

Fabbri-Destro, M., Cattaneo, L., Boria, S., and Rizzolatti, G. (2009). Planning actions in autism. *Exp. Brain Res.* 192, 521–525.

Falck-Ytter, T., and von Hofsten, C. (2011). How special is social looking in ASD: a review. *Prog. Brain Res.* 189, 209–222.

Flanagan, J., Landa, R., Bhat, A., and Bauman, M. (2012). Head lag in infants at risk for autism: a preliminary study. *Am. J. Occup. Ther.* 66, 1–9.

Fletcher-Watson, S., Leekam, S. R., Benson, V., Frank, M. C., and Findlay, J. M. (2009). Eye-movements reveal attention to social information in autism spectrum disorder. *Neuropsychologia* 47, 248–257.

Forti, S., Valli, A., Pergo, P., Nobile, M., Crippa, A., and Molteni, A. (2011). Motor planning and control in autism. A kinematic analysis of preschool children. *Res. Autism Spect. Disord.* 5, 834–842.

Goldman, S., Wang, C., Salgado, M. W., Greene, P. E., Kim, M., and Rapin, I. (2008). Motor stereotypies in children with autism and other developmental disorders. *Dev. Med. Child Neurol.* 51, 30–38.

Green, D., Baird, G., Barnett, A. L., Henderson, L., Huber, J., and Henderson, S. E. (2002). The severity and nature of motor impairment in Asperger's syndrome: a comparison with specific developmental disorder of motor function. *J. Child Psychol. Psychiatry* 43, 655–668.

Haas, R. H., Townsend, J., Courchesne, E., Lincon, A. J., Schreibman, L., and Yeung-Courchesne, R. (1996). Neurological abnormalities in infantile autism. *J. Child Neurol.* 11, 84–92.

Haswell, C. C., Izawa, J., Dowell, L. R., Mostofsky, S. H., and Shadmehr, R. (2009). Representation of internal models of action in the autistic brain. *Nat. Neurosci.* 8, 970–972.

Iacoboni, M., and Dapretto, M. (2006). The mirror neuron system and the consequences of its dysfunction. *Nat. Rev. Neurosci.* 7, 942–951.

Klin, A., Jones, W., Schultz, R., and Volkmar, F. (2003). The enactive mind, or from actions to cognition: lessons from autism. *Philos. Trans. R. Soc. Lond. B* 358, 345–360.

MacNeil, L., and Mostofsky, S. H. (2012). Specific dyspraxia in children with autism. *Neuropsychology* 26, 165–171.

Martineau, J., Cochin, S., Magne, R., and Barthelemy, C. (2008). Impaired cortical activation in autistic children: is the mirror neuron system involved? *Int. J. Psychophysiol.* 68, 35–40.

Miall, R. C. (2003). Connecting mirror neurons and forward models. *Neuroreport* 14, 2135–2137.

Mostofsky, S. H., Dubey, P., Jerath, V. K., Jansiewicz, E. M., Goldberg, M. C., and Denckla, M. B. (2006). Developmental dyspraxia is not limited to imitation in children with autism spectrum disorders. *J. Int. Neuropsychol. Soc.* 12, 314–326.

Mostofsky, S. H., and Ewen, J. B. (2011). Altered connectivity and action model formation in autism is autism. *Neuroscientist* 17, 437–448.

Oberman, L. M., Hubbard, E. M., McCleery, J. P., and Altschuler, E. L. (2005). EEG evidence for mirror neuron dysfunction in autism spectrum disorders. *Brain Res. Cogn. Brain Res.* 24, 190–198.

Oberman, L. M., Ramachandran, V. S., and Pineda, J. A. (2008). Modulation of mu suppression in children with autism spectrum disorders in response to familiar or unfamiliar stimuli: the mirror neuron hypothesis. *Neuropsychology* 46, 1558–1565.

Rizzolatti, G., and Craighero, L. (2004). The mirror neuron system. *Ann. Rev. Neurosci.* 27, 169–192.

Rizzolatti, G., and Sinigaglia, C. (2010). The functional role of the parieto-frontal mirror circuit: interpretations and misinterpretations. *Nat. Rev. Neurosci.* 11, 264–274.

Schmitz, C., Martineau, J., Barthélémy, C., and Assaiante, C. (2003). Motor control and children with autism: deficit of anticipatory function? *Neurosci. Lett.* 348, 17–20.

Siaperas, P., Ring, H. A., McAllister, C. J., Henderson, S., Barnett, A., Watson, P., et al. (2012). Atypical movement performance and sensory integration in Asperger's syndrome. *J. Autism Dev. Disord.* 42, 718–725.

Teitelbaum, P., Teitelbaum, O., Nye, J., Fryman, J., and Maurer, R. G. (1998). Movement analysis in infancy may be useful for early diagnosis of autism. *Proc. Natl. Acad. Sci. U.S.A.* 95, 13982–13987.

von Hofsten, C. (1993). Prospective control: a basic aspect of action development. *Hum. Dev.* 36, 253–270.

von Hofsten, C. (2004). An action perspective on motor development. *Trends Cogn. Sci.* 8, 266–272.

von Hofsten, C. (2007). Action in development. *Dev. Sci.* 10, 54–60.

von Hofsten, C., Uhlig, H., Adell, M., and Kochukhova, O. (2009). How children with autism look at events. *Res. Autism Spect. Disord.* 3, 556–569.

Wolff, J. J., Gu, H., Gerig, G., Elison, J. T., Styner, M., Gouttard, S., et al. (2012). Differences in white matter fiber tract development present from 6 to 24 months in infants with autism. *Am. J. Psychiatry* 169, 589–600.

Conflict of Interest Statement: The authors declare that the research was conducted in the absence of any commercial or financial relationships that could be construed as a potential conflict of interest.

13

Stereotypies in autism: a video demonstration of their clinical variability

Sylvie Goldman[1,2,3]* **and Paul E. Greene**[4]

[1] *Saul R. Korey Department of Neurology, Albert Einstein College of Medicine, Bronx, NY, USA*
[2] *Department of Pediatrics, Albert Einstein College of Medicine, Bronx, NY, USA*
[3] *Rose F. Kennedy Intellectual and Developmental Disabilities Research Center, Albert Einstein College of Medicine, Bronx, NY, USA*
[4] *Department of Neurology, Columbia University Medical Center, New York, NY, USA*

Edited by:
Elizabeth B. Torres, Rutgers University, USA

Reviewed by:
Adrian Rodriguez-Contreras, City College of New York, USA
Ruth Nass, NYU SOM, USA

Correspondence:
Sylvie Goldman, Department of Neurology, Albert Einstein College of Medicine, Kennedy Center, 807, 1300 Morris Park Avenue, Bronx, NY 10461, USA.
e-mail: sylviegold@aol.com

In autism, stereotypies are frequent and disabling, and whether they correspond to a hyperkinetic movement disorder, a homeostatic response aiming at sensory modulation, or a regulator of arousal remains to be established. So far, it has been challenging to distinguish among these different possibilities, not only because of lack of objective and quantitative means to assess stereotypies, but in our opinion also because of the underappreciated diversity of their clinical presentations. Herein, we illustrate the broad spectrum of stereotypies and demonstrate the usefulness of video-assisted clinical observations of children with autism. The clips presented were extracted from play sessions of 129 children with autism disorder. We conclude that compared to widely used questionnaires and interviews, systematic video observations provide a unique means to classify and score precisely the clinical features of stereotypies. We believe this approach will prove useful to both clinicians and researchers as it offers the level of detail from retrievable images necessary to begin to assess effects of age and treatments on stereotypies, and to embark on the type of investigations required to unravel the physiological basis of motor behaviors in autism.

Keywords: autism, motor stereotypies, video, classification, variability

INTRODUCTION

Autism Disorder is a neurodevelopmental disorder defined clinically by the presence of qualitative impairments in three core domains: social interaction, communication, and restricted repetitive and stereotyped patterns of behavior, interests and activities. Repetitive, purposeless, patterned, rhythmic movement called motor stereotypies belong to the third criterion and as such are the only motor deficits included in the DSM-IV-TR (American Psychiatric Association, 2000) for a diagnosis of Autism. Following the new wave of biology-based research in autism, motor anomalies are receiving increasing attention. Indeed, until recently deficient sociability and language and communication, the other two DSM-IV-TR and ICD-10 WHO (World Health Organization, 1992) criteria, were the focus of most studies. This new focus is reflected in the proposed upcoming DSM-5 diagnostic criteria for Autism Spectrum Disorders (ASD) which would be reduced to two criteria: persistent deficits in social communication and social interaction across contexts, and restricted, repetitive patterns of behavior, interests, or activities. The second criterion includes not only rituals and routines but also repetitive movements and sensory impairments. The inclusion of motor and sensory symptoms will require clinicians to develop the proper skills to identify and characterize these core symptoms.

Stereotypies do not only occur in the context of a neurodevelopmental disorder (i.e., secondary stereotypies) like autism, blindness, or intellectual disability, they are also observed in typically developing infants (i.e., primary stereotypies); the latter usually subside around age 3 years (Thelen, 1979) whereas secondary stereotypies tend to persist through life in various forms. The persistent motor stereotypies of autism encompass a broad range of simple and complex typically bilateral movements. They involve one or multiple body parts and can have a twisting or circular quality. Their duration, frequency and intensity are variable. Especially in children with limited cognitive abilities it is rarely possible to assess reliably the suppressibility or the presence of a premonitory urge, which contributes to the difficulty differentiating them from tics. If frequent, stereotypies can interfere with learning and with the quality of social interactions. Stereotypies are stigmatizing and may evolve into self-injurious behaviors which represent a major concern for parents who spend time and money on occupational therapy to try to alleviate them.

Much controversy surrounds the causes of stereotypies, and while no model has obtained overwhelming support, the currently predominant behavioral theory Applied Behavioral Analytic Approach (ABA) suggests that stereotyped movements are maintained by reinforcement associated with either automatic reinforcement or social interactions (Cunningham and

Schreibman, 2008). A second view, posited by homeostatic theories, assumes there is an optimal level of stimulation for an individual and that stereotypical motor movements serve a compensatory function to increase arousal in under-stimulating environments or reduce arousal in over-stimulating environments (Kinsbourne, 1980). A third sensory-equilibration view contends that individuals with ASD engage in stereotypical movements to modulate auditory, visual, vestibular, tactile, and/or proprioceptive stimulation (Gabriels et al., 2008) by dampening sensory stimulation or by inducing heightened sensory experience. Another approach is to view stereotypies as a *motor disorder* that does not depend on functional interpretation, but reflects involuntary output of a dysregulated motor control system, likely including the basal ganglia and dopaminergic pathways (Graybiel, 2008; Langen et al., 2011). To date, the pathophysiology of stereotypies remains undefined (Lewis and Kim, 2009; Langen et al., 2011). The highly diverse phenomenology of this behavior is an additional challenge for developing research programs to address its neurophysiologic basis. Limited effective behavioral management approaches and pharmacological treatment are direct consequences of this lack of understanding.

As a prerequisite to studying their physiology, we felt compelled to develop a classification based on our systematic characterization from video scoring (see **Table 1**). In a previous study, we reported the prevalence and characteristics of motor stereotypies in developmentally impaired preschool children with and without autism, using the scoring system we have developed (Goldman et al., 2009). Our approach was purely phenomenological and we purposefully kept away from any type of interpretation such as their putative function. We developed a fine-grained video coding to assist identification and provide clinicians and researchers with a systematic descriptive approach for classifying these disparate movements. This video coding has been applied in clinical (LeMonda et al., 2012) and imaging (Goldman et al., 2013) studies. Herein, we present a collection of videos to illustrate both the similarities and the variability of stereotypies observed in children with autism and how some of them evolve over time.

Table 1 | Types of stereotypies.

Body parts	Types of movements
Face	Grimacing, lips, tongue movements, opening the mouth
Head, trunk, shoulders	Head tilting, shaking, nodding; body rocking, bending, crunching; arching the back; shrugging the shoulders
Arm/leg	Flapping, crossing the arms on the chest, stamping the feet
Hand/finger	Shaking, tapping, waving, clapping, opening-closing, twirling the hand or fingers
Hand/finger with object	Shaking, tapping, twirling an object
Gait	Pacing, jumping, running, skipping, spinning
Self-directed	Covering the ears; mouthing; smelling; rubbing the eyes; tapping the chin; banging the arms against the body; slapping self or an object or surface; touching genitals
Visual	Staring at an object or the fingers "out of the corner of the eyes"

Reproduced with permission from Wiley-Blackwell.

METHODS

To define the spectrum of expression of stereotypies we undertook to study over 500 videos of standardized play sessions recorded between 1985 and 1992 as part of a multi-center, multidisciplinary, longitudinal, nosological study of children with autism, and other developmental disorders (Rapin, 1996). The patients and methods were described previously (Goldman et al., 2009). Briefly, we examined the videotapes of semi-structured play session of preschool children diagnosed with DSM–III-R (American Psychiatric Association, 1987) Autistic Disorder (AD or classical autism) (Rapin, 1996). Children were engaged in play using a uniform set of representational toys (e.g., cars, block, crayons, ball, and puppets). Examiners at four sites: Boston, MA; the Bronx, NY; Cleveland, OH; and Trenton, NJ were trained to interact and play with the children in a similar way. This paper focuses on the 129 children with AD recruited at preschool, of whom 76 were re-examined at age 7 years, and 77 at age 9 years. The mean age at recording was 4.5 years (54 months) (age range 35–97 months). Children with autism were divided in two groups based on nonverbal IQ (NVIQ): high functioning autism (HFA) with NVIQ $\geq$ 80 and low functioning autism (LFA) with NVIQ $<$ 80. Most of the children shown here were in the LFA group because, overall, this group exhibits higher numbers of stereotypies and thus has most teaching value. All clips were edited from the 30 min-play sessions. We identified as stereotypy any apparently purposeless movement seen at least twice to document its repetitive nature (Goldman et al., 2009). The video clips presented in this paper were selected for their didactic quality in order to best illustrate the *variety* of motor stereotypies in autism.

All the parents of children in the original study gave written informed consent approved by the Institutional Review Board of each institution to videotape their children for research. Parents of Bronx children whose videos are presented in this report signed an additional permission approved by the Institutional Review Board of the Albert Einstein College of Medicine for their children's videos to be shown at scientific meetings and included in scientific publications.

ILLUSTRATION AND LEGENDS TO THE VIDEOS

We selected from our video collection the following 32 clips to demonstrate the variety and co-occurrence of aberrant repetitive motor behaviors observed in our large cohort of children with autism. The segments are organized into eight categories (Movies 1 and 2). For clarity, children are numbered within each category. When available we present video clips of the same child over time to illustrate the evolution and also the constancy of a particular stereotypical movement over time. In order to document the qualitative differences among apparently similar movements usually lumped together under the common "stereotypy" label we present here several clips of the same stereotypy in different children.

MOVIE 1

1: Gait. These locomotion movements were all potentially normal movements but performed repetitively.
Segment #1: Child #1 circles endlessly around a table and cannot be distracted.
Segments #2, 3: Child #2 is seen at preschool spinning around a spot on the floor and then stamping.
Segment #4: Child #2 circles in place 5 years later. The hint of dystonic arm abduction seen in preschool has become a more obviously dystonic hand posturing with finger twiddling in this later clip.
Segment #5: Child #3 engages in brief complex movements involving jumping with arm movements and vocalizations.

2: Head trunk and shoulders. These axial movements were almost always rhythmic. These repetitive behaviors might be considered normal, but were performed beyond what might be considered a typical duration.
Segment #6: Child #1 shows repetitive head nodding.
Segment #7: Child #2 has sustained abnormal head position. Tonic positions, such as the neck extension in Child #2, were less common than repetitive movements in neck, trunk, and limbs.
Segment #8: Child #3 shows more complex axial movements.
Segment #9: Child #4 illustrates truncal rocking, sideways and back and forth.

3: Arm/hand/finger without objects. These types of movements, such as flapping, were the most common in the youngest group. The hand movements could be unilateral or bilateral.
Segments #10–12: Children #1, #2, and #3 are examples of clapping movements. Child #2 presented with clapping, leg swinging accompanied by vocalizations.
Segments #13–15: Children #3, #4, and #5 illustrate a common movement involving rapid shaking of the limb around a limp wrist (or elbow), which we have called twiddling. Both Child #1 in segment #10 (clapping and tonic head extension) and Child #3 in this segment (twiddling and tonic finger posturing) combined rhythmic and tonic movements.
Segments #16–17: Children #6 shows a brief rotation movement of the wrist and child #7 a unilateral more continuous shaking.

4: Hand/finger with objects. These movements involved repetitive, patterned manipulation of an object or part of an object. Some of these movements were similar to movements without objects described in the previous category, such as clapping objects together instead of clapping hands together. In other movements, the use of the object was an integral part of the movement (especially a peculiar form of playing with objects we call cluttering).
Segments #18, 19, 20: Child #1 illustrates rapid cluttering with objects at preschool and 4 years later. Child #2 clutters in a different more rhythmic way and with dystonic posturing of the thumbs.
Segment #21: Child #3 shakes objects with either hand.
Segment #22: Child #4 claps objects together.
Segment #23: Child #5 rolls objects.

MOVIE 2

5: Self-directed movements. These self-touching, repetitive movements in which children touched or hit themselves were especially common in LFA children and can be self-injurious. Segments #24, 25: Child #1 brings his face to the object while both Child #1 and Child #2 bring objects to their faces.
Segments #26, 27: Child #3 obsessively rubs his nose at ages 7 and 9, with either hand.
Segment #28: Child #4 claps and picks at his fingers.

6: Sustained posturing. Posturing stereotypies are characterized by short episodes of sustained dystonic posturing in the upper or lower limbs.
Segments #29, 30: Child #1 is a low functioning girl with autism seen at preschool and 5 years later. She exhibits a variety of briefly sustained postures, purely repetitive movements, and combinations of posturing with superimposed repetitive movements.

7: Complex movements. These more complex stereotypies combined motor and vocal repetitive patterned behaviors.
Segment #31: Child #1 is an example of a complex motor/vocal stereotypy.

8: Persistence of complex movements over time. This clip exemplifies the persistence over time of a very particular stereotyped movement which becomes the signature stereotypy for this child.
Segment #32: Child #1 shows a self-hugging stereotypy at ages 4 and 9.

CONCLUSION

Only a few studies have characterized stereotypies in detail (Symons et al., 2005). Our collection of 129 preschool children with a DSM–III-R (American Psychiatric Association, 1987) Autism Disorder diagnosis (the more severe classical form of autism) provided the opportunity to describe in depth each stereotypy observed over a fixed time interval (15 min) under standard play conditions (Goldman et al., 2009). The present report and the accompanying video clips illustrate the clinical variability of stereotypies in children with autism. We demonstrate that frequency, rhythmicity, tone, topography, and especially variety of movements can be characterized from video clips and can distinguish subgroups.

So far the main techniques for identifying the presence and the frequency of stereotypies are questionnaires/ interviews of parents/caretakers. These instruments allow for larger data collection and broader contexts, including age and cognitive ability. Direct observation (ideally from videos) and small sample case studies (DiGennaro Reed et al., 2012; Honey et al., 2012) provide detailed analysis and have often been limited to the study of environmental triggers. Despite advances in the validation of these instruments, none of them provides the necessary detailed description required for a differential diagnosis. Indeed, very few studies have developed methods for video coding to examine features of distinct stereotypies and compare them with the abnormal movements of other developmental disorders. Using this video-based clinical approach, Goldman and Temudo (2012) were able to identify striking differences in hand stereotypies of children with ASD and Rett syndrome (RTT) which prove to be important clinical signs for the differential diagnosis of RTT vs. ASD, especially when genetic testing for RTT is not an option.

A small number of longitudinal studies focus on the trajectories of stereotypies (Wetherby et al., 2004; Honey et al., 2006; Esbensen et al., 2008) and present relevant data about diagnostic outcome. For example, longitudinal evaluation of the younger at risk siblings of children with autism suggests that repetitive patterned behaviors may be early diagnostic markers for autism (Gamliel et al., 2007; Rogers, 2009; Zwaigenbaum et al., 2009). So far we are not aware of studies reporting data on trajectories of specific types of stereotypies.

Based on our video-analysis we found that among the 129 preschool children with AD the prevalence of stereotypies in the low functioning autism (LFA) group was 70.6%, marginally statistically higher than the 63.6% found in the high functioning autism group (HFA). In the larger cohort of 277 children that included children with autism and non-autism developmental disorders, statistical analysis comparing the autism to non-autism and cognitively competent to less competent (nonverbal IQ < 80) groups showed that the presence of stereotypies at preschool in the particular setting of our standardized play session was more strongly linked to autism than to cognitive incompetence. Moreover, the number of stereotypies per child and the variety of stereotypies was higher in the LFA group, with head/trunk, hand/finger, and gait (e.g., spinning, pacing) stereotypies being the most frequent in this group (Goldman et al., 2009).

Yet, our longitudinal observation shows that when stereotypies persist, they tend to remain essentially unchanged, at least over a period of several years (in preparation). The fact that the same involuntary movement is produced under a great variety of circumstances and over a long time span lends strength to the hypothesis that specific neuronal circuitry may be responsible for that particular stereotypy (i.e., *the motor disorder* view). Our follow-up clinical observational using objective computerized quantitative measures (i.e., body sensors, accelerometers) of the frequency, topography, complexity, duration, and amplitude of stereotypies in relation to electrophysiological and brain imaging measures are addressing this hypothesis. Another important factor that requires attention pertains to the potential effect of familiarity and context such as home vs. school or the laboratory.

We predict that our video-phenomenology-based approach will prove useful to clinicians and researchers to refine their observation and the analysis of the trajectory of repetitive movements as a function of age, cognitive ability and diagnosis. As such, we also believe that the kind of video-scoring that we have developed and that we discuss here may be instrumental in assessing efficacy of the treatments, which questionnaires or rating forms cannot provide reliably.

ACKNOWLEDGMENTS

We thank the children and their families for their participation. We are grateful to Isabelle Rapin for her insightful comments and continuous support. Sylvie Goldman was supported by the Einstein/Montefiore Autism Center and a LEND grant—Leadership Education in Neurodevelopmental and Related Disabilities from the Bureau of Maternal and Child Health in the Department of Health and Human Services. She was also supported by a grant from the Eunice Kennedy Shriver National Institute of Child Health and Human Development of the National Institutes of Health (NIH) under Award Number P30HD071593. The videos and clinical data on the children were supported by NINDS program project NS 20489.

SUPPLEMENTARY MATERIAL

The Supplementary Material for this article can be found online at: http://www.frontiersin.org/Integrative_Neuroscience/10.3389/fnint.2012.00121/abstract

REFERENCES

American Psychiatric Association. (1987). *Diagnostic and Statistical Manual of Mental Disorders, DSM III-R.* Washington, DC: American Psychiatric Association.

American Psychiatric Association. (2000). *Diagnostic and Statistical Manual of Mental Disorders, DSM IV-TR.* Washington, DC: American Psychiatric Association.

Cunningham, A., and Schreibman, L. (2008). Stereotypy in autism: the importance of function. *Res. Autism Spectr. Disord.* 2, 469–479.

DiGennaro Reed, F. D., Hirst, J. M., and Hyman, S. R. (2012). Assessment and treatment of stereotypic behavior in children with autism and other developmental disabilities: a thirty year review. *Res. Autism Spectr. Disord.* 6, 422–430.

Esbensen, A. J., Seltzer, M. M., Lam, K. S., and Bodfish, J. W. (2008). Age-related differences in restricted repetitive behaviors in autism spectrum disorders. *J. Autism Dev. Disord.* 39, 57–66.

Gabriels, R. L., Agnew, J., Miller, L. J., Gralla, J., Pan, Z., Goldson, E., et al. (2008). Is there a relationship between restricted, repetitive, stereotyped behaviors and interests and abnormal sensory response in children with autism spectrum disorders? *Res. Autism Spectr. Disord.* 2, 660–670.

Gamliel, I., Yirmiya, N., and Sigman, M. (2007). The development of young siblings of children with autism from 4 to 54 months. *J. Autism Dev. Disord.* 37, 171–183.

Goldman, S., O'Brien, L., Filipek, P. A., Rapin, I., and Herbert, M. A. (2013). Motor stereotypies and volumetric brain alterations in children with autistic disorder. *Res. Autism Spectr. Disord.* 7, 82–92.

Goldman, S., and Temudo, T. (2012). Hand stereotypies distinguish Rett syndrome from autism disorder. *Mov. Disord.* 27, 1060–1062.

Goldman, S., Wang, C., Salgado, M. W., Greene, P. E., Kim, M., and Rapin, I. (2009). Motor stereotypies in children with autism and other developmental disorders. *Dev. Med. Child Neurol.* 51, 30–38.

Graybiel, A. M. (2008). Habits, rituals, and the evaluative brain. *Annu. Rev. Neurosci.* 31, 359–387.

Honey, E., McConachie, H., Randle, V., Shearer, H., and Couteur, A. S. (2006). One-year change in repetitive behaviours in young children with communication disorders including autism. *J. Autism Dev. Disord.* 38, 1439–1450.

Honey, E., Rodgers, J., and McConachie, H. (2012). Measurement of restricted and repetitive behaviour in children with autism spectrum disorder: selecting a questionnaire or interview. *Res. Autism Spectr. Disord.* 6, 757–776.

Kinsbourne, M. (1980). Do repetitive movement patterns in children and animals serve a dearousing function? *J. Dev. Behav. Pediatr.* 1, 39–42.

Langen, M., Durston, S., Kas, M. J., van Engeland, H., and Staal, W. G. (2011). The neurobiology of repetitive behavior: ... and men. *Neurosci. Biobehav. Rev.* 35, 356–365.

LeMonda, B., Holtzer, R., and Goldman, S. (2012). Relationship between executive functions and motor stereotypies in children with autistic disorder. *Res. Autism Spectr. Disord.* 6, 1099–1106.

Lewis, M. H., and Kim, S. J. (2009). The pathophysiology of restricted repetitive behavior. *J. Neurodev. Disord.* 1, 114–132.

Rapin, I. (1996). *Preschool Children with Inadequate Communication.*

Developmental Language Disorder, Autism, Low IQ. London: Mac Keith.

Rogers, S. J. (2009). What are infant siblings teaching us about autism in infancy? *Autism Res.* 2, 125–137.

Symons, F. J., Sperry, L. A., Dropik, P. L., and Bodfish, J. W. (2005). The early development of stereotypy and self-injury: a review of research methods. *J. Intellect. Disabil. Res.* 49, 144–158.

Thelen, E. (1979). Rhythmical stereotypies in normal human infants. *Anim. Behav.* 27, 699–715.

Wetherby, A. M., Woods, J., Allen, L., Cleary, J., Dickinson, H., and Lord, C. (2004). Early indicators of autism spectrum disorders in the second year of life. *J. Autism Dev. Disord.* 34, 473–493.

World Health Organization. (1992). *International Classification of Mental and Behavioral Disorders: Clinical Descriptions and Diagnostic Guidelines.* Geneva.

Zwaigenbaum, L., Bryson, S., Lord, C., Rogers, S., Carter, A., Carver, L., et al. (2009). Clinical assessment and management of toddlers with suspected autism spectrum disorder: insights from studies of high-risk infants. *Pediatrics* 123, 1383–1391.

Conflict of Interest Statement: The authors declare that the research was conducted in the absence of any commercial or financial relationships that could be construed as a potential conflict of interest.

14

Motor abnormalities as a putative endophenotype for Autism Spectrum Disorders

Gianluca Esposito[1]* and Sergiu P. Paşca[2]*

[1] RIKEN Brain Science Institute, Unit for Affiliative Social Behavior, Wako-Shi, Saitama, Japan
[2] Department of Neurobiology, Stanford University School of Medicine, Stanford, CA, USA

Edited by:
Elizabeth B. Torres, Rutgers University, USA

Reviewed by:
Albino J. Oliveira-Maia, Champalimaud Foundation, Portugal
Stefanie Bodison, University of Southern California, USA

*Correspondence:
Gianluca Esposito, RIKEN Brain Science Institute, Unit for Affiliative Social Behavior, 2-1 Hirosawa, Wako-shi, Saitama, 351-0198, Japan
e-mail: gesposito@brain.riken.jp;
Sergiu P. Paşca, Department of Neurobiology, Stanford University School of Medicine, Fairchild Building, 299 Campus Drive West, D222 Stanford, CA 94305, USA
e-mail: spasca@stanford.edu

Autism Spectrum Disorders (ASDs) represent a complex group of behaviorally defined conditions with core deficits in social communication and the presence of repetitive and restrictive behaviors. To date, neuropathological studies have failed to identify pathognomonic cellular features for ASDs and there remains a fundamental disconnection between the complex clinical aspects of ASDs and the underlying neurobiology. Although not listed among the core diagnostic domains of impairment in ASDs, motor abnormalities have been consistently reported across the spectrum. In this perspective article, we summarize the evidence that supports the use of motor abnormalities as a putative endophenotype for ASDs. We argue that because these motor abnormalities do not directly depend on social or linguistic development, they may serve as an early disease indicator. Furthermore, we propose that stratifying patients based on motor development could be useful not only as an outcome predictor and in identifying more specific treatments for different ASDs categories, but also in exposing neurobiological mechanisms.

Keywords: Autism Spectrum Disorders, motor abnormalities, endophenotype, early assessment, early screening

Autism Spectrum Disorders (ASDs) comprise a complex group of behaviorally defined conditions with core deficits in social communication and the presence of repetitive and restrictive behaviors (American Psychiatric Association, 2000). ASDs are highly comorbid and notably heterogeneous in their clinical presentation. Multiple etiologies have been suggested, but no single genetic or environmental factor can account for more than a small fraction of all cases (Abrahams and Geschwind, 2008). Despite sustained efforts to identify the cell types and circuits that are impaired in ASDs, there remains a fundamental disconnection between the complex clinical features of ASDs and the underlying neurobiological mechanisms. Postmortem brain studies have failed to identify pathognomonic cellular features for ASDs (Pickett and London, 2005; Amaral et al., 2008). Despite reports of high heritability (Abrahams and Geschwind, 2008, 2010), large effect genetic events (copy number variants or *de novo* mutations) are rare, while common genetic variants can explain only a minute fraction of the phenotypic variability (Stein et al., 2013). In addition, environmental contributions have only rarely proved conclusive [e.g., rubella, thalidomide or valproic acid exposure in early pregnancy (Landrigan, 2010)]. While rodent models of ASDs have begun to provide pathophysiological and therapeutic clues, these models have been restricted to rare syndromic or Mendelian forms of ASDs, and have yet to address issues of specificity (i.e., the overlap between genes in ASDs, developmental delay, and schizophrenia) and cross-species clinical validity (Qiu et al., 2012). More recently, cellular reprogramming techniques have emerged as new tools for identifying neuronal phenotypes in cells derived *in vitro* from patients (Marchetto et al., 2010; Paşca et al., 2011; Novarino et al., 2012). However, these cellular investigations will have to be expanded considerably in order to identify common and divergent neuronal phenotypes in idiopathic ASDs cases.

These novel models, as well as the continued accumulation of clinical and genetic data in recent years, underscore a need to develop more reliable means of stratifying ASDs. The identification of discrete, genetically determined disease components, or endophenotypes (Gottesman and Gould, 2003), could prove essential in delineating biologically and therapeutically meaningful classes, adding power to genetic studies and guiding neurobiological investigations. One promising avenue in this direction is a more exhaustive and systematic investigation of motor abnormalities in ASDs.

Motor abnormalities in ASDs span a wide range of dysfunctions, including defects in gross and fine motor control, complex motor sequences (including dyspraxia and deficits in imitation), eye movement abnormalities and motor learning deficits. Pinpointed by Kanner (1943) and Asperger (1944) in their initial case series, these abnormalities were referred as "clumsiness in gait and motor performances" (Kanner and Lesser, 1958). Two decades later, Damasio and Maurer (1978) hypothesized mesolimbic dysfunction as a potential explanation for dyskinetic and dystonic movements observed in patients with ASDs, while others have either described a parkinsonian gait (Vilensky et al., 1981), an ataxic-cerebellar gait (Hallett et al., 1993; see also Nayate et al., 2012) or simply recognized asymmetric patterns of movement and infantile reflexes "gone astray"

(Teitelbaum et al., 1998, 2004; Esposito et al., 2009, 2011, 2012). Although a recent meta-analysis confirmed the presence of substantial motor coordination deficits in ASDs with a considerable effect size of 1.20 (Fournier et al., 2010), none of the studies to date have identified a single motor symptom as a universal sign or prodrome for ASDs (Yirmiya and Charman, 2010).

Though there may not be a single universal motor sign, several levels of evidence point toward the utility of motor assessments in ASDs, indicating that motor dysfunction may play a central role in elucidating pathophysiological mechanisms and facilitating diagnosis and treatment. We describe them here with an emphasis on highlighting specific commonalties and disparities in the presentation of motor abnormalities that could allow for ASDs stratification.

First, motor abnormalities in ASDs are present early, within the first year of life, and may precede social-communication deficits (Leary and Hill, 1996). For example, Flanagan et al. (2012), reported that head lag during pull-to-sit at the age of 6 months was associated with ASDs at 36 months and was more frequently observed in infants at high-risk for ASDs. Recently, two excellent prospective studies followed early motor symptoms in high-risk subjects. In the first longitudinal study, Landa et al. (2013) assessed 235 children with or without a sibling with ASDs to identify differential trajectories for normative versus early-onset or late-onset ASDs. Interestingly, although development was grossly intact by 6 months, fine motor delay was present as early as 14 months in the late-onset group, and only by 36 months in the early-onset ASDs group. In the second prospective study, Landa et al. (2012) followed ASDs siblings from 6 to 36 months and identified four main trajectory phenotypes: normal development, accelerated development, widespread skill acquisition delay, and receptive language and motor delay. Importantly, in the latter group, receptive language delay resolved by 24 months, while motor abnormalities persisted at 36 months. Taken together, these studies demonstrate that motor development is vulnerable to early delay in patients with ASDs and their siblings and could potentially inform subtype identification.

Second, motor symptoms in ASDs are persistent. Both fine and gross motor impairments are long-term deficits, whose severity is correlated with the degree of social impairment (Freitag et al., 2007). A recent large sample study (Lloyd et al., 2013) showed that in very young children with ASDs, these delays become more pronounced with age, even when controlling for non-verbal problem-solving skills. Additional reports have suggested that gross motor and fine motor symptoms may diminish over the course of life, but even in these cohorts oculomotor impairment and dyspraxia appear to persist (Freitag et al., 2007). These observations suggest that the persistence of motor symptoms could also assist with differential diagnosis. For instance, skill progression in Down syndrome is delayed, but the acquisition of developmental milestones occurs in an orderly manner and these deficits can significantly improve with therapeutic facilitation (Sacks and Buckley, 2003).

Third, there is preliminary evidence indicating that motor abnormalities in ASDs are heritable. For instance, motor delays are common among ASDs siblings and are predictive of communication delays in these individuals (Bhat et al., 2012), making them part of the broader autism phenotype. In addition, bivariate twin analyses indicate that physical clumsiness and autistic-like traits are highly correlated, an association that is most plausibly explained by genetic etiological overlap (Moruzzi et al., 2011). Moreover, a considerable proportion of the genetic variance in ASDs is shared with developmental coordination disorder, a childhood condition characterized by poor motor coordination and clumsiness (Lichtenstein et al., 2010). While not all studies have been able to detect motor skills impairments in unaffected siblings of children with ASDs (Hilton et al., 2012), future prospective studies should dissect more systematically and in larger cohorts the relative genetic contribution to motor abnormalities in ASDs.

Fourth, and perhaps the feature that best makes the case for the assessment of motor abnormalities for ASDs stratification, is the fact that motor development is relatively more quantitative in nature than communicative abilities or social traits. Multiple standardized test batteries that measure motor skills are currently available. For instance, the Mullen Scales of Early Learning evaluates gross motor development from 0 to 33 months, and the Griffiths Mental Development Scales quantify locomotor activity, including the ability to balance and to coordinate and control movements. Multiple studies have shown that these evaluations are reliable and easy to implement. Moreover, they have the potential for becoming screening tools especially if facilitated by video analyses (using computer vision tools as illustrated by Hashemi et al., 2012, for example). Coupled with the early onset of motor abnormalities, described above, the availability of reliable quantitative tools point toward the use of motor development as a more standard metric for patient stratification.

Fifth, is the suggestion that both motor and social-communicative deficits originate from a common etiology and that motor abnormalities would constitute an early window into the pathophysiology of ASDs. Although this assertion has not been tested systematically, we know a significant amount about the physiology of the motor system, and it is conceivable that neurobiological insights will be gained from investigating motor development in ASDs. Clinical and physiological studies indicate multiple levels of biological impairment in ASDs, from the vestibular brainstem nuclei to the cerebellum, basal ganglia and sensorimotor cortices. Therefore, involvement of individual structures, which are associated with specific subtypes of motor abnormalities, could be used as a stratification criterion. Postmortem brain findings have paved the way by reporting, in some ASDs patients, Purkinje cell deficits in the cerebellum (Bauman and Kemper, 1985; Arin et al., 1991; Bailey et al., 1998; Whitney et al., 2008; Fatemi et al., 2012) and hypoplasia of its vermal lobules VI–VII (Courchesne et al., 1994), an enlarged caudate nucleus (Langen et al., 2007) and a delayed functional specialization of the motor cortex (Nebel et al., 2012). One example of how motor abnormalities may inform a mechanistic understanding is the hypothesis of early damage to mirror neuron systems in ASD. According to this model, impairments in ASDs are rooted in the incapacity to assemble and directly grasp the intrinsic goal-directed organization of motor behavior (Cossu et al., 2012).

Sixth, motor abnormalities affect quality of life and correction is likely to improve functioning. Abnormal motor control can have pervasive consequences on the development of multiple skills. Delayed motor development constrains social interactions and impaired social interactions can further constrain motor skill development. Importantly, gross and fine motor skills can be learned and practiced, and although not tested prospectively, motor corrections may improve social-communicative functioning in ASDs (Baranek, 1999).

Lastly, recent studies indicate that motor abnormalities in ASDs may have predictive value. For instance, approximately 70% of high-risk infants (i.e., siblings of ASDs patients) who presented with early motor delays later developed deficits in communication (Bhat et al., 2012), while better motor outcome in 2-year-old children with ASDs correlates with better outcomes at 4 years (Sutera et al., 2007).

Taken together, these multiple lines of evidence underscore the need for more systematically assessing motor development in ASDs patients. With few exceptions (Provost et al., 2007; Ozonoff et al., 2008), most studies investigating motor development in ASDs report abnormalities at some levels (vestibular, fronto-striatal, cerebellar, cortical) and of a certain severity. Importantly, the standard deviations for the measured variables in these studies are always larger in the ASDs group, highlighting that at an individual level some children with ASDs are definitely atypical, while others are probably not remarkably different than their matching controls (Vernazza-Martin et al., 2005; Rinehart et al., 2006a,b,c; Esposito and Venuti, 2008). Depending on the task and the cohort, the proportion of ASDs children displaying motor development abnormalities varies. For instance Esposito et al. (2011), found that persistent postural asymmetries were present only in ~40% of children with ASDs. The variability in these deficits across the spectrum is a challenge that likely reflects the clinical and etiological heterogeneity of ASDs. At the same time, it constitutes a unique opportunity to identify disease subtypes.

Additional work is clearly needed to conclusively determine how motor abnormalities can contribute to understanding ASDs, while the limitations of existing studies also have to be addressed. For instance, cohorts that up until now have been restricted to high functioning patients should be expanded to reflect the full autism spectrum using objective disease measures (the Autism Diagnostic Observation Schedule—ADOS, Autism Diagnostic Interview, Revised—ADI-R). More prospective studies need to be developed, while retrospective studies should use well-matched controls and siblings. It is also important to explore motor disturbances in novel or cognitively demanding environments and combine these studies with genetic analyses and neuroimaging. Peculiar phenomena associated with ASDs, such as *kinesia paradoxa* during which motor function can appear smooth and seamless during fixation on one task, deserve more attention (Leary and Hill, 1996; Rinehart et al., 2006a,b,c). In addition, the confounding role of medications (antipsychotics, antidepressants, stimulants, mood stabilizers), which are so commonly prescribed in these patients, should be rigorously investigated in the context of behavioral and motor abnormalities. Benefits could also come from the development and implementation of novel, easy to use, standardized scales that could streamline the collection of motor developmental data and allow for large-scale analyses.

In conclusion, motor abnormalities in ASDs are early and persistent clinical signs, which, due to their heritability, can serve as disease endophenotypes. In addition, these abnormalities can be reliably quantified and, if improved, are likely to benefit the overall functioning of the patient. When viewed as an endophenotype, motor abnormalities have the potential to stratify ASDs into more tractable conditions leading to more productive etiological explorations, better clinical trials, and perhaps earlier detection and outcome prediction.

ACKNOWLEDGMENTS

The authors would like to thank Georgia Panagiotakos from the Department of Neurobiology at Stanford University School of Medicine, Stanford, USA for fruitful discussions and providing insightful comments on this manuscript, as well as Mariko Bennett, Chris Bennett, Carleton Goold, and Anca M. Pasca. This research was supported by the Japan Society for the Promotion of Science (Kakenhi, Wakate, B 24730563), the FPR Program for Gianluca Esposito, and the Tashia and John Morgridge Endowed Fellowship in Translational Pediatric Medicine and the NARSAD Young Investigator Award for Sergiu P. Paşca.

REFERENCES

Abrahams, B. S., and Geschwind, D. H. (2008). Advances in autism genetics: on the threshold of a new neurobiology. *Nat. Rev. Genet.* 9, 341–355. doi: 10.1038/nrg2346

Abrahams, B. S., and Geschwind, D. H. (2010). Connecting genes to brain in the autism spectrum disorders. *Arch. Neurol.* 67, 395–399. doi: 10.1001/archneurol.2010.47

Amaral, D. G., Schumann, C. M., and Nordahl, C. W. (2008). Neuroanatomy of autism. *Trends Neurosci.* 31, 137–145. doi: 10.1016/j.tins.2007.12.005

American Psychiatric Association. (2000). *Diagnostic and Statistical Manual of Mental Disorders, 4th edn (DSM-4).* Washington, DC: American Psychiatric Association.

Arin, D. M., Bauman, M. L., and Kemper, T. L. (1991). The distribution of Purkinje cell loss in the cerebellum in autism. *Neurology* 41, 307.

Asperger, H. (1944). Die "Autistischen Psychopathen" im Kindesalter. *Archiv für Psychiatrie und Nervenkrankheiten* 117, 132–135.

Bailey, A., Luthert, P., Dean, A., Harding, B., Janota, I., Montgomery, M., et al. (1998). A clinicopathological study of autism. *Brain* 121, 889–905. doi: 10.1093/brain/121.5.889

Baranek, G. T. (1999). Autism during infancy: a retrospective video analysis of sensory-motor and social behaviors at 9–12 months of age. *J. Autism Dev. Disord.* 29, 213–224. doi: 10.1023/A:1023080005650

Bauman, M., and Kemper, T. L. (1985). Histoanatomic observations of the brain in early infantile autism. *Neurology* 35, 866–874. doi: 10.1212/WNL.35.6.866

Bhat, A. N., Galloway, J. C., and Landa, R. J. (2012). Relation between early motor delay and later communication delay in infants at risk for autism. *Infant Behav. Dev.* 35, 838–846. doi: 10.1016/j.infbeh.2012.07.019

Cossu, G., Boria, S., Copioli, C., Bracceschi, R., Giuberti, V., Santelli, E., et al. (2012). Motor Representation of actions in children with autism. *PLoS ONE* 7:e44779. doi: 10.1371/journal.pone.0044779

Courchesne, E., Saitoh, O., Yeung-Courchesne, R., Press, G. A.,

Lincoln, A. J., Haas, R. H., et al. (1994). Abnormality of cerebellar vermian lobules VI and VII in patients with infantile autism: identification of hypoplastic and hyperplastic subgroups by MR imaging. *Am. J. Roentgenol.* 162, 123–130. doi: 10.2214/ajr.162.1.8273650

Damasio, A. R., and Maurer, R. G. (1978). A neurological model for childhood autism. *Arch. Neurol.* 35, 777–786.

Esposito, G., and Venuti, P. (2008). Analysis of toddlers' gait after six months of independent walking to identify autism: a preliminary study. *Percept. Mot. Skills* 106, 259–269. doi: 10.2466/pms.106.1.259-269

Esposito, G., Venuti, P., Apicella, F., and Muratori, F. (2011). Analysis of unsupported gait in toddlers with autism. *Brain Dev.* 33, 367–373. doi: 10.1016/j.braindev.2010.07.006

Esposito, G., Venuti, P., Maestro, S., and Muratori, F. (2009). An exploration of symmetry in early autism spectrum disorders: analysis of lying. *Brain Dev.* 31, 131–138. doi: 10.1016/j.braindev.2008.04.005

Esposito, G., Yoshida, S., Venuti, P., and Kuroda, K. (2012). Three lessons from Philip Teitelbaum and their application to studies of motor development in humans and mice. *Behav. Brain Res.* 231, 366–370. doi: 10.1016/j.bbr.2011.10.008

Fatemi, S. H., Aldinger, K. A., Ashwood, P., Bauman, M. L., Blaha, C. D., Blatt, G. J., et al. (2012). Consensus paper: pathological role of the cerebellum in autism. *Cerebellum* 11, 777–807. doi: 10.1007/s12311-012-0355-9

Flanagan, J. E., Landa, R., Bhat, A., and Bauman, M. (2012). Head lag in infants at risk for autism: a preliminary study. *Am. J. Occup. Ther.* 66, 577–585. doi: 10.5014/ajot.2012.004192

Freitag, C. M., Kleser, C., Schneider, M., and von Gontard, A. (2007). Quantitative assessment of neuromoto function in adolescents with high functioning autism and Asperger Syndrome. *J. Autism Dev. Disord.* 37, 948–959. doi: 10.1007/s10803-006-0235-6

Fournier, K., Hass, C., Naik, S., Lodha, N., and Cauraugh, J. (2010). Motor coordination in autism spectrum disorders: a synthesis and meta-analysis. *J. Autism Dev. Disord.* 40, 1227–1240. doi: 10.1007/s10803-010-0981-3

Gottesman, I. I., and Gould, T. D. (2003). The endophenotype concept in psychiatry: etymology and strategic intentions. *Am. J. Psychiatry* 160, 636–645.

Hallett, M., Lebiedowska, M. K., Thomas, S. L., Stanhope, S. J., Denckla, M. B., and Rumsey, J. (1993). Locomotion of autistic adults. *Arch. Neurol.* 50, 1304–1308.

Hashemi, J., Vallin Spina, T., Tepper, M., Esler, A., Morellas, V., Papanikolopoulos, N., et al. (2012). Computer vision tools for the non-invasive assessment of autism-related behavioral markers. Available online at: http://arxiv.org/pdf/1210.7014.pdf

Hilton, C. L., Zhang, Y., Whilte, M. R., Klohr, C. L., and Constantino, J. (2012). Motor impairment in sibling pairs concordant and discordant for autism spectrum disorders. *Autism* 16, 430–441. doi: 10.1177/1362361311423018

Kanner, L. (1943). Autistic disturbances of affective contact. *Nerv. Child* 2, 217–250.

Kanner, L., and Lesser, L. I. (1958). Early infantile autism. *Pediatr. Clin. North Am.* 5, 711–730.

Landa, R. J., Gross, A. L., Stuart, E. A., and Faherty, A. (2013). Developmental trajectories in children with and without autism spectrum disorders: the first 3 years. *Child Dev.* 84, 429–442. doi: 10.1111/j.1467-8624.2012.01870.x

Landa, R. J., Gross, A. L., Stuart, E. A., and Bauman, M. (2012). Latent class analysis of early developmental trajectory in baby siblings of children with autism. *J. Child Psychol. Psychiatry* 53, 986–996. doi: 10.1111/j.1469-7610.2012.02558.x

Landrigan, P. J. (2010). What causes autism? Exploring the environmental contribution. *Curr. Opin. Pediatr.* 22, 219–225. doi: 10.1097/MOP.0b013e328336eb9a

Langen, M., Durston, S., Staal, W. G., Palmen, S. J., and van Engeland, H. (2007). Caudate nucleus is enlarged in high-functioning medication-naïve subjects with autism. *Biol. Psychiatry* 62, 262–266. doi: 10.1016/j.biopsych.2006.09.040

Leary, M. R., and Hill, D. A. (1996). Moving on: autism and movement disturbance. *Ment. Retard.* 34, 39–53.

Lichtenstein, P., Carlström, E., Råstam, M., Gillberg, C., and Anckarsäter, H. (2010). The genetics of autism spectrum disorders and related neuropsychiatric disorders in childhood. *Am. J. Psychiatry* 167, 1357–1363. doi: 10.1176/appi.ajp.2010.10020223

Lloyd, M., MacDonald, M., and Lord, C. (2013). Motor skills of toddlers with autism spectrum disorders. *Autism* 17, 133–146. doi: 10.1177/1362361311402230

Marchetto, M. C., Carromeu, C., Acab, A., Yu, D., Yeo, G. W., Mu, Y., et al. (2010). A model for neural development and treatment of Rett syndrome using human induced pluripotent stem cells. *Cell* 143, 527–539. doi: 10.1016/j.cell.2010.10.016

Moruzzi, S., Ogliari, A., Ronald, A., Happé, F., and Battaglia, M. (2011). The nature of covariation between autistic traits and clumsiness: a twin study in a general population sample. *J. Autism Dev. Disord.* 41, 1665–1674. doi: 10.1007/s10803-011-1199-8

Nayate, A., Tonge, B. J., Bradshaw, J. L., McGinley, J., Iansek, R., and Rinehart, N. J. (2012). Differentiation of high-functioning autism and Asperger's disorder based on neuromotor behaviour. *J. Autism Dev. Disord.* 42, 707–717. doi: 10.1007/s10803-011-1299-5

Nebel, M. B., Joel, S. E., Muschelli, J., Barber, A. D., Caffo, B. S., Pekar, J. J., et al. (2012). Disruption of functional organization within the primary motor cortex in children with autism. *Hum. Brain Mapp.* Available online at: http://onlinelibrary.wiley.com/doi/10.1002/hbm.22188/full

Novarino, G., El-Fishawy, P., Kayserili, H., Meguid, N. A., Scott, E. M., Schroth, J., et al. (2012). Mutations in BCKD-kinase lead to a potentially treatable form of autism with epilepsy. *Science* 338, 394–397. doi: 10.1126/science.1224631

Ozonoff, S., Young, G. S., Goldring, S., Greiss-Hess, L., Herrera, A. M., Steele, J., et al. (2008). Gross motor development, movement abnormalities, and early identification of autism. *J. Autism Dev. Disord.* 38, 644–656. doi: 10.1007/s10803-007-0430-0

Paşca, S. P., Portmann, T., Voineagu, I., Yazawa, M., Shcheglovitov, A., Paşca, A. M., et al. (2011). Using iPSC-derived neurons to uncover cellular phenotypes associated with Timothy syndrome. *Nat. Med.* 17, 1657–1662. doi: 10.1038/nm.2576

Pickett, J., and London, E. (2005). The neuropathology of autism: a review. *J. Neuropathol. Exp. Neurol.* 64, 925–935.

Provost, B., Lopez, B. R., and Heimerl, S. (2007). A comparison of motor delays in young children: autism spectrum disorder, developmental delay, and developmental concerns. *J. Autism Dev. Disord.* 37, 321–328. doi: 10.1007/s10803-006-0170-6

Qiu, S., Aldinger, K. A., and Levitt, P. (2012). Modeling of autism genetic variations in mice: focusing on synaptic and microcircuit dysfunctions. *Dev. Neurosci.* 34, 88–100. doi: 10.1159/000336644

Rinehart, N. J., Bellgrove, M. A., Tonge, B. J., Brereton, A. V., Howells-Rankin, D., and Bradshaw, J. L. (2006a). An examination of movement kinematics in young people with high-functioning autism and Asperger's disorder: further evidence for a motor planning deficit. *J. Autism Dev. Disord.* 36, 757–767. doi: 10.1007/s10803-006-0118-x

Rinehart, N. J., Tonge, B. J., Bradshaw, J. L., Iansek, R., Enticott, P. G., and McGinley, J. (2006b). Gait function in high-functioning autism and Asperger's disorder: evidence for basal-ganglia and cerebellar involvement? *Eur. Child Adolesc. Psychiatry* 15, 256–264. doi: 10.1007/s00787-006-0530-y

Rinehart, N. J., Tonge, B. J., Iansek, R., McGinley, J., Brereton, A. V., Enticott, P. G., et al. (2006c). Gait function in newly diagnosed children with autism: cerebellar and basal ganglia related motor disorder. *Dev. Med. Child Neurol.* 48, 819–824. doi: 10.1017/S0012162206001769

Sacks, B., and Buckley, S. J. (2003). What do we know about the movement abilities of children with Down syndrome? *Down Syndrome News Update* 2, 131–141.

Stein, J. L., Parikshak, N. N., and Geschwind, D. H. (2013). Rare inherited variation in autism: beginning to see the forest and a few trees. *Neuron* 77, 209–211. doi: 10.1016/j.neuron.2013.01.010

Sutera, S., Pandey, J., Esser, E. L., Rosenthal, M. A., Wilson, L. B., Barton, M., et al. (2007). Predictors of optimal outcome in toddlers diagnosed with autism spectrum disorders. *J. Autism Dev. Disord.* 37, 98–107. doi: 10.1007/s10803-006-0340-6

Teitelbaum, O., Benton, T., Shah, P. K., Prince, A., Kelly, J. L., and Teitelbaum, P. (2004). Eshkol-Wachman movement notation in diagnosis: the early detection of Asperger's syndrome. *Proc. Natl. Acad. Sci. U.S.A.* 101, 11909–11914. doi: 10.1073/pnas.0403919101

Teitelbaum, P., Teitelbaum, O., Nye, J., Fryman, J., and Maurer, R. G. (1998). Movement analysis in infancy may be useful for early diagnosis of autism. *Proc. Natl. Acad. Sci. U.S.A.* 95, 13982–13987. doi: 10.1073/pnas.95.23.13982

Vernazza-Martin, S., Martin, N., Vernazza, A., Lepellec-Muller, A., Rufo, M., Massion, J., et al. (2005). Goal directed locomotion and balance control in autistic children. *J. Autism Dev. Disord.* 35, 91–102. doi: 10.1007/s10803-004-1037-3

Vilensky, J. A., Damasio, A. R., and Maurer, R. G. (1981). Gait disturbances in patients with autistic behavior. *Arch. Neurol.* 38, 646–649.

Whitney, E. R., Kemper, T. L., Bauman, M. L., Rosene, D. L., and Blatt, G. J. (2008). Cerebellar Purkinje cells are reduced in a subpopulation of autistic brains: a stereological experiment using calbindin-D28k. *Cerebellum* 7, 406–416. doi: 10.1007/s12311-008-0043-y

Yirmiya, N., and Charman, T. (2010). The prodrome of autism: early behavioral and biological signs, regression, peri- and post-natal development and genetics. *J. Child Psychol. Psychiatry* 51, 432–458. doi: 10.1111/j.1469-7610.2010.02214.x

Conflict of Interest Statement: The authors declare that the research was conducted in the absence of any commercial or financial relationships that could be construed as a potential conflict of interest.

15

Sensory-motor problems in autism

Caroline Whyatt * and Cathy Craig

Department of Psychology, Queen's University Belfast, Belfast, Antrim, UK

Edited by:
Elizabeth B. Torres, Rutgers University, USA

Reviewed by:
Elizabeth B. Torres, Rutgers University, USA
Lei Niu, Albert Einstein College of Medicine, USA

***Correspondence:**
Caroline Whyatt, Department of Psychology, Queen's University Belfast, 18-30 Malone Road, Belfast, BT7 1NN, Antrim, UK
e-mail: c.whyatt@qub.ac.uk

Despite being largely characterized as a social and cognitive disorder, strong evidence indicates the presence of significant sensory-motor problems in Autism Spectrum Disorder (ASD). This paper outlines our progression from initial, broad assessment using the Movement Assessment Battery for Children (M-ABC2) to subsequent targeted kinematic assessment. In particular, pronounced ASD impairment seen in the broad categories of manual dexterity and ball skills was found to be routed in specific difficulties on isolated tasks, which were translated into focused experimental assessment. Kinematic results from both subsequent studies highlight impaired use of perception-action coupling to guide, adapt and tailor movement to task demands, resulting in inflexible and rigid motor profiles. In particular difficulties with the use of temporal adaption are shown, with "hyperdexterity" witnessed in ballistic movement profiles, often at the cost of spatial accuracy and task performance. By linearly progressing from the use of a standardized assessment tool to targeted kinematic assessment, clear and defined links are drawn between measureable difficulties and underlying sensory-motor assessment. Results are specifically viewed in-light of perception-action coupling and its role in early infant development suggesting that rather than being "secondary" level impairment, sensory-motor problems may be fundamental in the progression of ASD. This logical and systematic process thus allows a further understanding into the potential root of observable motor problems in ASD; a vital step if underlying motor problems are to be considered a fundamental aspect of autism and allow a route of non-invasive preliminary diagnosis.

Keywords: autism spectrum disorders, perception-action coupling, prospective control, movement, developmental psychology

First identified in the seminal works of Leo Kanner (1943) and Hans Asperger (1944) Autism, also known as Autism Spectrum Disorder (ASD), is a developmental disorder characterized by impaired socialization, communication, and imagination (Wing and Gould, 1979; Wing, 1981; American Psychiatric Association, 2000). ASD research largely reflects this bias, with a strong focus on three core theories of Autism: Theory of Mind (Baron-Cohen et al., 1985), Weak Central Coherence theory (Frith, 1989), and Executive functioning theory (Ozonoff et al., 1991; Ozonoff and McEvoy, 1994).

This paper will provide a brief overview of these traditional theories, before outlining how research has attempted to profile and understand movement ability associated with a diagnosis of ASD. Combing specific examples, and discussing motor performance within the context of ecological psychology, we will draw well-defined links between standardized "norm" based assessment tools and in-depth kinematic movement analysis based studies. Specifically we will present sample studies that explore the role of timing and perception-action coupling in children with ASD who experience motor difficulties. These findings will then be discussed in light of the development of coherent movement control and its impact on social and cognitive ability, highlighting the potential role of a Theory of Sensory-motor control in ASD.

TRADITIONAL THEORIES OF AUTISM SPECTRUM DISORDER

First coined by Premack and Woodruff (1978) "Theory of Mind" (ToM) refers to the ability to make inferences regarding others' intentions and emotions. Impaired ToM results in the inability to attribute separate mental states to individuals, leading to difficulty understanding and predicting others' feelings and behaviors; classical social symptoms of ASD (Baron-Cohen et al., 1985). Despite early criticism (e.g., Hobson, 1991; Russell, 1992) ToM has received strong support (e.g., Baron-Cohen et al., 1997) and is often regarded as the predominant theory in ASD research. However, upon closer inspection fundamental difficulties adopting this theory become apparent. Initial evidence alluded to a preserved level of ToM in some individuals with ASD (Baron-Cohen et al., 1985; Happe, 1995; Bowler, 2006), whilst ToM as a construct fails to reliably differentiate individuals with ASD from those with Down's syndrome, sensory impairment or intellectual disability (Baron-Cohen et al., 1985; Russell et al., 1998; Yirmiya et al., 1998). Deconstructing this concept further highlights the strong cognitive basis of ToM, thought to be largely dependent on the capacity for complex thinking and metarepresentation (Boucher, 2012), which are reliant on language based strategies. These strong links to language ability (Happe, 1995) raises the question, is ToM truly implicated in ASD, or, by using impaired language ability as a diagnostic criterion is this level of impairment naturally inflated?

Weak Central Coherence theory (Frith, 1989) provides an explanation for "non-social" symptoms of ASD such as apparent difficulties with global processing and preference for local level detail. Referred to as a cognitive style, weak central coherence results in difficulties considering contextual information leading to cognitive detachment. This predisposition to the minutiae of a scene is thought to result in superior performance on low-level visual tasks and illusions (Happe, 1996). Yet, conflicting results implying intact levels of global visual processing in ASD (Motton et al., 1999; Edgin and Pennington, 2005) undermine the reliability of this theoretical framework.

Finally, *executive functioning theory* aims to explain behavioral characteristics of ASD including rigidity in regime, spontaneous unreserved actions, and the need for order. Strongly interwoven with main constructs of ToM (Joseph and Tager-Flusberg, 2004; Pellicano, 2007), executive functioning is thought to provide a route of higher level control over automatic responses to stimuli, an ability to switch mind-set as required for example in the Wisconsin card sorting task, and to help formulate novel ideas (Frith, 2003). Despite evidence for reduced levels of executive function in ASD (e.g., Russell, 1997) this construct also fails to reliably differentiate between ASD and other disorders such as ADHD (Pennington and Ozonoff, 1996).

Combined these largely cognitive driven theories of ASD are functionalist and fragmented (see also De Jaegher, 2013), and fail to encompass the diverse range of symptoms associated with ASD. The strong cognitive thread throughout all "traditional theories" largely reflects the characteristic cognitive and social symptoms of ASD (American Psychiatric Association, 2000) yet is questionable given the ability of some individuals with ASD to reach high levels of academic success. In addition, the use of restricted language as a diagnostic criterion may lead to individuals with ASD displaying a predisposition for such higher-level cognitive difficulties (e.g., Lewis and Osbourne, 1990; Happe, 1995). Moreover these complex levels of cognitive functioning do not emerge until approximately 4 years of age in typically developing children (Wimmer and Perner, 1983; Perner et al., 1987; Harris et al., 1989; Boucher, 2012). As such, a purely cognitive explanation for ASD fails to account for autistic symptoms within the first years of an infant's life (Gillberg et al., 1990; Osterling and Dawson, 1994; Dawson et al., 2000).

When viewed in light of evidence that shows how cognition and motor ability develop in parallel and are mutually dependent (Campos et al., 2000; Von Hofsten, 2007; Rakison and Woodward, 2008; Iverson, 2010), a purely cognitive explanation of ASD is short sighted. Indeed, evidence for cognitive-motor links in ASD have already been documented by Hilton et al. (2007), who identified a strong correlation between motor impairment and level of severity of ASD as measured using the social responsiveness scale (Constantino et al., 2003). Coupled with evidence for the presence of significant sensory-motor problems in ASD from a very early age (Teitelbaum et al., 1998; Sutera et al., 2007), we propose that a fundamental, developmental sensory-motor deficit may be the missing link in understanding core elements of ASD.

Indeed, although predominantly viewed as a social and cognitive disorder, mounting evidence suggests the presence of significant sensory-motor deficits across the entire ASD spectrum (Manjiviona and Prior, 1995; Ghaziuddin and Butler, 1998; Jansiewicz et al., 2006; Fournier et al., 2010). However, in spite of this mounting evidence and early recognition of sensory-motor problems in ASD (e.g., Asperger, 1944; Damasio and Maurer, 1978; Vilensky et al., 1981), they remain to be seen as secondary, "associated" symptoms (Ming et al., 2007). A recent review (Fournier et al., 2010) suggested discrepancies in controlling for underlying moderating variables (e.g., IQ) along with the inclusion of control groups with secondary impairments (e.g., Developmental Coordination Disorder) could be preventing sensory-motor symptoms from being viewed as a core component of ASD. If sensory-motor problems are to be considered a fundamental symptom of ASD, the nature of persistent motor problems *specific* to ASD must be identified.

OBSERVABLE MOVEMENT PROBLEMS IN ASD

Standardized tests of movement coordination are used by clinicians and researchers to assess the development of a broad range of motor skills. By comparing standardized scores, these tests are often the first step in identifying pronounced, observable motor deficits. A number of studies have used a range of standardized tests of motor performance to assess levels of motor proficiency in ASD (Manjiviona and Prior, 1995; Miyahara et al., 1997; Ghaziuddin and Butler, 1998; Green et al., 2002, 2009; Hilton et al., 2007; Provost et al., 2007; Staples and Reid, 2010; Siaperas et al., 2012). Although the number of research studies in this area is arguably limited, they provide preliminary evidence for persistent and significant observable motor difficulties across the Autistic Spectrum, with notable impairment in the sub-categories of manual dexterity and ball skills (Manjiviona and Prior, 1995; Miyahara et al., 1997; Green et al., 2002, 2009; Hilton et al., 2007). However, scoring methods commonly used in such standardized tests may inevitably mask underlying variation in performance. In particular, sub-category scores often rely on the summing of performance on multiple individual tasks. For example, performance in the sub-category of *'Ball Skills'* in the Movement Assessment Battery for Children (M-ABC, Henderson and Sugden, 1992, 2nd Edition, Henderson and Sugden (2007)) relies on the summing of performance on two distinct tasks; a *'Throwing'* and *'Catching'* task (see **Table 1**). This is often further complicated by the scoring parameters included in individual tasks, with accuracy and speed used interchangeably (see **Table 1**).

To maximize the potential use of such standardized assessment batteries, we suggest deconstructing performance to consider ability at the individual task level, and viewing performance in light of differentiating factors (Whyatt and Craig, 2012). Comparing performance on the M-ABC2 (Henderson and Sugden, 2007), our recent study provided further evidence for persistent motor deficits in ASD in relation to age-matched children, with *no* secondary impairments (Whyatt and Craig, 2012). Moreover, supporting results from other studies, the breakdown of performance into specific sub-categories indicated the presence of significant difficulty in the areas of both *manual dexterity* and *ball skills* (Manjiviona and Prior, 1995; Miyahara et al., 1997;

Table 1 | Table outlining the construction of the movement assessment battery for children 2 (Henderson and Sugden, 2007).

M-ABC Sub-tasks and scoring				
	Sub-Categories	**Sub-tasks**	**Accuracy**	**Timed**
Overall movement assessment battery (M-ABC2)	Manual dexterity	Peg-board	✓	✓
		Assembly task	✓	✓
		Trace task	✓	
	Balance	Static	✓	✓
		Dynamic	✓	
		Heel-toe walk	✓	
	Ball skills	Catching	✓	
		Throwing	✓	

As shown, overall movement performance is assessed via the sub-categories; manual dexterity, balance and ball skills. Each sub-category is then further divided into performance on sub-tasks, each measuring individual levels of performance and scored according to either spatial accuracy and/or timed performance.

Green et al., 2002, 2009; Hilton et al., 2007; Provost et al., 2007; Staples and Reid, 2010; Siaperas et al., 2012). However, taking the deconstruction of performance to the individual task level revealed a specific pattern of impairment on a single task in each sub-category; *peg-board* task and *catching* task. Viewing the pattern of performance at this individual level, and in light of differentiating factors, suggests an underlying difficulty with the spatial-temporal control of movement. More specifically, catching requires the person catching the ball to prospectively control the movement of their catching hand as a function of the movement of the approaching ball. Therefore, performance on *catching* tasks is driven by externally imposed spatial and temporal constraints, where the dynamics of the moving object should guide the control of the action. Conversely, performance on the *throwing* task is predominantly internally driven, as the external contextual variables are stationary (i.e., no temporal constraints). Whilst questions are also raised over the reliability of the *peg-board* task, due to dual scoring using both spatial accuracy and age-related temporal parameters (see **Table 1**). Evidence for poor temporal awareness in ASD (Boucher, 2001) suggests this dual scoring component may artificially inflate levels of ASD impairment.

Moreover, given the body of evidence that suggests a significant relationship between IQ, specifically verbal ability (e.g., Leary and Hill, 1996; Chaix et al., 2007; Dziuk et al., 2007), and movement, both non-verbal and receptive language ability were independently controlled for (Whyatt and Craig, 2012). When these control group comparisons were carried out, further differences in ASD performance were noted. Overall impairment in the sub-category of *ball skills* and the underlying individual *catching* task was found in relation to both the non-verbal and receptive language control groups ($p < 0.01$). However, impaired levels of *manual dexterity* were seen to vary. Specifically, overall impairment in the sub-category was found when ASD performance was compared to the control group matched on receptive language ability only ($p < 0.05$). Yet underlying variation in performance on the individual *peg-board* task was isolated to comparisons with the non-verbal IQ control group ($p < 0.05$). This pattern of results highlights the difficulties encountered when using standardized tests, specifically their ability to reliably 'mark' variation, reinforcing the need to tease apart levels of performance, and implies a cognitive element to difficulties with *manual dexterity*.

Combined, these results may suggest a specific difficulty using external sensory information to prospectively guide and control action. However, despite this systematic deconstruction of performance, standardized product orientated tests still lack the sensitivity in measurement to unpick subtle variations in real-time patterns of performance.

INTERNAL vs. EXTERNAL TIMING: THE ROLE OF PERCEPTION ACTION COUPLING

Internal timing, mediated by the basal ganglia (Graybiel et al., 1994; Gowen and Miall, 2005), is critical in the initiation of self-timed actions, for example reaching for a stationary object. However, despite being internally generated, unfolding temporal control over the movement will be directly modulated by external spatial parameters, for example as a function of target width (Fitts, 1954) or degree of curvature of the movement required (Viviani and Schneider, 1991). Conversely actions that require one to successfully couple movements onto that of the environment are driven and guided by externally imposed spatial and temporal constraints. For example, when catching a moving ball an individual needs to visually pick up information from the moving ball to anticipate where and when the ball will arrive and subsequently control the movement of the catching limb to arrive in the right place at the right time. Although largely taken for granted, this intricate relationship between the perception of the spatial and temporal characteristics of the moving ball and the control of the moving limb is critical to successful interception and is often described as *perception-action coupling*.

Information in the environment is thought to be continuously available from the eye in the form of the optic array (Gibson, 1969). Our movement through the environment then provides a time-varying optic array otherwise known as the optic flow field (Gibson, 1979; Lee, 1980) from which sensory invariants can be picked up and used to guide action (Gibson, 1969). These optical invariants are non-linear algorithms (Fajen, 2005), directly linking perception and action (Richardson, 2000) from which information can be extrapolated to provide prospective spatial and temporal control (Lishman and Lee, 1973; Lee, 1980). More specifically, research suggests that through maturity and perceptual attunement infants converge on the use of Time to contact information (Tau; Kayed and van der Meer, 2009) to allow them to prospectively control their movements. Tau in the visual domain is traditionally specified as the inverse of the rate of expansion of the image on the retina, whilst changes in the spectral and temporal characteristics of an auditory-based stimulus have also been shown to provide reliable time to contact information (Neuhoff and McBeath, 1996). Mathematically, tau is specified as the time to gap closure at its current closure rate (see Lee, 1980). In the example of catching an oncoming ball, Tau (τ) is calculated as the ratio between the distance gap separating the catcher and the ball (x) and the rate of closure ($\dot{x}$) of that gap so that:

$$\tau(x) = x/\dot{x} \qquad (1)$$

Extending this specification of temporal information further, other research has shown how the taus of two or more gaps can be closed synchronously to arrive at the right place at the right time (known as tau coupling—see Lee, 1998; Lee et al., 2001). Encompassing both temporal and spatial characteristics of the moving target, Tau provides reliable, robust information that the actor can tune into and use to successfully perform the task. Using tau-based information is therefore indicative of mature levels of prospective control. The gradual progression to this level of control would be evidenced in a person's ability to tailor the temporal characteristics of their movement, such as initiation time, to the event related information in the environment (e.g., the time to arrival of a moving target), resulting in higher levels of spatial/temporal accuracy of the movement and a reduction in the number of corrective sub movements (e.g., Von Hofsten, 1991; Van der Meer et al., 1994; Caljouw et al., 2004; Van Hof et al., 2008).

Studies that have examined movement kinematics in the ASD population have frequently documented pronounced difficulty with movement initiation (preparation), online control and smooth sequential actions (Hughes and Russell, 1993; Hughes, 1996; Rinehart et al., 2001; Mari et al., 2003; Schmitz et al., 2003; Glazebrook et al., 2006; Rinehart et al., 2006a; Cattaneo et al., 2007; Fabbri-Destro et al., 2009; Papadopoulos et al., 2012);. These difficulties emerge as an inability to prospectively control one's own movements (e.g., Hughes, 1996; Schmitz et al., 2003), but also a deficit in anticipating outcomes of others actions (e.g., Cattaneo et al., 2007). These underlying problems appear to reside in fundamental problems with the temporal control of movement, with both akinesia and hyperdexterity also being documented (e.g., Muller et al., 2001; Mari et al., 2003; Kleinhans et al., 2005; Rinehart et al., 2006a; Price et al., 2012a,b). This variability in movement timing is further significantly correlated with poor motor coordination (Price et al., 2012b), implying that spatial movement difficulties in ASD are in fact rooted in a more fundamental temporal deficit. In addition recent qualitative first hand reports provide rich evidence for temporal underpinnings, with reported difficulties "controlling movements," "problems with starting or stopping movements," and a tendency to "lose the rhythm" (Robledo et al., 2012. p. 6). Despite this, results are often attributed to an underlying difficulty with *motor programming;* specifically motor programme selection, re-programming and degradation (e.g., Rinehart et al., 2001, 2006a,b; Mari et al., 2003; Glazebrook et al., 2006, 2008; Nazarali et al., 2009). This implied motor programming deficit draws an explicit link between ASD and Parkinson's disease (PD), with distinguishing characteristics of PD such as akinesia and bradykinesia long considered the by-product of "an inability to select and/or maintain *internal* control over the algorithms" needed to generate actions (Robertson and Flowers, 1990, p. 591). This is of particular interest given recent evidence of patients with PD using external sensory information to improve the synchronization and timing of movements (Majsak et al., 1998, 2008). Comparing performance on a reach-to grasp task with a stationary and moving ball, Majsak et al. (1998, 2008) demonstrated how a dynamic moving target can act as an external 'cue' to time movement. By exploiting the perception-action link, the dynamic target provides *external* temporal information, which removes the emphasis on using *internal* temporal processes. The use of external temporal information therefore allows patients with PD to successfully overcome akinesia and bradykinesia to produce smooth sequential actions, implying a common underlying timing mechanism (Majsak et al., 1998, 2008). Given repeated evidence for a potential link between ASD and PD (Damasio and Maurer, 1978; Vilensky et al., 1981; Mari et al., 2003; Rinehart et al., 2006a; Vernazza-Martin et al., 2005; Hollander et al., 2009) such results highlight the potential importance of explicitly assessing levels of perception-action coupling in individuals with ASD.

Unfortunately, sensory-motor tasks used in ASD research to date are largely abstract, requiring mental retention and/or rotation to predict task outcome, which may artificially lower ASD performance (e.g., Leekman and Perner, 1991). Further, as noted by Van der Weel et al. (1996) goal-directed, concrete tasks which are controlled in such a way that sensory information (e.g., visual and auditory) is picked up from the environment and used to achieve the desired goal, are "true" sensory-motor tasks. Therefore, these abstract tasks fail to provide a true sensory-motor assessment and prevent results from being easily viewed within the context of observable motor problems such as those seen with standardized tests. To further unpick the potential role of external environmental constraints, namely sensory information on ASD temporal control, previous results (Whyatt and Craig, 2012) were used as a basis to design two targeted experimental paradigms which aimed to understand performance on a manual dexterity and interceptive task, in a more systematic way.

PERCEPTION-ACTION COUPLING STUDIES

MANUAL DEXTERITY STUDY (SAMPLE)

Manual dexterity refers to fine motor control of the small muscles in the hands and fingers to adequately manipulate objects and produce skillful performance. Although standardized testing has repeatedly implied poor levels of manual dexterity in ASD (Miyahara et al., 1997; Green et al., 2002, 2009; Hilton et al., 2007; Provost et al., 2007; Staples and Reid, 2010; Whyatt and Craig, 2012; Siaperas et al., 2012), recent evidence suggests this impairment is based on *specific* tasks scored using both *time* and *accuracy* parameters (e.g., peg-board), raising questions over the validity and reliability of this impairment (Whyatt and Craig, 2012). In particular, inherent variability in temporal production (e.g., Price et al., 2012b) and awareness (Boucher, 2001) may underpin poor performance on such dual-scored tasks.

To provide participants with a controlled manual dexterity task, the original trace task from the M-ABC2 was digitized and presented on a tablet PC (see **Figure 1** for example trace recordings). Performance was recorded with real-time visual feedback on the position of the line participants were drawing being instantly provided. Although not identified as a key task from the M-ABC2 (Whyatt and Craig, 2012), this task requires high levels of precision and perception-action coupling

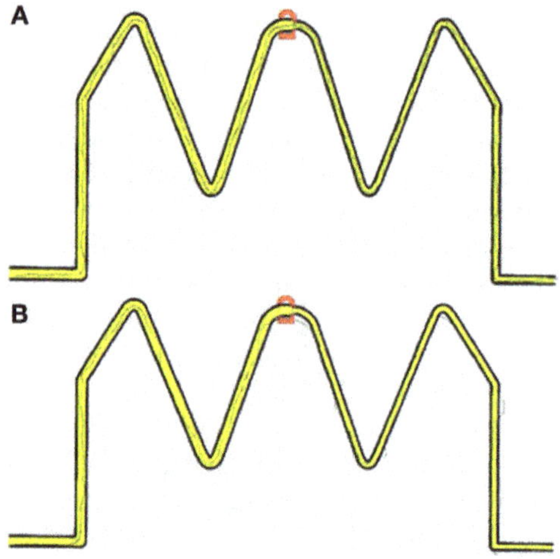

FIGURE 1 | Example of recorded traces produced by (A) a Non-verbal control participant (B) an age matched autistic participant.

to prospectively control the movement to accurately navigate the pen between the boundaries of the drawing. Therefore, this task provides a strong test of fine motor control, yet is scored using accuracy parameters only. By digitizing the stimulus, sequentially deconstructing performance and viewing this in light of perceptual information (i.e., perceived width of tracks), a fuller understanding of true spatial-temporal control during fine motor tasks is achievable. Despite being internally generated, unfolding temporal control as the movement progresses will be directly modulated by external spatial parameters, for example target width (Fitts, 1954) or degree of curvature of the movement required (Viviani and Schneider, 1991). One would therefore expect high levels of spatial accuracy to be reflected in high levels of temporal or prospective control, for example an ability to prospectively control line drawing movement to avoid errors such as sufficient deceleration when approaching the corner sections. Data were filtered offline, from which displacement and temporal information were calculated. As before performance was compared between a group of children with a formal diagnosis of ASD and two age-matched control groups of typically developing children (non-verbal IQ and receptive language).

Initial results of spatial accuracy imply significant ASD impairment throughout the task. However, in line with previous results (Whyatt and Craig, 2012) this impairment was only found to be significant when compared with the non-verbal IQ control group ($p < .05$; see **Figure 2** for sample data). These high levels of spatial error observed in the ASD group were mirrored in high levels of temporal variability. Specifically, the ASD group displayed significantly faster performance times across the trace compared to the non-verbal control group ($p < .05$; see **Figure 2** for sample data). Despite apparent similarities between the ASD and receptive language control group, an analysis of prospective control, namely deceleration when approaching corners, successfully distinguished between the ASD

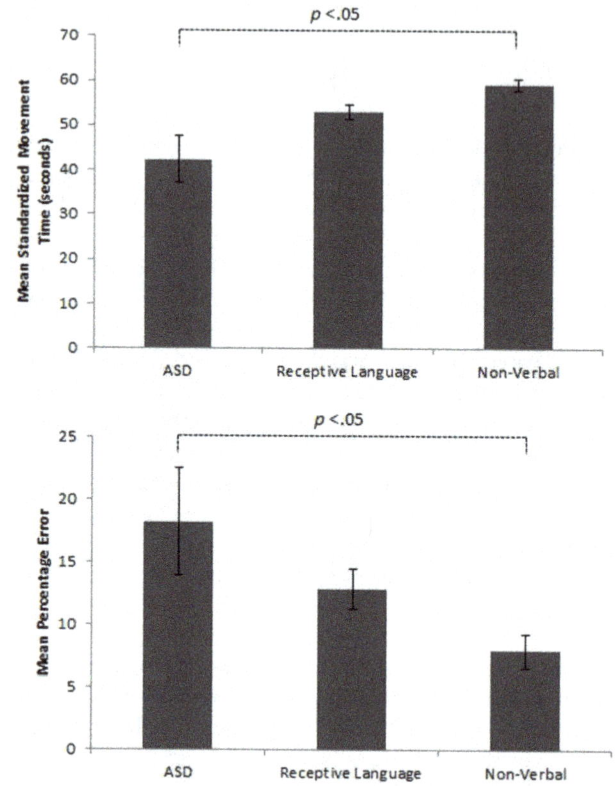

FIGURE 2 | Example summary graphs showing mean level of overall percentage error and associated standardized times (seconds) for the three different experimental groups.

and *both* control groups, with significantly shorter phases of corner deceleration being observed in the ASD group (see **Figure 3** for sample data). This inability to adequately anticipate the upcoming corner and sufficiently 'brake' or decelerate in order to meet the spatial requirements of the task (i.e., stay within the boundaries) implies a specific difficulty with the spatial-temporal control of movement in ASD, which could in turn suggest an underlying problem with perception-action coupling.

INTERCEPTIVE SKILLS STUDY (SEE WHYATT AND CRAIG, 2013)

In line with qualitative reports (Frith, 2003; Glazebrook et al., 2006), a deconstruction of performance on the M-ABC2 highlighted specific ASD difficulties with catching tasks (Whyatt and Craig, 2012). As previously mentioned, catching is a dynamic action that requires a tight link between one's own movement and the spatial-temporal constraints being imposed by the moving target i.e., the ball. Sufficient levels of movement coupling will ensure the participant synchronizes their movement to the movement of the external target, so they move sufficiently ahead of time to catch the ball. One would therefore expect that initiation times are tailored as a function of the speed of the moving ball toward the target zone, with skilled movement showing a decrease in corrective sub movements and increased successful interception. Apparent difficulties with underlying spatial-temporal control previously demonstrated in the levels of manual dexterity in children with ASD may therefore be further exaggerated when catching a ball, reflecting the persistent results previously found using standardized tests (Whyatt and Craig, 2012).

To further explore potential underlying difficulties with perception-action coupling a controlled catching task was designed, where participants were asked to catch a ball that was rolled down a ramp, in a target zone at the end of the ramp (a task similar to Majsak et al., 1998; see Whyatt and Craig, 2013). Starting and catching areas were fixed for all trials, resulting in a task where all individuals had to move the same distance but adjust how and when they moved as a function of the velocity of the moving ball (adjusted by raising or lowering the ramp between 14 cm (low) and 21 cm (high) settings). To effectively 'catch' the ball, participants had to 'tune into' or pick up timing information from the movement of the ball to guide their movement to the catching zone so they arrive at the right time. In other words, they have to tailor the temporal characteristics of their movements to the task demands (ball velocity) by coupling perceptual information specifying time to ball arrival to their own actions. Performance in each trial was recorded using Qualisys motion capture infrared cameras, which tracked the movement of the ball (covered in reflective tape) and the hand of the participant (a reflective marker placed on top). Accuracy (number of successful 'catches') was measured, and also the ability to modulate initiation time as a function of ball velocity. As before performance was compared between a group of children with ASD and two groups of age-matched controls (receptive language and non-verbal IQ controls).

Mirroring ASD performance found in the manual dexterity study, significantly impaired levels of spatial performance (as measured via successful 'catches') were observed when comparing results to those of both the non-verbal and receptive language control groups ($p < 0.05$; see **Figure 4** for sample data; also see Whyatt and Craig, 2013). When viewing levels of temporal control, both the ASD and receptive language control groups failed to adequately adapt their initiation times to meet the task demands. For instance, trials using the lower ramp setting, thus lower ball velocity will result in a longer arrival time for the ball. If participants are adequately using sensory information to guide movement, one would therefore expect a longer initiation time. However, the ASD and receptive language groups fail to adapt initiation time to task demands (i.e., ball velocity). In contrast, the non-verbal control group were able to significantly monitor and tailor initiation time to ball velocity ($p < 0.05$), resulting in this group displaying highest levels of overall task success (see **Figure 4** for sample data; Whyatt and Craig, 2013). Supporting results from the manual dexterity study, this profile suggests a common underlying difficulty in the ASD and receptive language control group in spatial-temporal control of movement. However, further analysis implies that an ability to guide online necessary temporal modifications to the movement in the receptive language control group compensate for these difficulties with movement initiation (similar to intact corner deceleration profiles shown in the manual dexterity case study). In contrast, the ASD group fails to utilize any sensory information for compensatory strategies, resulting in poor performance.

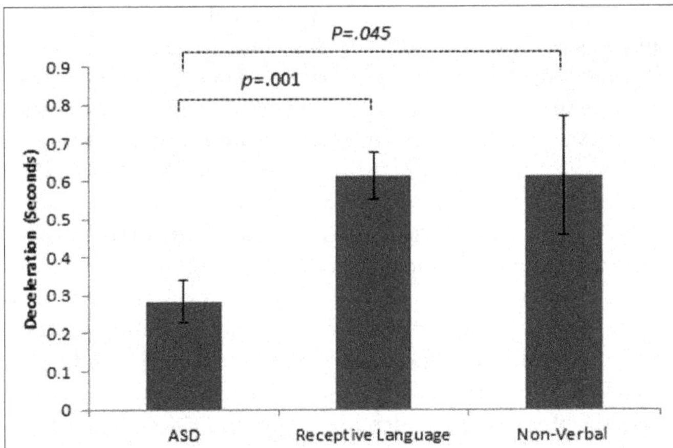

FIGURE 3 | Example summary graph for deceleration patterns when approaching a *single* comer section of the track task. Combined analysis of performance on *all* comer sections highlights significantly shorter phases of deceleration in the ASD group than both the receptive language ($p < 0.05$) and non-verbal ($p < 01$) *control groups.*

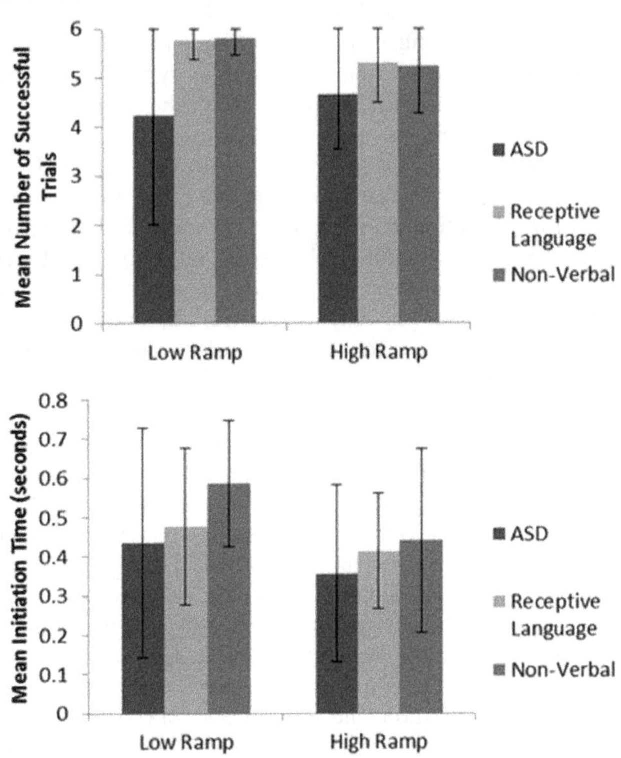

FIGURE 4 | Example summary graphs for spatial accuracy (measured via number of successful catches), and mean initiation time. For full data please see Whyatt and Craig (2013).

AUTISM: THEORY OF SENSORY-MOTOR DEVELOPMENT

Combined with mounting evidence for the presence of significant sensory-motor difficulties in ASD (Fournier et al., 2010), these studies further suggest such lower level problems are a fundamental core symptom of ASD. More specifically this body of work suggests reoccurring prominent difficulties with *manual dexterity* and *ball skills* (e.g., Green et al., 2002, 2009), may be due to underlying variation in the ability to temporally control movement. In particular, the children diagnosed with ASD are found to display an inability to adapt the temporal characteristics of their movement to conform to external spatial constraints. This difficulty emerges as an inability to slow the movement down in complex sections of the manual dexterity task, (e.g., tight turns in corner sections) and an inability adapt to initiation times when intercepting a ball travelling at different speeds to a goal zone. In both cases the children with ASD show higher levels of spatial error than both control groups. Whilst supporting previous studies that suggest an underlying difficulty using visual information to guide movement (Masterson and Biederman, 1983; Gepner and Mestre, 2002; Mari et al., 2003; Minshew et al., 2004; Glazebrook et al., 2006, 2009; Gowen et al., 2008; Dowd et al., 2012), the studies presented above explicitly highlight underlying spatial-temporal control problems which further suggest motor difficulties may be due to a fundamental perception-action coupling deficit.

Although largely taken for granted, perception-action coupling is honed through maturity and experience, and is dependent on the gradual filtering of sensory information to identify sensory invariants to facilitate the establishment of coherent motor control. This filtering or attunement process is dependent on afferent feedback from early exploratory behavior during infancy, which helps teach the infant about the intrinsic properties of the environment, their own abilities, and the relationship between these (Thelen, 1979; Von Hofsten, 2004). These initial explorations are therefore thought to provide the foundations for perception-action coupling, thereby facilitating the progression of meaningful, goal-directed interactions between infants and their surroundings (Von Hofsten, 2004) and the simultaneous decline in early rhythmical exploratory behavior (Thelen, 1979). Reduced levels of goal-directed exploratory behavior during infancy (Pierce and Courchesne, 2001; Ozonoff et al., 2008), the persistence of rhythmical "stereotypies" (Pierce and Courchesne, 2001; Richler et al., 2007), and delayed sensorimotor skill acquisition in ASD (Teitelbaum et al., 1998; Zwaigenbaum et al ., 2005), may therefore suggest specific a fundamental problem with perception-action coupling as a consequence of impaired perceptual attunement. Combined, this evidence implies a fundamental difficultly with sensory-motor development in Autism Spectrum Disorders, which may precede later social and cognitive symptoms. Indeed, sensory-motor difficulties may even underline classical symptoms of ASD such as cognition, socialization, and communication (Leary and Hill, 1996; Von Hofsten, 2007; Haswell et al., 2009). Strong links have been repeatedly demonstrated between cognition and motor ability (e.g., Chaix et al., 2007; Dziuk et al., 2007) with both developing in parallel and being mutually dependent (Campos et al., 2000; Von Hofsten, 2007; Rakison and Woodward, 2008; Iverson, 2010). Whilst, a poor internal sense of time in ASD (Boucher, 2001) and variable temporal production may extend to difficulties with the social "dance" such as turn taking and eye contact (Leary and Hill, 1996; Wimpory, 2002). Moreover, growing evidence for substantial links between motor ability and intensity of classical ASD symptoms (Dewey et al., 2007; Freitag et al., 2007; Hilton et al., 2007; Fuentes and Bastian, 2009) further suggest sensory-motor difficulties are potentially a fundamental, core symptom of ASD, which are currently being overlooked.

This inability for children with ASD to use sensory information to guide and time action also suggests that despite similarities between ASD and PD (e.g., Mari et al., 2003; Rinehart et al., 2006a; Hollander et al., 2009) a fundamental difference exists. In particular, PD may be seen as the by-product of a systematic degeneration of the sensory-motor control system, thus reflecting the gradual loss of motor control. In contrast, recent longitudinal and retrospective studies have demonstrated movement problems in children diagnosed with ASD from birth (Teitelbaum et al., 1998; Zwaigenbaum et al ., 2005). As such, emerging difficulties with internal temporal control in PD can be successfully minimized by exploiting the pre-established perception-action loop to harness external temporal information (Majsak et al., 1998, 2008). Recent research at the Movement Innovation Lab at Queen's University Belfast has provided additional evidence for the ability of individuals with PD to harness the perception-action loop to maximize movement performance. In particular, this research has demonstrated the use of rich audio and visual temporal 'cues' to guide walking performance, balance rehabilitation and reach-grasp movements (Bieńkiewicz, 2011). It is hoped that this research will result in practical implementations to improve quality of life and overall well-being in individuals with PD.

In contrast, movement problems inherent with ASD often encompass both internal and external temporal control issues, thus potentially reflecting a difficulty with the fundamental establishment of coherent and controlled movement. Combined with evidence for persistent sensory-motor difficulties across the spectrum, this suggests the need for early interventions to promote early engaged, exploratory behavior in infants at risk of or with a preliminary diagnosis of ASD. Breaking research has explicitly demonstrated the potential for sensory-motor therapy in ASD (Woo and Leon, 2013), with sensory enrichment (including movement) leading to improved perceptual, social and cognitive functioning in children aged 3–12 years. Sensitivity to the particular sensory preferences and difficulties of an individual, may allow tailored sensory enrichment to facilitate this exploratory process at later stages of development. For instance, advanced motion capture technology can now allow real-time feedback to be presented in relation to positional information. By targeting feedback to the specific sensory preference of the individual, these feedback loops may directly facilitate this exploratory behavior and body mapping by the explicit nature of this perception-action loop.

Moreover, progressive PD includes a battery of 'non-motor symptoms', which bear a striking resemblance to classical ASD e.g., pronounced difficulties with ToM, executive functioning tasks, and obsessive compulsive behaviors (Saltzman et al., 2000; Mengelberg and Siegert, 2003; Peron et al., 2009). The dominance of motor symptoms in PD is in stark contrast to the characterization of ASD, in which cognitive and social symptoms are seen as core aspects, with sensory-motor difficulties often referred to as secondary by-products. Substantial evidence for behavioral similarities (Damasio and Maurer, 1978; Vilensky et al., 1981; Mari et al., 2003; Vernazza-Martin et al., 2005; Hollander et al., 2009), coupled with this characterization of PD as a "motor" or "movement" disorder further highlights the importance of sensory-motor problems in ASD, and the need for more objective measurement.

Although the underlying etiology of ASD is still unknown, persistent difficulties with internal timing and preparatory processes imply underlying cerebellar and/or basal ganglia deficits (Paulin, 1993; Graybiel et al., 1994; Courchesne, 1997; Gowen and Miall, 2005). These behavioral manifestations are supported by neuroanatomical research implying reduced basal ganglia and cerebellar activation and neuroanatomical abnormalities in ASD (Allen and Courchesne, 2003; Palmen et al., 2004; Amaral et al., 2008; see also Allen, 2006). The cerebellum is also known to play a critical role in the development and maturation of the sensory integration processes, including visuo-motor integration (Glickstein, 1998). Underlying abnormalities within the cerebellum, commonly present in individuals with ASD (Courchesne et al., 1993; Bauman, 1996; Courchesne, 1997), may therefore emerge as potential problems with sensory integration resulting in a lack of perception-action coupling. This is further supported by evidence for cerebellar hyperactivity in PD, compensating for hypoactivity of the basal ganglia (Yu et al., 2007). This pattern would imply the cerebellum plays a vital role in the exploiting of external sensory temporal information to compensate for underlying difficulties with internal timing, which is moderated by the basal ganglia. This is of particular interest as weak perception-action coupling has previously been shown to be a potential indicator of underlying neurological integrity (Van der Meer et al., 1995; Craig et al., 2000).

However, the question still remains; can these symptoms provide a route of early, non-invasive diagnosis? Initial research implies inherent ASD difficulties with predictive gaze (Von Hofsten et al., 2009), one of the earliest indicators of prospective control (Von Hofsten, 2007), whilst anticipatory deficits are now thought to be a precursor of classical cognitive and social symptoms (Brisson et al., 2011). This is a crucial avenue of future research, as the predictive validity of the social precursors of ASD seems to be questionable prior to 18 months of age (Baranek, 1999). Although not all infants with sensory-motor difficulties will later be formally diagnosed with ASD, the specific nature of sensory-motor difficulties in ASD may be an essential factor. Prominent social and cognitive symptoms may be the measureable, observable product of an underlying difficulty establishing coherent goal-directed, interactive behavior. A new Theory of Sensory-motor control development in ASD may play a critical role in heightening awareness of sensory-motor problems in ASD, whilst providing avenues for preliminary diagnosis. However, for the role of sensory-motor difficulties in ASD to be fully understood it is vital that this particular area of research attracts further support, and a holistic approach is taken. As highlighted, there is an intricate relationship between perception and action, with a need to "move to perceive and perceive to move" (Gibson, 1979), thus neither perception nor motor control can be viewed in isolation. By progressing from abstract tasks, to true, goal-directed tests of sensory-motor control a fuller understanding of the role, and underpinnings of motor deficits may be achieved. Furthermore, examination of motor control through the analysis of kinematic profiles allows an objective assessment of difficulties, removed from product orientated and subjective methods currently adopted in standardized tests and correlational analyses. Given repeated evidence for parallels between ASD and PD, comparing and contrasting kinematic and cognitive performance between these populations may further reveal the relationship between cognitive and motor symptoms. In particular, the disparity in the classification between populations despite strong etiology and behavioral similarities demonstrates the need to explore the complex relationship between motor, cognitive, and social ability.

CONCLUSION

In summary, repeated evidence for the presence of significant sensory-motor symptoms across the Autistic Spectrum suggests a traditional cognitive and social view of ASD is short sighted. This work simultaneously highlights both the potential and the limitations of using standardized "norm" based tests commonly used in clinical and research settings. These easy to use standardized tests may provide a gross overview of areas where the motor deficits may reside and can then act as a stepping-stone to unpick sensory-motor difficulties using goal directed tasks with kinematic based analyses. However, if performance was further deconstructed to consider ability at the individual task level additional information may be gained. Moreover the sequential breakdown of performance on a standardized assessment tool (M-ABC2, Henderson and Sugden, 2007) has allowed clear links to be drawn between measurable motor difficulties and underlying kinematic variation. Results also demonstrate the importance of considering both facets of ability when comparing performance across the Autistic spectrum. These results are particularly pertinent given the persistence of significant language delay in ASD, and potential similarities between children with ASD and those with receptive language difficulties (Bartak et al., 1975; Howlin et al., 2000). Such results explicitly highlight the need for this moderating variable to be adequately controlled. Overall it can be seen that motor difficulties are potentially a key component of ASD, rooted in an underlying difficulty with temporal control, due to specific difficulties with perception-action coupling.

ACKNOWLEDGMENTS

This research was supported by the TEMPUS-G project funded by the European Research Council (210007 StIG).

REFERENCES

Allen, G. (2006). Cerebellar contributions to autism spectrum disorders. *Clin. Neurosci. Res.* 6, 195–207. doi: 10.1016/j.cnr.2006.06.002

Allen, G., and Courchesne, E. (2003). Differential effects of developmental cerebellar abnormality on cognitive and motor functions in the cerebellum: an fMRI study of autism. *Am. J. Psychol. 160*, 262–273. doi: 10.1176/appi.ajp.160.2.262

Amaral, D. G., Schumann, C. M., and Nordahl, C. W. (2008). Neuroanatomy of autism. *Trends Neurosci. 31*, 137–145. doi: 10.1016/j.tins.2007.12.005

American Psychiatric Association. (2000). *Diagnostic and Statistical Manual of Mental Disorders, 4th Edn., DSM-IV-TR (Text Revision).* Washington, DC: American Psychiatric Association.

Asperger, H. (1944). *'Autistic Psychopathy' in Children. Translated in U. Frith (1991). Autism and Asperger's Syndrome.* Cambridge: Cambridge University Press.

Baranek, G. T. (1999). Autism during infancy: a retrospective video analysis of sensory – motor and social behaviours at 9 – 12 months of age. *J. Autism Dev. Disord. 29*, 213–224. doi: 10.1023/A:1023080005650

Baron-Cohen, S., Jolliffe, T., Mortimore, C., and Robertson, M. (1997). Another advanced test of theory of mind: evidence from very high functioning adults with Autism and Asperger's syndrome. *J. Child Psychol. Psychiatry* 38, 813–822. doi: 10.1111/j.1469-7610.1997.tb01599.x

Baron-Cohen, S., Leslie, A., and Frith, U. (1985). Does the autistic child have a theory of mind. *Cognition* 21, 37–46. doi: 10.1016/0010-0277(85)90022-8

Bartak, L., Rutter, M., and Cox, A. (1975). A comparative study of infantile Autism, and specific developmental receptive language disorder. I: the children. (1975). *Br. J. Psychiatry* 126, 127–145. doi: 10.1192/bjp.126.2.127

Bauman, M. L. (1996). Brief report: neuroanatomic observations of the brain in pervasive developmental disorders. *J. Autism Dev. Disord. 26*, 199–203. doi: 10.1007/BF02172012

Bieńkiewicz, M. M. N. (2011). *Parkinson's – Is Time on Your Side. Temporal Enhancement of Motor Performance Using Sensory Guides.* Belfast: Queen's University of Belfast.

Boucher, J. (2001). "Lost in a sea of time: time parsing and Autism," in *Time and Memory*, eds T. McCormack and C. Hoerl (Oxford: Oxford University Press), 111–135.

Boucher, J. (2012). Putting theory of mind in its place: psychological explanations of the socio-emotional-communicative impairments in autistic spectrum disorder. *Autism* 16, 226–246. doi: 10.1177/1362361311430403

Bowler, D. M. (2006). "Theory of Mind" in Asperger's Syndrome Dermot, M. Bowler. *J. Child Psychol. Psychiatry 33*, 877–893. doi: 10.1111/j.1469-7610.1992.tb01962.x

Brisson, J., Varreyn, P., Serres, J., Foussier, S., and Adrein, L. (2011). Motor anticipation failure in infants with Autism: a retrospective analysis of feeding situations. *Autism* 16, 420–429. doi: 10.1177/1362361311423385

Caljouw, S. R., Van der Kamp, J., and Savelsbergh, G. J. P. (2004). Catching optical information for the regulation of timing. *Exp. Brain Res.* 155, 427–438. doi: 10.1007/s00221-003-1739-3

Campos, J. J., Anderson, D. I., Barbu-Roth, M. A., Hubbard, E. M., Hertenstein, M. J., and Witherington, D. (2000). Travel broadens the mind. *Infancy* 1, 149–219. doi: 10.1207/S15327078IN0102_1

Cattaneo, L., Fabbri-Destro, M., Boria, S., Pieraccini, C., Monti, A., Cossu, G., et al. (2007). Impairment of actions chains in Autism and its possible role in intention understanding. *Proc. Natl. Acad. Sci. U.S.A. 104*, 17825–17830. doi: 10.1073/pnas.0706273104

Chaix, Y., Albaret, J.-M., Brassard, C., Cheuret, E., de Castelnau, P., Benesteau, J., et al. (2007). Motor impairment in Dyslexia: the influence of attention disorders. *Eur. J. Paediatr. Neurol.* 11, 368–374. doi: 10.1016/j.ejpn.2007.03.006

Constantino, J. N., Davis, S. A., Reich, W., Schindler, M. K., Gross, M. M., Brophy, S. L., et al. (2003). Validation of a brief quantitative measure of autistic traits: comparison of the social responsiveness scale with the autism diagnostic interview-revised. *J. Autism Dev. Disord.* 33, 427–433. doi: 10.1023/A:1025014929212

Courchesne, E. (1997). Brainstem, cerebellar and limbic neuroanatomical abnormalities in Autism. *Curr. Opin. Neurobiol. 7*, 269–278. doi: 10.1016/S0959-4388(97)80016-5

Courchesne, E., Press, G. A., and Yeung-Courchesne, R. (1993). Parietal lobe abnormalities detected with MR in patients with infantile autism. *Am. J. Roentgenol.* 160, 387–393. doi: 10.2214/ajr.160.2.8424359

Craig, C. M., Grealy, M. A., and Lee, D. N. (2000). Detecting motor abnormalities in preterm infants. *Exp. Brain Res.* 131, 359–365. doi: 10.1007/s002219900227

Damasio, A. R., and Maurer, R. G. (1978). A neurological model for childhood Autism. *Arch. Neurol.* 35, 777–786. doi: 10.1001/archneur.1978.00500360001001

Dawson, G., Osterling, J., Meltzoff, A. N., and Kuhl, J. (2000). Case study of the development of an infant with Autism from birth to two years of age. *J. Appl. Dev. Psychol.* 21, 299–313. doi: 10.1016/S0193-3973(99)00042-8

De Jaegher, H. (2013). Embodiment and sense-making in autism. *Front. Integr. Neurosci.* 7:15. doi: 10.3389/fnint.2013.00015

Dewey, D., Cantell, M., and Crawford, S. G. (2007). Motor and gestural performance in children with Autism spectrum disorders, developmental coordination disorder and/or attention deficit hyperactivity disorder. *J. Int. Neuropsychol. Soc.* 13, 246–256. doi: 10.1017/S1355617707070270

Dowd, A. M., McGinley, J. L., Tafee, J. R., and Rinehart, N. J. (2012). Do planning and visual integration difficulties underpin motor dysfunction in Autism. A kinematic study of young children with Autism. *J. Autism Dev. Disord.* 42, 1539–1548. doi: 10.1007/s10803-011-1385-8

Dziuk, M. A., Larson, J. C. G., Apostu, A., Mahone, E. M., Denckla, M. B., and Mostofsky, S. H. (2007). Dyspraxia in Autism: association with motor, social, and communicative deficits. *Dev. Med. Child Neurol.* 49, 734–739. doi: 10.1111/j.1469-8749.2007.00734.x

Edgin, J. O., and Pennington, B. F. (2005). Spatial cognition in Autism Spectrum Disorders: superior, impaired, or just intact. *J. Autism Dev. Disord.* 35, 729–745. doi: 10.1007/s10803-005-0020-y

Fabbri-Destro, M., Cattaneo, L., Boria, S., and Rizzolatti, G. (2009). Planning actions in Autism. *Exp. Brain Res.* 192, 521–525. doi: 10.1007/s00221-008-1578-3

Fajen, B. R. (2005). Perceiving possibilities for action: on the necessity of calibration and perceptual learning for the visual guidance of action. *Perception* 34, 717–740. doi: 10.1068/p5405

Fitts, P. M. (1954). The information capacity of the human motor system in controlling the amplitude of movement. *J. Exp. Psychol.* 47, 381–391. doi: 10.1037/h0055392

Fournier, K. A., Hass, C. J., Naik, S. K., Lodha, N., and Cauraugh, J. H. (2010). Motor coordination in Autism Spectrum Disorders: a synthesis and meta-analysis. *J. Autism Dev. Disord.* 40, 1227–1240. doi: 10.1007/s10803-010-0981-3

Freitag, C. M., Klesser, C., Schneider, M., and von Gontard, A. (2007). Quantitative assessment of neuromotor function in adolescents with high functioning Autism and Asperger Syndrome. *J. Autism Dev. Disord.* 37, 948–959. doi: 10.1007/s10803-006-0235-6

Frith, U. (1989). *Autism: Explaining the Enigma*. Oxford, UK: Blackwell.

Frith, U. (2003). *Autism: Explaining the Enigma, 2nd Edn.* Oxford UK: Blackwell.

Fuentes, C. T., and Bastian, A. J. (2009). 'Motor Cognition'- what is it and is the cerebellum involved. *Cerebellum* 6, 232–236. doi: 10.1080/14734220701329268

Gepner, B., and Mestre, D. R. (2002). Brief Report: postural reactivity to fast visual motion differentiates autistic from children with Asperger's syndrome. *J. Autism Dev. Disord.* 32, 231–238. doi: 10.1023/A:1015410015859

Ghaziuddin, M., and Butler, E. (1998). Clumsiness in autism and Asperger Syndrome: a further report. *J. Intellect. Disabil. Res.* 42, 43–48. doi: 10.1046/j.1365-2788.1998.00065.x

Gibson, E. J. (1969). "Trends in perceptual development," in *An Odyssey in Learning and Perception*, ed E. J. Gibson (Cambridge, MA: MIT Press), 450–472.

Gibson, J. J. (1979). *The Ecological Approach to Visual Perception.* Boston, MA: Houghton Mifflin.

Gillberg, C., Ehlers, S., Schaumann, H., Jakobsson, G., Dahlgren, S. O., Lindblom, R., et al. (1990). Autism under age 3 years: a clinical study of 28 Cases referred for Autistic Symptoms in infancy. *J. Child Psychol. Psychiatry* 31, 921–934. doi: 10.1111/j.1469-7610.1990.tb00834.x

Glazebrook, C., Eillot, D., and Szatmari, P. (2008). How do individuals with autism plan their movements. *J. Autism Dev. Disord.* 38, 114–126. doi: 10.1007/s10803-007-0369-1

Glazebrook, C., Elliott, D., and Lyons, J. (2006). A kinematic analysis of how young adults with and without Autism plan and control goal-directed movements. *Mot. Control* 10, 244–264.

Glazebrook, C., Gonzalez, D., Hanson, S., and Eillot, D. (2009). The role of vision for online control of manual aiming movements in persons with Autism Spectrum Disorders. *Autism* 13, 411–433. doi: 10.1177/1362361309105659

Glickstein, M. (1998). Cerebellum and the sensory guidance of movement. *Novartis Found. Symp.* 218, 252–266.

Gowen, E., and Miall, R. C. (2005). Behavioural aspects of cerebellar function in adults with Asperger Syndrome. *Cerebellum* 4, 1–11. doi: 10.1080/14734220500355332

Gowen, E., Stanley, J., and Miall, R. C. (2008). Movement interference in Autism-Spectrum Disorder. *Neuropsychologia* 46, 1060–1068. doi: 10.1016/j.neuropsychologia.2007.11.004

Graybiel, A. M., Aosaki, T., Flaherty, A. W., and Kimura, M. (1994). The basal ganglia and adaptive motor control. *Science* 265, 1826–1831. doi: 10.1126/science.8091209

Green, D., Baird, G., Barnett, A. L., Henderson, L., Huber, J., and Henderson, S. E. (2002). The severity and nature of motor impairment in Asperger's Syndrome: a comparison with specific developmental disorder of motor function. *J. Child Psychol. Psychiatry* 43, 655–668. doi: 10.1111/1469-7610.00054

Green, D., Charman, T., Pickles, A., Chandler, S., Loucas, T., Simonoff, E., et al. (2009). Impairment in movement skills of children with Autistic Spectrum Disorders. *Dev. Med. Child Neurol.* 51, 311–316. doi: 10.1111/j.1469-8749.2008.03242.x

Happe, F. (1995). The role of age and verbal ability in the theory of mind task performance of subjects with Autism. *Child Dev.* 66, 843–855. doi: 10.2307/1131954

Happe, F. (1996). Studying weak central coherence at low levels: children with Autism do not succumb to visual illusions. *J. Child Psychol. Psychiatry* 37, 873–877. doi: 10.1111/j.1469-7610.1996.tb01483.x

Harris, P. L., Johnson, C. N., Hutton, D., Andrews, G., and Cooke, T. (1989). Young children's Theory of mind and emotion. *Cogn. Emot.* 3, 379–400. doi: 10.1080/02699938908412713

Haswell, C., Izawa, J., Dowell, L., Mostofsky, S., and Shadmehr, R. (2009). Representation of internal models of action in the Autistic brain. *Nat. Neurosci.* 12, 970–972. doi: 10.1038/nn.2356

Henderson, S., and Sugden, D. (1992). *The Movement Assessment Battery for Children*. London: The Psychological Corporation.

Henderson, S., and Sugden, D. (2007). *The Movement Assessment Battery for Children, 2nd Edn*. London: The Psychological Corporation.

Hilton, C., Wente, L., LaVesser, P., Ito, M., Reed, C., and Herzberg, G. (2007). Relationship between motor skill impairment and severity in children with Asperger Syndrome. *Res. Autism Spectr. Disord.* 1, 339–349. doi: 10.1016/j.rasd.2006.12.003

Hobson, R. P. (1991). Against the theory of mind. *Br. J. Dev. Psychol.* 9, 33–51. doi: 10.1111/j.2044-835X.1991.tb00860.x

Hollander, E., Wang, A. T., Braun, A., and Marsh, L. (2009). Neurological considerations: Autism and Parkinson's Disease. *Psychiatry Res. 170*, 43–51. doi: 10.1016/j.psychres.2008.07.014

Howlin, P., Mawhood, L., and Rutter, M. (2000). Autism and Developmental Receptive Language Disorder- a follow-up comparison in early adult life. II: social, behavioural, and psychiatric outcomes. *J. Child Psychol. Psychiatry* 41, 561–578. doi: 10.1111/1469-7610.00643

Hughes, C. (1996). Brief report: planning problems in Autism at the level of motor control. *J. Autism Dev. Disord.* 26, 99–107. doi: 10.1007/BF02276237

Hughes, C., and Russell, J. (1993). Autistic children's difficulty with mental disengagement from an object: its implications for theories of Autism. *Dev. Psychol.* 29, 498–510. doi: 10.1037/0012-1649.29.3.498

Iverson, J. M. (2010). Developing language in a developing body: the relationship between motor development and language development. *J. Child Lang.* 37, 229–261. doi: 10.1017/S0305000909990432

Jansiewicz, E. M., Goldberg, M. C., Newschaffer, C. J., Denckla, M. B., Landa, R., and Mostofsky, S. H. (2006). Motor signs distinguish children with high functioning Autism and Asperger's Syndrome from controls. *J. Autism Dev. Disord.* 36, 613–621. doi: 10.1007/s10803-006-0109-y

Joseph, R. M., and Tager-Flusberg, H. (2004). The relationship of theory of mind and executive functions to symptom type and severity in children with Autism. *Dev. Psychopathol.* 16, 137–155. doi: 10.1017/S095457940404444X

Kanner, L. (1943). Autistic disturbances of affective contact. *Nerv. Child* 2, 217–250.

Kayed, N. S., and van der Meer, A. L. H. (2009). A longitudinal study of prospective control in catching by full-term and preterm infants. *Exp. Brain Res.* 149, 245–258. doi: 10.1007/s00221-008-1692-2

Kleinhans, N., Akshoomoff, N., and Delis, D. C. (2005). Executive functions in Autism and Asperger's Disorder: flexibility, fluency, and inhibition. *Dev. Neuropsychol.* 27, 379–401. doi: 10.1207/s15326942dn2703_5

Leary, M. R., and Hill, D. A. (1996). Moving on: autism and movement disturbance. *Ment. Retard.* 34, 39–53.

Lee, D. N. (1980). The optic flow field: the foundation of vision. *Philos. Trans. R. Soc. Lond. B Biol. Sci.* 290, 169–179. doi: 10.1098/rstb.1980.0089

Lee, D. N. (1998). Guiding movement by coupling Taus. *Ecol. Psychol.* 10, 221–250.

Lee, D. N., Georgopoulos, A. P., Clark, M. J. O., Craig, C., and Port, N. L. (2001). Guiding contact by coupling Taus of gaps. *Exp. Brain Res.* 139, 151–159. doi: 10.1007/s002210100725

Leekman, S. R., and Perner, J. (1991). Does the Autistic child have a metarepresentational deficit. *Cognition* 40, 203–218. doi: 10.1016/0010-0277(91)90025-Y

Lewis, C., and Osbourne, A. (1990). Three-year-olds' problems with False Belief: conceptual deficit or Linguistic Artifact. *Child Dev.* 61, 1514–1519. doi: 10.2307/1130760

Lishman, J. R., and Lee, D. N. (1973). The autonomy of visual kinaesthesis. *Perception* 2, 287–294. doi: 10.1068/p020287

Majsak, M. J., Kaminski, T., Gentile, A. M., and Gordon, A. M. (2008). Effects of moving target versus a temporal constraint on reach and grasp in patients with Parkinson's Disease. *Exp. Neurol.* 210, 479–488. doi: 10.1016/j.expneurol.2007.11.023

Majsak, M. J., Kaminski, T., Gentile, M., and Flanagan, J. R. (1998). The reaching movements of patients with Parkinson's Disease under self-determined maximal speed and visually cued conditions. *Brain* 121, 755–766. doi: 10.1093/brain/121.4.755

Manjiviona, J., and Prior, M. (1995). Comparison of Asperger syndrome and high-functioning autistic children on a test of motor impairment. *J. Autism Dev. Disord.* 25, 23–29. doi: 10.1007/BF02178165

Mari, M., Castiello, U., Marks, D., Marraffa, C., and Prior, M. (2003). The reach-to-grasp movement in children with autism spectrum disorder. *Philos. Trans. R. Soc. B Biol. Sci.* 358, 393–403. doi: 10.1098/rstb.2002.1205

Masterson, B. A., and Biederman, G. B. (1983). Proprioceptive versus visual control in autistic children. *J. Autism Dev. Disord.* 13, 141–152. doi: 10.1007/BF01531815

Mengelberg, A., and Siegert, R. (2003). Is theory of mind impaired in Parkinson's Disease. *Cogn. Neuropsychiatry* 8, 191–209. doi: 10.1080/13546800244000292

Ming, X., Brimacombe, M., and Wagner, G. (2007). Prevalence of motor impairment in Autism Spectrum Disorders. *Brain Dev.* 29, 565–570. doi: 10.1016/j.braindev.2007.03.002

Minshew, N. J., Sung, K., Jones, B. L., and Furman, J. M. (2004). Underdevelopment of the postural control system in Autism. *Neurology* 63, 2056–2061. doi: 10.1212/01.WNL.0000145771.98657.62

Miyahara, M., Tisujii, M., Hori, M., Nakanishi, K., Kageyama, H., and Sugiyama, T. (1997). Brief report: Motor incoordination in children with Asperger Syndrome and learning disabilities. *J. Autism Dev. Disord.* 27, 595. doi: 10.1023/A:1025834211548

Motton, L., Burack, J. A., Stauder, J. E. A., and Robaey, P. (1999). Perceptual processing among high-functioning persons with Autism. *J. Child Psychol. Psychiatry* 40, 203–211. doi: 10.1111/1469-7610.00433

Muller, R.-A., Pierce, K., Ambrose, J. B., Allen, G., and Courshesne, E. (2001). Atypical patterns of cerebral motor activation in autism: a functional magnetic resonance study. *Biol. Psychiatry* 49, 665–676. doi: 10.1016/S0006-3223(00)01004-0

Nazarali, N., Glazebrook, C., and Eillot, D. (2009). Movement planning and reprogramming in individuals with autism. *J. Autism Dev. Disord.* 39, 1401–1411. doi: 10.1007/s10803-009-0756-x

Neuhoff, J. G., and McBeath, M. K. (1996). The Doppler illusion: the influence of dynamic intensity change on perceived pitch. *J. Exp. Psychol. Hum. Percept. Perform.* 71, 970–985. doi: 10.1037/0096-1523.22.4.970

Osterling, J., and Dawson, G. (1994). Early recognition of children with Autism: a study of first birthday home videotapes. *J. Autism Dev. Disord.* 24, 247–257. doi: 10.1007/BF02172225

Ozonoff, S., Macari, S., Young, G. S., Goldring, S., Thompson, M., and Rogers, S. L. (2008). Atypical object exploration at 12 months of age is associated with autism in a prospective sample. *Autism* 12, 457–472. doi: 10.1177/1362361308096402

Ozonoff, S., and McEvoy, R. (1994). A longitudinal study of executive function and theory of mind development in autism. *Dev. Psychopathol.* 6, 415–431. doi: 10.1017/S0954579400006027

Ozonoff, S., Pennington, B., and Rogers, S. (1991). Executive function deficits in high-functioning autistic children: relationship to theory of mind. *J. Child Psychol. Psychiatry* 32, 1081–1106. doi: 10.1111/j.1469-7610.1991.tb00351.x

Palmen, S. J., van Engeland, H., Hof, P. R., and Schmitz, C. (2004). Neuropathological findings in autism. *Brain* 127, 2572–2583. doi: 10.1093/brain/awh287

Papadopoulos, N., McGinley, J., Tonge, B. J., Bradshaw, J. L., Saunders, K., and Rinehart, N. J. (2012). An investigation of upper limb motor functioning in high functioning Autism and Asperger's Disorder using a repetitive Fitt's aiming task. *Res. Autism Spectr. Disord.* 6, 286–292. doi: 10.1016/j.rasd.2011.05.010

Paulin, M. G. (1993). The role of the cerebellum in motor control and perception. *Brain Behav. Evol.* 41, 39–50. doi: 10.1159/000113822

Pellicano, E. (2007). Links between Theory of Mind and executive function in young children with Autism: clues to developmental primacy. *Dev. Psychol.* 43, 974–990. doi: 10.1037/0012-1649.43.4.974

Pennington, B. F., and Ozonoff, S. (1996). Executive functions and developmental psychopathology. *J. Child Psychol. Psychiatry* 37, 51–87. doi: 10.1111/j.1469-7610.1996.tb01380.x

Perner, J., Leekman, S. R., and Wimmer, H. (1987). Three-year olds' difficulty with false belief: the case for a conceptual deficit. *Br. J. Dev. Psychol.* 5, 125–137. doi: 10.1111/j.2044-835X.1987.tb01048.x

Peron, J., Vicente, S., Leray, E., Drapier, S., Drapier, D., Cohen, R., et al. (2009). Are dopaminergic pathways involved in theory of mind. A study in Parkinson's disease. *Neuropsychologia* 47, 406–414. doi: 10.1016/j.neuropsychologia.2008.09.008

Pierce, K., and Courchesne, E. (2001). Evidence for a cerebellar role in reduced exploration and stereotyped behaviour in autism. *Soc. Biol. Psychiatry* 49, 655–664. doi: 10.1016/S0006-3223(00)01008-8

Premack, D., and Woodruff, G. (1978). Does the chimpanzee have a 'theory of mind'. *Behav. Brain Sci.* 4, 515–526. doi: 10.1017/S0140525X00076512

Price, K. J., Shiffrar, M., and Kerns, K. A. (2012a). Movement perception and movement production in Asperger's Syndrome. *Res. Autism Spectr. Disord.* 6, 391–398. doi: 10.1016/j.rasd.2011.06.013

Price, K. J., Edgell, D., and Kerns, K. A. (2012b). Timing deficits are implicated in motor dysfunction in Asperger's Syndrome. *Res. Autism Spectr. Disord.* 6, 857–860. doi: 10.1016/j.rasd.2011.11.007

Provost, B., Heimerl, S., and Lopez, B. R. (2007). Levels of gross and fine motor development in young children with Autism Spectrum Disorder. *Phys. Occup. Ther. Paediatr.* 27, 21–36. doi: 10.1080/J006v27n03_03

Rakison, D. H., and Woodward, A. L. (2008). New perspectives on the effects of action on perceptual and cognitive development. *Dev. Psychol.* 44, 1209–1213. doi: 10.1037/a0012999

Richardson, K. (2000). *Developmental Psychology: How Nature and Nurture Interact.* Mahwah, NJ: Lawrence Erlbaum Associates.

Richler, J., Bishop, S. L., Kleinke, J. R., and Lord, C. (2007). Restricted and repetitive behaviours in young children with Autism Spectrum Disorders. *J. Autism Dev. Disord.* 37, 73–85. doi: 10.1007/s10803-006-0332-6

Rinehart, N., Bradshaw, J., Brereton, A., and Tonge, B. (2001). Movement preparation in high-functioning Autism and Asperger Disorder: a serial choice reaction time task involving motor reprogramming. *J. Autism Dev. Disord.* 31, 79–88. doi: 10.1023/A:1005617831035

Rinehart, N. J., Bellgrove, M. A., Tonge, B. J., Brereton, A. V., Howells Rankin, D., and Bradshaw, J. L. (2006a). An examination of movement kinematics in young people with high-functioning autism and Asperger's Disorder: further evidence for a motor planning deficit. *J. Autism Dev. Disord.* 36, 757–767. doi: 10.1007/s10803-006-0118-x

Rinehart, N. J., Tonge, B. J., Bradshaw, J. L., Iansek, R., Enticott, P. G., and Johnson, K. A. (2006b). Movement- related potentials in high-functioning Autism and Asperger's Disorder. *Dev. Med. Child Neurol.* 48, 272–277. doi: 10.1017/S0012162206000594

Robertson, C., and Flowers, K. A. (1990). Motor sets in Parkinson's Disease. *J. Neurol. Neurosurg. Psychiatr.* 53, 583–592. doi: 10.1136/jnnp.53.7.583

Robledo, J., Donnellan, A. M., and Strandt-Conroy, K. (2012). An exploration of sensory and movement differences from the perspective of individuals with Autism. *Front. Integr. Neurosci.* 6:107. doi: 10.3389/fnint.2012.00107

Russell, J. (1992). The theory-theory: so good they named it twice. *Cogn. Dev.* 7, 485–519. doi: 10.1016/0885-2014(92)80005-Z

Russell, J. (1997). *Autism as an Executive Disorder.* Oxford: Oxford University Press.

Russell, P., Hoise, J., Gray, C., Scott, C., Hunter, N., Banks, J., et al. (1998). The development of theory of mind in deaf children. *J. Child Psychol. Psychiatry* 40, 859–868. doi: 10.1111/1469-7610.00504

Saltzman, J., Strauss, E., Hunter, M., and Archibald, S. (2000). Theory of Mind and executive functions in normal human aging and Parkinson's Disease. *J. Int. Neuropsychol. Soc.* 6, 781–788. doi: 10.1017/S1355617700677056

Schmitz, C., Martineau, J., Barthélémy, C., and Assaiante, C. (2003). Motor control and children with Autism: deficit of anticipatory function. *Neurosci. Lett.* 348, 17–20. doi: 10.1016/S0304-3940(03)00644-X

Siaperas, P., Ring, H. A., McAllister, C. J., Barnett, A., Watson, P., and Holland, A. J. (2012). Atypical movement performance and sensory integration in Asperger's Syndrome. *J. Autism Dev. Disord.* 42, 718–725. doi: 10.1007/s10803-011-1301-2

Staples, K. L., and Reid, G. (2010). Fundamental movement skills and Autism Spectrum Disorders. *J. Autism Dev. Disord.* 40, 209–217. doi: 10.1007/s10803-009-0854-9

Sutera, S., Pandey, J., Esser, E., Rosenthal, M. A., Wilson, L. B., Barton, M., et al. (2007). Predictors of optimal outcome in toddlers diagnosed with autism spectrum disorders. *J. Autism Dev. Disord.* 37, 98–107. doi: 10.1007/s10803-006-0340-6

Teitelbaum, P., Teitelbaum, O., Nye, J., Fryman, J., and Maurer, R. G. (1998). Movement Analysis in infancy may be useful for early diagnosis of Autism. *Proc. Natl. Acad. Sci. U.S.A.* 95, 13982–13987. doi: 10.1073/pnas.95.23.13982

Thelen, E. (1979). Rhythmical stereotypes in normal human infants. *Anim. Behav.* 27, 699–715. doi: 10.1016/0003-3472(79)90006-X

Van der Meer, A. L. H., Van der Weel, F. R., and Lee, D. N. (1994). Prospective control in catching by infants. *Perception* 23, 287–302. doi: 10.1068/p230287

Van der Meer, A. L. H., Van der Weel, F. R., Lee, D. N., Laing, I. A., and Lin, J. P. (1995). Development of prospective control of catching moving objects in preterm at risk infants. *Dev. Med. Child Neurol.* 37, 145–158. doi: 10.1111/j.1469-8749.1995.tb11984.x

Van der Weel, F. R., van der Meer, A. L. H., and Lee, D. N. (1996). Measuring dysfunction of basic movement control in Cerebral Palsy. *Hum. Mov. Sci.* 15, 253–283. doi: 10.1016/0167-9457(95)00046-1

Van Hof, P., Van der Kamp, J., and Savelsbergh, G. J. P. (2008). The relation between infants' perception of catchableness and control of catching. *Dev. Psychol.* 44, 182–194. doi: 10.1037/0012-1649.44.1.182

Vernazza-Martin, S., Martin, N., Vernazza, A., Leper-Muller, A., Rufo, M., Massio, J., et al. (2005). Goal Directed locomotion and balance control in Autistic children. *J. Autism Dev. Disord.* 35, 91–102. doi: 10.1007/s10803-004-1037-3

Vilensky, J. A., Damasio, A. R., and Maurer, R. G. (1981). Gait disturbance in patients with Autistic behaviour. *Arch. Neurol.* 38, 646–649. doi: 10.1001/archneur.1981.00510100074013

Viviani, P., and Schneider, R. (1991). A developmental study of the relationship between geometry and kinematics in drawing movements. *J. Exp. Psychol. Hum. Percept. Perform.* 17, 198–218. doi: 10.1037/0096-1523.17.1.198

Von Hofsten, C. (1991). Structuring of early reaching movements: a longitudinal study. *J. Mot. Behav.* 23, 280–292. doi: 10.1080/00222895.1991.9942039

Von Hofsten, C. (2004). An action perspective on motor development. *Trends Cogn. Sci.* 8, 266–272. doi: 10.1016/j.tics.2004.04.002

Von Hofsten, C. (2007). Action in development. *Dev. Sci.* 10, 54–60. doi: 10.1111/j.1467-7687.2007.00564.x

Von Hofsten, C., Uhlig, H., Adell, M., and Kochukhova, O. (2009). How children with autism look at events. *Res. Autism Spectr. Disord.* 3, 556–569. doi: 10.1016/j.rasd.2008.12.003

Whyatt, C., and Craig, C. M. (2012). Motor skills in children aged 7-10 years, diagnosed with Autism Spectrum Disorder. *J. Autism Dev. Disord.* 42, 1799–1809. doi: 10.1007/s10803-011-1421-8

Whyatt, C., and Craig, C. M. (2013). Interceptive skills in children aged 9-11 years, diagnosed with Autism Spectrum Disorder. *Res. Autism Spectr. Disord.* 7, 613–623. doi: 10.1016/j.rasd.2013.01.003

Wimmer, H., and Perner, J. (1983). Beliefs about beliefs: representation and the constraining function of wrong beliefs in young children's understanding of deception. *Cognition* 13, 103–128. doi: 10.1016/0010-0277(83)90004-5

Wimpory, D. (2002). Social timing, clock genes and Autism: a new hypothesis. *J. Intellect. Disabil. Res. 46*, 352–358. doi: 10.1046/j.1365-2788.2002.00423.x

Wing, L. (1981). Language, social and cognitive impairments in autism and severe mental retardation. *J. Autism Dev. Disord.* 11, 31–44. doi: 10.1007/BF01531339

Wing, L., and Gould, J. (1979). Severe Impairments of social interaction and associated abnormalities in children: epidemiology and classification. *J. Autism Dev. Disord.* 9, 11–29. doi: 10.1007/BF01531288

Woo, C. C., and Leon, M. (2013). Environmental enrichment as an effective treatment for Autism: a randomized controlled trial. *Behav. Neurosci.* Advanced online publication, Available online at: http://www.apa.org/pubs/journals/releases/bne-ofp-woo.pdf. doi: 10.1037/a0033010

Yirmiya, N., Erel, O., Shaked, M., and Solomonica-Levi, D. (1998). Meta-analyses comparing theory of mind abilities of individuals with Autism, individuals with mental retardation and normally developing individuals. *Psychol. Bull.* 124, 283–307. doi: 10.1037/0033-2909.124.3.283

Yu, H., Sternad, D., Corcos, D. M., and Vaillancourt, D. E. (2007). Role of hyperactive cerebellum and motor cortex in Parkinson's Disease. *Neuroimage* 35, 222–233. doi: 10.1016/j.neuroimage.2006.11.047

Zwaigenbaum, L., Bryson, S., Rogers, T., Roberts, W., Brian, J., and Szatmari, P. (2005). Behavioural manifestations of autism in the first year of life. *Int. J. Dev. Neurosci.* 23, 143–152. doi: 10.1016/j.ijdevneu.2004.05.001

Conflict of Interest Statement: The authors declare that the research was conducted in the absence of any commercial or financial relationships that could be construed as a potential conflict of interest.

16

Autism and social disconnection in interpersonal rocking

Kerry L. Marsh[1,2]*, Robert W. Isenhower[1,2]*, Michael J. Richardson[3], Molly Helt[2], Alyssa D. Verbalis[2], R. C. Schmidt[4] and Deborah Fein[2]

[1] *Center for the Ecological Study of Perception and Action, University of Connecticut, Storrs, CT, USA*
[2] *Department of Psychology, University of Connecticut, Storrs, CT, USA*
[3] *Department of Psychology, University of Cincinnati, Cincinnati, OH, USA*
[4] *Department of Psychology, College of the Holy Cross, Worchester, MA, USA*

Edited by:
Caroline Whyatt, Queen's University Belfast, UK

Reviewed by:
Lynden Miles, University of Aberdeen, UK
Emma Gowen, The University of Manchester, UK

****Correspondence:***
Kerry L. Marsh, Department of Psychology, University of Connecticut, Unit 1020, 406 Babbidge Road, Storrs, CT 06269-1020, USA.
e-mail: kerry.l.marsh@uconn.edu
Robert W. Isenhower, Douglass Developmental Disabilities Center, Rutgers University, 151 Ryders Lane, New Brunswick, NJ 08901, USA.
e-mail: risenhow@rci.rutgers.edu

Individuals with autism spectrum disorders (ASDs) have significant visuomotor processing deficits, atypical motoric behavior, and often substantial problems connecting socially. We suggest that the perceptual, attentional, and adaptive timing deficiencies associated with autism might directly impact the ability to become a socially connected unit with others. Using a rocking chair paradigm previously employed with typical adults, we demonstrate that typically-developing (TD) children exhibit spontaneous social rocking with their caregivers. In contrast, children diagnosed with ASD do not demonstrate a tendency to rock in a symmetrical state with their parents. We argue that the movement of our bodies is one of the fundamental ways by which we connect with our environment and, especially, ground ourselves in social environments. Deficiencies in perceiving and responding to the rhythms of the world may have serious consequences for the ability to become adequately embedded in a social context.

Keywords: ASD, movement coupling, rocking synchrony, synchrony, rocking chair

AUTISM AND SOCIAL DISCONNECTION IN INTERPERSONAL ROCKING

A defining characteristic of autism spectrum disorder (ASD) involves impairments in connecting with others, including impaired verbal and non-verbal communication, and lack of imitation and social reciprocity (APA, 2000). Early accounts of explaining such deficits seemed to partition off such deficits from perceptuo-motoric problems that also frequently occur (i.e., unusual attention processes, poor praxis and balance, and difficulty coordinating perception with action, and one limb with another; see Bhat et al., 2011), focusing instead on cognitive or motivational accounts of the social deficits. Because many social abilities such as pretend play with others can involve complex skills (e.g., joint attention, joint action, and understanding of intentions), it has been suggested that children with ASD might have a theory of mind deficit (Baron-Cohen et al., 1985; Rogers and Pennington, 1991; Williams et al., 2004). Although embodied simulation accounts that arose from research on mirror neuron processes (Rizzolatti and Craighero, 2004; Williams et al., 2004; Oberman et al., 2005) seem to give credence to theory of mind accounts, empirical evidence has failed to corroborate the role of deficiencies in these processes in the emergence of social deficits (Carpenter et al., 2001; Sebanz et al., 2005).

An adequate theoretical grounding of ASD sociality deficits is urgent in light of the increasing numbers of children being diagnosed with ASD, and the considerable resources being employed in autism interventions. Such research might have significant implications for whether the current dominant theoretical framework for developing interventions for children with ASD should continue to focus exclusively on social, cognitive, and communication skills or whether new approaches might fruitfully be added that focus on the development of a better perceptuo-motor grounding in the social world. Since communication requires movement and timing, it may well be that motoric difficulties link in crucial ways to being socially connected with others (Gernsbacher et al., 2008). In the current study, we examine whether low-level motoric processes that occur normally during social interaction—the tendency to synchronize the incidental movements of our bodies with others—is deficient in children with ASD.

Our perspective to understanding potential synchrony deficits in children with ASD starts with the assumption that humans are grounded in an environment that includes others (e.g., Marsh, 2010; Semin and Echterhoff, 2010), and that even trivial non-goal-directed movements are foundational for allowing us to be embedded in that world, to be of the world rather than standing apart from it. Crucial to a sense of connection to one's world (non-social or social) is first the ability to be able to entrain perceptually—to be able to follow and track the world. If sensory systems operate in such a way that rhythms of the world flow unexpectedly fast or slow, that one does not have sensory systems properly attuned to detect and thus synchronize with the flow of information at the proper rate, it could be uncomfortable, frightening, frustrating, or excessively arousing, which could ultimately lead one to shut off from such excessive or unpredictable stimulation.

There is substantial evidence that sensory and visual perception (e.g., timing) processes can be disrupted in children with ASD (Grossberg and Seidman, 2006). Coordination between an individual with ASD and an environmental rhythm has been examined (Gepner et al., 1995; Gepner and Mestre, 2002a,b). Typically-developing (TD) children show spontaneous entrainment of their postural sway motions to oscillatory stimuli presented on a screen; children with ASD did not exhibit such spontaneous coupling. Adults with Asperger syndrome have also been found to show impaired performance on tapping tasks that involve timing their movements to auditory stimuli (Gowen and Miall, 2005). Additionally, general deficits in motion perception have been found in children with ASD (Gepner et al., 2005; Milne et al., 2005).

As evidence from research on postural sway suggests, perceptual responses to the world are often reflected in one's movements. However, even if perceptual and visual timing systems are intact but individuals are motorically unable to be embedded in the world, and cannot properly partake in the rhythms of the world by moving their own bodies to pace themselves to it, it would be like catching a merry-go-round when we cannot run fast enough to jump on. If our bodies do not work in the regular rhythmic and symmetrical patterns that are signatures of normal rhythmic behavior (Schmidt and Richardson, 2008), a crucial and necessary condition for social connection is missing. We have hypothesized that a minimal condition for becoming a social synergy with others—a coordinated perception-action system with another (Marsh et al., 2006)—is that one is pulled into the natural orbit of another's movement rhythms—responsive to the speed of their movement and pulled to move in ways that match them temporally.

A Gibsonian ecological theory of perception (Gibson, 1979) and a dynamical systems approach to action (Warren, 2006) both posit that action is crucial for learning properly about the world, about the flow of the world, and our relationship to that world. For instance, developing proper perceptual attunement to the visual cliff comes with having crawled sufficiently to experience the optic flow in connection with our movement. Children who develop new physical capabilities encounter new possibilities for action, or affordances, particularly social affordances (Campos et al., 2000; Karasik et al., 2012). From an ecological and dynamical perspective, a child would have increased difficulty in properly developing new skills to be embedded and situated in the world, if motoric processes were off kilter.

There is substantial evidence that motoric deficiencies are often common in children with ASD. These can include fine and gross motor coordination, postural control and balance deficiencies, as well generalized difficulties performing gestures and complex movement sequences, along with bilateral arm coordination difficulties (Henderson and Sugden, 1992; Ghaziuddin et al., 1994; Ghaziuddin and Butler, 1998; Minshew et al., 2004; Jansiewicz et al., 2006; Mostofsky et al., 2006; Isenhower et al., 2012). Severity of ASD has also been linked to deficiencies synchronizing one's gestures with one's speech (de Marchena and Eigsti, 2010). Recent narrative (Bhat et al., 2011) and meta-analytic reviews (Fournier et al., 2010) of the pervasiveness of motoric difficulties in ASD suggest that motoric coordination deficits might be considered cardinal features of ASD. If perceptuo-motor deficits are integral to the social deficits of children with ASD such as deficiencies in imitation, in joint attention, and engaging in physical cooperative or verbal communication tasks (turn-taking and reciprocity) that reflect joint action (e.g., Baron-Cohen, 1989; Williams et al., 2004; Kelley et al., 2006), what might be reasonable tasks for beginning to look at such links? Many of these social tasks can require a high level of complex coordination involving attention (e.g., gaze), gesture and other complex behaviors, as well as the production of words in cognitive demanding circumstances (e.g., verbalizing thoughts). Moreover, focusing on motoric skills in the context of overtly social tasks requires that the task be one for which the child has adequate interest. Otherwise, if motoric deficiencies occur in the course of performing such a task, one could falsely assume that because the child does not perform the correct motoric behavior, they are not *able* to do so even if social interest was sufficient (Kinsbourne and Helt, 2011).

In the current paper, we focus instead on understanding the more minimal conditions that are involved in social responsiveness, focusing not on goal-directed action and all of the challenges (e.g., adequate interest in the goals) that such tasks require, but instead on inadvertent movement patterns that occur automatically under natural social interactions. An ideal task would be one in which the motoric behavior is not constrained by whether a child has shared overt goals. One approach, for example, has been to look at inadvertent social influence (movement interference) when another person (vs. an environmental stimulus) is moving in a different plane while one rhythmically moves one's arm back and forth (Gowen et al., 2008). Intriguingly, high functioning adults with ASD showed relatively limited differences in interference patterns, relative to control adults—both groups showed the typical interference effect, enhanced when the stimuli moved in a biological style of motion, and maximally impactful if the stimulus was another person's arm moving.

Whereas Gowen et al.'s task involved overt, intentional movement in the context of some other stimulus obviously moving congruently or incongruently, in our study we examined spontaneous coordination of less overt, and more incidental movement as it occurs in a social context. Focusing on simple periodic rhythmic movements is useful not only because many important movements (solitary as well as social) involve rhythmic behavior (e.g., walking or clapping), but also because considerable past research provides insight into natural dynamics of interpersonal coordination even when such movements are incidental or irrelevant to goal state (Schmidt and Richardson, 2008). The natural tendency to display such dynamics, we suggest, might be particularly informative about an individual's foundation for being socially grounded in the environment. In the current study, we use the task of spontaneously synchronizing a rocking chair to that of an adult. We use this task for two reasons. First, rocking in a chair is a natural behavior that is familiar to both children who have ASD and those who do not. Second, unlike many other tasks that may require relatively complex motor skills, or motor skills of some particular type, steadily moving a rocking chair can be achieved equally well using a variety of different methods (e.g., by pushing off with one's feet, or by merely moving one's trunk back and forth). A rocking chair is an external prop that can simultaneously amplify and simplify movement.

Although this particular paradigm has not been previously used with children, researchers have demonstrated the usefulness of a social collaborator for improving rhythmic coordination in children. For example, children's unilateral or bilateral drumming performance can be facilitated by having an adult drum with the child (Kirschner and Tomasello, 2009; Kleinspehn-Ammerlahn et al., 2011). We hypothesize that if deficiencies in the interpersonal coordination of rhythmic incidental movements occur in ASD, it may provide a window into understanding some of the minimal underlying motoric dynamic deficiencies that might restrain a child from being solidly grounded in a social world. Moreover, research with adults importantly links such interpersonal synchrony to creation of social bonds and increased susceptibility to others' influence (e.g., Hove and Risen, 2009; Miles et al., 2009; Wiltermuth and Heath, 2009; Wiltermuth, 2012).

To examine interpersonal synchrony, in the current study an adult was asked to rock at a set rhythm and children's tendency to spontaneously rock in synchrony with the adult was assessed. The synchronization model we use here is one proposed by Haken et al. (1985; HKB model) for understanding rhythmic interlimb coordination. Its modeling of the entrainment dynamics of coupled oscillators (Kugler and Turvey, 1987; Kelso, 1995) has provided an important framework for studying rhythmic coordination in adults (cf. Turvey, 1990; Amazeen et al., 1998) and children (Fitzpatrick et al., 1996; Robertson, 2001; Lantero and Ringenbach, 2007). Moreover, the model applies to both the coordination of limb movements within individuals as well as the coupling of different individuals' movements, under circumstances involving both intentional (Schmidt et al., 1990, 1998) as well as spontaneous (Schmidt and O'Brien, 1997; Richardson et al., 2005) conditions. For example, the model has been used to explain the spontaneous rocking coordination of pairs of adults in studies purportedly about rocking chair ergonomics (Richardson et al., 2007).

In the rocking chair paradigm used with adults, participants are merely asked to focus their attention on their partner's chair while each rocks at their own individual pace. Sensors tracking participants' chair movements during brief trials (e.g., 90 s) reveal that participants spontaneously synchronize rocking in a symmetrical state called in-phase behavior. In-phase rocking means that both individuals are at their maximum point forward (or backward) in their rocking cycle *relative* to each other (i.e., they are at 0° relative phase). Spontaneous synchrony in adults is evidenced by in-phase rocking at rates above 11% of a trial, with the lower range of synchronous states (e.g., 20% of a trial) occurring during spontaneous synchrony while participants are simultaneously engaged in a filler task such as mentally rehearsing memory words or forming impressions of a picture (Demos et al., 2012). When the cover story of the experiment (e.g., "rocking chair ergonomics") does not necessitate participants doing a simultaneous task, rates of in-phase behavior can be substantially higher (e.g., 45%, Richardson et al., 2007).

In the current study we extended the rocking chair paradigm to children by assessing rocking behavior during a natural interaction with their caregiver. We predicted that children without ASD would show significantly more in-phase rocking behavior than children with ASD.

METHOD

OVERVIEW

We individually assessed children with and without ASD in their spontaneous tendency to synchronize the movement of their rocking chairs with those of a parent. The parent read a storybook to the child, while sitting in her own rocking chair and rocking throughout to a set tempo.

PARTICIPANTS

Eleven children receiving a clinical diagnosis of ASD and 19 TD children participated in the study. Seven children (3 with ASD and 4 without) did not rock in the trials, leaving a sample of 8 children with ASD and 15 TD children. Participants with ASD were recruited from the ongoing University of Connecticut Early Detection ASD study (Kleinman et al., 2008). Clinicians administered the *Autism Diagnostic Observation Scale* (ADOS; Lord et al., 1999) to determine that the child met the cutoffs for and ASD. The ADOS is a semi-structured standardized assessment of communication, social interaction, and play behaviors in which a trained evaluator induces social situations that are designed to encourage the child to initiate and respond to socially. The ADOS currently has four modules corresponding to varying expressive language levels from pre-verbal/single words to fluent speech. A licensed clinician at the University of Connecticut and a doctoral student both assessed the child's score on the ADOS. A diagnosis of ASD was given if the licensed clinician determined that the child met the necessary diagnostic criteria. TD participants were a convenience sample recruited from the local university community; none of these children showed developmental delays in any domain.

Of the TD children (chronological age: 33–98 months), eight were female, the other seven were male. Children diagnosed with ASD ranged from 46 to 103 months in chronological age; two of these participants were female; the other six were male. Some analyses involved a subset of the sample matched for intellectual age. The Mullen Scales of Early Learning (Mullen, 1995), administered to all participants, assessed intellectual development on five scales: gross motor, visual reception, fine motor, receptive language, and expressive language. Fourteen children in the ASD and TD sample who could be matched to within 6 months on the visual reception subscale of the Mullen were retained as an age-equivalent-matched subsample; see **Table 1** for details on this sample.

PROCEDURE

A rocking chair methodology that has been used to assess spontaneous synchrony in adults (Richardson et al., 2007) was modified to examine spontaneous synchrony in children. To provide baseline rocking data, children were induced to rock continuously for 30 s in a child-sized rocking chair. For the test trials, the parent sat to the right of the child's chair, in an adult-sized rocking chair

Table 1 | Characteristics of subsample of children: ASD and matched TD controls.

ASD				TD			
Child	Gender	Chronological age (months)	Mullen visual reception (months)	Child	Gender	Chronological age (months)	Mullen visual reception (months)
1	M	47	27	1	F	35	27
2	F	47	29	2	F	34	33
3	M	45	30	3	M	53	34
4	M	46	46	4	M	45	40
5	F	48	48	5	F	40	42
6	M	49	60	6	M	53	60
7	M	49	61	7	M	55	66
Mean		47.4	43.0			45.2	43.1

Note: Matching within 6 months on visual reception subscale of Mullen. The groups did not differ significantly in chronological age or visual reception scores, $|t|s < 1$.

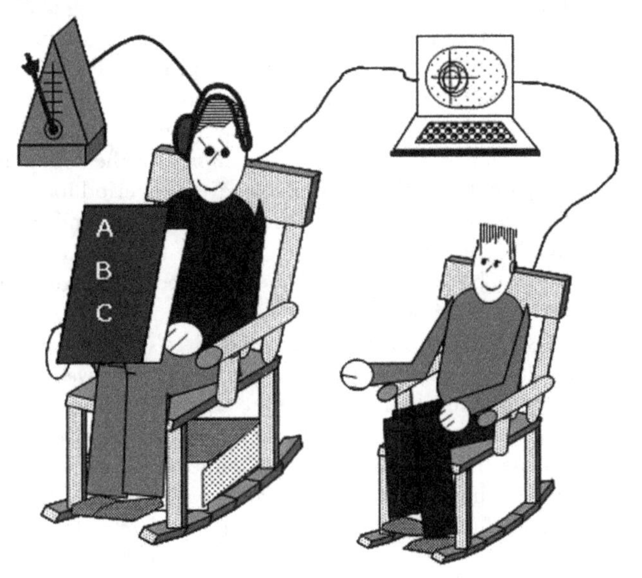

FIGURE 1 | The experimental set up. Parents and children sat in rocking chairs. The parent read the child a story while rocking at a pace prescribed by a metronome only they can hear. Rocking movements of the parents and children were recorded via motion-tracking sensors attached unobtrusively to each chair.

reading the child a book, and rocking at a prescribed tempo (see **Figure 1**). Two trials were conducted when the child's patience permitted. Each trial took between 2 and 5 min depending on the length of the book. During the trial, the parent held a children's book so that they could read it and the child could see it. Rocking chairs have a natural frequency that is determined by their construction, size, overall mass, and center of mass; the natural period of a chair's "inverted pendulum" movement can be adjusted by attaching additional weights below the center of mass. Thus, lead weights (36.3 Kg) were attached to the base of the parent's chair to allow it to rock easily at a frequency comparable to the typical rocking frequency of the child's rocking chair. In order to keep the parent rocking at a period typical of children's preferred rocking (determined to be 1.2 s in pilot testing), parents wore an earphone on one ear through which they heard a double metronome set to that period (i.e., a beep occurred every 0.6 s). Having the periods of the adult's chair move at a frequency within the range of what is natural for children allows the greatest opportunity for interpersonal synchrony to occur (Lopresti-Goodman et al., 2008). Moreover, any synchrony that occurred would be due to the child's spontaneous, unidirectional entrainment with the parent; children were not explicitly told to rock their chair during the test trials. Sensors attached to the back of each chair's headrest recorded the movement data of each rocking chair at 60 Hz (i.e., 60 samples per second) using a Polhemus Fastrak magnetic tracking system. A subsample of children also completed a bimanual drumming task alone; those data have been presented elsewhere (Isenhower et al., 2012). At the end of the session, participants received a children's book or equivalent monetary compensation for their participation.

COORDINATION PREDICTIONS

Predictions regarding coordinated rocking behavior were based on assumptions that if a child and adult become coordinated in their rocking, those coordination states can be understood in terms of the HKB equation for two coupled oscillators (Haken et al., 1985).

The motion equation for the HKB model (Haken et al., 1985) is as follows:

$$\dot{\phi} = \Delta\omega - a\sin\phi - 2b\sin 2\phi + \sqrt{Q}\xi_t \quad (1)$$

Relative phase (ϕ) is the collective variable that captures the spatio-temporal relationship between the two component oscillators (i.e., rocking chairs in the present study). $\dot{\phi}$ is the rate of change of relative phase. The detuning parameter, $\Delta\omega$, captures the difference in the natural, uncoupled, frequency of the two oscillators (Sternad et al., 1995). ξ_t is a Gaussian noise process that dictates a stochastic force of strength Q (Schöner et al., 1986). The relationship of the sine functions ($a\sin\phi$ and $2b\sin 2\phi$) index the relative strength of the two stable fixed point attractors of the coupled oscillators—in-phase ($\phi = 0°$) and anti-phase ($\phi = 180°$). At 0° relative phase, both individuals in a pair are at the same phase in their rocking cycle (e.g., both forward or backward at the same time). With rocking chair movement, spontaneous coordination is typically indicated by the amount of time that a dyad's movements are 0° relative phase. Anti-phase (being at the forward-most point in one's rocking cycle while the other is at their backward-most point) is also a stable coordination pattern that adult dyads can intentionally maintain when instructed (Richardson et al., 2007), but the HKB equation predicts that in-phase is a much stronger attractor (Haken et al., 1985).

RESULTS

To test the hypothesis that TD children would show stronger in-phase coordination of their rocking chair movement with their parents than ASD children would exhibit with their parents, continuous relative phase (CRP) was analyzed on the forward/backward dimension of each dyad's movements. Children did not rock continuously throughout the trials. Children with ASD rocked an average of 42.0% ($SD = 27.1\%$) of the time whereas TD children rocked an average of 47.9% of the time ($SD = 26.8\%$). This difference was not significant, $t_{(21)} = 0.51$, $p = 0.62$, nor were differences (46.4% vs. 56.3%) significant in the matched sample, $|t| < 1$. Thus, comparable amounts of data were available in both groups of children to allow for analysis of bouts of continual rocking. CRP was used to calculate the average amount of time the dyad spent in a given relative phase in these bouts (with each rocking segment weighted by its relative length) using 9 bins in 20° increments arrayed from in-phase (10° either side of 0°) to anti-phase (10° either side of 180°). A 2 (Group) × 9 (Phase Region) mixed analysis of variance conducted on CRP for the full sample with phase region as a within-subjects factor revealed only a significant interaction between group and phase region, [$F_{(8, 168)} = 5.49, p < 0.01$]. As **Figure 2** indicates, relative to children with ASD, TD children spent more time rocking in-phase with their parent. The pattern that occurred is illustrated by a significant linear contrast for the phase × group interaction, [$F_{(1, 21)} = 9.11$, $p < 0.01$]. The linear contrast tests the prediction of a continual decrease in occurrence of behavior for each relative phase region, as that region shifts further away from 0°. The linear trend of phase bin was significant for TD children only and revealed the typical pattern found for relative interpersonal coordination in adults: As relative phase values shifted away from in-phase, there was a linear decrease in the percentage of time this occurred throughout the trial.

Repeating the 2 × 9 mixed ANOVA for the age-equivalent-matched subsample alone revealed similar results. The phase region × group interaction was again significant, [$F_{(8, 96)} = 3.17$, $p < 0.05$]. As **Figure 3** indicates, the pattern was the same as with the full sample. TD children showed significantly more in-phase coordination (0°) than children with ASD, $t_{(12)} = 2.66, p < 0.05$.

EXPLORATORY ANALYSES

To explore whether children's rocking period was affected by the parent's rocking period, we compared the child's rocking period on the baseline trial and on the test trial (for the age-matched subsample) to the parent's rocking period on the test trial. Shifts in rocking period toward the parent's period would mean that the child was mimicking the speed of the parent, regardless of whether the child was coordinating the *timing* of their rocking cycle to the parent's. **Table 2** presents the average period for each child and parent in the matched sample. As the table indicates, parents were successful rocking at a rate close to their intended period of 1.2 s. Children's baseline rocking periods (when rocking alone) were sometimes longer and sometimes shorter than that of their parents. To determine whether the children's rocking period in the test trial (i.e., when they rocked with the parent) was closer to the parent's period than happened to occur by chance in the baseline trial, the parent's rocking period was subtracted from the child's baseline trial period and the absolute value of each pair was taken (|Baseline—Parent|). This value was compared to the absolute value of the parent's rocking period subtracted from the

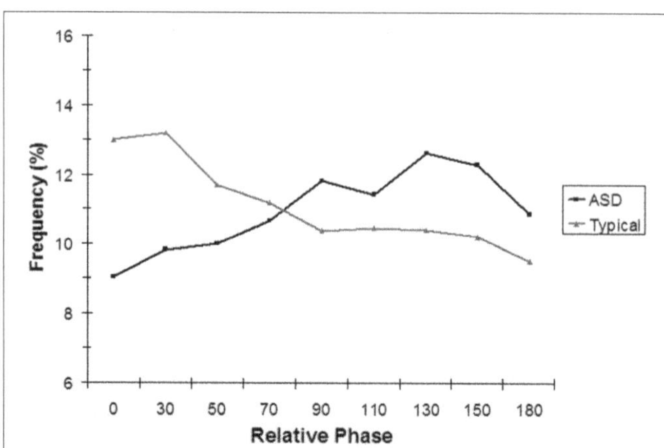

FIGURE 2 | Analysis of continuous relative phase (CRP), binned into nine equal intervals, for the complete sample.

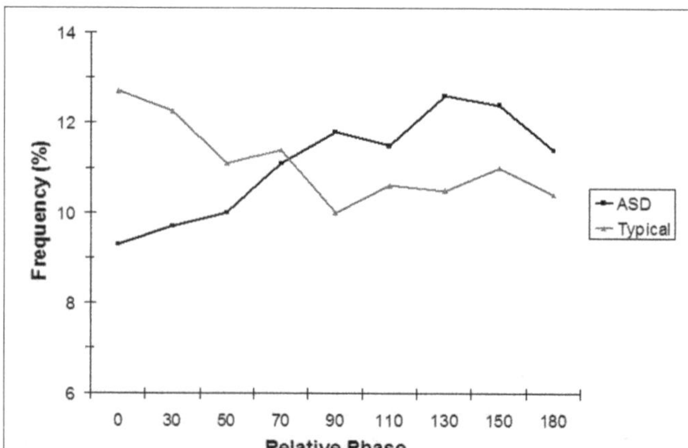

FIGURE 3 | Analysis of continuous relative phase (CRP), binned into nine equal intervals, for seven ASD and seven typically developing children, age-matched on the visual reception subscale of the Mullen. For the in-phase (0°) bin only, the effects of group were statistically significant.

Table 2 | Average periods of child and parent rocking for the matched sample of children.

ASD				TD			
Child no.	**Baseline**	**W/Parent**	**Parent**	**Child no.**	**Baseline**	**W/Parent**	**Parent**
1	1.10	1.13	1.21	1	1.46	1.13	1.22
2	1.27	1.16	1.34	2	1.52	1.38	1.23
3	1.64	1.12	1.34	3	1.04	1.15	1.20
4	1.05	1.05	1.14	4	1.53	1.30	1.33
5	1.57	1.58	1.30	5	1.16	1.26	1.21
6	1.23	1.38	1.30	6	1.33	1.23	1.23
7	1.17	1.29	1.34	7	1.14s	1.21	1.23
M	1.29	1.25	1.28	*M*	1.31	1.24	1.24
SD	0.23	0.19	0.08	*SD*	0.20	0.08	0.04

Note: Children's average periods when rocking alone and rocking with their parents, as well as the parents' average periods, are presented in seconds.

Table 3 | Differences between parent and child rocking periods, for the matched sample.

ASD			TD		
Pair no.	**|Baseline—Parent|**	**|W/Parent—Parent|**	**Pair no.**	**|Baseline—Parent|**	**|W/Parent—Parent|**
1	0.117	0.082	1	0.238	0.092
2	0.072	0.183	2	0.292	0.153
3	0.303	0.222	3	0.161	0.051
4	0.093	0.087	4	0.197	0.031
5	0.266	0.280	5	0.048	0.048
6	0.069	0.080	6	0.097	0.006
7	0.167	0.047	7	0.091	0.020
M	0.156	0.140	*M*	0.161	0.057
SD	0.095	0.088	*SD*	0.088	0.051

Note: The absolute values of the difference between each child's average period (rocking alone, and rocking with parent) and that of his or her parent are presented in seconds.

child's rocking period in the test trial (|Test—Parent|). **Table 3** presents these values for each pair. A 2 (Group: Typical vs. ASD) × 2 (Trial: |Baseline—Parent| vs. |Test—Parent|) mixed ANOVA was conducted, with trial as a within-subjects factor. There was no effect of Group, $F < 1$, but there was a significant effect of Trial, $[F_{(1,\ 12)} = 11.36, p < 0.01]$. This effect was moderated by a significant Trial × Group interaction, $[F_{(1,\ 12)} = 6.21, p < 0.05]$. As **Figure 4** indicates, although the periods of both groups of children's movements shifted toward their parents' periods during the course of the study, this effect was weaker in children with ASD.

For exploratory purposes, the percentage of time a child spent in symmetrical rocking (in-phase) with their caregiver was correlated with chronological age and intellectual age. Chronological age was not correlated with spontaneous coordination of rocking, $r = 0.08$, *ns*. However, intellectual age, as assessed by Mullen scores, was significantly correlated with in-phase rocking, $r = 0.54, p < 0.05$, a pattern that was stable within both groups.

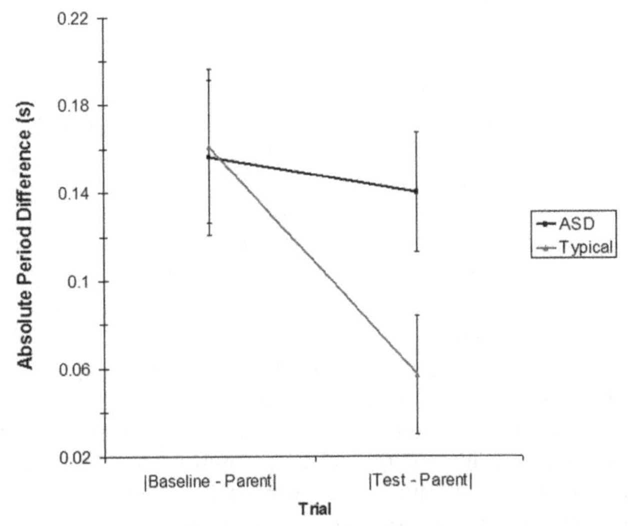

FIGURE 4 | The absolute value of the children's rocking period for the baseline condition and the test condition compared to the parent's rocking period in the test condition for the ASD and TD groups. Error bars represent the standard error of the mean.

DISCUSSION

The present study used a rocking chair paradigm to examine the dynamics of uninstructed social coordination of children with ASD and those with no history of developmental disabilities. Not surprisingly, overall interpersonal coordination levels in children were much lower than seen in previous adult studies using rocking chairs (Richardson et al., 2007). Nevertheless, TD children exhibited significantly more in-phase rocking behavior with their parents than did children with ASD matched using the age equivalent on the visual reception subscale of the Mullen. Furthermore, examining the overall period of children's rocking movements against their parents' revealed that TD children shifted their period to that of their parent to a greater degree than did children in the age-matched sample who were diagnosed with ASD. These differences do not appear likely to be a consequence of the parents' rocking tempo being too dissimilar, on average, to the children's tempo—and therefore in dynamical systems terms, were not outside a natural period basin of entrainment. Parents were able to keep their movements close to the instructed frequency, and as a consequence, the period difference between children and parents was less than 4%. Previous research has shown that this period difference is within the basin of entrainment (Lopresti-Goodman et al., 2008) that allows for unintentional interpersonal coordination to emerge. Given that children in both groups had an equal opportunity to unintentionally coordinate with their parents, it is likely that differences between the two groups of children in their perceptual or motoric processes underlies the differences in observed coordination. However, further research is required to be able to rule out the rival possibility that children with ASD merely paid less attention globally to their parent.

With research failing to support key tenets of a theory of mind account of autism (Carpenter et al., 2001; Sebanz et al., 2005), it is a critical time to look how the motoric deficiencies that underlie autism (Bhat et al., 2011; Gowen and Hamilton, 2013; Grossberg and Seidman, 2006; Isenhower et al., 2012) could link to children's inability to engage in joint attention, joint action, and mimicry of others (e.g., Helt et al., 2010; Kinsbourne and Helt, 2011). The results of the current study suggest that at rather fundamental, low-level of motoric behavior that does not depend on intentional, goal-directed action, there are deficiencies in the social grounding of ASD children's movements. Previous research has provided only limited evidence of a link between deficits of synchrony between parent and child; evidence was lacking that synchrony could be due to a unidirectional coupling of the child to the parent (Kinsbourne and Helt, 2011). The current paradigm, examining children's propensity to be pulled into the orbit of their parents' movement patterns during an engaging interpersonal exchange (i.e., reading a book together), provides evidence that children with ASD do not show movement dynamics comparable to what a coupled oscillator account of the coordination of incidental, non-purposive movements would predict. Clues to deficiencies in sociality in ASD may lie in understanding more basic perceptual, attentional (e.g., Liss et al., 2006), and movement abnormalities that often may be the earliest detectable clue that a child has ASD (Grossberg and Seidman, 2006). Marsh et al. (2006) suggest that the ability to time, coordinate, and flexibly adapt our movements with others, may underlie or contribute significantly to our ability to engage others socially. Deficits in intra-personal (within a person) coordination, therefore, may reduce the ability to coordinate interpersonally (between people) and to become moored in a social environment.

Further research is required before such conclusions can be definitively drawn, however. A primary limitation of the current study is its small sample. Future research should replicate and extend these findings, using a wider range of synchrony behaviors across more participants. In the current study, intellectual age was correlated with how much synchrony occurred. Further research would also be needed to rule out differences in the ASD group's degree of overall attention to the adult, or differences in their ability to attend simultaneously to the story and the rocking rate. Recent evidence suggests that for some passive mimicry tasks (e.g., facial movement when viewing a face dynamically expressing emotions), ASD are not impaired in automatic imitation, provided attention is carefully controlled (Press et al., 2010). Whether similar success of ensuring attention could occur for imitation that also requires *temporal* coordination of one's movements with another (as in rocking synchrony) is a critical issue.

Moreover, intervention research is needed to explore the conditions under which interventions will impact interpersonal coordination of movement, and to determine whether motoric-based interventions can have an impact on the sociality deficits of children with ASD. The rationale of this approach is that by focusing the child's attention on the adult's movements, and facilitating simple motoric movement synchrony, individuals can be pulled into the orbit of another, becoming a social unit of perceiving and acting. This is a necessary condition, we suggest, for becoming a fully functional and responsive social actor in more complex interactions with others.

ACKNOWLEDGMENTS

This research was funded by an Autism Speaks Innovative Technology for Autism Bridge Grant awarded to Kerry L. Marsh. The children with ASD were participating in an NICHD-funded project on early detection of autism (RO1 HD039961 to Deborah Fein). We thank Paula Silva for assistance with data collection.

REFERENCES

Amazeen, P., Amazeen, E., and Turvey, M. T. (1998). "Dynamics of intersegmental coordination: theory and research," in *Timing of Behavior: Neural, Computational, and Psychological Perspectives*, eds D. Rosenbaum and C. Collier (Boston, MA: MIT Press), 237–259.

American Psychological Association. (2000). *Diagnostic and Statistical Manual of Mental Disorders: DSM-IV-TR.* Washington, DC: American Psychiatric Press, Inc.

Baron-Cohen, S. (1989). The autistic child's theory of mind: the case of specific developmental delay. *J. Child Psychol. Psychiatry* 30, 285–298.

Baron-Cohen, S., Leslie, A. M., and Firth, U. (1985). Does the autistic child have a "theory of mind"? *Cognition* 21, 37–46.

Bhat, A. N., Landa, R. J., and Galloway, J. C. (2011). Current perspectives on motor functioning in infants, children, and adults with autism spectrum disorders. *Phys. Ther.* 91, 1116–1129.

Campos, J. J., Anderson, D. I., Barbu-Roth, M. A., Hubbard, E. M., and Witherington, D. (2000). Travel broadens the mind. *Infancy* 1, 149–219.

Carpenter, M., Pennington, B. F., and Rogers, S. J. (2001). Understanding of others' intentions in children with autism and children with developmental delays. *J. Autism Dev. Disord.* 31, 589–599.

de Marchena, A., and Eigsti, I. (2010). Conversational gestures in Autism Spectrum Disorders: asynchrony but not decreased frequency. *Autism Res.* 3, 311–322.

Demos, A. P., Chaffin, R., Begosh, K. T., Daniels, J. R., and Marsh, K. L. (2012). Rocking to the beat: effects of music and partner's movements on spontaneous interpersonal coordination. *J. Exp. Psychol. Gen.* 141, 49–53.

Fitzpatrick, P. A., Schmidt, R. C., and Lockman, J. J. (1996). Dynamical patterns in the development of clapping. *Child Dev.* 67, 2691–2708.

Fournier, K. A., Hass, C. J., Naik, S. K., Lodha, N., and Cauraugh, J. H. (2010). Motor coordination in autism spectrum disorders: a synthesis and meta-analysis. *J. Autism Dev. Disord.* 40, 1227–1240.

Gepner, B., Lainé, F., and Tardif, C. (2005). E-Motion mis-sight and other temporal processing disorders in autism. *Curr. Psychol. Cogn.* 23, 104–121.

Gepner, B., and Mestre, D. R. (2002a). Brief report: postural reactivity to fast visual motion differentiates autistic from children with asperger syndrome. *J. Autism Dev. Disord.* 32, 231–238.

Gepner, B., and Mestre, D. R. (2002b). Rapid visual motion integration deficit in autism. *Trends Cogn. Sci.* 6, 455.

Gepner, B., Mestre, D. R., Masson, G., and de Schonen, S. (1995). Postural effects of motion vision in young autistic children. *Neuroreport* 6, 1211–1214.

Gernsbacher, M. A., Stevenson, J. L., Khandakar, S., and Hill-Goldsmith, H. (2008). Why does joint attention look atypical in autism? *Child Dev. Perspect.* 2, 38–45.

Ghaziuddin, M., and Butler, E. (1998). Clumsiness in autism and Asperger syndrome: a further report. *J. Intellect. Disabil. Res.* 42, 43–48.

Ghaziuddin, M., Butler, E., Tsai, L., and Ghaziuddin, N. (1994). Is clumsiness a marker for Asperger syndrome? *J. Intellect. Disabil. Res.* 38, 519–527.

Gibson, J. J. (1979). *The Ecological Approach to Visual Perception.* Hillsdale, NJ: Lawrence Erlbaum Associates.

Gowen, E., and Hamilton, A. (2013). Motor abilities in autism: a review using a computational context. *J. Autism Dev. Disord.* 43, 323–344.

Gowen, E., and Miall, R. C. (2005). Behavioural aspects of cerebellar function in adults with Asperger syndrome. *Cerebellum* 4, 279–289.

Gowen, E., Stanley, J., and Miall, R. C. (2008). Movement interference in autism-spectrum disorder. *Neuropsychologia* 46, 1060–1068.

Grossberg, S., and Seidman, D. (2006). Neural dynamics of autistic behaviors: cognitive, emotional, and timing substrates. *Psychol. Rev.* 113, 483–525.

Haken, H., Kelso, J. A. S., and Bunz, H. (1985). A theoretical model of phase transition in human hand movements. *Biol. Cybern.* 51, 347–356.

Helt, M. S., Eigsti, I.-M., Snyder, P. J., and Fein, D. A. (2010). Contagious yawning in autistic and typical development. *Child Dev.* 81, 1620–1631.

Henderson, S. E., and Sugden, D. A. (1992). *Movement Assessment Battery for Children*. London: Psychological Corporation.

Hove, M. J., and Risen, J. L. (2009). It's all in the timing: interpersonal synchrony increases affiliation. *Soc. Cogn.* 27, 949–961.

Isenhower, R. W., Marsh, K. L., Richardson, M. J., Helt, M., Schmidt, R. C., and Fein, D. (2012). Rhythmic bimanual coordination is impaired in young children with autism spectrum disorder. *Res. Autism Spectr. Disord.* 6, 25–31.

Jansiewicz, E. M., Goldberg, M. C., Newschaffer, C. J., Denckla, M. B., Landra, R., and Mostofsky, S. H. (2006). Motor signs distinguish children with high functioning autism and Asperger's syndrome from controls. *J. Autism Dev. Disord.* 36, 613–621.

Karasik, L. B., Adolph, K. E., Tamis-LeMonda, C. S., and Zuckerman, A. L. (2012). Carry on: spontaneous object carrying in 13-month-old crawling and walking infants. *Dev. Psychol.* 48, 389–397.

Kelley, E., Paul, J., Fein, D., and Naigles, L. R. (2006). Residual language deficits in optimal outcome children with a history of autism. *J. Autism Dev. Disord.* 36, 807–828.

Kelso, J. A. S. (1995). *Dynamic Patterns*. Cambridge, MA: MIT press.

Kinsbourne, M., and Helt, M. (2011). "Entrainment, mimicry, and interpersonal synchrony," in *The Neuropsychology of Autism*, ed D. A. Fein (New York, NY: Oxford University press), 339–365.

Kirschner, S., and Tomasello, M. (2009). Joint drumming: social context facilitates synchronization in preschool children. *J. Exp. Child Psychol.* 102, 299–314.

Kleinman, J. M., Robins, D. L., Ventola, P. E., Pandey, J., Boorstein, H. C., Esser, E. L., et al. (2008). The modified checklist for autism in toddlers: a follow-up study investigating the early detection of autism spectrum disorders. *J. Autism Dev. Disord.* 38, 827–839.

Kleinspehn-Ammerlahn, A., Riediger, M., Schmiedek, F., Oertzen, T. V., Li, S. C., and Lindenberger, U. (2011). Dyadic drumming across the lifespan reveals a zone of proximal development in children. *Dev. Psychol.* 4, 632–644.

Kugler, P. N., and Turvey, M. T. (1987). *Information, Natural Law, and the Self-Assembly of Rhythmic Movements*. Hillsdale, NJ: Lawrence Erlbaum Associates.

Lantero, D. A., and Ringenbach, S. D. (2007). Factors influencing children's performances of a steady-state bimanual coordination task. *Res. Q. Exerc. Sport* 80, 205–212.

Liss, M., Saulnier, C., Fein, D., and Kinsbourne, M. (2006). Sensory and attention abnormalities in autistic spectrum disorders. *Autism* 10, 155–172.

Lopresti-Goodman, S. M., Richardson, M. J., Silva, P., and Schmidt, R. C. (2008). Period basin of entrainment for unintentional visual coordination. *J. Mot. Behav.* 40, 3–10.

Lord, C., Rutter, M., DiLavore, P. C., and Risi, S. (1999). *Autism Diagnostic Observation Schedule*. Los Angeles, CA: Western Psychological Services.

Marsh, K. L. (2010). "Sociality from an ecological, dynamical perspective," in *Grounding Sociality: Neurons, Minds, and Culture*, eds G. R. Semin and G. Echterhoff (London: Psychology Press), 43–71.

Marsh, K. L., Richardson, M. J., Baron, R. M., and Schmidt, R. C. (2006). Contrasting approaches to perceiving and acting with others. *Ecol. Psychol.* 18, 1–37.

Miles, L. K., Nind, L. K., and Macrae, C. N. (2009). The rhythm of rapport: interpersonal synchrony and social perception. *J. Exp. Soc. Psychol.* 45, 585–598.

Milne, E., Swettenham, J., and Campbell, R. (2005). Motion perception and autistic spectrum disorder: a review. *Curr. Psychol. Cogn.* 23, 3–34.

Minshew, N. J., Sung, K. B., Jones, B. L., and Furman, J. M. (2004). Underdevelopment of the postural control system in autism. *Neurology* 63, 2056–2061.

Mostofsky, S. H., Dubey, P., Jerath, V. K., Jansiewicz, E. M., Goldberg, M. C., and Denckla, M. B. (2006). Developmental dyspraxia is not limited to imitation in children with autism spectrum disorders. *J. Int. Neuropsychol. Soc.* 12, 314–326.

Mullen, E. M. (1995). *Mullen Scales of Early Learning, AGS Edn*. Circle Pines, MN: American Guidance Service, Inc.

Oberman, L. M., Hubbard, E. M., McCleery, J. P., Altschuler, E. L., Ramachandran, V. S., and Pineda, J. A. (2005). EEG evidence for mirror neuron dysfunction in autism spectrum disorders. *Cogn. Brain Res.* 24, 190–198.

Press, D., Richardson, D., and Bird, G. (2010). Intact imitation of emotional facial actions in autism spectrum conditions. *Neuropsychologia* 48, 3291–3297.

Richardson, M. J., Marsh, K. L., Isenhower, R. W., Goodman, J. R. L., and Schmidt, R. C. (2007). Rocking together: dynamics of intentional and unintentional interpersonal coordination. *Hum. Mov. Sci.* 26, 867–891.

Richardson, M. J., Marsh, K. L., and Schmidt, R. C. (2005). Effects of visual and verbal interaction. *J. Exp. Psychol. Hum. Percept. Perform.* 31, 62–79.

Rizzolatti, G., and Craighero, L. (2004). The mirror-neuron system. *Annu. Rev. Neurosci.* 27, 169–192.

Robertson, S. D. (2001). Development of bimanual skill: the search for stable patterns of coordination, *J. Mot. Behav.* 33, 114–126.

Rogers, S. J., and Pennington, B. F. (1991). A theoretical approach to the deficits in infantile autism. *Dev. Psychopathol.* 3, 137–162.

Schmidt, R. C., Bienvenu, M., Fitzpatrick, P. A., and Amazeen, P. G. (1998). A comparison of intra- and interpersonal interlimb coordination: coordination breakdowns and coupling strength. *J. Exp. Psychol. Hum. Percept. Perform.* 24, 884–900.

Schmidt, R. C., Carello, C., and Turvey, M. T. (1990). Phase transitions and critical fluctuations in the visual coordination of rhythmic movements between people. *J. Exp. Psychol. Hum. Percept. Perform.* 16, 227–247.

Schmidt, R. C., and O'Brien, B. (1997). Evaluating the dynamics of unintended interpersonal coordination. *Ecol. Psychol.* 9, 189–206.

Schmidt, R. C., and Richardson, M. J. (2008). "Dynamics of interpersonal coordination," in *Coordination: Neural, Behavioural and Social Dynamics*, eds A. Fuchs and V. Jirsa (Heidelberg: Springer-Verlag), 281–308.

Schöner, G., Haken, H., and Kelso, J. A. S. (1986). A stochastic theory of phase transitions in human movement. *Biol. Cybern.* 53, 247–257.

Sebanz, N., Knoblich, G., Stumpf, L., and Prinz, W. (2005). Far from action blind: action representation in individuals with autism. *Cogn. Neuropsychol.* 22, 433–454.

Semin, G. R., and Echterhoff, G. (eds.). (2010). *Grounding Sociality: Neurons, Minds, and Culture*. London: Psychology Press.

Sternad, D., Collins, D., and Turvey, M. T. (1995). The detuning factor in the dynamics of interlimb rhythmic coordination. *Biol. Cybern.* 73, 27–35.

Turvey, M. T. (1990). Coordination. *Am. Psychol.* 45, 938–953.

Warren, W. H. (2006). The dynamics of perception and action. *Psychol. Rev.* 113, 358–389.

Williams, J., Whiten, A., and Singh, T. (2004). A systematic review of action imitation in autistic spectrum disorder. *J. Autism Dev. Disord.* 34, 285–296.

Wiltermuth, S. S. (2012). Synchrony and destructive obedience. *Soc. Influence* 7, 78–89.

Wiltermuth, S. S., and Heath, C. (2009). Synchrony and cooperation. *Psychol. Sci.* 20, 1–5.

Conflict of Interest Statement: The authors declare that the research was conducted in the absence of any commercial or financial relationships that could be construed as a potential conflict of interest.

17

Visuomotor resonance in autism spectrum disorders

Cristina Becchio[1] and Umberto Castiello[2*]

[1] Dipartimento di Psicologia, Centro di Scienza Cognitiva, Università di Torino, Turin, Italy
[2] Dipartimento di Psicologia Generale, Università di Padova, Padova, Italy

Edited by:
Elizabeth B. Torres, Rutgers University, USA

Reviewed by:
Antonio Pereira, Federal University of Rio Grande do Norte, Brazil
Raffaella I. Rumiati, Scuola Internazionale Superiore di Studi Avanzati, Italy

***Correspondence:**
Umberto Castiello, Dipartimento di Psicologia Generale, Università di Padova, Via Venezia, 8, Padova 35131, Italy.
e-mail: umberto.castiello@unipd.it

When we observe the actions performed by others, our motor system "resonates" along with that of the observed agent. Is a similar visuomotor resonant response observed in autism spectrum disorders (ASD)? Studies investigating action observation in ASD have yielded inconsistent findings. In this perspective article we examine behavioral and neuroscientific evidence in favor of visuomotor resonance in ASD, and consider the possible role of action-perception coupling in social cognition. We distinguish between different aspects of visuomotor resonance and conclude that while some aspects may be preserved in ASD, abnormalities exist in the way individuals with ASD convert visual information from observed actions into a program for motor execution. Such abnormalities, we surmise, may contribute to but also depend on the difficulties that individuals with ASD encounter during social interaction.

Keywords: autism, visuomotor resonance, motor facilitation, mirror system, social cognition

INTRODUCTION

When we observe the actions performed by others, our motor system "resonates" along with that of the observed agent. The prevalent assumption in the literature is that this motor resonance to others' actions depends on a common coding for action execution and observation: observing the actions of others activates, within the observer's motor system, the same motor programs used to execute the observed actions (see Blakemore and Frith, 2005, for a review). Is a similar visuomotor resonant response observed in autism spectrum disorders (ASD)? In the following, we review evidence in favor of visuomotor resonance in neurotypical and participants with ASD. First, we consider evidence stemming from behavioral and neuroscientific methods. Following this groundwork, we examine some of the factors that, by modulating visuomotor resonance, may help integrating apparently divergent findings. Finally, we consider the possible role of visuomotor resonance in social cognition. We speculate that, in accordance with associative proposals, abnormalities in visuomotor resonance may contribute to, but also depend on the difficulties that individuals with ASD encounter during social interaction.

MOTOR FACILITATION AND INTERFERENCE BY ACTION OBSERVATION

WHEN ACTION OBSERVATION FACILITATES ACTION EXECUTION

Interactions between action observation and action execution can be tested by looking at compatibility effects during movement execution and observation paradigms. If action execution and observation share a common coding, then observing an action should *facilitate* motor performance of a similar action. In accordance with this hypothesis, in neurotypical participants reaction times to initiate a tapping action have been shown to be faster in response to the observation of a task-irrelevant congruent movement (tapping a finger) than in response to the observation of a task-irrelevant incongruent movement (lifting a finger; e.g., Brass et al., 2000, 2001). Similarly, reaction times to initiate a grasping action have been demonstrated to be faster following the observation of a photograph of the final hand posture necessary for the grasping action relative to an incompatible hand posture (Craighero et al., 2002). These compatibility effects have been replicated for various pairs of actions, with both static action stimuli (stills depicting the end of the movement) and dynamic action stimuli (videos), in choice and simple reaction time tasks (for review, see Heyes, 2011). Using a choice reaction time task, Bird et al. (2007) report that ASD participants show an equivalent compatibility effect: responses on compatible trials (e.g., performing an opening hand movement after observing a hand in an opening position) were faster than those on incompatible trials (e.g., performing an opening hand movement after observing a hand in a closing position). As for typically developing controls, the compatibility effect was greater when responses were made to human than to robotic hand postures. These findings have been interpreted as motor facilitation in terms of faster response initiation when there is high compatibility of topographical features of task-irrelevant action stimuli and the prepared action; however, an equally plausible interpretation is that response initiation is delayed when the topographical features of task-irrelevant action stimuli are incompatible with the movement being prepared (Blakemore and Frith, 2005; Heyes, 2011). Evidence that compatibility effects are due, at least in part, to interference rather than facilitation comes from studies showing that responding is slower in imitatively incompatible trials than in baseline trials where the task-relevant cue is presented in the absence of a task-irrelevant movement stimulus (Brass et al., 2000; Bertenthal et al., 2006; Gillmeister et al., 2008).

An alternative approach to motor facilitation, taken by Castiello et al. (2002) and Edwards et al. (2003), has been to investigate motor priming by observation of prehensile movements. Neurotypical participants observed a grasping action directed to an object (e.g., a small object) and then had to grasp either the same object (small object) or a different object (large object). Results revealed a reliable priming effect on the kinematics of the reach-to-grasp movements. Reaching was faster and grasping was more precise when the observed object was the same size as the object to be reached, suggesting that observation of an action facilitated subsequent execution of a matching action.

Using a similar visuomotor priming paradigm, Pierno et al. (2006) found that motor facilitation is impaired in participants with ASD. Whereas typically developing children showed facilitation effects in terms of movement speed following the observation of the model grasping or simply gazing at an object, children with autism did not show any motor facilitation from action or gaze (Pierno et al., 2006). These findings suggest that, in contrast to typically developing children, in children with ASD information from others' gaze and action fails to automatically modulate motor execution. A subsequent study by Pierno et al. (2008) reports motor facilitation for robotic but not for human hand movements: children with autism were facilitated—as revealed by a faster movement duration and an anticipated peak velocity—when primed by a robotic but not by a human arm movement. The opposite pattern was found for typically developing controls (see **Figure 1**).

WHEN ACTION OBSERVATION INTERFERES WITH ACTION EXECUTION

If the motor system is geared up to execute observed movement, this should result in *interference* when the observed movement is qualitatively different from the performed movement. This has been demonstrated for simultaneous movement performance-observation (Kilner et al., 2003; see also, Stanley et al., 2007; Hardwick and Edwards, 2012). Kilner et al. (2003) asked participants to make either horizontal or vertical intransitive and continuous arm movements in time with the movements of an experimenter so that the two peoples' movements were either congruent (i.e., both moving in the same plane) or incongruent (i.e., participant moving their arm in plane perpendicular to that of experimenter). Finger tip movement variability (as measured in the orthogonal plane) was greater in the orthogonal plane for incongruent than for congruent conditions. A similar pattern of interference has been reported during observation of moving dot stimuli when the participants were informed that they were observing prerecorded human movement (Stanley et al., 2007).

Using the same paradigm, Gowen et al. (2008) found an equivalent interference effect in control participants and participants with ASD: both groups displayed greater error plane deviation during incongruent compared to congruent trials. Compared to control participants, however, ASD participants showed a different pattern of movement variability (calculated by summing congruent and incongruent error plane deviation). Whereas control participants made generally more variable movements during observation of biological dot motion stimuli than during observation of arm movements, the reverse was true for ASD participants. These results may indicate reduced visuomotor integration in ASD so that the visual properties of the observed dot motion are less efficiently integrated into the

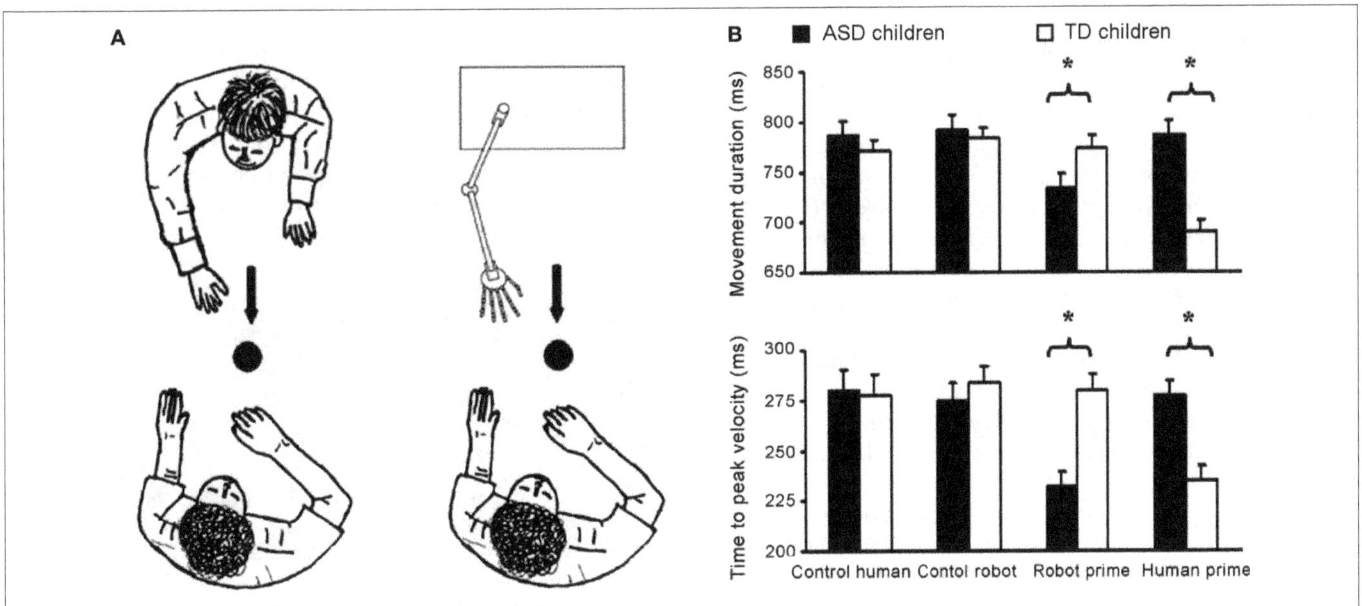

FIGURE 1 | Motor facilitation for robotic but not for human hand movements. (A) Experimental set up. Participants were requested to observe either a human or a robotic arm model performing a reach-to-grasp action toward a spherical object. Subsequently, they were asked to perform the same action toward the same object. Two "control" conditions in which participants performed the movement in the presence of either the static human or robot model were also included. **(B)** Graphical representation of the significant interaction between group (autistic children, typically developing children) and condition (control human, control robot, robot prime, and human prime) for movement duration and time to peak velocity. For the normally developing children movement duration was shorter and the time to peak velocity was reached earlier for the "human prime" than for the "robot prime" and the two "control" conditions ($ps < 0.001$). For the children with ASD movement duration was shorter and time to peak velocity was earlier for the "robot prime" than for the "human" and the two "control" conditions ($ps < 0.001$). Bars represent the standard errors of the means. Asterisks indicate significance for the main contrasts of interest (adapted from Pierno et al., 2008).

executed movement during continuous movement execution and observation paradigms.

Becchio et al. (2007) found that in comparison with matched, typically developing controls, children with ASD are immune to motor interference in the form of transfer of distractor-mediated effects. In a series of experiments, participants observed a model reaching toward an object presented in isolation or flanked by a distractor object. Immediately after the completion of the model's action, they were asked to perform the same action on the same object, but in absence of the distractor object. Despite the distractor being removed, distractor-mediated effects were evident in the kinematics of typically developing children. Consistent with prior evidence, transfer of interference was also present when the model simply looked at the target in the presence of the distractor object, suggesting that, even in the absence of any overtly executed action, motor intentions read in other's people gaze may cause interference effects (Castiello, 2003). In contrast, children with ASD did not show any interference effect either from action or from gaze observation.

Immunity from the effects of a gaze-based social context is further confirmed by Schilbach et al. (2011) showing that individuals with ASD are not susceptible to the modulatory effect of gaze cues in a stimulus response compatibility paradigm. Participants were asked to generate spatially congruent or incongruent motor responses to changes in a face, a face-like and an object stimulus. Whereas in the comparison group being looked at by a virtual other led to a reduction of reaction time costs associated with generating a spatially incongruent response, this effect was not observed in the ASD group.

MIRROR EFFECTS TO ACTION OBSERVATION

At a neural level support for the common coding hypothesis comes from studies showing that action observation recruits the observer's motor system. Evidence for common coding has been found at the level of single neurons, the so-called mirror neurons, in the premotor cortex of macaque monkeys (for review, see Rizzolatti and Sinigaglia, 2010). In humans, the first demonstration of covert motor activation during action observation was provided by Fadiga et al. (1995) using transcranial magnetic stimulation (TMS). TMS was applied to the sector of primary motor cortex (M1) that represents the hand, and motor-evoked potentials (MEPs) were recorded from contralateral hand muscles during the passive observation of hand movements. Observing hand actions determined an enhancement of MEPs in the same muscular groups used in executing those actions (for review, see Fadiga et al., 2005). Corticospinal facilitation during action observation has since been replicated in numerous studies, and it is now well-established that in neurotypical observers the mere observation of others' actions modulates the excitability of the observer's corticospinal circuitry involved in the execution of the same movements (e.g., Strafella and Paus, 2000; Aziz-Zadeh et al., 2002; Maeda et al., 2002; Urgesi et al., 2006; Cavallo et al., 2012). Applying TMS over M1 during observation of intransitive, meaningless finger movements, Théoret et al. (2005) found that overall modulation of M1 excitability during action observation is significantly lower in individuals with ASD compared with matched controls.

Along the same lines, abnormalities in the neural mechanism matching action observation and execution in ASD have been reported using electroencephalography (EEG; Oberman et al., 2005, 2008; Martineau et al., 2008), magnetoencephalography (MEG; Nishitani et al., 2004) and functional magnetic resonance imaging (fMRI; Williams et al., 2006; Martineau et al., 2010). Oberman et al. (2005) found that in comparison to typically developing controls, mu wave suppression—an index of mirror neuron activity—is reduced in ASD during action observation. Nishitani et al. (2004) report abnormalities in the cortical activation chain of ASD participants while they imitate orofacial gestures. MEG responses were normal in strength and timing at the early steps of the sequence, that is, in occipital and superior temporal sulcus regions. The main abnormality was observed in mirror areas including the inferior frontal gyrus. Inferior frontal gyrus activations were spatially more scattered in ASD than control participants, and the signals were delayed and reduced in strength. Using fMRI, Martineau et al. (2010) found atypical activation in ASD during observation of human movement in various cerebral areas, including the motor cortex, the inferior frontal gyrus (pars opercularis), the parietal lobule, and the precuneus. There is also evidence that ASD adults exhibit structural abnormalities in cortical thickness in areas related to action observation (Hadjikhani et al., 2006; see **Figure 2**).

Other studies, however, fail to report functional abnormalities to action observation. Using EEG, Raymaekers et al. (2009) found significant mu wave suppression to self and observed movements in both high-functioning ASD children and typically developing children. Similarly, Fan et al. (2010) report that mu suppression over sensorimotor cortex when watching hand actions did not significantly differ in ASD and control participants. Oberman et al. (2008) found that mu suppression is sensitive to the degree of familiarity: in contrast to typically developing children, children with ASD show mu suppression but only when they can identify in some personal way with the observed movements

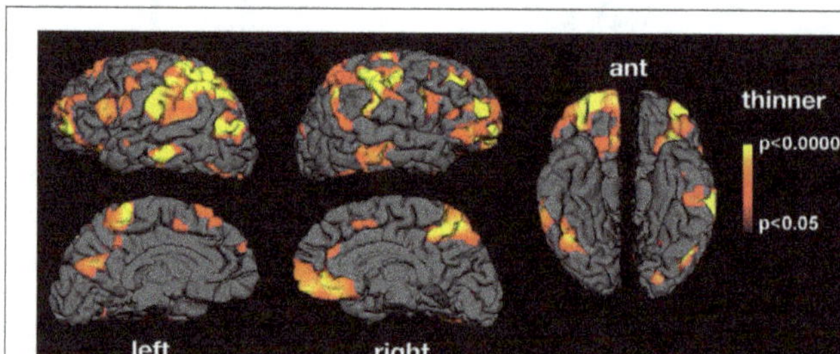

FIGURE 2 | Mean thickness difference significance maps. Lateral, medial, and ventral views of the brain showing areas presenting cortical thinning in the autism group compared with neurotypical controls. Significant thinning was found in areas belonging to the MNS (inferior frontal gyrus, inferior parietal lobule, and superior temporal sulcus) as well as in areas involved in facial expression production and recognition (face regions in sensory and motor cortex and in middle temporal gyrus), imitation (superior parietal lobule), and social cognition (prefrontal cortex, anterior cingulate, medial parietal cortex, supramarginal gyrus, and middle and inferior temporal cortex; from Hadjikhani et al., 2006).

(i.e., when observing their own movement or the movement of a familiar person).

ON AND BEYOND THE BROKEN MIRROR HYPOTHESIS

Do individuals with ASD resonate to others' actions? The research discussed above identifies a number of effects that are preserved in ASD: individuals with ASD show compatibility effects to task-irrelevant action stimuli, demonstrate motor interference for simultaneous execution-observation of meaningless arm-movements, exhibited mu suppression when watching others actions (but see Oberman et al., 2005). Other features of the visuomotor resonant response, however, appear to be absent or abnormal. Below we consider some of the factors that modulate visuomotor resonance in neurotypical individuals and that, in our opinion, can be of help in interpreting apparently divergent results in ASD.

MOTOR HIERARCHY

In accordance with the idea that the motor system is hierarchically organized (Grafton and Hamilton, 2007), motor resonance has been proposed to operate at different levels (Blakemore and Frith, 2005). At the lowest level there is resonance to movements as long as these are made (or believed to be made, see Stanley et al., 2007) by biological entities. At a higher level there is resonance to specific goal-directed actions. At an even higher level, motor resonance may be caused by intentions. Observer with ASD may resonate to others' action at some levels (goal, e.g., Bird et al., 2007), but not at other levels (intention; Pierno et al., 2006; Becchio et al., 2007).

BIOLOGICAL TUNING

A number of studies have demonstrated that, in neurotypical observers, human movements produce larger visuomotor resonance than artificial, impossible, or robotic movements (Castiello et al., 2002; Tai et al., 2004; Longo et al., 2008; Longo and Bertenthal, 2009; Liepelt and Brass, 2010). This been proposed to reflect tuning to both the form and kinematic profile of human movements (Press, 2011). Apparently divergent results in ASD may be interpreted assuming that observers with ASD are sensitive to the form (Bird et al., 2007), but not by the kinematics of the human movement (Pierno et al., 2006; Becchio et al., 2007). The finding of robotic tuning (Pierno et al., 2008) raise the interesting possibilities that observers with ASD might be more responsive to robotic than human kinematics.

INPUT/OUTPUT MODULATION

Visuomotor resonance is modulated by changes in spatial attention and feature selection (input modulation), as well as by social cognitive processes influencing the extent to which motor activation is inhibited or allowed to influence overt behavioral performance (output modulation; for review, see Heyes, 2011). Differences in the way observers with ASD distribute their attentional resources and process social stimuli may help to explain differences in motor resonance to different features of actions. For example, differences in output modulation by emotional cues have been observed for imitative movements (Grecucci et al., in press). Whereas typically developing controls showed a strong modulation (i.e., faster responses) of imitative responses when primed by social/emotional cues, children with ASD did not. The finding that gaze does not modulate motor facilitation and interference effects in ASD (Pierno et al., 2006; Becchio et al., 2007; Schilbach et al., 2011) adds to this view, suggesting that inability to read motor intention from gaze direction might contribute to abnormalities in the way visual information from observed actions is converted into a program for motor execution. It remains unclear whether the degree of familiarity is critical for the visuomotor resonant response to occur (Oberman et al., 2008).

HETEROGENEITY OF THE ASD POPULATION

We know little about whether and how visuomotor resonance varies across the different diagnostic subcategories of ASDs. Some aspects of motor functioning and motion perception appear to vary across different clinical subpopulations within the autism spectrum (for review, see Kaiser and Shiffrar, 2009; Bhat et al., 2011). For example, there is evidence that, during the perception of locally oriented patterns, observers with high functioning autism show elevated motion coherence thresholds relative to typical observers, whereas observers with Asperger Syndrome do not (Spencer and O'Brien, 2006; Tsermentseli et al., 2008). Moreover, although both children with ASD and typically developing children show decreasing motion coherence thresholds with increasing age, this trend appears to be more pronounced for observers with ASD (Kaiser and Shiffrar, 2009). Diagnostic heterogeneity between subjects as well as age related differences might thus contribute to some of the variability of results across studies investigating visuomotor resonance.

VISUOMOTOR RESONANCE IN THE CONTEXT OF SOCIAL INTERACTION

To date, researchers have specifically emphasized the potential contribution of visuomotor abnormalities to deficits in social cognition associated with autism. Dysfunction of visuomotor resonance mechanisms early in development may give rise to deficits in imitation (Iacoboni and Dapretto, 2006). It may underlie deficits in intention recognition (Cattaneo et al., 2007) and empathy (Gallese, 2006). Finally, by disrupting embodied simulation, dysfunction of visuomotor resonance may contribute to deficits related to more sophisticated mental abilities such as theory of mind and language (Oberman and Ramachandran, 2007). All these potential functions consider the role of visuomotor integration in social and communicative deficits in ASD. However, to the extent that the visuomotor resonance is forged by experience, abnormalities in visuomotor resonance may not only contribute to, but also depend on the difficulties that individuals with ASD encounter during social interaction.

This hypothesis is supported by recent findings suggesting that sensorimotor experience can enhance (Press et al., 2007), abolish (Heyes et al., 2005), and even reverse (Catmur et al., 2007, 2008) visuomotor resonance in human subjects. For example, training to perform one action (e.g., little finger movement) while observing another action (index finger movement) can reverse TMS-induced muscle-specific activation, so that after training the observation of index finger movement produces more activity in little finger than in index finger muscles (Catmur et al., 2007). In line with associative sequence learning models, this suggests that visuomotor resonance can be readily transformed by sensorimotor experience (Heyes, 2010).

Because in naturalistic settings much of sensorimotor experience is obtained through interaction with others, experiences that differ from those typically encountered during life may reconfigure the sensory-motor integration and change the way it operates. In this view, social deficits in ASD may play a constitutive role in abnormalities in visuomotor resonance. If abnormalities exist in the way individuals with ASD connect observed and executed movements, this might be, at least in part, because deficits in social interaction hinder sensorimotor learning.

ACKNOWLEDGMENTS

Cristina Becchio was supported by a grant from the Regione Piemonte, bando Scienze Umane e Sociali 2008, L.R. n.4/2006. Umberto Castiello was supported by a grant from the (MIUR).

REFERENCES

Aziz-Zadeh, L., Maeda, F., Zaidel, E., Mazziotta, J., and Iacoboni, M. (2002). Lateralization in motor facilitation during action observation: a TMS study. *Exp. Brain Res.* 144, 127–131.

Becchio, C., Pierno, A., Mari, M., Lusher, D., and Castiello, U. (2007). Motor contagion from gaze: the case of autism. *Brain* 130, 2401–2411.

Bertenthal, B. I., Longo, M. R., and Kosobud, A. (2006). Imitative response tendencies following observation of intransitive actions. *J. Exp. Psychol. Hum. Percept. Perform.* 32, 210–225.

Bhat, A. N., Landa, R. J., and Galloway, J. C. (2011). Current perspectives on motor functioning in infants, children, and adults with autism spectrum disorders. *Phys. Ther.* 91, 1116–1129.

Bird, G., Leighton, J., Press, C., and Heyes, C. (2007). Intact automatic imitation of human and robot actions in autism spectrum disorders. *Proc. Biol. Sci.* 274, 3027–3031.

Blakemore, S.-J., and Frith, C. D. (2005). The role of motor contagion in the prediction of action. *Neuropsychologia* 43, 260–267.

Brass, M., Bekkering, H., and Prinz, W. (2001). Movement observation affects movement execution in a simple response task. *Acta Psychol.* 106, 3–22.

Brass, M., Bekkering, H., Wohlschlager, A., and Prinz, W. (2000). Compatibility between observed and executed finger movements: comparing symbolic, spatial, and imitative cues. *Brain Cogn.* 44, 124–143.

Castiello, U. (2003). Understanding other's people actions: intention and attention. *J. Exp. Psychol. Hum. Percept. Perform.* 29, 416–430.

Castiello, U., Lusher, D., Mari, M., Edwards, M. G., and Humphreys, G. W. (2002). "Observing a human or a robotic hand grasping an object: differential motor priming effects," in *Common Mechanisms in Perception and Action: Attention and Performance XIX*, eds W. Prinz and B. Hommel (New York, NY: Oxford University Press), 315–333.

Catmur, C., Gillmeister, H., Bird, G., Liepelt, R., Brass, M., and Heyes, C. (2008). Through the looking glass: counter-mirror activation following incompatible sensorimotor learning. *Eur. J. Neurosci.* 28, 1208–1215.

Catmur, C., Walsh, V., and Heyes, C. (2007). Sensorimotor learning configures the human mirror system. *Curr. Biol.* 17, 1527–1531.

Cattaneo, L., Fabbri-Destro, M., Boria, S., Pieraccini, C., Monti, A., Cossu, G., et al. (2007). Impairment of actions chains in autism and its possible role in intention understanding. *Proc. Natl. Acad. Sci. U.S.A.* 104, 17825–17830.

Cavallo, A., Becchio, C., Sartori, L., Castiello, U. (2012). Grasping with tools: corticospinal excitability reflects observed hand movements. *Cereb. Cortex* 22, 710–716.

Craighero, L., Bello, A., Fadiga, L., and Rizzolatti, G. (2002). Hand action preparation influences the response to hand pictures. *Neuropsychologia* 40, 492–502.

Edwards, M. G., Humphreys, G. W., and Castiello, U. (2003). Motor facilitation following action observation: a behavioural study in prehensile action. *Brain Cogn.* 53, 495–502.

Fadiga, L., Craighero, L., and Olivier, E. (2005). Human motor cortex excitability during the perception of others' action. *Curr. Opin. Neurobiol.* 15, 213–218.

Fadiga, L., Fogassi, L., Pavesi, G., and Rizzolatti, G. (1995). Motor facilitation during action observation: a magnetic stimulation study. *J. Neurophysiol.* 73, 2608–2611.

Fan, Y.-T., Decety, J., Yang, C.-Y., Liu, J.-L., and Chen, Y. (2010). Unbroken mirror neurons in autism spectrum disorders. *J. Child Psychol. Psychiatry* 51, 981–988.

Gallese, V. (2006). Intentional attunement: a neurophysiological perspective on social cognition and its disruption in autism. *Brain Res. Rev.* 1079, 15–24.

Gillmeister, H., Catmur, C., Liepelt, R., Brass, M., and Heyes, C. M. (2008). Experience-based priming of body parts: a study of action imitation. *Brain Res.* 1217, 157–170.

Gowen, E., Stanley, J., and Miall, R. C. (2008). Movement interference in autism-spectrum disorder. *Neuropsychologia* 46, 1060–1068.

Grafton, S. T., and Hamilton, A. F. de C. (2007). Evidence for a distributed hierarchy of action representation in the brain. *Hum. Mov. Sci.* 26, 590–616.

Grecucci, A., Siugzdaite, R., Londero, D., Fabbro, F., Brambilla, P., and Rumiati, R. I. (in press). Emotional resonance deficits in autistic children. *J. Autism Dev. Disord.*

Hadjikhani, N., Joseph, R. M., Snyder, J., and Tager-Flusberg, H. (2006). Anatomical differences in the mirror neuron system and social cognition network in autism. *Cereb. Cortex* 16, 1276–1282.

Hardwick, R. M., and Edwards, M. G. (2012). Motor interference and facilitation arising from observed movement kinematics. *Q. J. Exp. Psychol.* 65, 840–847.

Heyes, C. (2010). Where do mirror neurons come from? *Neurosci. Biobehav. Rev.* 34, 575–583.

Heyes, C. (2011). Automatic imitation. *Psychol. Bull.* 137, 463–483.

Heyes, C., Bird, G., Johnson, H., and Haggard, P. (2005). Experience modulates automatic imitation. *Cogn. Brain Res.* 22, 233–240.

Iacoboni, M., and Dapretto, M. (2006). The mirror neuron system and the consequences of its dysfunction. *Nat. Rev. Neurosci.* 7, 942–951.

Kaiser, M. D., and Shiffrar, M. (2009). The visual perception of motion by observers with autism spectrum disorders: a review and synthesis. *Psychon. Bull. Rev.* 16, 761–777.

Kilner, J. M., Paulignan, Y., and Blakemore, S. J. (2003). An interference effect of observed biological movement on action. *Curr. Biol.* 13, 522–525.

Liepelt, R., and Brass, M. (2010). Top-down modulation of motor priming by belief about animacy. *Exp. Psychol.* 57, 221–227.

Longo, M. R., and Bertenthal, B. I. (2009). Attention modulates the specificity of automatic imitation to human actors. *Exp. Brain Res.* 192, 739–744.

Longo, M. R., Kosobud, A., and Bertenthal, B. I. (2008). Automatic imitation of biomechanically possible and impossible actions: effects of priming movements versus goals. *J. Exp. Psychol. Hum. Percept. Perform.* 34, 489–501.

Maeda, F., Kleiner-Fisman, G., and Pascual-Leone, A. (2002). Motor facilitation while observing hand actions: specificity of the effect and role of observer's orientation. *J. Neurophysiol.* 87, 1329–1335.

Martineau, J., Andersson, F., Barthélémy, C., Cottier, J. P., and Destrieux, C. (2010). Atypical activation of the mirror neuron system during perception of hand motion in autism. *Brain Res.* 1320, 168–175.

Martineau, J., Cochin, S., Magné, R., and Barthélémy, C. (2008). Impaired cortical activation in autistic children: is the mirror neuron system involved? *Int. J. Psychophysiol.* 68, 35–40.

Nishitani, N., Avikainen, S., and Hari, R. (2004). Abnormal imitation-related cortical activation sequences in Asperger's syndrome. *Ann. Neurol.* 55, 558–562.

Oberman, L. M., Hubbard, E. M., McCleery, J. P., Altschuler, E. L., Ramachandran, V. S., and Pineda, J. A. (2005). EEG evidence for mirror neuron dysfunction in autism spectrum disorders. *Cogn. Brain Res.* 24, 190–198.

Oberman, L. M., and Ramachandran, V. S. (2007). The simulating social mind: the role of simulation in the social and communicative deficits of autism spectrum disorders. *Psychol. Bull.* 133, 310–327.

Oberman, L. M., Ramachandran, V. S., and Pineda, J. A. (2008). Modulation of mu suppression in children with autism spectrum disorders in response to familiar or unfamiliar stimuli: the mirror neuron hypothesis. *Neuropsychologia* 46, 1558–1565.

Pierno, A. C., Mari, M., Georgiou, I., Glover, S., and Castiello, U. (2006). Failure to read motor intentions from gaze in children with autism. *Neuropsychologia* 44, 1483–1488.

Pierno, A. C., Mari, M., Lusher, D., and Castiello, U. (2008). Robotic movement elicits visuomotor priming in children with autism. *Neuropsychologia* 46, 448–454.

Press, C. (2011). Action observation and robotic agents: learning and anthropomorphism. *Neurosci. Biobehav. Rev.* 35, 1410–1418.

Press, C., Gillmeister, H., and Heyes, C. (2007). Sensorimotor experience enhances automatic imitation of robotic action. *Proc. Biol. Sci.* 274, 2509–2514.

Raymaekers, R., Wiersema, J. R., and Roeyers, H. (2009). EEG study of the mirror neuron system in children with high functioning autism. *Brain Res.* 1304, 113–121.

Rizzolatti, G., and Sinigaglia, C. (2010). The functional role of the parieto-frontal mirror circuit: interpretations and misinterpretations. *Nat. Rev. Neurosci.* 11, 264–274.

Schilbach, L., Eickhoff, S. B., Cieslik, E. C., Kuzmanovic, B., and Vogeley, K. (2011). Shall we do this together? Social gaze influences action control in a comparison group, but not in individuals with high-functioning autism. *Autism* 16, 151–162.

Spencer, J. V., and O'Brien, J. M. D. (2006). Visual form-processing deficits in autism. *Perception* 35, 1047–1055.

Stanley, J., Gowen, E., and Miall, R. C. (2007). Effects of agency on movement interference during observation of a moving dot stimulus. *J. Exp. Psychol. Hum. Percept. Perform.* 33, 915–926.

Strafella, A. P., and Paus, T. (2000). Modulation of cortical excitability during action observation: a transcranial magnetic stimulation study. *Neuroreport* 11, 2289–2292.

Tai, Y. F., Scherfler, C., Brooks, D. J., Sawamoto, N., and Castiello, U. (2004). The human premotor cortex is 'mirror' only for biological actions. *Curr. Biol.* 14, 117–120.

Théoret, H., Halligan, E., Kobayashi, M., Fregni, F., Tager-Flusberg, H., and Pascual-Leone, A. (2005). Impaired motor facilitation during action observation in individuals with autism spectrum disorder. *Curr. Biol.* 15, R84–R85.

Tsermentseli, S., O'Brien, J. M., and Spencer, J. V. (2008). Comparison of form and motion coherence processing in autistic spectrum disorders and dyslexia. *J. Autism Dev. Disord.* 38, 1201–1210.

Urgesi, C., Moro, V., Candidi, M., and Aglioti, S. M. (2006). Mapping implied body actions in the human motor system. *J. Neurosci.* 26, 7942–7949.

Williams, J. H., Waiter, G. D., Gilchrist, A., Perrett, D. I., Murray, A. D., and Whiten, A. (2006). Neural mechanisms of imitation and 'mirror neuron' functioning in autistic spectrum disorder. *Neuropsychologia* 44, 610–621.

Conflict of Interest Statement: The authors declare that the research was conducted in the absence of any commercial or financial relationships that could be construed as a potential conflict of interest.

18

Gait analysis of teenagers and young adults diagnosed with autism and severe verbal communication disorders

Michael J. Weiss[1]*, Matthew F. Moran[2], Mary E. Parker[3] and John T. Foley[4]

[1] Department of Psychology, Fairfield University, Fairfield, CT, USA
[2] Department of Physical Therapy and Human Movement Science, Sacred Heart University, Fairfield, CT, USA
[3] Department of Physical Therapy, Texas State University, San Marcos, TX, USA
[4] Physical Activity Laboratory, Department of Physical Education, State University of New York at Cortland, Cortland, NY, USA

Edited by:
Anne M. Donnellan, University of San Diego, USA

Reviewed by:
Antonio Pereira, Federal University of Rio Grande do Norte, Brazil
A. Blythe LaGasse, Colorado State University, USA

***Correspondence:**
Michael J. Weiss, Department of Psychology, Fairfield University, Bannow Hall, 1073 North Benson Road, Fairfield, CT 06824, USA.
e-mail: mweiss@fairfield.edu

Both movement differences and disorders are common within autism spectrum disorders (ASD). These differences have wide and heterogeneous variability among different ages and sub-groups all diagnosed with ASD. Gait was studied in a more homogeneously identified group of nine teenagers and young adults who scored as "severe" in both measures of verbal communication and overall rating of Autism on the Childhood Autism Rating Scales (CARS). The ASD individuals were compared to a group of typically developing university undergraduates of similar ages. All participants walked a distance of 6-meters across a GAITRite (GR) electronic walkway for six trials. The ASD and comparison groups differed widely on many spatiotemporal aspects of gait including: step and stride length, foot positioning, cadence, velocity, step time, gait cycle time, swing time, stance time, and single and double support time. Moreover, the two groups differed in the percentage of the total gait cycle in each of these phases. The qualitative rating of "Body Use" on the CARS also indicated severe levels of unusual body movement for all of the ASD participants. These findings demonstrate that older teens and young adults with "severe" forms of Verbal Communication Impairments and Autism differ widely in their gait from typically developing individuals. The differences found in the current investigation are far more pronounced compared to previous findings with younger and/or less severely involved individuals diagnosed with ASD as compared to typically developing controls. As such, these data may be a useful anchor-point in understanding the trajectory of development of gait specifically and motor functions generally.

Keywords: autism spectrum disorders, gait, motor control, verbal communication disorders, movement disorders

INTRODUCTION

Movement disorders among individuals with an Autism Spectrum Disorder (ASD) have been gaining greater attention over recent years. Historically, movement disorders have been considered from two diagnostic perspectives. Primarily, forms of unusual movement have been characterized as one of the fundamental characteristics of ASD as a "narrow range of actions or interests" [Diagnostic and Statistical Manual of the American Psychiatric Association, 4th Edition—Revised, (DSM-4-R, 2000)]. Secondarily, "odd" movements have been described as an "associated feature" of ASD or in more extreme presentations a diagnosis of catatonia has been rendered (Wing and Shah, 2000, 2006). In either instance, little has been understood or studied in relation to *why* individuals diagnosed with ASD present with a wide array of differences in their movement and what relation these movement patterns may have to understanding the underlying etiology of the disorders.

The presentation of aberrant movements in ASD has been apparent from the first inception of the diagnosis (Kanner, 1943). Movement disorders have included a wide range of differences such as greater clumsiness, motor coordination abnormalities, postural control impairments and instability, hypotonia, muscle rigidity, akinesia, and bradykinesia, and more (Damasio and Maurer, 1978; Jones and Prior, 1985; Bauman, 1992; Kohen-Raz et al., 1992; Leary and Hill, 1996; Rogers et al., 1996; Rapin, 1997; Ghaziuddin and Butler, 1998; Molloy et al., 2003; Minshew et al., 2004; Donnellan et al., 2006, 2010). However, there is a growing number of researchers who have characterized disorders of movement as fundamental aspects of ASD (Leary and Hill, 1996; Donnellan et al., 2010; Fournier et al., 2010). This is a non-trivial distinction implying that differences in movement may offer clues to the underlying etiology of ASD, rather than simply being "associated" with the diagnosis.

The study of gait has been one domain of movement that has drawn interest for a number of years in this population. However, the relatively small numbers of empirical studies of gait that have been reported have varied in the methodologies and technologies used, participant ages, sample sizes, and ASD subtypes that have been studied (Vilensky et al., 1981; Hallett et al., 1993; Vernazza-Martin et al., 2005; Rinehart et al., 2006a,b; Calhoun et al., 2011; Esposito et al., 2011). Hence, it is not surprising that these reports have offered mixed findings in the extent and types of movement differences that have been found across these different individuals.

In considering some of the differing accounts of gait in this population, we are struck by two trends. First, every group of individuals diagnosed with an ASD who have participated in studies of gait show some form of movement differences as compared to typically developing control participants. This is consistent with Leary and Hill's (1996); Fournier et al.'s (2010) and Donnellan et al.'s (2010) similar conclusions that movement differences are pervasive among the entire population and as such should be thought of as a core deficit or difference in ASD.

Second, preliminary considerations indicate possible trends regarding the types of differences found in gait patterns correlating with the type of ASD that participants present with. Fournier et al. (2010) concluded that the pervasive differences in motor functions are not related to intelligence, to which we agree. However, there may be a correlation between the extent or type of differences found in gait as a function of the form or severity of the ASD diagnosis. By "severity" we are referring to the extent of difficulties in the so called "core deficits" of Autism—disorders or differences in communication, social interactions and range of actions and interests. Bear in mind that cognitive status has never been considered a "core deficit," though ability to perform on any standardized cognitive test will co-vary with communication, social interaction and range of action skills (Zelazo et al., 1989; Zelazo and Weiss, 1990). Hence, we should be considering relations between the criteria of ASD such as the type of communication disorders a person presents with and movement patterns, rather than cognition, *per se*.

The few studies of gait that have been reported to date raise a question of whether a relation exists between types of movement differences shown by differing sub-groups of individuals on the Autism Spectrum and the extent of communication impairments. Vilensky et al. (1981) reported significant differences in a number of spatial and temporal parameters of gait between ASD and control participants. ASD participants in this study were described as having profound disorders of communication and social relatedness. Alternatively, Vernazza-Martin et al. (2005), whose participants' also presented with significant communication differences, found only relatively minor differences in spatiotemporal parameters of gait, *per se*. However, they found significant and meaningful variations or "oscillations" of the head, shoulders and trunk causing less stability and greater variability in posture as they walked. A series of other studies of individuals diagnosed with "High Functioning" Autism and/or Asperger Syndrome reported only minor variations in spatiotemporal parameters of gait, but reported significant variations in coordination, smoothness, consistency, and posture of the arms, head and trunk (Rinehart et al., 2006a,b), other parameters of posture and hypotonia associated with gait (Calhoun et al., 2011), or a generalized "clumsiness" among ASD participants as they walked (Hallett et al., 1993).

It is indeed likely that we will learn much from differentiating the gait patterns associated with differences among subtypes of ASD. Hence, it would be useful to segregate more precise descriptors of participants in the study of movement differences in those aspects of development associated with the diagnosis, such as specific descriptors of their social and language skills, or the types of narrow or repetitive range of actions and interests that these individuals show. Terms such as "high functioning" are routinely used in reference to cognitive status, which does not characterize the ASD diagnosis, *per se*. Similarly, the inclusion of an array of participants who share an ASD diagnosis, but have widely varied measures of communication, social or intellectual functions, needs to be differentiated if we are to tease out precise correlations with movement functions.

It is parenthetically interesting that Kern et al. (2010) demonstrated that the degree of "severity" in the ASD diagnosis has been shown to correlate with muscle strength. Similarly, Travers et al. (2012) found a correlation between ASD symptom severity and postural stability. These reports, coupled with the variations in reports of gait described above, indicate a need to differentiate the movement patterns of individuals who differ in their specific forms of ASD. Clearly, there is a need to unpack both the different aspects of movement that can be characterized, as well as clarifying the developmental presentations across the range of individuals who have an ASD diagnosis.

The intention of our current study was to evaluate gait patterns among a group of individuals diagnosed with ASD using narrowly defined *a priori* selection criteria of "severe" presentations of ASD in general and severe impairments in Verbal Communication specifically, among a group of older teenagers and young adults. We singled out the criteria of severe Verbal Communication impairments precisely because it is fundamental to the ASD diagnosis and because we wanted to look at the most extreme form of that criterion. We hypothesized that individuals with severe forms of Verbal Communication disorders would show widespread quantitative and qualitative aberrations in gait and other movement patterns reflected in CARS "body use" ratings, as compared to control participants of similar age and gender.

MATERIALS AND METHODS

Sacred Heart University's Institutional Review Board (IRB) approved all study protocols and procedures for this study.

PARTICIPANTS

As shown in **Table 1**, nine participants with a prior diagnosis of autism (age range 16-years, 9-months to 22 years, 4-months of age, mean 19-years; one female and eight males) were recruited for the study. The Childhood Autism Rating Scale (CARS) was used to establish the appropriateness of the "severe autism" diagnosis for each participant, and that each participant presented with severe impairments of Verbal Communication. The CARS is a criterion-referenced diagnostic tool routinely used in the research literature (Perry et al., 2005; Mayes et al., 2009) as a standardized assessment of the degree of autism symptomatology across 15 developmental domains, e.g., "relating to people" and "object use." Each domain is scored on a seven point Likert Scale with lower ratings, e.g., a score of 1 or 1.5 indicative of developmentally appropriate levels in each subscale, and high ratings, e.g., a score of 3.5 or 4 indicative of "severely abnormal" levels of each subscale. The subscales are then added together to form a "total score." Scores from 15 to 30 indicate a "non-autistic" rating, 30–37 indicates a "mild-moderately autistic" rating, and 37 to 60 indicate a "severely

Table 1 | Participants.

	Gender	Age (in years and months)	Height (inches)	Weight (pounds)	CARS total rating	CARS "Verbal Communication" subscale rating	CARS "Body Use" subscale rating
ASD PARTICIPANTS							
E1	M	18-y, 7-m	75	195	51.5	4	4
E2	M	17-y, 3-m	71	199	49.5	4	4
E3	F	19-y, 1-m	69	148	52	4	4
E4	M	16-y, 11-m	70	205	59.5	4	4
E5	M	22-y, 4-m	70	240	41.5	4	4
E6	M	21-y, 6-m	71	162	48.5	4	4
E7	M	18-y, 3-m	70	172	50.5	4	4
E8	M	17-y, 6-m	73	170	59	4	4
E9	M	19-y, 10-m	70	165	48	4	4
ASD Group Means		19-y, 0-m	71.00	184.00	51.11	4	4
CONTROL PARTICIPANTS							
C1	F	19-y, 7-m	67	126	n/a	n/a	n/a
C2	F	19-y, 11-m	67	134	n/a	n/a	n/a
C3	F	20-y, 7-m	62	134.1	n/a	n/a	n/a
C4	M	19-y, 10-m	67	126.3	n/a	n/a	n/a
C5	M	16-y, 9-m	75	158.7	n/a	n/a	n/a
C6	M	20-y, 0-m	72	178.5	n/a	n/a	n/a
C7	M	19-y, 10-m	68	156.1	n/a	n/a	n/a
C8	M	20-y, 2-m	70	203.7	n/a	n/a	n/a
C9	M	19-y, 8-m	71	160	n/a	n/a	n/a
C10	M	20-y, 6-m	69.25	178.8	n/a	n/a	n/a
Control Group Means		19-y, 8-m	68.825	155.62			

autistic" rating. For the current study, the CARS ratings were performed by a psychologist experienced in developmental evaluations of the population diagnosed with Autism spectrum disorders. Following a standardized protocol, these ratings were done through observations of the potential participants and parental interviews within 1-month prior to participation in the study protocol.

Participants were selected to participate in this study if they met the following two criteria on the CARS: (1) a rating of "severely autistic" on their overall rating; and (2) at least a rating of 3 out of 4 on Sub-Scale XI "Verbal Communication," which indicates a severe disorder of verbal behavior (i.e., not speaking in more than a few words or phrases; routinely not using verbally produced sentences as a principal mode of communication). As shown in **Table 1**, all of the experimental participants met the "severely autistic" criteria (mean ± *SD*; 51.11 ± 5.54), and all presented with severe disorders of Verbal Communication (indicated by a rating of "4" out of 4).

Ten control group participants of similar ages to the ASD participants (18–20 years of age, mean 19.5 ± 0.5 years; three females and seven males) were also recruited under IRB approval and with their consent. None of the participants in the control group had a known developmental or other health problem that would interfere with their performance. A series of *t*-tests revealed that the groups were not significantly different for age, height, and weight (**Table 1**). The CARS ratings were not conducted with the participants in the control group.

EXPERIMENTAL PROTOCOL

The GAITRite (GR) Walkway System (CIR Systems Inc., Sparta, NJ) was used to collect spatiotemporal gait data. The GR is an electronic walkway (700 × 90 cm), with pressure sensors embedded in a horizontal grid. The recordable area of the mat is approximately 610 cm long × 61 cm wide. Sensors are separated at a distance of 1.27 cm, with a frequency of 80 Hz and temporal resolutions of 11 ms. The walkway is connected by a serial interface cable to a desktop computer running MS Windows XP.

For each individual trial, the participant walked along the length of the GR walkway. Participants completed six trials of preferred gait consecutively with about 30–60 s between each trial. Prior to the first trial, participants were given a demonstration and were then required to show their understanding of the instructions by walking down the mat. The participants were simply directed to walk to a research assistant who was standing approximately 2 m beyond the end of the GR mat. No participant required more than one demonstration and practice trial. The quantitative dependent variables collected via the GR Walkway System included both Spatial and Temporal measurements of gait and are described in **Table 2**.

QUALITATIVE DATA COLLECTION

As indicated above, we used the CARS ratings to preselect participants as presenting with "severe" levels of global Autism and Verbal Communication only. We did not use any of the other sub-scales as criteria for inclusion in the study, other than how they contributed to the overall rating. That said, a reliable and

Table 2 | Temporal and spatial measures of gait recorded by the GAITRite walkway system.

SPATIAL MEASURES	
Step length (cm)	Measurement along the line of progression, from the heel center of the current footprint to the heel center of the previous footprint on the opposite foot.
Stride length (cm)	Measurement on the line of progression between the heel points of two consecutive footprints of the same foot (left to left, right to right).
Heel-to-heel base of support or base width (cm)	Vertical distance from heel center of one footprint to the line of progression formed by two footprints of the opposite foot.
Toe in/out (degrees from midline)	Angle between the line of progression and the midline of the footprint. The Toe in/out angle is zero if the geometric mid-line of the footprint is parallel to the line of progression; positive, toe-out, when the mid-line of the footprint is outside the line of progression and negative, toe-in, when inside the line of progression.
TEMPORAL MEASURES	
Cadence (steps/min)	Number of steps per minute across the walkway.
Gait cycle time (s)	Elapsed time between the first contacts of two consecutive footfalls of the same foot.
Velocity (cm/s)	Obtained after dividing the distance traveled by the Ambulation time.
Step time (s)	Time elapsed from first contact of one foot to first contact of the opposite foot.
Stride time (s)	Time elapsed between the first contacts of two consecutive footfalls of the same foot.
Heel contact (s)	Time that the first sensor appears in the heel quadrilateral of the foot.
Last contact (s)	Time that the last sensor goes off in any quadrilateral.
Toe off (s)	The time that the last sensor turns off in the forefoot quadrilateral of the foot.
Stance time (s) and percent of stance time (% of gait cycle)	The Stance Phase is the weight-bearing portion of each gait cycle. It is initiated by heel contact and ends with toe off of the same foot. It is the time elapsed between the first contact and the last contact of two consecutive footfalls on the same foot.
Swing time (s) and percent swing time (% of gait cycle)	Initiated with toe off and ends with heel strike. It is the time elapsed between the Last Contact of the current footfall to the First Contact of the next footfall on the same foot. It is expressed in seconds (s) and it is also presented as a percent of the Gait Cycle of the same foot. The Swing Time is equal to the Single Support time of the opposite foot.
Single support (s) and percent single support (% of Gait Cycle)	Time elapsed between the last contact of the current footfall to the first contact of the next footfall of the same foot. Single Support time is equal to the Swing Time of the opposite foot.
Initial double support (s) and percent initial double support (% of gait cycle)	The first period in the Gait Cycle in which both feet are on the floor. Initial double support occurs from heel contact of one footfall to toe-off of the opposite footfall.
Terminal double support (s) and percent terminal double support (% of gait cycle)	The second period in the Gait Cycle when both feet are on the floor. Terminal Double Support occurs from opposite footfall heel strike to support footfall toe-off.
Total double support (s) and percent total double support (% of gait cycle)	Total double support is the sum of the Initial added to the Terminal Double Support.

valid qualitative index of movement abnormalities is included in the CARS on the sub-scale of sub-scale IV "Body Use." This sub-scale is characterized by the authors (Schopler et al., 1988) as "representing both coordination and appropriateness of body movements. It includes such deviations as posturing, spinning, tapping, and rocking, toe-walking, and self-directed aggression…Consider such activities as cutting with scissors, drawing, or putting together puzzles in addition to active physical games. Evaluate the frequency and intensity of bizarre body use…" (p. 13). Hence, the scale is a collection of aberrations in movement and actions. All of the sub-scales of the CARS are rated on a seven point scale from 1 to 4 (including "0.5" measures

1.5, 2.5, and 3.5). The characterizations for the Body Use ratings include a rating of:

(1) *Age appropriate body use*—The child moves with the same ease, agility, and coordination of a normal child of the same age.
(2) *Mildly abnormal body use*—Some minor peculiarities may be present, such as clumsiness, repetitive movements, poor coordination, or the rare appearance of more unusual movements.
(3) *Moderately abnormal body use*—Behaviors that are clearly strange or unusual for a child of this age are noted. These may include strange finger movements, peculiar finger or body posturing, staring or picking at the body, self-directed aggression, rocking, spinning, finger-wiggling, or toe-walking.
(4) *Severely abnormal body use*—Intense or frequent movements of the type listed above are signs of severely abnormal body use. These behaviors may persist despite attempts to discourage them or involve the child in other activities.

Where there was no pre-selection criteria used regarding the Body Use sub-scale, these ratings represented a valid qualitative dependent measure of each ASD participant's movement.

STATISTICAL ANALYSIS

All dependent measures were calculated as the average across the six repeated trials for each measure described above. Cadence and velocity were compared with Student's t-test's between the ASD and Control participants. All other analyses were performed as 2 (group) × 2 (Left and Right) Analysis of Variance (ANOVA).

RESULTS

HOMOGENEITY OF VARIANCES

All of the following parameters were assessed to determine if the variances in each between group analyses were homogeneous, using Levene's Test of Equality of Error Variances. Only two of the following analyses were found to have significant group differences in their respective variances—the analyses of Double Support Load Time and Double Support Unload Time (F-values are presented with those analyses below). No other analyses revealed a statistical lack of homogeneity of variances.

Table 3 | Summary of ASD and control participants' means (standard deviations) and *p*-values compared on spatial and temporal parameters of the gait cycle.

	Control group	ASD group	*p*-value <
SPATIAL PARAMETERS			
Step length left (cm)	78.13 (5.47)	67.96 (9.18)	0.016
Step length right (cm)	78.265 (7.07)	69.93 (8.68)	0.016
Stride length left (cm)	156.5 (12.22)	139.09 (17.16)	0.019
Stride length right (cm)	156.44 (12.2)	138.12 (18.17)	0.019
Support base left (cm)	10.74 (1.96)	10.04 (1.98)	n.s.
Support base right (cm)	9.94 (1.7)	9.75 (1.74)	n.s.
Toe in/out angle left (degree)	0.87 (4.82)	14.67 (11.93)	0.002
Toe in/out angle right (degree)	4.02 (3.39)	15.03 (8.95)	0.002
TEMPORAL PARAMETERS			
Cadence (steps/min)	112.52 (5.02)	100.11 (11.18)	0.0055
Cycle time (s)	1.07 (0.025)	1.22 (0.0065)	0.004
Velocity (cm/s)	146.5 (9.81)	116.11 (26.66)	0.009
Step time left (s)	0.5347 (0.02)	0.6142 (0.07)	0.004
Step time right (s)	0.5323 (0.03)	0.6017 (0.06)	0.004
Left stance (s)	0.659 (0.03)	0.783 (0.1)	0.001
Right stance (s)	0.663 (0.03)	0.785 (0.1)	0.001
Left swing (s)	0.41 (0.02)	0.427 (0.04)	0.1
Right swing (s)	0.40 (0.03)	0.43 (0.04)	0.1
Single support left (s)	0.40 (0.03)	0.43 (0.04)	0.1
Single support right (s)	0.41 (0.02)	0.427 (0.04)	0.1
Heel off/on left (s)	0.1697 (0.09)	0.1242 (0.1)	n.s.
Heel off/on right (s)	0.1667 (0.07)	0.1305 (0.1)	n.s.
Double support left (s)	0.2569 (0.02)	0.3479 (0.07)	0.001
Double support right (s)	0.2565 (0.02)	0.344 (0.06)	0.001
Double support load left (s)	0.1288 (0.01)	0.1684 (0.03)	0.001
Double support load right (s)	0.129 (0.01)	0.1799 (0.04)	0.001
Double support unload left (s)	0.1282 (0.01)	0.1797 (0.04)	0.001
Double support unload right (s)	0.1292 (0.01)	0.1642 (0.03)	0.001

SPATIAL PARAMETERS

As shown in **Table 3**, a number of spatial parameters differentiated the ASD and control participants. Step length was longer for the control's ($F = 7.12, p < 0.016$), with no differences between Left or Right legs or Group × Leg (Left vs. Right) interactions. Similarly, the groups also differed in Stride Length, with the Controls being significantly longer than those in the ASD group ($F = 6.72; p < 0.019$), with no difference found in Left vs. Right sides or Group by Leg interactions.

The two groups also differed in the extent to which their feet positions varied, indexed by the toes pointing In or Out. As exemplified in **Figure 1**, the ASD group showed a positive index, indicating that their Left foot was pointed outward from the line of progression by 14.67° and right foot by 15.03°, compared to the control participants who showed an average of 0.87° on the left and 4.02° on the right feet ($F = 13.94, p < 0.002$). Though the orientation of the feet implied a subtly wider base of support for the ASD participants, there was no significant difference found in the Heel-to-Heel Base of Support between the two groups ($F = 0.31, p < 0.59$). Again, no differences were found in any of these analyses in Left vs. Right Leg or a Group by Leg interaction.

TEMPORAL PARAMETERS

Widespread temporal gait differences were found between groups (**Table 3**). The participants in the control group walked with a greater Cadence [$t = 3.18$ ($df = 17$), $p < 0.0055$], Velocity [$t = 3.23(df = 17)$, $p < 0.009$], and Gait Cycle Time ($F = 11.29$, $p < 0.004$) as compared to the ASD group. The ASD participants also showed longer time durations for their step time ($F = 11.26$, $p < 0.004$) and stance phase ($F = 14.37$, $p < 0.001$). There was also a trend for a significantly longer swing phase for the ASD participants compared to controls ($F = 2.94$, $p < 0.1$), with a correspondingly identical trend for Single Support Time ($F = 2.94$, $p < 0.1$; which is occurring concurrently with the opposite Leg Swing Times). No significant differences were found in any of these analyses for Left vs. Right Leg Differences or Group × Leg interactions. There were also no differences found in the duration of Heel Off and On for either Leg or Group ($F = 0.901$, $p < 0.36$).

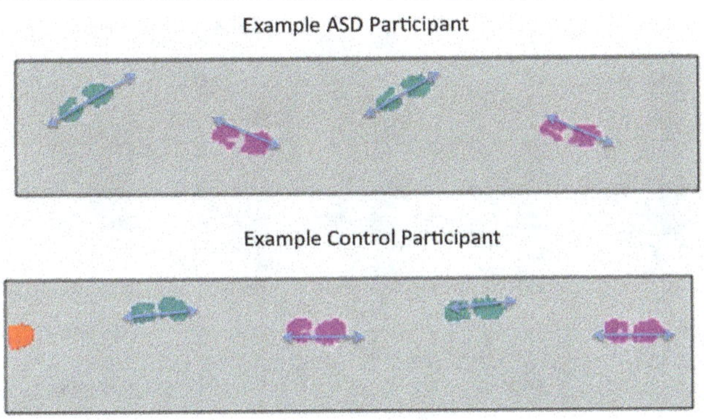

FIGURE 1 | Example of foot positioning of ASD and Control Group participants.

The groups also differed with the ASD participants having both feet on the ground simultaneously as indicated by Initial Double Support time ($F = 16.48$, $p < 0.001$), Terminal Double Support time ($F = 16.56$, $p < 0.001$) and the corresponding Total Double Support time ($F = 17.09$, $p < 0.001$). An analysis with Levene's Test of Equality of Error Variances did reveal group differences in the homogeneity of variance for both the Initial [left leg ($F = 4.36$, $p < 0.052$) and right leg ($F = 5.53$, $p < 0.031$)] and Terminal Double Support [left leg ($F = 6.37$, $p < 0.022$) and right leg ($F = 8.38$, $p < 0.01$)]. As stated above, these were the only analyses that revealed a lack of homogeneous variances across all other tests.

TEMPORAL PARAMETERS: PERCENTAGE OF GAIT CYCLE

As shown in **Figure 2**, the ASD participants spent a greater percentage of the total Gait Cycle in the Stance phases and less time in the Swing phase relative to controls. The percentage of Swing Time (and corresponding alternate leg Single Support percentage shown on **Figure 3**) was larger for the control compared to ASD participants ($F = 14.99$, $p < 0.001$). Alternatively, the percentage of Stance Time was larger for the ASD participants ($F = 14.95$, $p < 0.001$). **Figure 3** shows the distribution of Gait Cycle elements, which differ between groups on all but one element across the entire cycle. Each element that contributes to Total Stance time differs between groups in the percentage of time spent in Initial Double Support Load ($F = 11.96$, $p < 0.003$), Terminal Double Support Unload ($F = 11.45$, $p < 0.004$) and Total Double Support ($F = 14.8$, $p < 0.001$). There were no

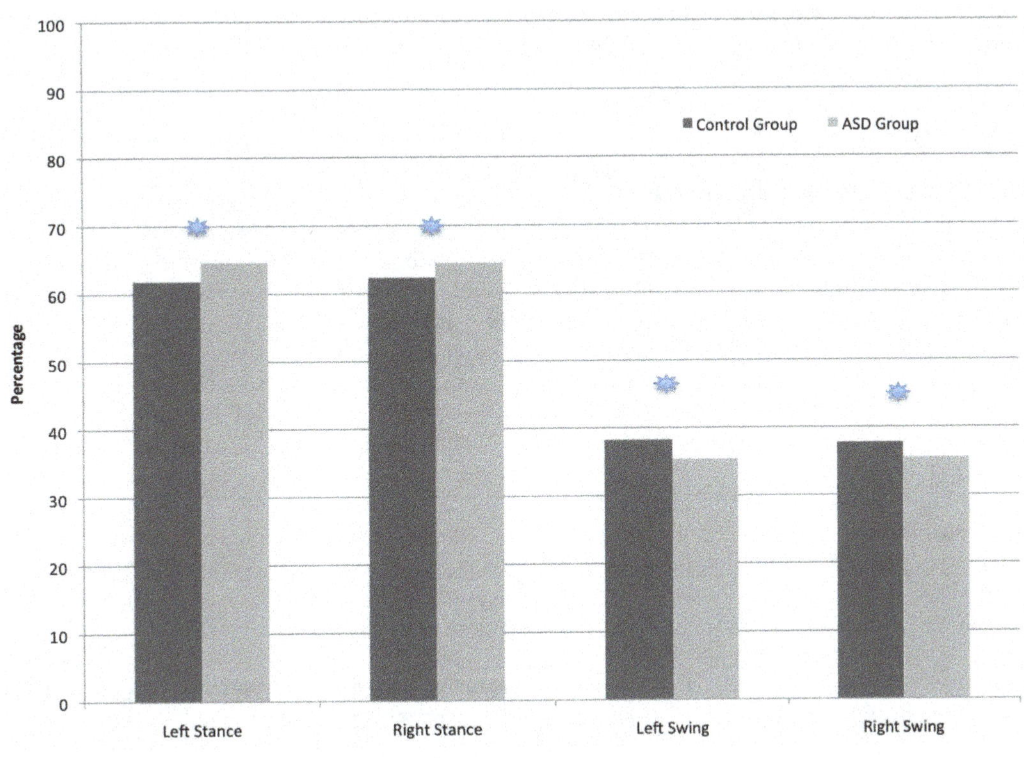

FIGURE 2 | Comparison of the two groups in the percentage of time spent in the Stance and Swing Phases of the Gait Cycle. $p < 0.001$ (✱).

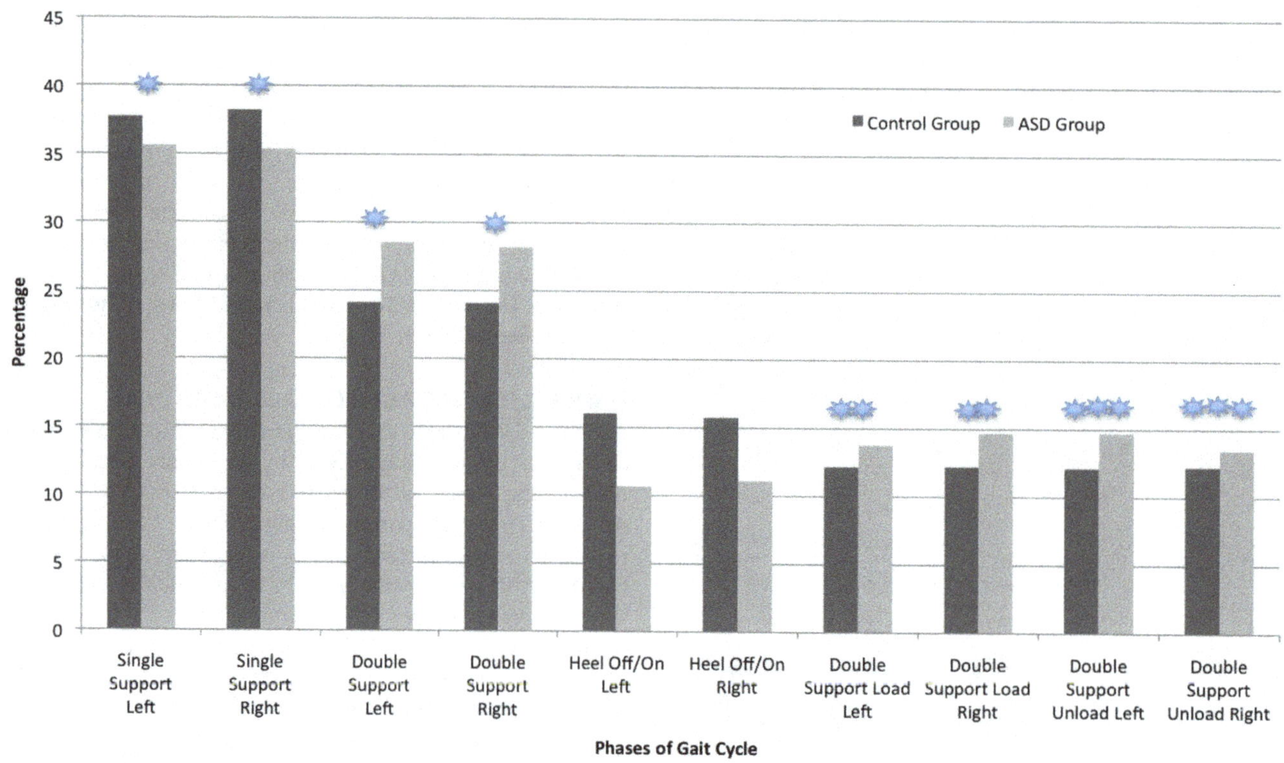

FIGURE 3 | Comparison of the two groups in the percentage of time spent in each Gait Cycle phase. $p < 0.001$ (*); $p < 0.003$ (**); $p < 0.004$ (***).

differences found in the percentages of Single Support, Stance Time or Double Support elements comparing Left vs. Right Legs or Group × Leg interactions. The only percentage of the Gait Cycle in which between group difference were not found was in the percentage of Heel Contact ($F = 1.78, p < 0.2$).

QUALITATIVE PRESENTATION OF MOVEMENT: CARS RATINGS OF "BODY USE"

All nine participants in this study diagnosed with ASD showed the highest rating—4 out of 4—on the sub-scale of sub-scale IV "Body Use" (see **Table 1**). These ratings were predicated upon an array of unusual and otherwise inappropriate actions demonstrated by each of the ASD participants such as finger waving or contorting, hand and/or arm flapping, halting or ballistic movements of the hands, arms or legs, seemingly uncontrolled rocking or jumping movements, a "skipping" gait, stilted, stiff or "freezing" body postures, repetitive actions such as touching or poking at objects, various unusual facial contortions, peculiar grasp patterns, difficulty either moving from a standing to a seated position or visa-versa, and more.

DISCUSSION

SUMMARY OF FINDINGS

In this study, we found that older teenagers and young adults diagnosed with globally "severe" forms of ASD that included severe ratings of Verbal Communication disorders, quantitatively walked slower, taking shorter steps, are in a stance position longer and swing their limbs for a shorter percentage of their spontaneous gait cycle. Though there is not a difference found in the Groups' Bases of Support *per se*, individuals with ASD show a significant variance in their foot positions relative to Controls vis-à-vis Toe Out positioning relative to their gait line of progression.

Though these individuals were selected to participate in this study due to both global ratings of the severity of their Autism and severity of their Verbal Communication, participants were also rated to engage in the most severe forms of movement abnormalities as indexed by the CARS rating scale. Hence, as we predicted individuals who have severe forms of Autism and low Verbal Communication will also have significant variations in gait and other qualitative aspects of their movement.

These findings are consistent with a number of studies that report movement differences between individuals diagnosed with ASD as compared to typically developing individuals. However, a number of differences also exist between our study sample, and their associated results, compared to other samples previously reported (cf., Fournier et al., 2010), which will be considered below.

IS THERE A RELATION BETWEEN DIFFERENCES OF MOVEMENT AND LEVEL OF "SEVERITY" OF ASD?

In reviewing the range of studies that have been reported to date there are some meaningful differences in gait that may correlate with the severity of the ASD diagnosis. All of the studies report differences between individuals diagnosed with ASD as compared to typically developing comparison groups. However, these differences are reflected in different parameters related to gait. In our current study, all of the participants presented with severe forms of the ASD diagnosis and showed widespread differences in both quantitative and qualitative aspects of gait and movement, respectively. Our findings are in contrast to the data reported by Rinehart et al. (2006a,b); Calhoun et al. (2011), and Hallett et al. (1993) who reported only limited or no differences in spatiotemporal parameters of gait among individuals diagnosed with "High Functioning" forms of ASD. Rinehart et al. reported that young children diagnosed with High Functioning Autism (HFA) and Asperger Syndrome (AS) showed greater *variability* in stride length, though the average stride length was comparable to that of the typically developing children. They did find meaningful differences between groups in qualitative indexes of movement (e.g., upper body postural variations, smoothness of movement, etc.), but little in the way of quantitative differences in temporal and spatial parameters of gait, *per se*.

Similarly, Calhoun et al. (2011) reported data from "high functioning" children (mean age of 6.3-years) in which they found that the ASD individuals had a significantly higher cadence compared to controls, but there were few other temporal and spatial parameters of gait that differentiated the ASD from control participants. For example, Calhoun et al., like Rinehart et al. found no significant differences in stride length, or in the percentage of the gait cycle time spent in the stance phase. However, Calhoun et al. (2011) found widespread and significant differences between an Autism group compared to typically developing children (mean age of 6.3-years) in peak hip and ankle kinematics and kinetics. Significant differences were found for sagittal ankle and hip components, indicative of reduced plantarflexor moments and increased dorsiflexion angles, which may be associated with hypotonia. Furthermore, decreased hip extensor moments were found for the autism group compared to the control group. Indeed, independent clinical evaluation of the ASD participants in that study resulted in 33% of the group being diagnosed with hypotonia and gross motor delays were reported in 25% of the participants.

The only prior data regarding adults that utilized three dimensional kinematic data acquisition with synchronously processed kinetic information (force plate data) was reported by Hallett et al. (1993). Participants in that study were 25 to 38-years of age and described as "high functioning and had good language ability" and were reported to have Wechsler Adult Intelligence Scale-Revised (WAIS-R) full-scale scores ranging from 78 to 107 (mean of 88, SD ± 12). Though the authors reported "mild clumsiness" in four of five ASD participants and differences in upper limb posturing during gait in three of the five participants, there were few specific aspects of gait that the groups differed on as compared to typically developing age-matched adults. The velocity of gait, step length, cadence, step width, stance time, and vertical ground reaction forces were comparable to the control participants. The ASD participants did show decreased range of motion of the ankle and decreased knee flexion in early stance reminiscent of the data reported subsequently by Calhoun et al. (2011). Moreover, their "awkwardness" was similar to the qualitative findings reported by Rinehart et al. (2006a,b).

Alternatively, Vilensky et al. (1981)—similar to the data that we report here—found variations between their ASD group compared to typically developing age-matched controls on temporal and spatial elements such as reduced stride lengths and increased stance times not found by Rinehart et al. (2006a,b); Calhoun et al. (2011), or Hallett et al. (1993). Vilensky et al. did report increased hip flexion at toe-off, and decreased knee extension and ankle dorsiflexion at ground contact, all similar to data reported by Calhoun et al. and consistent with the qualitative ratings reported by Rinehart et al. Also related to level of function, Vilensky et al. (1981) reported a significant negative correlation between level of Intelligence and the ankle joint angle at initial contact with the floor. Hence the authors concluded, "Thus the more intelligent children had heel strikes that more closely resembled those of the normal children."

The one exception that we have found in relation to severity of ASD and type of movement anomalies was reported by Vernazza-Martin et al. (2005). These authors characterized their study group as presenting with "pronounced alteration of social interactions, a lack of verbal communication (p. 93)," and children diagnosed with Asperger Syndrome were excluded from the study. These authors found only relatively minor differences in spatiotemporal parameters of gait between age-matched 4-to-6-year old children diagnosed with ASD as compared to typically developing controls. However, these authors report significant "oscillations" of the head, shoulders and trunk stability among the children diagnosed with ASD. These findings indicated meaningfully reduced stability and greater variability in posture as they walked similar to Rinehart et al. (2006a,b) and Calhoun et al. (2011), despite the fact that the participants are seemingly "lower" functioning compared to these other reports.

Finally, any consideration of a possible relation between level of function and aspects of gait also must include the findings reported by Kern et al. (2010) who demonstrated that the degree of "severity" in the ASD diagnosis correlates with muscle strength. Similarly, Travers et al. (2012) found a correlation between ASD symptom severity and postural stability.

Though we clearly need to be cautious in any direct comparison from our data to those reported above, we find it informative to consider the possibility that there is a relation between the level of severity in the ASD diagnosis of the participants and their corresponding characteristics of movement. Those studies reporting data from "high functioning" participants showed only mild variations in their temporal and spatial gait patterns, with more prevalent differences in the smoothness of movement and postural controls. There are unmistakable differences in the movement patterns of these individuals. However, their findings are in marked contrast to our report of severe levels of functioning in our population, who also show far more significant variations in the temporal and spatial gait patterns as compared to the control participants.

When these few studies are taken together, they beg the question for further study to address the relation between severity of the ASD diagnosis and movement aberrations. The hypothesis that we are left with is that children, teenagers and young adults that have more severe forms of the ASD—as those described in our current study and by Vilensky et al. (1981)—may be more likely to show differences in spatiotemporal parameters of gait, as well as postural differences and increases in aberrant movements (e.g., hand flapping, ballistic movements, etc.). Alternatively, individuals diagnosed as "high functioning Autism" or Asperger Syndrome—as described by Hallett et al. (1993); Rinehart et al. (2006a,b) and Calhoun et al. (2011)—will show less evident variations in spatiotemporal parameters, but meaningful variations in balance and posture contributing to these individuals qualitatively seeming "awkward" in their movement.

IS THERE A RELATION BETWEEN DIFFERENCES IN GAIT AND SEVERE VERBAL COMMUNICATION DISORDERS?

It was not surprising to us that we confirmed out hypothesis of widespread variations in the gait patterns of individuals diagnosed with severe forms of ASD and low Verbal Communication as compared to typically developing university undergraduate students. As indexed by the qualitative ratings in our study sample and as indicated by the very criteria of Autism in the DSM-IV-R (2000), movement disorders are rife within this population. However, our data raises the question of whether the differences in movement may be more acute in a group of young adults who present with profoundly low Verbal Communication.

What has been surprising to us is that there are so few questions being asked in the literature on ASD and movement about the "chicken and egg" aspects of the relation between disorders of movement, disorders of verbal expression and global ratings of "severe" forms of Autism (cf., Donnellan et al., 2010). Our study does not answer questions about the relation between different facets of movement in individuals diagnosed with ASD *per se*, other than to show that individuals with highly impaired verbal expression also have significantly different gait patterns compared to typically developing young adults. What this study should do is to raise further questions about what the interrelations among different aspects of movement dysregulation may be. Is there more than just a correlation between aberrant gait and inability to speak verbally? Or, may it be the case that aberrations in movement patterns can manifest in a variety of ways both across different individuals with the ASD diagnosis or among different movement systems for a single individual? We suspect that differences in walking have an analogous etiological and developmental trajectory as does the emergence of aberrations in speech and language.

GENERAL CONCLUSIONS

In comparing our data to that reported by others (Vilensky et al., 1981; Hallett et al., 1993; Vernazza-Martin et al., 2005; Rinehart et al., 2006a,b; Calhoun et al., 2011), it would appear that there are greater and more widespread differences in spatiotemporal parameters of gait among individuals who present with more severe forms of ASD and verbal communication disorders. Though the current study does not allow for more than a correlational coupling of gait and verbal expression, we believe the next steps in this research will require asking questions about the interrelation of movement systems within individuals. We need to consider the fundamentally circular etiological question of "which comes first," disorders of communication and social interaction, or aberrations in movement? We propose that greater attention must be paid to hypotheses that Autism is primarily a disorder of movement first. This is clearly consistent with the neuro-anatomical and neuro-imaging data demonstrating significant aberrations of the cerebellum (Courchesne et al., 1999; Allen et al., 2004; Bauman and Kemper, 2005a,b) and the Basal Ganglia (Hollander et al., 2005; Langen et al., 2007). There is clear evidence that differences in the cerebellum must have gone awry during early embryological development (Bauman and Kemper, 1994, 2003, 2005a,b; Rodier et al., 1996; Rodier and Arndt, 2005). As such, disorders of verbal expression, disorders of social interaction and hence the global diagnosis of ASD may be secondary to the primary disorder—or core deficit in ASD—of developmental anomalies of movement. It is clearly time to advance questions that consider the etiology of ASD as it relates to the trajectory of movement across development.

ACKNOWLEDGMENTS

This work was supported by a Sacred Heart University Research and Creativity Grant. The authors wish to thank Marissa DeFede and Herb Kemp for their assistance during data collection and Nicole Fogliano for assistance with data analysis.

REFERENCES

Allen, G., Müller, R. A., and Courchesne, E. (2004). Cerebellar function in autism: functional magnetic resonance image activation during a simple motor task. *Biol. Psychiatry* 56, 269–278.

American Psychiatric Association. (2000). *Diagnostic and Statistical Manual of Mental Disorders: DSM-IV-TR*. Washington, DC: American Psychiatric Association.

Bauman, M. L. (1992). "Motor dysfunction in autism," in *Movement Disorders in Neurology and Neuropsychiatry*, eds A. Joseph and R. R. Young (Boston, MA: Blackwell Publishers), 660–663.

Bauman, M. L., and Kemper, T. L. (1994). *The Neurobiology of Autism*. Baltimore: Johns Hopkins University Press.

Bauman, M. L., and Kemper, T. L. (2003). The neuropathology of the autism spectrum disorders: what have we learned? *Novartis Found. Symp.* 251, 112–122.

Bauman, M. L., and Kemper, T. L. (2005a). Neuroanatomic observations of the brain in autism: a review and future directions. *Int. J. Dev. Neurosci.* 23, 183–187.

Bauman, M., and Kemper, T. (2005b). "Structural brain anatomy in autism: what is the evidence?" in *The Neurobiology of Autism*, eds M. Bauman and T. Kemper (Baltimore, ML: Johns Hopkins University Press), 121–135.

Calhoun, M., Longworth, M., and Chester, V. (2011). Gait patterns in children with autism. *Clin. Biomech.* 26, 200–206.

Courchesne, C., Townsend, J., and Saitoh, O. (1999). The brain in infantile autism: posterior fossa structures are abnormal. *Neurology* 44, 214–223.

Damasio, A. R., and Maurer, R. G. (1978). A neurological model for childhood autism. *Arch. Neurol.* 35, 777–786.

Donnellan, A. M., Leary, M., and Robledo, J. (2006). "I can't get started: stress and the role of movement differences for individuals with the autism label," in *Stress and Coping in Autism*, eds M. G. Baron, J. Groden, G. Groden, and L. Lipsitt (Oxford: Oxford University Press), 205–245.

Donnellan, A. M., Hill, D. A., and Leary, M. R. (2010). Rethinking autism: implications of sensory and movement differences. *Disabil. Stud. Q.* 30, 1–25.

Esposito, G., Venuti, P., Apicella, F., and Muratori, F. (2011). Analysis of unsupported gait in toddlers with autism. *Brain Dev.* 33, 367–373.

Fournier, K., Hass, C., Naik, S., Lodha, N., and Cauraugh, J. (2010). Motor coordination in autism spectrum disorders: a synthesis and meta-analysis.

J. Autism Dev. Disord. 40, 1227–1240.

Ghaziuddin, M., and Butler, E. (1998). Clumsiness in autism and asperger syndrome: a further report. *J. Intellect. Disabil. Res.* 42, 43–48.

Hallett, M., Lebiedowska, M. K., Thomas, S. L., Stanhope, S. J., Denckla, M. B., and Rumsey, J. (1993). Locomotion of autistic adults. *Arch. Neurol.* 50, 1304–1308.

Hollander, E., Anagnostou, E., Chaplin, W., Esposito, K., Haznedar, M., Licalzi, E., et al. (2005). Striatal volume on magnetic resonance imaging and repetitive behaviors in autism. *Biol. Psychiatry* 58, 226–232.

Jones, V., and Prior, M. (1985). Motor imitation abilities and neurological signs in autistic children. *J. Autism Dev. Disord.* 15, 37–46.

Kanner, L. (1943). Autistic disturbances of affective contact. *Nerv. Child* 2, 217–250.

Kern, J., Geier, D., Adams, J., Troutman, M., Davis, G., King, P., et al. (2010). Autism severity and muscle strength: a correlation analysis. *Res. Autism Spectr. Disord.* 5, 1011–1015.

Kohen-Raz, R., Volkmar, F., and Cohen, D. (1992). Postural control in children with autism. *J. Autism Dev. Disord.* 22, 419–432.

Langen, M., Durston, S., Staal, W. G., Palmen, S., and van Engeland, H. (2007). Caudate nucleus is enlarged in high-functioning medicated-naïve subjects with Autism. *Biol. Psychiatry* 62, 262–266.

Leary, M. R., and Hill, D. A. (1996). Moving on: autism and movement disturbance. *Ment. Retard.* 34, 39–53.

Mayes, S., Calhoun, S., Murray, M., Morrow, J., Yurich, K., Mahr, F., et al. (2009). Comparison of scores on the checklist for autism spectrum disorder, childhood autism rating scale, and Gilliam Asperger's disorder scale for children with low functioning autism, high functioning autism, Asperger's disorder, ADHD, and typical development. *J. Autism Dev. Disord.* 39, 1682–1693.

Minshew, N. J., Sung, K., Jones, B. L., and Furman, J. M. (2004). Underdevelopment of the postural control system in autism. *Neurology* 63, 2056–2061.

Molloy, C. A., Dietrich, K. N., and Bhattacharya, A. (2003). Postural stability in children with autism spectrum disorder. *J. Autism Dev. Disord.* 33, 643–652.

Perry, A., Condillac, R. A., Freeman, N. L., Dunn-Geier, J., and Belair, J. (2005). Multi-site study of the Childhood Autism Rating Scale (CARS) in five clinical groups of young children. *J. Autism Dev. Disord.* 35, 625–634.

Rapin, I. (1997). Autism. *New Engl. J. Med.* 337, 97–104.

Rinehart, N. J., Tonge, B. J., Bradshaw, J. L., Iansek, R., Enticott, P. G., and McGinley, J. (2006a). Gait function in high-functioning autism and Asperger's disorder. *Eur. Child Adolesc. Psychiatry* 15, 256–264.

Rinehart, N. J., Bruce, J., Tonge, B. J., Iansek, R., McGinley, J., Brereton, A. V., et al. (2006b). Gait function in newly diagnosed children with autism: cerebellar and basal ganglia related motor disorder. *Dev. Med. Child Neurol.* 48, 819–824.

Rodier, P., and Arndt, T. (2005). "The brainstem in autism," in *The Neurobiology of Autism,* eds M. Bauman and T. Kemper (Baltimore: Johns Hopkins University Press), 136–149.

Rodier, P. M., Ingram, J. L., Tisdale, B., Nelson, S., and Romano, J. (1996). Embryological origin for autism: developmental anomalies of the cranial nerve motor nuclei. *J. Comp. Neurol.* 370, 247–261.

Rogers, S. J., Bennetto, L., McEvoy, R., and Pennington, B. F. (1996). Imitation and pantomime in high-functioning adolescents with autism spectrum disorders. *Child Dev.* 67, 2060–2073.

Schopler, E., Reichler, R. J., and Renner, B. R. (1988). *The Childhood Autism Rating Scale (CARS).* Los Angeles, CA: Western Psychological Services.

Travers, B., Powell, P., Klinger, L., and Klinger, M. (2012). Motor difficulties in autism spectrum disorder: linking symptom severity and postural stability. *J. Autism Dev. Disord.* doi: 10.1007/s10803-012-1702-x. [Epub ahead of print].

Vernazza-Martin, S., Martin, N., Vernazza, A., Lepellec-Muller, A., Rufo, M., Massion, J., et al. (2005). Goal directed locomotion and balance control in autistic children. *J. Autism Dev. Disord.* 35, 91–102.

Vilensky, J. A., Damasio, A. R., and Maurer, R. G. (1981). Gait disturbances in patients with autistic behavior: a preliminary study. *Arch. Neurol.* 38, 646–649.

Wing, L., and Shah, A. (2000). Catatonia in Autism Spectrum Disorders. *Br. J. Psychiatry,* 176, 357–362.

Wing, L., and Shah, A. (2006). "A systematic examination of catatonia-like clinical pictures in Autism Spectrum Disorders," in *Catatonia in Autism Spectrum Disorders, International Review of Neurobiology,* Vol. 72, eds D. M. Dhossche, L. Wing, M. Ohita, and K.-L. Neumarker (London: Academic Press/Elsevier), 21–39.

Zelazo, P. R., and Weiss, M. J. (1990). "Measures of infant attention: an alternative approach to assessment," in *Interdisciplinary Assessment of Infants,* eds B. Gibbs and D. Teti (Baltimore, ML: Paul Brookes), 129–144.

Zelazo, P. R., Weiss, M. J., and Leonard, E. (1989). "Acquisition of early motor competence: the interaction of cognition, behavioral and maturational influences," in *Challenges to Developmental Paradigms,* eds P. R. Zelazo and R. Barr (Hilsdale, NJ: Lawrence Erlbaum Associates), 139–166.

Conflict of Interest Statement: The authors declare that the research was conducted in the absence of any commercial or financial relationships that could be construed as a potential conflict of interest.

19

Meta review of systematic and meta analytic reviews on movement differences, effect of movement based interventions, and the underlying neural mechanisms in autism spectrum disorder

Motohide Miyahara*

Movement Development Clinic, School of Physical Education, University of Otago, Dunedin, New Zealand

Edited by:
Anne M. Donnellan, University of Wisconsin-Madison, Uzbekistan

Reviewed by:
Nandakumar Narayanan, Yale University, USA
Elizabeth B. Torres, Rutgers University, USA

Correspondence:
Motohide Miyahara, Movement Development Clinic, School of Physical Education, University of Otago, 46 Union Street, PO Box 56, Dunedin 9054, New Zealand.
e-mail: motohide.miyahara@otago.ac.nz

Purposes: To identify and appraise evidence from published systematic and meta analytic reviews on (1) movement differences of individuals with autism spectrum disorders (ASD); (2) the effects of movement based interventions for ASD; (3) hypothesized underlying neural mechanisms for the movement characteristics.

Methods: A meta review of published systematic and meta analytic reviews on movement differences, structural, and functional brain anomalies in ASD and the effects of movement based interventions for individuals with ASD between 1806 and October 2012. The methodological quality of the identified systematic and meta analytic reviews was independently assessed by two assessors with the assessment of multiple systematic reviews (AMSTAR).

Results: The search yielded a total of 12 reviews that met the inclusion/exclusion criteria. The methodological quality of the reviews varied, but the review conclusions were similar. Although individuals with ASD generally perform less well than age-matched controls in developmental movement tasks, there are few exceptions whose movement abilities are intact. Most movement based interventions report their efficacies. However, all existing studies employ the research design that is inherently incapable of providing strong evidence, and they often fail to report the extent of psychosocial interactions within the movement interventions. The hypothesized neural mechanisms are still under development and speculative in nature.

Conclusions: It is premature to designate movement disturbance as a core symptom of ASD. The effects of movement based interventions on the present ASD core symptoms need to be further validated by stronger evidence and verified theoretical mechanisms linking ASD with movement disorders.

Keywords: autism, movement, developmental coordination disorder, motor development, MRI and fMRI

INTRODUCTION

The core symptoms of autism spectrum disorders (ASD) encompass impairments in social interaction and communication, as well as circumscribed interest and fixed behaviors (American Psychiatric Association, 2012). A cross-cutting dimension of these clinical signs is the development of movement skills that are observable, functional, goal-oriented, and acquired as a result of practice. For example, the movements of the vocal cord and the other body parts are essential for communicative speech, gesture, writing, and typing. Stereotypies and preoccupation can be only inferred from observed physical movement patterns. Thus, movement disturbances seem to co-exist with ASD, but the relations between the two disorders have not been critically appraised or adequately synthesized from the previous reviews.

In this meta review, I will evaluate the methodological quality of reviews, re-examine the strength of evidence, the homogeneity of studies and research designs, and integrate the findings to answer my three research questions: movement differences, effect of movement based interventions, and the underlying neuronal mechanisms that link ASD with movement disturbance.

METHODS

My search was based on the electronic databases available at the University of Otago, Dunedin, New Zealand: Web of Knowledge (1898–2012), Medline (1950–2012), PsychINFO (1806–2012), EMBASE (1980–2012), and ERIC (1987–2012) on June 12, 2012. I used the combinations of three or four keywords from the following inclusion criteria: (1) type of paper: systematic review or meta analysis; (2) population or comparison: autism, pervasive developmental disorders, autism spectrum disorder, Asperger disorder; (3) intervention: sport, exercise, physical exercise, physical activity; (4) primary outcome: movement skills, motor skills, motor coordination, physical fitness, imitation; secondary outcome: social skills, autistic behaviors, self-perception, and academics; (5) magnetic resonance imaging (MRI). I included only published studies in English, and excluded "gray" and "figitive" literature. To conduct duplicate study selection, a reference librarian served as a reviews search coordinator. Any inconsistencies in our results were resolved through subsequent collaborative search, reading of respective journal articles, and discussion.

The content of identified review studies was assessed with respect to the professional field of reviewers, type and topic of reviews, numbers of reviewed studies, year range of the studies, total number of subjects, level of evidence, review method, outcome variables, and theoretical interpretation. The methodological quality of the reviews was assessed by two independent assessors with the assessment of multiple systematic review (AMSTAR) tool (Shea et al., 2007). Disagreements were resolved by discussion.

RESULTS

Our search yielded a total of 12 studies. As shown in **Table 1**, four studies examined the existing evidence of movement differences, the other four evaluated the evidence of movement based treatment effects, and the remaining four studies synthesized the foregoing studies that investigated the neuronal mechanisms that link ASD and movement disturbance. I excluded three studies (Redcay and Courchesne, 2005; Sugranyes et al., 2011; Ipser et al., 2012) from further analysis because they did not address my research questions directly. The AMSTAR methodological quality scores of the 12 reviewed studies ranged from 20 (Emck et al., 2009) to 67% (Petrus et al., 2008; Stanfield et al., 2008) of the relevant criteria (**Table 2**).

MOVEMENT DIFFERENCES OF ASD

Of the four objective reviews available on this topic, Fournier et al.'s study (2010) is the only standard meta analytic review on movement differences between individuals with ASD and controls. The remaining three systematic reviews consist of Emck et al.'s (2009) examination of gross motor performance and self-perceived motor competence in ASD, Downey and Rapport's (2012) examination of the movement differences that limit motor activity, and Williams et al.'s (2004) investigation into the differential imitation ability in which they attempted to quantify the movement differences based on p-values. Thus, the four reviews analyzed different yet partially overlapping aspects of movements with each distinctive method.

Fournier et al. (2010) provide the only standard meta analysis that examines motor difference in ASD. As evident on the relatively high AMSTAR score (**Table 2**), their methodological procedures are fairly meticulous. They found a large effect ($ES = 1.20$) which they called *motor coordination deficit* in ASD. Upon scrutiny, however, the variables included in the meta analysis were not only standard assessment of motor coordination, but also sensory motor measures, the measures of letter height (Beversdorf et al., 2001), neurological soft signs (Tani et al., 2006), and even an indicator of the cognitive executive function (Coldren and Halloran, 2003).

Inheritant to meta analysis is the "apples and oranges" problem in that data of different nature are analyzed together, and this criticism may be overruled if the analysis aims to generalize to a higher-order class as "fruit" (Matt and Cook, 2009). Though Fournier et al. name the higher-order class of meta analysed dependent variables "motor coordination," specific sensory motor measures are not usually considered as the indicators of motor coordination in assessing developmental coordination disorder (DCD). Because the proposed DSM-5 (American Psychiatric Association, 2012) allows dual diagnoses of ASD and DCD, it is more meaningful and clinically practical to exclusively use the standard assessment of motor coordination. Fournier et al.'s moderator variable analyses were limited to subtypes of ASD, without including the types of movement measures as a moderator variable. Hence, I computed a random effects model meta analysis on the six comparisons in the five studies that had used standard motor coordination measures. The aggregated standardized mean difference effect was significant, 2.91 ($SE = 0.581$; $p < 0.001$; $Z = 5.01$; $I^2 = 93.48$; 95% $CI = 1.774 - 4.051$), larger than 1.20, the effect size of the all 51 studies, suggesting a high degree of comorbidity of ASD with DCD.

Emck et al.'s (2009) systematic review only covered gross motor performance and perceived competence. The authors concluded that children with ASD were clearly impaired in gross motor development. It is noteworthy that they acknowledge the existence of children with ASD whose gross motor performance fell within the normal range. Because this review neither evaluated the strength of evidence nor attempted quantitative synthesis, their conclusions need to be interpreted with caution.

Downey and Rapport (2012) categorized the movement differences into early motor development, gesture and motor imitation, postural control, and dyspraxia. The strategy for their literature search was described clearly, but the strength of evidence was not evaluated in this systematic review. The movement differences were summed up as *activity limitations* (World Health Organization, 2001) which should take both biological and social aspects into account. However, the authors focused on individual functional adaptation, and recommended physical therapists to promote functional intervention without adequately addressing the needs for social and environmental accommodation. It is open to question whether all aspects of movement differences actually reflect the limitations in motor activity.

Williams et al. (2004) conducted a review on the difference in action imitation between individuals with ASD and matched controls. Although the levels of evidence were not specifically evaluated, the authors ensured the quality of reviewed studies by only including those studies that had employed control groups into their review. Out of thus selected 21 studies, 17 studies were pooled into a meta analysis. The combined logit p-value <0.0005 indicated a significant group difference.

In summary, a meta review of the four review studies indicates substantial movement differences between young people

Table 1 | Characteristics of reviews which met the inclusion criteria ($N = 12$).

First author (Year)	Professional field of the reviewers	Type of review	Topic of review	No. of reviewed studies	Year range of the studies	Total no. of subjects	Levels of reviewed studies	Method used in reviewed studies	Outcome variables	Theoretical interpretations offered
Williams (2004)	Pediatrics, Psychology	Systematic	Imitation difference	21	1966–2002	281	Not assessed	Comparative	Action imitation	Yes
Emck (2009)	Kinesiology, Psychiatry	Systematic	Movement difference	5*	1997–2007	Not reported	Not assessed	Comparative	Gross motor performance, self-perception	Yes
Fournier (2010)	Kinesiology	Meta analytic	Movement difference	51	1980–2009	Not reported	Not assessed	Comparative	Motor coordination	Yes
Downey (2012)	Physicla Therapy	Systematic	Movement difference	49	Not reported	Not reported	Level 2–3	Comparative	Motor development, imitation, posture, dyspraxia	Yes
Baranek (2002)	Education	Systematic	Treatment effect	4^	1980–1993	Not reported	Level 3–4	Case series	Sensory motor functions, behavior	Yes
Petrus (2008)	Physicla Therapy	Systematic	Treatment effect	7	1982–2003	25	Level 2–5	Case series	Stereotypic behaviors	No
Lang (2010)	Education	Systematic	Treatment effect	18	1974–2007	64	Not assessed	Case series	Behavior, academics, physical fitness	Yes
Sowa (2012)	Neuroscience	Meta analytic	Treatment effect	16	1991–2011	133	Not assessed	Case series	Motor skills, social skills	No
Stanfield (2008)	Psychiatry	Meta analytic	Structural difference	46	1984–2006	Over 1600	Not assessed	Comparative	Brain volume	Yes
Müller (2011)	Psychology, Neuroscience	Systematic	Connectivity difference	32	2004–2010	Not reported	Not assessed	Comparative	Functional connectivity	Yes
Philip (2012)	Psychiatry	Meta analytic	Brain activation difference	3†	1984–2009	24	Not assessed	Comparative	Brain activation	Yes
Nickl-Jockschat (2012)	Psychiatry, Neuroscience	Meta analytic	Structural difference	16	1999–2009	580	Not assessed	Comparative	Structural changes	Yes

Note: All Meta analytic reviews included systematic reviews.

No. of movement difference studies only; ^No. of movement intervention studies only; †No. of movement task studies only.

Table 2 | Methodological quality evaluated by the assessment of multiple systematic reviews tool (AMSTAR) (Shea et al., 2007).

First author (Year)	1. Was an "a priori" design provided?	2. Was there duplicate study selection and data extraction?	3. Was a comprehensive literature search performed?	4. Was the status of publication (i.e., gray literature) used as an inclusion criterion?	5. Was a list of studies (included and excluded) provided?	6. Were characteristics of included studies provided?	7. Was the scientific quality of the included studies assessed and documented?	8. Was the scientific quality of the included studies used appropriately in formulating conclusions?	9. Were the methods used to combine the findings of studies appropriate?	10. Was the likelihood of publication bias assessed?	11. Were potential conflicts of interest included?	Total score	Percent
Williams (2004)	CA	CA	Yes	CA	No	Yes	Yes	Yes	NA	NA	No	4/9	44
Emck (2009)	CA	CA	CA	CA	No	Yes	Yes	No	NA	No	No	2/10	20
Fournier (2010)	CA	Yes	Yes	Yes	Yes	Yes	Yes	No	No	Yes	No	7/11	64
Downey (2012)	CA	CA	No	No	No	Yes	Yes	No	NA	NA	No	2/9	22
Baranek (2002)	CA	No	Yes	CA	No	Yes	Yes	Yes	NA	NA	No	4/9	44
Petrus (2008)	CA	Yes	Yes	Yes	No	Yes	Yes	Yes	NA	NA	No	6/9	67
Lang (2010)	CA	Yes	Yes	No	No	Yes	Yes	Yes	NA	NA	No	5/9	56
Sowa (2012)	CA	CA	No	CA	No	Yes	No	No	No	Yes	No	2/11	18
Stanfield (2008)	CA	Yes	Yes	Yes	No	Yes	NA	NA	Yes	Yes	No	6/9	67
Müller (2011)	CA	Yes	No	No	No	Yes	NA	NA	Yes	No	No	3/9	33
Philip (2012)	CA	CA	Yes	Yes	No	Yes	NA	NA	Yes	No	No	4/9	44
Nickl-Jockschat (2012)	CA	CA	CA	No	No	Yes	NA	NA	Yes	No	No	2/9	22

Note: CA, can't answer; NA, not applicable.

with ASD and their typically developing counterparts through a limited quality and quantity of data synthesis. However, not all individuals with ASD have DCD (Emck et al., 2009). Therefore, movement disturbance cannot constitute a *core* symptom of ASD. If present, a comorbid diagnosis of DCD should be given in accordance with the proposed DSM-5 (American Psychiatric Association, 2012).

EFFECTS OF MOVEMENT BASED INTERVENTIONS

Four studies (Baranek, 2002; Petrus et al., 2008; Lang et al., 2010; Sowa and Meulenbroek, 2012) examined the effects of movement based interventions in individuals with ASD. Only Sowa and Meulenbroek (2012) conducted a meta analysis, and the other studies reviewed foregoing studies systematically. All four studies included the effects of physical exercise on ASD symptoms and movement functions.

In addition to the effects of physical exercise, which will be elaborated later with more recent reviews, Baranek (2002) covered sensory- and motor-based interventions, such as sensory integration therapy and sensory stimulation techniques, which have decreased in popularity recently. Although slightly outdated, her review is comprehensive for the covered range of movement based interventions. She also pointed out the issue of internal validity, particularly the degree of psychosocial interaction that occurred during physical exercise. This information is crucial to determine whether physical exercise alone or a combination of exercise and interpersonal interaction altered dependent variables. She maintained that the effect of physical exercise would be specific to the context of physical exercise, and it would not be generalized or transferred to social play.

Petrus et al.'s (2008) systematic review on exercise intervention effects targeted the outcome variable of stereotypic behaviors in children with ASD. They reviewed seven studies which used either the case series or case study design with small sample sizes ($N < 6$). Petrus et al. classified the studies by Kern et al. (1982) and Kern et al. (1984) as Level II: smaller RCT. However, these studies had no control group, and therefore, should be reclassified as Level IV: case series. Given the weak evidence of the reviewed studies, Petrus et al.'s claim of "weak to moderately strong evidence" (p. 142) should be revised to *weak* evidence.

Lang et al.'s (2010) systematic review overlaps with Petrus et al.'s (2008) review, but included wider outcome variables other than stereotypic behaviors. As in the case of Petrus et al.'s (2008) review, the appraised studies were characterized by small sample sizes ($N < 9$) and the use of time-series analysis to evaluate the intervention outcome (7 of the 18 studies). This review provided critical information that 15 of the 18 studies had involved teaching exercise, mostly jogging, to individuals with ASD by modeling, physical guidance, verbal reinforcement and contingency management. One study even used jogging in social plays, such as follow-the-leader and tag. Such a psychosocial component in the "physical" intervention could explain the improvement in the behavioral and academic domains, as well as in the physical domain. The authors narratively evaluated the research methodologies and the intervention outcomes, but neither categorical classification of evidence levels nor meta analysis was performed. Yet Lang et al. (2010) acknowledged the limitations of reviewed research being the fact that no research employed the experimental design, but depended on time-series analysis. An advantage of time-series analysis lies in its capability to infer the effect of intervention on an individual without considering inter-individual differences. The inevitable corollary of the advantage reduces generalizability. Hence, the reported benefits of physical exercises from the time-series data need to be confirmed by randomized control trials.

Sowa and Meulenbroek (2012) searched movement based intervention studies published between 1991 and 2011 with respect to the effects of the interventions on the physical and psychosocial domains in people with ASD. Of the 16 studies they identified, seven studies conducted individual physical exercise programs and nine studies administered group programs. All activity programs yielded significant progress on the assessed measures, but the individual programmes elicited significantly more improvement than the group interventions not only in the movement domain, but also in the social domain. A question may be raised as to whether physical exercise indirectly triggered the improvement in social functions through a yet unknown mechanism, or the psychosocial interactions that occurred during the physical exercise programs directly enhanced the social skills. Unfortunately, a majority of the original studies cited in the review failed to report the extent of psychosocial interactions in the "physical" exercises, making it difficult to determine the cause of the improvement in the social domain.

As the analytic method of the improvement rates indicates, Sowa and Meulenbroek's analysis examines only the differences before and after the interventions without considering the control groups. Indeed, this is still a meta analysis in the sense of aggregating studies, such an analytic method falls in Grade III-3 to IV level of evidence, which is regarded as either satisfactory or poor (NHMRC, 2000). The absence of the control groups in the analysis does not allow us to tease out the intervention effects from confounding factors, such as Hawthorne effect. No matter how large the combined sample size may be, no definite conclusion can be drawn from Sowa and Meulenbroek's meta analysis with regard to the causal effects of the individual or group motor interventions on the motor or the psychosocial domain. On an additional note, the authors seem to be unfamiliar with the difficulties that individuals with ASD face while engaging in complex team sports in which the environment changes constantly, as the authors wonder why there is no "naturalistic group-based sport intervention like soccer" (p. 56).

Thus, all four reviews reported the benefit of movement based interventions, physical exercise, in particular, on the physical and psychosocial domains. On closer scrutiny however, the extent of psychosocial intervention within the movement based interventions has not been quantified or partialed out, but confounded. Coupled with the limited generalizability of time-series analysis employed by a majority of the reviewed studies, the reported effects need to be interpreted cautiously with understanding of these limitations.

THEORETICAL MODELS LINKING MOVEMENT DISORDERS AND ASD

Six out of the eight reviews on motor differences or motor interventions offered theoretical insights into the relations between ASD and motor functions, ranging from causal directions between the motor and the social domains to underlying neural structures and functions (**Table 1**).

In their systematic review, Downey and Rapport (2012) raised a question whether limited social behaviors of individuals with ASD prevented them from learning motor skills, or poor motor functions impoverished social life. This is a curious question, but it is extremely difficult to establish clear-cut causalities for methodological reasons.

Four review studies speculated the underlying mechanism between movement and autistic disorders. On the functional level, Williams et al. (2004) attributed the movement difference to an ASD specific deficit in self-other mapping ability particularly for the imitation tasks that have low congruence between semantic and visuomotor couplings. On the physiological level, Baranek (2002) cited Kern et al. (1982) and Kern et al. (1984) to explain the benefit of physical exercise in term of physiological responses, such as the secretion of neurotransmitters, beta-endorphins, and acetylcholine. Emck et al. (2009) attributed the co-occurrence of the multiple impairments to "an abnormal connectivity of brain system" (p. 512) based on functional correlations between motor, cognitive, and socio-emotional impairments. More specifically, Fournier et al. (2010) attribute motor dysfunctions to abnormalities in fronto-striatal connections and basal ganglia, based on the foregoing neurophysiological studies. Four reviews on actual neurophysiological studies provide us with the "state of art" hindsight of structural and functional MRI studies.

Stanfield et al. (2008) meta analyzed 46 volumetric MRI studies on regional brain size in ASD by adjusting age and IQ. The cerebrum and the cerebellum (vermal lobules VI-VII and VIII-X) of the ASD were larger than the control, whereas the corpus callosum was smaller in size. The authors related the enlarged cerebellum and its presumably disorganized connection with the cerebral regions to motor dysfunction, as well as cognitive and socio-emotional dysfunctions in ASD. Thus, the authors ascribed the link between movement disturbance and ASD to morphological changes in the brain.

In their systematic review and meta analysis of functional MRI research on ASD, Philip et al. (2012) identified three studies which had employed motor tasks of button pressing in MRI scanners. Compared to controls, individuals with ASD showed significantly different activation patterns (either hyper- or hypo-activation) in the motor regions (e.g., the cerebellum, the precentral gyrus, the basal ganglia) and attentional systems (the basal ganglia, the superior and inferior parietal lobules). The authors related the ASD groups' hyper-activation in the right inferior frontal gyrus and the hypo-activation in the left inferior parietal lobule to the *mirror neuron system hypothesis* in that these regions were involved in observation and execution of model movements. Note that Philip et al. were conservative in that they made no link between the differential brain activation patterns and the movement difference in ASD or the effect of movement based intervention on ASD.

Müller et al. (2011) reviewed 32 functional connectivity MRI studies of ASD, and found 22 studies supported the general underconnectivity hypothesis, whereas 11 studies did not support the hypothesis. The authors recognized the diversity in data analysis, suggesting that the discrepant findings might depend on each study's methodology. They interpreted underconnectivity as decreased efficiency of network interactions, and the increased functional connectivity as a malformation in experience-driven network. Müller et al. (2011) believed that all results represented the anomaly in white matter development which resulted in ASD symptomatology encompassing social, communicative, and movement disorders.

Nickl-Jockschat et al. (2012) meta analyzed 16 morphometric MRI studies and linked disturbances in the left pericental region, the left putamen, the right caudate, and the right parietal operculum with sensorymotor impairment in ASD.

The theoretical links between movement disorder and ASD have been explored in terms of the directions of influence and the neurophysiological levels. It is difficult to establish the direction of causalities. None of the neurophysiological evidence sufficiently accounts for the movement differences in ASD or why movement based interventions result in the improvement in the motor and psychosocial domains in ASD.

CONCLUSIVE REMARKS

Accumulated studies indicate significant movement differences between ASD and control groups. However, the existence of individuals with ASD, who are free from movement problems, does not warrant the designation of movement disturbance as a core symptom of ASD. There is moderate to low quality evidence for the effects of movement based intervention on the motor, behavior, and psychosocial domains. Coupled with the limited descriptions on the psychosocial interactions during the movement based interventions, future research on the process and the outcome of movement based intervention needs to control and examine the interactions more precisely. Neurophysiological accounts for the movement differences and the effects of movement based intervention range from the size of brain regions, differential brain activation patterns during motor tasks, and functional connectivity. While none of these theoretical hypotheses can directly explain the movement differences or the effects of movement based interventions, they serve as useful theoretical models to be refined and tested in further research.

ACKNOWLEDGMENTS

I would like to thank Justin Farquhar for severing as a reviews search coordinator, and Losia Lagisz for independently assessing the selected review studies with the AMSTAR.

REFERENCES

American Psychiatric Association. (2012). *DSM-5 Development*. [Online]. American Psychiatric Association. Available online at: http://www.dsm5.org (Accessed October 29, 2012).

Baranek, G. T. (2002). Efficacy of sensory and motor interventions for children with autism. *J. Autism Dev. Disord.* 32, 397–422.

Beversdorf, D. Q., Anderson, J. M., Manning, S. E., Anderson, S. L., Nordgren, R. E., Felopulos, G. J., et al. (2001). Brief report: macrographia in high-functioning adults with autism spectrum disorder. *J. Autism Dev. Disord.* 31, 97–101.

Coldren, J. T., and Halloran, C. (2003). Spatial reversal as a measure of executive functioning in children with autism. *J. Genet. Psychol.* 164, 29–41.

Downey, R., and Rapport, M. J. K. (2012). Motor activity in children with autism: a review of current literature. *Pediatr. Phys. Ther.* 24, 2–20.

Emck, C., Bosscher, R., Beek, P., and Doreleijers, T. (2009). Gross motor performance and self-perceived motor competence in children with emotional, behavioural, and pervasive developmental disorders: a review. *Dev. Med. Child Neurol.* 51, 501–517.

Fournier, K. A., Hass, C. J., Naik, S. K., Lodha, N., and Cauraugh, J. H. (2010). Motor coordination in autism spectrum disorders: a synthesis and meta-analysis. *J. Autism Dev. Disord.* 40, 1227–1240.

Ipser, J. C., Syal, S., Bentley, J., Adnams, C. M., Steyn, B., and Stein, D. J. (2012). 1H-MRS in autism spectrum disorders: a systematic meta-analysis. *Metab. Brain Dis.* 27, 275–287.

Kern, L., Koegel, R. L., and Dunlap, G. (1984). The influence of vigorous versus mild exercise on autistic stereotyped behaviors. *J. Autism Dev. Disord.* 14, 57–67.

Kern, L., Koegel, R. L., Dyer, K., Blew, P. A., and Fenton, L. R. (1982). The effects of physical exercise on self-stimulation and appropriate responding in autistic-children. *J. Autism Dev. Disord.* 12, 399–419.

Lang, R., Koegel, L. K., Ashbaugh, K., Regester, A., Ence, W., and Smith, W. (2010). Physical exercise and individuals with autism spectrum disorders: a systematic review. *Res. Autism Spectr. Dis.* 4, 565–576.

Matt, G. E., and Cook, T. D. (2009). "Threats to the validity of generalized inferences," in *The Handbook of Research Synthesis and Meta-Analysis, 2nd Edn.*, eds H. Cooper, L. V. Hedges, and J. C. Valentine (New York, NY: Russell Sage Foundation), 537–560.

Müller, R. A., Shih, P., Keehn, B., Deyoe, J. R., Leyden, K. M., and Shukla, D. K. (2011). Underconnected, but how? A survey of functional connectivity MRI studies in autism spectrum disorders. *Cereb. Cortex* 21, 2233–2243.

NHMRC. (2000). *How to Use the Evidence: Assessment and Application of Scientific Evidence*. Canberra, ACT: National Health and Medical Research Council.

Nickl-Jockschat, T., Habel, U., Michel, T. M., Manning, J., Laird, A. R., Fox, P. T., et al. (2012). Brain structure anomalies in autism spectrum disorder—a meta-analysis of VBM studies using anatomic likelihood estimation. *Hum. Brain Mapp.* 33, 1470–1489.

Petrus, C., Adamson, S. R., Block, L., Einarson, S. J., Sharifnejad, M., and Harris, S. R. (2008). Effects of exercise interventions on stereotypic behaviours in children with autism spectrum disorder. *Physiother. Can.* 60, 134–145.

Philip, R. C. M., Dauvermann, M. R., Whalley, H. C., Baynham, K., Lawrie, S. M., and Stanfield, A. C. (2012). A systematic review and meta-analysis of the fMRI investigation of autism spectrum disorders. *Neurosci. Biobehav. Rev.* 36, 901–942.

Redcay, E., and Courchesne, E. (2005). When is the brain enlarged in autism? A meta-analysis of all brain size reports. *Biol. Psychiatry* 58, 1–9.

Shea, B. J., Grimshaw, J. M., Wells, G. A., Boers, M., Andersson, N., Hamel, C., et al. (2007). Development of AMSTAR: a measurement tool to assess the methodological quality of systematic reviews. *BMC Med. Res. Methodol.* 7:10. doi: 10.1186/1471-2288-7-10

Sowa, M., and Meulenbroek, R. (2012). Effects of physical exercise on autism spectrum disorders: a meta-analysis. *Res. Autism Spectr. Disord.* 6, 46–57.

Stanfield, A. C., McIntosh, A. M., Spencer, M. D., Philip, R., Gaur, S., and Lawrie, S. M. (2008). Towards a neuroanatomy of autism: a systematic review and meta-analysis of structural magnetic resonance imaging studies. *Eur. Psychiatry* 23, 289–299.

Sugranyes, G., Kyriakopoulos, M., Corrigall, R., Taylor, E., and Frangou, S. (2011). Autism spectrum disorders and schizophrenia: meta-analysis of the neural correlates of social cognition. *PLoS ONE* 6:e25322. doi: 10.1371/journal.pone.0025322

Tani, P., Lindberg, N., Appelberg, B., Nieminen-von Wendt, T., von Wendt, L., and Porkka-Heiskanen, T. (2006). Clinical neurological abnormalities in young adults with Asperger syndrome. *Psychiatry Clin. Neurosci.* 60, 253–255.

Williams, J. H. G., Whiten, A., and Singh, T. (2004). A systematic review of action imitation in autistic spectrum disorder. *J. Autism Dev. Disord.* 34, 285–299.

World Health Organization. (2001). *International Classification of Functioning, Disability and Health (ICF).* Geneva: World Health Organization.

Conflict of Interest Statement: The author declares that the research was conducted in the absence of any commercial or financial relationships that could be construed as a potential conflict of interest.

Permissions

All chapters in this book were first published in ATMP, by Frontiers Media SA; hereby published with permission under the Creative Commons Attribution License or equivalent. Every chapter published in this book has been scrutinized by our experts. Their significance has been extensively debated. The topics covered herein carry significant findings which will fuel the growth of the discipline. They may even be implemented as practical applications or may be referred to as a beginning point for another development.

The contributors of this book come from diverse backgrounds, making this book a truly international effort. This book will bring forth new frontiers with its revolutionizing research information and detailed analysis of the nascent developments around the world.

We would like to thank all the contributing authors for lending their expertise to make the book truly unique. They have played a crucial role in the development of this book. Without their invaluable contributions this book wouldn't have been possible. They have made vital efforts to compile up to date information on the varied aspects of this subject to make this book a valuable addition to the collection of many professionals and students.

This book was conceptualized with the vision of imparting up-to-date information and advanced data in this field. To ensure the same, a matchless editorial board was set up. Every individual on the board went through rigorous rounds of assessment to prove their worth. After which they invested a large part of their time researching and compiling the most relevant data for our readers.

The editorial board has been involved in producing this book since its inception. They have spent rigorous hours researching and exploring the diverse topics which have resulted in the successful publishing of this book. They have passed on their knowledge of decades through this book. To expedite this challenging task, the publisher supported the team at every step. A small team of assistant editors was also appointed to further simplify the editing procedure and attain best results for the readers.

Apart from the editorial board, the designing team has also invested a significant amount of their time in understanding the subject and creating the most relevant covers. They scrutinized every image to scout for the most suitable representation of the subject and create an appropriate cover for the book.

The publishing team has been an ardent support to the editorial, designing and production team. Their endless efforts to recruit the best for this project, has resulted in the accomplishment of this book. They are a veteran in the field of academics and their pool of knowledge is as vast as their experience in printing. Their expertise and guidance has proved useful at every step. Their uncompromising quality standards have made this book an exceptional effort. Their encouragement from time to time has been an inspiration for everyone.

The publisher and the editorial board hope that this book will prove to be a valuable piece of knowledge for researchers, students, practitioners and scholars across the globe.

List of Contributors

Elizabeth B. Torres
Psychology Department, Rutgers Center for Cognitive Science, Center for Computational Biomedicine Imaging and Modeling (Computer Science), Movement Disorders, Neurology, Rutgers University School of Medicine, Rutgers University, New Brunswick, NJ, USA
Movement Disorders, Neurology Department, Indiana University School of Medicine, Indianapolis, IN, USA

Maria Brincker
Philosophy Department, University of Massachusetts, Boston, MA, USA

Robert W. Isenhower
Psychology Department, Rutgers University, Piscataway, NJ, USA

Polina Yanovich
Computer Science Department, Rutgers University, Piscataway, NJ, USA

Kimberly A. Stigler
Department of Psychiatry, Indiana University School of Medicine, Indiana University, Indianapolis, IN, USA

John I. Nurnberger
Department of Psychiatry, Christian Sarkine Autism Treatment Center, Riley Hospital for Children, Indiana University School of Medicine, Indiana University, Indianapolis, IN, USA

Dimitris N. Metaxas
Computer Science Department, Center for Computational Biomedicine Imaging and Modeling, Rutgers Center for Cognitive Science, Rutgers University, Piscataway, NJ, USA

Jorge V. José
Physics Department Bloomington, Department of Cellular and Integrative Physiology, Indiana University School of Medicine, Indiana University, Bloomington, IN, USA

Joseph P. McCleery, Natasha A. Elliott, Dimitrios S. Sampanis and Chrysi A. Stefanidou
School of Psychology, University of Birmingham, West Midlands, Birmingham, UK

Jodi Robledo
School of Education, California State University San Marcos, San Marcos, CA, USA

Anne M. Donnellan
School of Leadership and Education Sciences, University of San Diego, San Diego, CA, USA

Karen Strandt-Conroy
Parkview School District, Orfordville, WI, USA

David A. Hill
Tri-County Regional School Board, Yarmouth, NS, Canada

Martha R. Leary
Private Practice, Halifax, NS, Canada

Michelle W. Hardy and A. Blythe LaGasse
Center for Biomedical Research in Music, Colorado State University, Fort Collins, CO, USA

Sudha M. Srinivasan
Department of Kinesiology, Neag School of Education, University of Connecticut, Storrs, CT, USA
Center for Health, Intervention, and Prevention, University of Connecticut, Storrs, CT, USA

Anjana N. Bhat
Department of Kinesiology, Neag School of Education, University of Connecticut, Storrs, CT, USA
Center for Health, Intervention, and Prevention, University of Connecticut, Storrs, CT, USA
Center for the Ecological Study of Perception and Action, University of Connecticut, Storrs, CT, USA

Pat Amos
Training and Private Consultation, Ardmore, PA, USA

Hanne De Jaegher
Department of Logic and Philosophy of Science, IAS-Research Centre for Life, Mind, and Society, University of the Basque Country, San Sebastián, Spain
Department of Informatics, Centre for Computational Neuroscience and Robotics, Centre for Research in Cognitive Science, School of Life Sciences, University of Sussex, Brighton, UK

Colwyn Trevarthen
Department of Psychology, College of Humanities and Social Sciences, University of Edinburgh, Edinburgh, UK

Jonathan T. Delafield-Butt
Early Years, School of Education, Faculty of Humanities and Social Sciences, University of Strathclyde, Glasgow, UK

Matthew K. Belmonte
The Groden Center, Providence, RI, USA
Division of Psychology, Nottingham Trent University, Nottingham, UK
Center for the Study of Human Development, Brown University, Providence, RI, USA

Tanushree Saxena-Chandhok, Ruth Cherian, Reema Muneer, Lisa George and Prathibha Karanth
The Com DEALL Trust, Bangalore, India

Claes von Hofsten and Kerstin Rosander
Department of Psychology, Uppsala University, Uppsala, Sweden

Sylvie Goldman
Saul R. Korey Department of Neurology, Albert Einstein College of Medicine, Bronx, NY, USA
Department of Pediatrics, Albert Einstein College of Medicine, Bronx, NY, USA
Rose F. Kennedy Intellectual and Developmental Disabilities Research Center, Albert Einstein College of Medicine, Bronx, NY, USA

Paul E. Greene
Department of Neurology, Columbia University Medical Center, New York, NY, USA

Gianluca Esposito
RIKEN Brain Science Institute, Unit for Affiliative Social Behavior, Wako-Shi, Saitama, Japan

Sergiu P. Paşca
Department of Neurobiology, Stanford University School of Medicine, Stanford, CA, USA

Caroline Whyatt and Cathy Craig
Department of Psychology, Queen's University Belfast, Belfast, Antrim, UK

Kerry L. Marsh and Robert W. Isenhower
Center for the Ecological Study of Perception and Action, University of Connecticut, Storrs, CT, USA
Department of Psychology, University of Connecticut, Storrs, CT, USA

Michael J. Richardson
Department of Psychology, University of Cincinnati, Cincinnati, OH, USA

Molly Helt, Alyssa D. Verbalis and Deborah Fein
Department of Psychology, University of Connecticut, Storrs, CT, USA

R. C. Schmidt
Department of Psychology, College of the Holy Cross, Worchester, MA, USA

Cristina Becchio
Dipartimento di Psicologia, Centro di Scienza Cognitiva, Università di Torino, Turin, Italy

Umberto Castiello
Dipartimento di Psicologia Generale, Università di Padova, Padova, Italy

Michael J. Weiss
Department of Psychology, Fairfield University, Fairfield, CT, USA

Matthew F. Moran
Department of Physical Therapy and Human Movement Science, Sacred Heart University, Fairfield, CT, USA

Mary E. Parker
Department of Physical Therapy, Texas State University, San Marcos, TX, USA

John T. Foley
Physical Activity Laboratory, Department of Physical Education, State University of New York at Cortland, Cortland, NY, USA

Motohide Miyahara
Movement Development Clinic, School of Physical Education, University of Otago, Dunedin, New Zealand

Index

S

T

V

W

www.ingramcontent.com/pod-product-compliance
Lightning Source LLC
LaVergne TN
LVHW060526210926
848485LV00005B/1157
* 9 7 8 1 6 3 9 2 7 2 8 3 9 *